Psychopathology *and* Function

Fifth Edition

Psychopathology *and* Function

Fifth Edition

Bette Bonder, PhD, OTR/L, FAOTA
Professor Emerita
Cleveland State University
Cleveland, Ohio

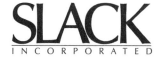

www.Healio.com/books

ISBN: 978-1-61711-884-5

Psychopathology and Function, Fifth Edition includes ancillary materials specifically available for faculty use. Included are PowerPoint slides. Please visit www.efacultylounge.com to obtain access.

Dr. Bette Bonder and *Dr. Chris Paxos* have no financial or proprietary interest in the materials presented herein. *Dr. Sara E. Dugan* is on the Clinical Advisory Panel for Ohio College of Pharmacy Government Resource Center.

The procedures and practices described in this publication should be implemented in a manner consistent with the professional standards set for the circumstances that apply in each specific situation. Every effort has been made to confirm the accuracy of the information presented and to correctly relate generally accepted practices. The authors, editors, and publisher cannot accept responsibility for errors or exclusions or for the outcome of the material presented herein. There is no expressed or implied warranty of this book or information imparted by it. Care has been taken to ensure that drug selection and dosages are in accordance with currently accepted/recommended practice. Off-label uses of drugs may be discussed. Due to continuing research, changes in government policy and regulations, and various effects of drug reactions and interactions, it is recommended that the reader carefully review all materials and literature provided for each drug, especially those that are new or not frequently used. Some drugs or devices in this publication have clearance for use in a restricted research setting by the Food and Drug and Administration or FDA. Each professional should determine the FDA status of any drug or device prior to use in their practice.

Any review or mention of specific companies or products is not intended as an endorsement by the author or publisher.

SLACK Incorporated uses a review process to evaluate submitted material. Prior to publication, educators or clinicians provide important feedback on the content that we publish. We welcome feedback on this work.

Published by: SLACK Incorporated
                   6900 Grove Road
                   Thorofare, NJ 08086 USA
                   Telephone: 856-848-1000
                   Fax: 856-848-6091
                   www.Healio.com/books

Contact SLACK Incorporated for more information about other books in this field or about the availability of our books from distributors outside the United States.

Library of Congress Cataloging-in-Publication Data

Bonder, Bette, author.
  Psychopathology and function / Bette Bonder. -- Fifth edition.
      p. ; cm.
  Includes bibliographical references and index.
  ISBN 978-1-61711-884-5 (alk. paper)
  I. Title.
  [DNLM: 1. Mental Disorders--diagnosis. 2. Mental Disorders--classification. 3. Mental Disorders--therapy. 4. Occupational Therapy--methods. WM 141]
  RC454
  616.89--dc23
                              2014033008

Printed in the United States of America.

Last digit is print number: 10 9 8 7 6 5 4

Dedication

To my colleagues at Cleveland State University, who have been consistently supportive and who are both friends and role models.

Contents

Acknowledgments

This book is the result of the efforts of many individuals. I am grateful to Sheerli Ratner, PhD, who provided insight into the many changes to the systems of care in which mental disorders are treated. I am particularly appreciative of the efforts of my colleagues, Chris Paxos and Sara Dugan, who undertook a wholesale (and very effective) revision of the psychopharmacology chapter. Jordan Bray provided excellent copyediting assistance.

I am grateful to my students over the years for their critical review of the material and to the reviewers of this most recent manuscript. They had a major task, given the substantial changes required for the new edition, and they provided thoughtful and helpful comments.

Many individuals at SLACK Incorporated have been supportive of my projects over the years. In particular, I thank Brien Cummings, who has shepherded this edition—like those before it—into production. His consistent interest and assistance over the years and through numerous projects has been extraordinary. April Billick, Dani Malady, Kat Rola, and Michelle Gatt have also provided assistance in bringing this project to fruition and making sure that people know about it. John Bond has provided invaluable assistance and support through our many years of association.

As always, my family—Patrick, Aaron, and Jordan Bray, Lisa Gomersall, and Rebecca Devens—deserve thanks and recognition. They provided moral support throughout this effort and offered a variety of helpful insights as the manuscript emerged. For this and for many other reasons, they have my profound gratitude.

About the Author

Bette Bonder, PhD, OTR/L, FAOTA is Professor Emerita, School of Health Sciences and Department of Psychology, Cleveland State University. Dr. Bonder is the former Dean of the College of Sciences and Health Professions at Cleveland State University. Dr. Bonder is the author of numerous papers on mental health, aging, and cultural competence, and former editor of the *Occupational Therapy Journal of Research* (now *OTJR: Occupation, Participation, and Health*). Dr. Bonder is also the coauthor of *Culture in Clinical Care: Strategies for Competence* (2nd ed., with Laura Martin) and a coeditor of *Functional Performance in Older Adults* (3rd ed.). Dr. Bonder has served on the Board of Directors of the Occupational Therapy Foundation, as well as many other community and professional boards.

Contributing Authors

Sara E. Dugan, PharmD (Chapter 21) is Associate Professor of Pharmacy Practice, Northeast Ohio Medical University. Dr. Dugan is board certified in psychiatric pharmacy (BCPP) and pharmacotherapy (BCPS). Dr. Dugan's research focuses on psychopharmacology in the outpatient setting. Dr. Dugan is an active member of the College of Psychiatric and Neurological Pharmacists and the Ohio Pharmacists Association.

Chris Paxos, PharmD (Chapter 21) is Assistant Professor of Psychiatry and Associate Professor of Pharmacy Practice, Northeast Ohio Medical University. Dr. Paxos is board certified in psychiatric pharmacy (BCPP) and pharmacotherapy (BCPS) and has a geriatrics certification (CGP) as well. Dr. Paxos' current research focuses on antipsychotic polypharmacy in inpatient settings. He is an active member of the College of Psychiatric and Neurological Pharmacists (CPNP) and the Ohio Society of Health-System Pharmacists (OSHP).

Introduction

When the first edition of this book was published, the *Diagnostic and Statistical Manual of Mental Disorders* (DSM) was in its third edition (actually its fourth, as it was a revision of the DSM-III; American Psychiatric Association [APA], 1987). The third edition marked a turning point for diagnosis in mental health. It had vastly expanded both the number of diagnoses and the specificity of the criteria for making determinations, and although the DSM-III asserted that it was atheoretical, the structure was clearly influenced by the growing understanding of mental disorders as being biologically based. At the same time, the guiding document in occupational therapy practice was the *Uniform Terminology Checklist* (American Occupational Therapy Association [AOTA], 1989). It was, as the name implies, a list of terms that had been developed with the simple goal of having all occupational therapists use consistent terminology to describe their diagnostic system, evaluation strategies, intervention approaches, and outcome measurements.

Both publications were groundbreaking at the time, and both generated more than a little controversy. In the world of psychiatry, there were concerns about the increasing complexity of its diagnostic system, and, in occupational therapy, there were concerns about the creation of a terminology structure that was separate and different from other classification systems, such as the DSM and the World Health Organization's (WHO) *International Classification of Impairments, Disabilities, and Handicaps* (ICIDH; 1980).

Sure enough, each of these documents has been revised substantially. Only the DSM has kept its name, as the ICIDH is now called the *International Classification of Functioning, Disability and Health* (ICF; WHO, 2001), and the *Uniform Terminology Checklist* is now called the *Occupational Therapy Practice Framework: Domain and Process* (AOTA, 2008).

It is no surprise that these documents would require modification over time. The world of health and health care has changed dramatically in the 25 years since the first edition of *Psychopathology and Function*. Much of the change is the result of a substantial focus on research to better understand how to ameliorate disease, disability, and dysfunction, including those disorders whose symptoms are primarily emotional or cognitive. In addition, particularly in the United States but around the world as well, changes in patterns of care provision, policies about reimbursement, and societal values about health have altered the landscape as well. From today's perspective, those early documents look almost quaint, although the thoughtful work that went into their development should not be discounted. At the time of publication, each document was innovative.

It is also no surprise that each change is accompanied by controversy. Some of the controversy reflects the simple fact that change is difficult. This is particularly true in the large and complex (some would argue, convoluted) health care system. Particularly in the United States, many interacting organizational structures—hospitals, clinics, insurers, employers, schools—must adjust to changes in diagnostic and treatment systems. However, it is worth noting that the ferocity of the controversy surrounding the DSM-5 seems substantially greater than what has been seen in the past. There are even some calls in the mental health community to ignore it or to resist the more drastic changes (Frances, 2012).

The publication of the DSM-5 (APA, 2013) and this edition of *Psychopathology and Function* come at a particularly interesting and challenging time in US health care. The enactment of the *Affordable Care Act* represents a major change in the health care system. It is much too early to know what will be the overall impact. The Affordable Care Act's goals of increasing access and quality while managing costs are ambitious, but the law, like all major legislation, reflects a series of compromises to win the support needed to pass the legislation.

Nevertheless, it is inevitable that it will have a major impact. Not the least of these is yet another attempt to ensure that individuals with mental disorders are provided the same access to care that is available for individuals with other kinds of illnesses and disabilities.

The specific nature of the changes in the documents mentioned will be described in the chapters of this book. Two major threads can be seen—one that has clearly affected the development of the DSM-5 (APA, 2013) and one that is directly relevant to the practice of occupational therapy—in mental health and in practice more generally. The first is the growing understanding of and emphasis on the biological nature of mental disorders (Stetka & Correll, 2014). Because research has increasingly identified genetic, inflammatory, and other biological sources of cognitive and emotional difficulties, medical treatment has moved toward increased use of psychopharmacological agents. This emphasis can be seen throughout the DSM-5, which no longer purports to be atheoretical.

The second thread is a growing awareness of the importance of quality of life. Occupational therapy is not alone in its focus on ensuring that individuals live meaningful lives. Psychology has developed a significant emphasis on positive psychology (cf. Seligman and Csikszentmihalyi, 2000) and medicine, as well as recognizing that health is much more than the absence of illness. This means that occupational therapy has a tremendous opportunity to increase its impact in serving its clients, as this focus has always been at the core of its professional values.

To function effectively in providing mental health services, occupational therapists must have a clear understanding of the needs of the individual, the system in which they are providing care, the roles of other professionals, and their own potential contributions to treatment. They must be able to communicate effectively across disciplinary lines, hence the importance of knowing the DSM diagnostic structure well. Therapists must also understand payment sources because payment for services is almost always provided, at least in part, by someone other than the identified client. This may be an insurance company, the government, or an employer; someone whose interests may be different from those of the client. These entities are interested in care that is effective but also cost effective. While acknowledging these factors, occupational therapists must also clearly understand that their perspectives on health and wellness differ from other disciplines and that they have a unique and vital contribution to make to their clients' well-being.

This book is designed to guide occupational therapists in providing effective attention to psychological factors, understanding their clients, communicating with other professionals, providing care to individuals in real-life situations, and ensuring that quality of life is maintained or enhanced for those being served. The text is not intended to provide comprehensive coverage of the occupational therapy process in mental health. Many other books discuss that subject from a variety of perspectives. Rather, it is designed as an overview of the kinds of clients with whom occupational therapists and other health care providers are likely to work and to give therapists an understanding of the ways in which other mental health professionals view these individuals. Understanding the context for service and the diagnostic conceptualizations of other professionals enables occupational therapists to enhance their interventions and define their unique contribution to mental health.

References

American Occupational Therapy Association (1989). *Uniform terminology checklist*. Rockville, MD: Author.

American Occupational Therapy Association (2008). Occupational therapy practice framework: Domain & process, 2nd edition. *American Journal of Occupational Therapy, 62*(6), 625-683.

American Psychiatric Association (1987). *Diagnostic and statistical manual of mental disorders* (3rd ed., revised). Washington, DC: Author.

American Psychiatric Association (2013). *Diagnostic and statistical manual of mental disorders* (5th ed.). Washington, DC: Author.

Frances, A. (2012, December 2). DSM-5 is a guide, not a bible—Ignore its 10 worst changes [Web log post]. *Psychology Today*. Retrieved from http://www.psychologytoday.com/blog/dsm5-in-distress/201212/dsm-5-is-guide-not-bible-ignore-its-ten-worst-changes.

Seligman, M.E.P., & Csikszentmihalyi, M. (2000). Positive psychology: An introduction. *American Psychologist, 55*(1), 5-14.

Stetka, B.S., & Correll, C.U. (2014, January 16). 7 advances in schizophrenia. *Medscape.* Retrieved from http://www.medscape.com/viewarticle/819068_1.

World Health Organization (1980). *International classification of impairments, disabilities, and handicaps.* Geneva, Switzerland: Author.

World Health Organization (2001). *International classification of functioning, disability and health* (ICF). Geneva, Switzerland: Author.

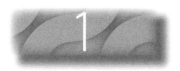

Psychiatric Diagnosis and the Classification System

Learning Outcomes

By the end of this chapter, readers will be able to:

- Discuss the reasons for having a classification system for psychiatric disorders
- Describe the history of the development of the American Psychiatric Association's (APA) *Diagnostic and Statistical Manual of Mental Disorders* (DSM) editions
- Compare and contrast the DSM; the World Health Organization's (WHO) *International Classification of Diseases* (ICD); and the WHO's *International Classification of Functioning, Disability and Health* (ICF)
- Discuss the reasons for the revision of the DSM and the process that was undertaken to develop the DSM-5
- Describe the controversies that surround the changes in the newest edition of the DSM

Bonder B.
Psychopathology and Function, Fifth Edition (pp 1-19).
© 2015 SLACK Incorporated.

KEY WORDS

- Mental disorder
- Etiology
- Dementia
- Interrater reliability
- Reliable
- Reliability coefficients
- Operational criteria
- Descriptive psychopathology

- Atheoretical
- Multiaxial classification
- Hierarchical
- Spectrum disorders
- Prevalence
- Evidence-based practice
- Medicalization
- Comorbid

CASE VIGNETTE

Enid Sanderson is an 82-year-old widow who lives alone in a second floor apartment in a large inner city neighborhood. She has lived in that community for 50 years, raised her three children there, and has been involved in many community organizations. Recently, the pastor at her church and the president of the sisterhood have become concerned because Mrs. Sanderson, who always attended regularly, had missed several Sunday services. When she does go the services, she is frequently dressed in dirty, disheveled, or peculiar clothing, which is a significant change from her usual immaculate dress. She seems confused about where she is and who the pastor and sisterhood president are.

Ralph Livingston is a 68-year-old former car salesman who recently had open heart surgery. Since the surgery, he has been confused, lethargic, sad, and tearful. He has difficulty motivating himself to get out of bed in the morning and has days when he does not get dressed or leave the house.

Maude Brown is a 44-year-old manicurist who was recently brought to the emergency department of a large urban hospital following a suicide attempt. She is well known to both the emergency department and the emergency medical personnel, as this is her fourth suicide attempt in the past 6 months. During this time, she had also switched jobs three times and had five different boyfriends.

Tyler Anderson is a 6-year-old first grader whose teacher sends him to the principal's office at least twice per day. Tyler is unable to sit still during class, frequently blurts out "jokes" that disrupt the lesson, and pulls books and toys randomly off shelves, dropping them on the floor as he moves on to the next object. He seems bright enough to manage the work, having learned to read along with the class. But his attention span is very brief, and his physical activity level exhausts the teacher and many of his classmates.

THOUGHT QUESTIONS

1. In your view, do any of these individuals have a condition that might be considered a mental disorder?
2. For those who you think do have mental disorders, what factors in the descriptions led to your conclusion?

(continued)

CASE VIGNETTE (CONTINUED)

3. Do you see any characteristics in these descriptions that you believe affect the individuals' daily activities?
4. If so, are they the same factors that led to your decision about whether the individuals described have mental disorders? How are they the same? How are they different? Based on your prior knowledge of the role of occupational therapy, can you think of ways in which occupational therapy intervention might be able to make a difference?

When we think about health conditions labeled as "physical," most of us have a pretty clear idea of what is meant. We probably think of symptoms (sore throat, stomach pain), causes (virus, trauma), and perhaps consequences (pain, physical disability). So, although the range of such conditions is vast, most people would probably agree on a set of criteria for delineating the majority of them.

Although physical ailments are not always easy to define (i.e., is multiple chemical sensitivity a disease?), psychiatric or mental disorders are more difficult to classify. It may seem evident that an individual who cries several times a day has a problem, but knowing what the precise problem is (e.g., a person working in a hospice setting who has empathy for his clients or someone with major depression) and, more importantly, knowing whether the person has a condition that requires treatment, is much more difficult. We know that a head cold is caused by a virus, that its symptoms can be treated by decongestants and chicken soup, and that it will remit within 10 days or so. What level of unhappiness deserves a label of depression? What causes it? How long will it last? How should we treat it? For that matter, is it really a health-related condition, or is it simply a consequence of living?

Conceptualizing mental disorders is not a new challenge. For hundreds, perhaps thousands of years, there have been efforts to understand and categorize psychiatric conditions (Millon, 2004). Demon possession, humoral imbalance resulting in melancholia, evil spirits, and other characterizations of behavioral disorders appear in the Old Testament, early Greek texts, and many other written documents through the ages.

As health care in general and mental health care more specifically developed a more scientific, data-based framework over time, the American Psychiatric Association (APA) set out to provide guidance for physicians, especially psychiatrists, and other health professionals working with clients with emotional and behavioral conditions. The result of such guidance was the DSM, currently in its fifth edition (APA, 2013). As you will see in this chapter, the development of that guide reflects not only advances in science but also changes in the societal circumstances in which behavior and emotion are evaluated.

For the purposes of this book, we will adopt the definition of mental disorder that is provided in the DSM. According to the fifth edition of the *Diagnostic and Statistical Manual of Mental Disorders* (DSM-5; APA, 2013; A note on citing the new DSM: During the development process for the DSM-5, a change from Roman numerals [V] to Arabic numerals was made to allow for more frequent updates [e.g., DSM-5.1, 5.2, and so on]. Where this book mentions a specific reference, you will see the Roman numeral used if this is how the manual is listed in that particular reference), **a mental disorder** is:

> a syndrome characterized by clinically significant disturbance in an individual's cognition, emotion regulation, or behavior that reflects a dysfunction in the

psychological, biological, or developmental processes underlying mental functioning. Mental disorders are usually associated with significant distress or disability in social, occupational, or other important activities. An expectable or culturally approved response to a common stressor or loss, such as the death of a loved one, is not a mental disorder. Socially deviant behavior (e.g., political, religious, or sexual) and conflicts that are primarily between the individual and society are not mental disorders unless the deviance or conflict results from a dysfunction in the individual, as described above. (p. 20)

As one can see, this definition is quite general. It might (and arguably does) allow for considerable latitude in labeling a particular set of beliefs, behaviors, or thoughts as mental disorders.

This definition does not provide an explanation of what leads to mental disorders. This can be problematic when trying to assert that the label is valid and meaningful, even though for some physical disorders there are also ongoing differences of opinion about **etiology**, that is, the cause of the disorder. As just one example—about which you will read more later in this book—the etiology of Alzheimer's disease, a common disorder characterized by **dementia** (significant cognitive decline), is not yet known. Dementia is associated with changes in brain structure and chemistry, but no one can yet explain why these changes occur. As is true for many of the disorders in the DSM-5 (APA, 2013), it can be construed as a mental disorder, but it is also often clustered with other neurological (i.e., physical) diseases.

Although some mental disorders, such as Alzheimer's disease, are recognized as having a biological origin—even if we don't know the precise mechanism—for others, this is less certain. Numerous theories exist about mental disorders, such as depression and anxiety, with varying implications for intervention. Biological, behavioral, analytical, developmental, and neuropsychological approaches differ greatly in terms of their postulates about the origins of mental disorders, methods for intervening, and language for describing the disorders and their treatment.

This variation creates a dilemma for service providers. Without a common ground for understanding, communication among professionals becomes impossible, as noted by Moriyama, Loy, and Robb-Smith (2011):

The purpose of a disease nomenclature is to promote the use of the most appropriate diagnostic term to describe a particular disease. A generally accepted standard or authoritative medical vocabulary comprised of unambiguous medical terminology is essential for precise and effective communication about disease and medical entities. (p. 5)

The resolution of the dilemma has been the development of a widely used system of classifications created by the APA—the DSM. Since its first appearance in 1952, the guide has undergone repeated revisions, most recently the fifth edition, the DSM-5 (APA, 2013). A crucial purpose of this system is to provide a way for professionals to communicate through a common classification of labels for which the criteria are clear and to communicate the expectations about the client's circumstances (Mezzich & Berganza, 2005).

Communication is a vital function of a classification system, but there are others. According to the APA (2012c), the purposes of the DSM are to "provide a common language among clinicians—professionals who treat clients with mental disorders" (para. 1), ensure that diagnosis is both "accurate and consistent" (para. 1), "establish criteria that can be used in research on psychiatric disorders" (para. 2), serve as "the basis for treatment indications by the FDA or and for clinical Practice Guidelines" (para. 2), and as a mechanism for reporting to insurers for purposes of payment and to public health officials who need reliable data on trends in health.

To understand the extent to which the APA's DSM is successful in achieving these very challenging goals, it is helpful to first consider its history.

Emergence of the *Diagnostic and Statistical Manual of Mental Disorders*

In 1840, the United States had a one-category classification system for mental illness: "idiocy/insanity" (Williams, 1988). By 1880, the system had increased to eight categories. As understanding and awareness increased over time, the classification system was refined and was eventually formalized both as a chapter in the World Health Organization's (WHO) 1992 *International Classification of Diseases, 10th edition* (ICD-10; Moriyama et al., 2011), the diagnostic system for all diseases used around the world, and as the DSM.

The *Diagnostic and Statistical Manual, Mental Disorders*, later to be known as DSM-I, was published in 1952 by the APA. It was a major breakthrough for the field of mental health, as it provided the first comprehensive volume describing a range of mental disorders. However, the descriptions were quite general, making diagnosis unreliable. As psychiatric knowledge grew, it became clear that a revision was needed.

The DSM-II appeared in 1968, following 3 years of work by the APA. It coincided with the eighth revision of the ICD. The differences between the DSM-I (APA, 1952) and the DSM-II (APA, 1968) were minor, with some changes in the names of syndromes and minor modifications in descriptive language. However, similar to the DSM-I (APA, 1952), descriptions were general and often vague. A major criticism of both the DSM-I and DSM-II was the poor reliability of diagnosis (Klerman, 1988). Professionals were unable to consistently identify the same disorder in a specific client, the extent to which two different clinicians make the same diagnosis, reflecting poor **interrater reliability**. Also, the diagnosis might change over time, even if nothing had happened to alter the behavior or symptoms of the individual, which is further evidence of poor "test–retest" reliability.

The DSM-III, released by the APA in 1980, represented a major change in the nature of the diagnostic process (Blacker & Tsuang, 1999). As with DSM-II (APA, 1968), its development coincided with a revision of the ICD. American psychiatrists and other mental health care providers were concerned that the ICD lacked many specific diagnoses that were well-accepted in the United States on the basis of research data. There was also concern that the glossary of the ICD was inadequate in the area of mental health (Williams, 1988).

Furthermore, in the 1960s and 1970s, there was heated debate about the nature, and even the existence, of mental illness (Szasz, 1974; Walker, 2006). Szasz argued that mental illness was a societal phenomenon, rather than a disease. He suggested that mental illness was used as a label to explain deviant, and therefore socially unacceptable, behavior and that the purpose of the label was to provide an excuse to control such behavior. The poor reliability of diagnoses supported his contention. If two professionals were unlikely to make the same diagnosis, perhaps it was because they were responding to societal expectations about proper behavior, rather than to any real problem with the individual's health. The idea that there are serious issues in understanding mental disorders based on social and political considerations, rather than the well-being of the individual, appears regularly in the literature (cf. Greenberg, 2013).

In the 1970s, several advances contributed to the discussion. Foremost among these was the vastly increased knowledge about biology and psychopharmacology. For the first time, biological factors in mental disturbance could be identified in terms of both genetic and biochemical characteristics. Research capabilities were enhanced through development of new methodologies and clinical instruments that were found to be **reliable** (Klerman, 1988).

This meant that, based on clearer description of each disorders and improved training, professionals became more consistent in their views of specific clients and that diagnoses were more stable over time if the client's behaviors and emotions did not change. One instrument developed during this time was the Research Diagnostic Criteria (RDC; Spitzer, Endicott, & Robins, 1975). The emergence of this measure and others (e.g., the Diagnostic Interview Schedule and Structured Clinical Interview for the DSM-III-R [Taylor & Jason, 1998]) demonstrated that it was possible to provide clear, consistent guidelines to allow discrimination among symptom groupings.

In 1974, the APA appointed a committee to begin development of the DSM-III, a task that ultimately took 6 years. Both the process of development and the product were novel, representing a significant departure from the DSM-II (APA, 1968). The process involved not only a great deal of committee work to develop descriptions and diagnostic criteria but also a major research effort to validate diagnoses and determine reliability in a systematic fashion. During the research phase, more than 12,000 individuals were evaluated (Spitzer, Forman, & Nee, 1979). Clinicians around the United States completed reports and commented on any difficulties they had while using the system.

Interrater reliability studies, focused on ensuring that there would be agreement among professionals evaluating the same client, involved 796 clients, each of whom was evaluated by two clinicians. Because these were field studies, some variables were poorly controlled; however, the new classification system had **reliability coefficients** ranging from 0.7 (Axis I) to 0.6 (Axis II; Williams, 1985). This means, roughly, that professionals agreed 60% to 70% of the time. The attempt to confirm reliability was itself novel, even though some studies have found lower reliability, especially for Axis II (Mellsop, Varghese, Joshua, & Hicks, 1982). The notion of an axial system of classification (with five different axes) was another innovation in the DSM-III and will be described in the paragraph that follows (APA, 1980).

The DSM-III product was notably different than the DSM-II. First, the number of diagnoses was expanded to more than 150. In addition, descriptions were designed to be as specific and concrete as possible, with criteria about constellations of symptoms, onset of the disorder, duration, and probable course. This was the first classification to provide operational criteria as a means to assure reliability (Klerman, 1988). **Operational criteria** are specific, observable characteristics that describe a particular syndrome or disorder. It is also noteworthy that the DSM-III (APA, 1980) provided **descriptive psychopathology,** rather than inferred etiology. In other words, the guide described what clinicians saw, not the causation of what they observed. In addition, descriptions were intended to be **atheoretical** (i.e., without reference to particular theories or points of view). The intent was to make the product an effective mechanism for communication among therapists subscribing to divergent philosophies about cause and treatment (Williams, 1988).

The DSM-III (APA, 1980) also reflected a realization that a diagnosis alone might not provide sufficient data to implement treatment. As a result, several new categories were developed to provide additional information, making it the first **multiaxial classification** system for psychiatric disorders (Klerman, 1988). These axes made it possible not only to name a syndrome but also to identify disordered personality characteristics, accompanying medical conditions of significance to treatment and prognosis, levels of stress encountered by the individual, and recent level of function.

Inclusion of this last axis was of particular importance to occupational therapists, as it represented an acknowledgment that diagnosis alone does not adequately describe a person's ability to accomplish daily tasks. It is also noteworthy that Axis V (level of function) appeared to be the most reliable of the axes, with a correlation coefficient between 0.7 and 0.8 of a possible 1.0 (Williams, 1988).

In the DSM-III (APA, 1980), categories were **hierarchical**, based on the assumption that disorders higher on the hierarchy had symptoms that were also found in those of lower hierarchy but not the opposite. For example, major depressive disorder was conceptualized to be at one end of a spectrum that included dysthymia—a less severe but more persistent form of depression. Subsequent research challenged the assumption of hierarchies (Boyd, Burke, Grundberg, Holzer, & Rae, 1984), one of the many findings that led to the almost immediate effort to revise the DSM-III. The DSM-III-R was published by the APA in 1987 and reflected advances in scientific knowledge at that time. One change was the deletion of the assumption of hierarchies (Williams, 1988), although this assumption has been replaced with a focus on **spectrum disorders** (Stetka & Correll, 2013). The spectrum conceptualization reflects the belief that related disorders fall along a continuum from more severe to less severe, so that, for example, anxiety is thought to fall on a scale from most severe to less severe (APA, 2013). Although changes in the DSM-III-R were minor, they reflected an effort to resolve the problems with the DSM-III and to disseminate new knowledge as quickly as possible.

Before the DSM-III-R (APA, 1987) was completed, discussion had turned to the development of the DSM-IV (APA, 1994). As with other editions of the DSM, this revision was timed to coincide with a revision of the IDC (Kendall, 1991). The 10th edition of the WHO's ICD appeared in 1992, at which point the DSM-IV was nearing completion.

The process by which the DSM-IV (APA, 1994) was developed was intended to be careful, thoughtful, and largely empirical. Task groups of experts for each existing and proposed diagnostic category began by undertaking massive reviews of research literature (Widiger, Frances, Pincus, & Davis, 1990). These reviews were to serve as meta-analyses to guide the working groups about whether or not to include each diagnosis and what criteria would be listed. A series of field trials of the proposed criteria was also undertaken (APA, 1994). Twelve trials, including more than 6,000 research participants, were designed to examine the reliability and clinical utility of the proposed categories.

Decisions were ultimately guided by a set of standards that the development committee had agreed to in advance. Criteria for the addition of a new category or exclusion of an existing category were to be more stringent than those to retain what existed (APA, 1994). This was done to avoid unnecessary changes that would confuse practitioners and reduce researchers' ability to track long-term consequences of mental disorders and treatment. In addition, an effort was made, where possible, to conform categories to those in the ICD-10 (WHO, 1992), which was completed just prior to publication of the DSM-IV (Kendall, 1991).

According to the APA and to individuals involved in the development of this new DSM, the best possible scientific evidence was used in delineating criteria (Frances et al., 1991). Issues of reliability, validity, and utility were considered, with an eye to assuring the highest possible standards.

Several new factors were included in the DSM-IV. Among these was recognition of cultural differences in psychiatric constructs (Fabrega, 1992). Cultural factors clearly influence both the kinds of symptoms an individual may be having and his or her help-seeking behaviors (Hwang, Myers, Abe-Kim, & Ting, 2008). For example, some Hispanic cultures expect a high degree of emotional expressiveness that might seem excessive, and therefore disordered, in mainstream U.S. culture. Recognizing that externalized expression of emotion is culturally appropriate for some individuals, a clinician might be less likely to misdiagnose such an individual with histrionic personality disorder, for example. Among the factors that vary based on culture are as follows:

- **Prevalence**—the proportion of the population identified as having a particular disorder at a particular time—of mental disorders in general and specific conditions

- Perceived etiology

- Phenomenology
- Diagnostic and assessment considerations
- Coping styles and help-seeking behaviors
- Intervention choices and strategies

The DSM-IV (APA, 1994) includes an appendix that lists terms applied to mental disorders in other cultures, which might be encountered by practitioners in the United States. For example, *nervios* (which translates roughly to "nerves" and is a hybrid of depression and anxiety) and *zar* (a form of spirit possession) are briefly explained in their cultural context. This strategy works less well as the United States becomes more culturally diverse. And, of course, the DSM is used in many other countries, where cultural variations likewise exist. The presence of an appendix, as opposed to incorporating conditions such as *nervios* in the body of the text implies that the diagnoses in the main body of the text are somehow not culturally mediated—an assumption that can certainly be questioned. In a multicultural society, the assumption that one set of culturally mediated syndromes is "real," whereas another is an artifact of group values, sets up the potential for conflict among care providers, clients, institutions, and the communities they wish to serve. There have been increasing calls for more culturally inclusive understanding of normal and dysfunctional behavior (Arnett, 2008).

Another factor that was newly considered is recognition of the relationship among spiritual difficulties and mental disorders (APA, 1994). According to Frey, Daaleman, and Peyton (2005), spirituality "may be tied to attributes of personal meaning that may or may not be tied to religious traditions" (p. 556). Personal meaning is thought to be relevant in the development of mental disorders. For example, depression may be related to a person's feeling that his or her life lacks meaning. There is also evidence that emphasizing spirituality has implications for outcomes of care (Wilding, May, & Muir-Cochrane 2005). For this reason, a number of diagnoses listed, now indicate spiritual considerations as factors in the diagnostic process.

One issue that seems quite basic has generated considerable debate and discussion. While there appears to be considerable agreement that diagnoses are dimensional, there is also recognition that a dimensional classification system may be too complicated to use and that such a system presents significant challenges in terms of data management and research. As indicated in the paragraphs that follow, the DSM-5 (APA, 2013) moves in the direction of greater acknowledgement of the dimensional nature of mental disorders with, for example, the inclusion of autism spectrum disorder.

As noted previously, one of the important purposes of a diagnostic system is to facilitate research. To be able to study a disorder and its causes, course, and outcomes of various treatments, one must be able to consistently identify and label the condition of interest. A current major emphasis in health care, including psychosocial health care, is a focus on **evidence-based practice** (EBP; Painter, 2012). Evidence-based practice is practice that is based on findings in the research literature that validate particular interventions. The goal is to provide care that is known to work. For example, Weisz, Jensen-Doss, and Hawley (2006) used meta-analysis techniques to identify evidence-based treatments for young people aged 3 to 18 years and to compare these interventions with what they labeled as "usual care." They explored the treatment of delinquency, substance abuse, conduct problems, depression, and anxiety and found that the evidence-based interventions were superior to usual care. Without a diagnostic system, that kind of study would be impossible, and it would be much more difficult to know what interventions are useful.

In mental health, the move toward EBP has been ongoing for some time and is closely associated with the changes in the DSM structure. As described previously, the DSM-IV was developed based on the best available literature at the time, and the DSM-5 has made substantial efforts to continue this trend (Kupfer, First, & Regier, 2002). Nevertheless, a great

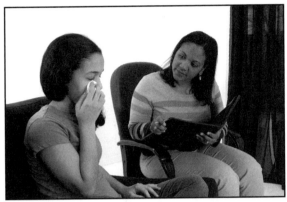

Figure 1-1. Psychotherapy can be valuable in helping many individuals with mental disorders. (©2014 Shutterstock.com.)

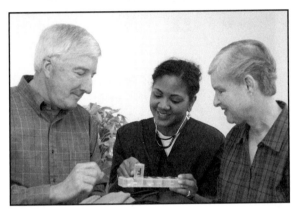

Figure 1-2. Another common, and often helpful, intervention is medication. (©2014 Shutterstock.com.)

deal of research is needed to ascertain whether psychotherapy (Figure 1-1), psychopharmacology (Figure 1-2), a combination of the two, or one of the many other possible intervention strategies has the greatest chance for success in treating a particular individual with a particular condition.

There are reasons to be concerned about EBP. In particular, research inevitably focuses on group averages, rather than on individuals. Thus, although EBP may identify effective interventions based on analyses of large numbers of interventions with large numbers of people, individuals vary greatly, and it can be difficult to discern when they differ enough to make the evidence-based intervention less helpful (APA Presidential Task Force on Evidence-Based Practice, 2006). Strategies to remedy this problem are being sought (cf. Borckardt et al., 2008), but the dilemma remains. Nevertheless, for the foreseeable future, EBP is a reality. This issue will be discussed further in Chapter 2 because it has clear implications for occupational therapy interventions.

From the perspective of occupational therapists, one of the many unresolved concerns is the appropriate strategy for identifying the functional factors that may (or may not) accompany psychiatric diagnoses. Both the DSM-IV (APA, 1994) and the ICD-10 (WHO, 1992) attempted to capture this information, with the DSM-IV introducing an axis to provide an operational assessment of impairment in functioning. Even though it had relatively good reliability and validity, the axis for describing function, Axis V, was not as well developed as the other axes and it frequently went unused. The WHO, by comparison, has an additional classification to supplement and complement the ICD-10 (1992). The *International Classification of Functioning, Disability and Health* (ICF; WHO, 2001), includes 10 areas of functioning (e.g., interpersonal interactions, social, civil life). The ICF (WHO, 2001) certainly ties more closely with occupational therapy concepts of mental health and mental illness, as noted in Chapter 2. The DSM-5 (APA, 2013) has eliminated the axis that specifically focused on function, including instead the functional criteria in various diagnostic categories. From the perspective of occupational therapy, this is a move in the right direction in the sense that it acknowledges function as a central component of well-being. However, the general statements in the diagnostic criteria are, as demonstrated in the chapters that follow, insufficient to really capture the details of occupational performance and individual satisfaction within occupational constellations.

As is always true for the establishment of diagnostic systems, the development of the DSM-IV (APA, 1994) was a political, as well as scientific, process with numerous and sometimes heated arguments about the following:

- Inclusion and exclusion of categories (Caplan, 1991)
- Criteria for existing categories
- Concern that the atheoretical stance of the DSM-IV led to elimination of important constructs
- Whether to have multiple axes and, if so, what they should be
- Concern that the DSM is excessively focused on biologically based explanations of disorders (Rogers, 2001)
- Exclusion of disciplines, other than psychiatry, in the development process (DeAngelis, 1991)

These political disputes reflect the reality that "acceptance of the person into (or exclusion from) the mental health system invariably involves ethical and political judgments" (Horsfall, 2001, p. 425). Such judgments may lead to overdiagnosis for those who do not conform to societal expectations or to the **medicalization** of problems that could also be considered as simply problems of living (Johnson, 2013; PLOS Medicine Editors, 2013). Underdiagnosis can likewise result from decisions to include or exclude particular factors from the diagnostic structure. Decisions about spending for mental health care may well be based on the view of a psychiatric disorder as either serious and enduring or less serious and more temporary, depending on criteria in the diagnostic guide rather than on the subjective experience of the individual (Perkins & Repper, 1998).

Some felt that the development of the DSM-IV was premature (Zimmerman, Jampala, Sierles, & Taylor, 1991). Critics suggested that although the DSM-III and DSM-III-R were gaining acceptance, they were not yet fully implemented in clinical settings (Maser, Kaelber, & Weise, 1991) and that change would be resisted (Morey & Ochoa, 1989). These critics also suggested that rapid change in diagnostic categories would reduce the ability of researchers to follow outcomes longitudinally or to compare research results for a specific disorder. Certainly, these criticisms have been reflected in the long wait for the DSM-5.

Due to the difficulties inherent in the development of the DSM-IV and because of concerns about excessively rapid change in the diagnostic structure, publication of the APA's DSM-5, originally planned for 2006, was delayed for 7 years, until its release in 2013. As a temporizing measure to bridge the gap in time between editions, a text revision of the DSM-IV was published in 2000. The DSM-IV-TR (APA, 2000) did not alter any of the diagnostic criteria. Rather, it provided an update of epidemiological and other information designed to clarify understanding of each category. For example, in the discussion of Asperger's syndrome, a newly included category in the DSM-IV (APA, 1994), information about specific examples of behavior that would assist in diagnosis, clarification of the possibility of communication deficits, and other relevant information had been added to the text, even though the criteria themselves remain unchanged. As described later, Asperger's syndrome, after considerable debate and discussion, was not included in the DSM-5 (APA, 2013).

Clearly, the development of the classification system is a complex scientific and political process that has involved physicians, psychologists, social workers, and political or special interest groups. This remains true for the DSM-5 (APA, 2013), although efforts have been made to recognize and respond to the many criticisms of previous classification systems. As you will see, the DSM-5 is no less controversial, in spite of these efforts.

Toward the *Diagnostic and Statistical Manual of Mental Disorders-5*

As the APA began to discuss a new edition of the DSM, there was general agreement that no new classification system should be published unless it improved on the existing one (Kendler, Kupfer, Narrow, Phillips, & Faucett, 2009). Each new version brings both improvements and problems, and the former must outweigh the latter if the change is to be worthwhile. Kendler et al. (2009) noted that the APA was guided by the following four principles (p. 2):

1. The DSM is above all a manual to be used by clinicians, and changes made for DSM-V must be implementable in routine specialty practices.

2. Recommendations should be guided by research evidence.

3. Continuity with previous editions should be maintained when possible (i.e., to avoid unnecessary disruption for clinicians, we should use research evidence to support maintaining the good qualities of DSM-IV, as well as to make revisions that will lead to better clinical diagnostic practice).

4. Unlike in DSM-IV, there will be no *a priori* constraints on the degree of change between DSM-IV and DSM-V.

The last two conditions are, obviously, in tension with each other, but the various individuals working on the manual felt that although continuity was important and valuable, changes that were clearly warranted on the basis of utility and/or research should be incorporated.

The process of developing the DSM-5 (APA, 2012a) was lengthy, complex, and, as has been the case with prior versions of the manual, contentious. The revision began with the convening of a global task force charged with overseeing a process of discussion and data collection intended to consider every aspect of the manual. These included examination of specific diagnoses, but also included consideration of the structure of the manual, how to deal with symptoms that might not be part of the diagnostic criteria but co-occur frequently, and how best to reflect the severity of the condition, as well as the specific label. The task force appointed 13 working groups to examine a wide array of questions they identified as being important to the thoughtful development of an improved classification system. Among these working groups were those that focused on, for example, eating disorders, mood disorders, and psychotic disorders (APA, 2012b). The task forces were charged with determining, on the basis of their clinical expertise and research findings, what worked and didn't work in the DSM-IV-TR (APA, 2000), evaluating research findings since its publication, and developing a research plan to study issues and resolve dilemmas. They were to examine the literature, undertake any needed secondary data analyses, and reconfigure diagnostic structures on the basis of all this evidence (Kendler et al., 2009).

The working groups and the task force held a number of conferences, posted materials for comment, and met regularly, both in person and virtually, over the course of a 12-year process. A total of 13 conferences, each of which had representatives from around the world, including individuals from the WHO and the World Psychiatric Association, were held during the course of the revision process (APA, 2012b). As was true for the development of the DSM-IV, disciplines other than psychiatry were also represented throughout the process.

Nevertheless, the new classification system was the target of considerable criticism even before it was on bookshelves. Among the concerns is the potential that millions of people will now be added to the rolls of those with mental illness and will be affected by the accompanying stigma (Brauser, 2012; Crocker, 2013; Rosenberg, 2013). As Rosenberg (2013) pointed out, "the odds will probably be greater than 50 percent, according to the new manual, that you'll have a mental disorder in your lifetime" (para. 1). The inclusion of new and controversial diagnoses like disruptive mood dysregulation disorder, which some feel applies a mental disorder to normal, age-appropriate temper tantrums, and binge eating disorder, perceived by many to be common overeating, rather than a mental disorder, led some commentators to suggest that everyday life has been pathologized (Deibler, 2013). The countervailing argument is to ensure that individuals get the help they need, it is important to be inclusive. Evidence has also suggested that, if anything, the prevalence of mental disorders is understated (Takayanagi et al., 2014). Of course, no one argues about "physical" diagnoses, for which lifetime prevalence, in combination, is almost certainly 100%.

Figure 1-3 shows the prevalence of serious mental disorders, both in total and by gender, age, and race. Note that gender, age, and race are all associated with differential rates of psychiatric disorder—a fact that we will return to regularly throughout this text. These data predate the DSM-5 (APA, 2013), and researchers will be paying close attention as it is used in clinical practice to distinguish whether concerns about skyrocketing rates of mental disorders are warranted.

A further criticism is that the process had been a closed and secretive one, a perception fueled by the requirement that members of the task force and working groups must sign a "member acceptance form" (Carey, 2008), which APA indicated was intended to protect intellectual property. Others perceived the form as a confidentiality agreement that prevented access by those not on the working groups. The chair of the DSM-III task force, Robert Spitzer, said the following:

> When I first heard about this agreement, I just went bonkers. Transparency is necessary if the document is to have credibility, and, in time, you're going to have people complaining all over the place that they didn't have the opportunity to challenge anything. (cited in Carey, 2008, para. 26)

Those on the task force dispute the contention that the process was closed, emphasizing that the acceptance form was not intended to create a closed system.

The issue of cultural variation in psychiatric disorders is one that the DSM has only begun to address, which is another source of dissatisfaction with the DSM-5 (APA, 2013). Cultural factors influence both the kinds of symptoms an individual may experience and their help-seeking behavior (Bonder & Martin, 2013). Examples abound of misunderstanding caused by misinterpretation of such culturally mediated syndromes. An individual from a culture holding a belief in the spirit world might find himself or herself diagnosed with schizophrenia. An individual from a culture that prescribes reticence and avoidance of eye contact might be diagnosed with depression. The simple problem of language difference can lead to misunderstanding and inappropriate diagnosis (see Bonder & Martin, 2013, for a comprehensive discussion of cultural factors in health care). Efforts were made in the development of the DSM-5 to be more inclusive of cultural (and gender) factors (Clay, 2013). The manual now has a brief section accompanying each diagnosis that indicates what cultural factors should be considered before making the diagnosis. It also includes tools for cultural assessment and a

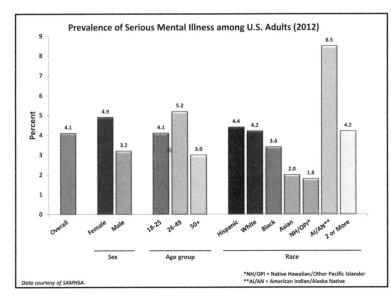

Figure 1-3. Prevalence of serious mental illness among U.S. adults by sex, age, and race in 2012 (National Institute of Mental Health, http://www.nimh.nih.gov/statistics/SMI_AASR.shtml).

section describing common culturally defined syndromes. However, according to some, this manual falls short in its efforts to incorporate culture in a more comprehensive and robust fashion (deJong, 2012).

Another focus of criticism is the extent to which the DSM-5 (APA, 2013) shifts from a supposedly atheoretical stance to a biomedical focus. There are those who have been very critical of the manual's emphasis on symptoms, rather than on underlying biology (Friedman, 2013). Such individuals point to the growing evidence of genetic causes for mental disorders (DeAngelis, 2013), the impact of maternal nutritional status or illness during pregnancy (Brown, 2011), and other evidence of biological etiology. The concern of these individuals, according to Dr. Thomas Insel (cited in Belluck & Carey, 2013) is that "as long as the research community takes the D.S.M. to be a bible, we'll never make progress" (para. 4) in identifying and thereby treating the underlying causes of mental disorders. One of the dilemmas of labeling that is based on symptom clusters is it ignores the fact that there is evidence they may be biologically heterogeneous (Friedman, 2013). For example, some people with a diagnosis of depression respond to antidepressants that enhance the neurotransmitter serotonin, whereas others respond to medication that increases dopamine. This makes it likely that different biological processes are at work within a single diagnosis. In response to these concerns, the National Institute of Mental Health (n.d.) has indicated plans to move away from the DSM and toward the Research Domain Criteria, which is a classification system being developed specifically to improve categorization for research purposes.

On the other side of this argument are those who feel that the biological research does not yet exist to support a fully biologically based diagnostic system (Brooks, 2013). Brooks noted that "mental diseases are not really understood the way, say, liver diseases are understood, as a pathology of the body and its tissues and cells. Researchers understand the structure of very few mental ailments" (para. 7).

Regardless of these controversies, care providers must use the generally accepted system, while remaining aware of its limitations. Currently, in the United States and via the ICD, globally, that system is the DSM-5. We will now turn our attention to a description of the structure of that guide.

Format of the *Diagnostic and Statistical Manual of Mental Disorders, Fifth Edition*

One of the most significant changes found in the DSM-5 (APA, 2013) is the elimination of the multiaxial system found in the DSM-IV and DSM-IV-TR. For occupational therapists, deletion of Axis IV (degree of stress within the 12 months preceding diagnosis) and Axis V (level of function) are particularly unfortunate, as these axes (although never extensively used) reflected the emphasis of occupational therapy intervention. Instead of these two axes, the new classification system focuses on cross-cutting dimensional assessment (Phillips, 2011). It allows for the rating of severity of symptoms as *very severe, severe, moderate,* or *mild,* as well as for rating other factors, such as accompanying personality traits and symptoms that do not fit the specified criteria. For many diagnoses, functional limitations are included as criteria supporting the label, although when such criteria are included they are typically stated in general terms. For example, criterion B for a diagnosis of intellectual disability indicates the following:

> Deficits in adaptive functioning that result in failure to meet developmental and sociocultural standards for personal independence and social responsibility. Without ongoing support, the adaptive deficits limit functioning in one or more activities of daily life such as communication, social participation, and independent living across multiple environments, such as home, school, work, and community. (APA, 2013, p. 33)

In addition, this system has been developed with an eye toward the National Institutes of Health (2010) Patient-Reported Outcome Measurement Information System (PROMIS). The PROMIS is intended to be a reliable and precise measurement of patient outcomes for all forms of health status: physical, psychosocial, and social. Its goal is to facilitate understanding of what really works in treatment as a way to improve outcomes. Clearly, this is an important goal for mental health care; the extent to which the DSM-5 (APA, 2013) diagnostic criteria assist in evaluating outcomes will be an important measure of the success of the new classification system.

That edition of the DSM is divided into three main sections. The first—DSM-5 Basics (APA, 2013)—describes the use of the manual. In particular, this section emphasizes that multiple diagnoses can be applied in a single situation and that subtypes and specifiers are included to assist in increasing the specificity of the disorder's presentation in a particular client. It discusses the use of principal (main) and provisional (temporary) diagnoses and includes a discussion of the development of assessment and monitoring mechanisms.

Section II comprises the bulk of the text. Its 22 chapters focus on specific diagnoses, clustered "based on underlying vulnerabilities as well as symptom characteristics" (APA, 2012b, n.p.). Section II includes general categories, such as neurodevelopmental, emotional, and somatic disorders, and, within these general categories, individual chapters focus on more specific categorizations. Many diagnoses are similar to those that appeared in the DSM-IV-TR (APA, 2000), with only minor modifications in diagnostic criteria. In some cases, the greatest change is in the reorganization that was undertaken to try to cluster similar diagnoses. For instance, Conduct Disorder, which was previously in the section on Disorders Usually First Diagnosed in Infancy, Childhood, or Adolescence (APA, 2000), is now included in the chapter on Disruptive, Impulse-Control, and Conduct Disorders (APA, 2013). In addition, some disorders, such as schizophrenia and autism, are specifically noted as spectrum disorders. This emphasizes the reality that their presentation occurs along a continuum of severity.

Individual diagnostic categories include an array of specifiers, modifying information intended to provide greater clarity about the unique presentation of the disorder in a specific individual (APA, 2013). For example, the specifiers for schizophrenia include an option to indicate that the disorder has presented with mood-congruent or mood-incongruent psychotic features, with catatonia, peripartum onset, or seasonal pattern, in partial or full remission, and whether it is mild, moderate, or severe. Therefore, an individual diagnosed with schizophrenia could have the diagnosis further described as *moderate, with catatonia, in partial remission.*

Each diagnostic category also includes a discussion of conditions that need to be considered in the differential diagnosis process, as well as those that might be **comorbid**; that is, they accompany the diagnosis under consideration (APA, 2013). For example, an individual might have both an anxiety disorder and a depressive disorder or a personality disorder and an anxiety disorder.

There are several additional factors included for each diagnostic category (APA, 2013). These will be described here and will not be repeated in subsequent chapters. However, it is important to keep in mind that they apply to every diagnosis. One of these factors is that for almost all diagnoses there are criteria indicating that the diagnosis applies only if another diagnosis does not better fit the symptoms. For example, one would not diagnose posttraumatic stress disorder if generalized anxiety disorder symptoms are a better fit for the individual's situation. Some diagnoses are relatively similar; and clinicians responsible for diagnosis must take those minor differences into account. There is also a criterion for most diagnoses that note they should be made only if they are not accounted for by a medical condition. This means that if an individual's anxiety is the result of a hyperthyroid condition, it would not be diagnosed as generalized anxiety disorder. Of course, an individual with a hyperthyroid condition might also have a generalized anxiety disorder; again, the diagnosing clinician must make a thoughtful judgment in such a case.

One set of options make clear the extent to which individuals' symptoms deviate from the defined criteria for a particular diagnosis (APA, 2013). Each diagnostic category includes an "other specified" choice and an "unspecified" choice.

The third section (APA, 2013) includes a great deal of supplemental information, including assessment and cross-cutting symptom measures, discussion of cultural formulations, and the appendices that provide information about changes to this edition of the DSM and a list of conditions for further study. This last set of discussions sets the stage for the DSM-5.1, 5.2, and so on. Finally, it contains appendices that include a description of changes from the DSM-IV to the DSM-5, glossaries of technical terms and cultural concepts, and listings of DSM codes that correlate with the ICD-9 and ICD-10.

This book presents a discussion of the relationship of diagnosis to occupational therapy and the consideration of major diagnostic categories, with emphasis on what is known or theorized about etiology and course of the disorders, the types of treatments currently being used, and the efficacy of those treatments. For the most part, the chapter structure mirrors the chapters in DSM-5 (APA, 2013). In a few cases, information has been combined to minimize duplication. Information about the various diagnoses is linked to probable effects on the occupational performance of the individual and recommendations about potential occupational therapy interventions. Here, you will find a fair amount of repetition. As you read, consider why the information about occupational therapy interventions might be so repetitive if the mental disorder diagnoses are so varied. An answer will be forthcoming in Chapters 22 and 23.

CASE STUDY

Siobhan McLain is a 35-year-old psychology graduate student who lives alone in graduate student housing in a large eastern city. She is in her second semester of graduate school after graduating from a California state university near her home. She is an attractive and typically well-groomed young woman who has always been a good student and who enjoys academic challenges. She has a large network of friends, participates weekly in a study group with several other students, and works as a tutor for undergraduate students at her institution.

In the past 2 weeks, Ms. McLain has had difficulty getting out of bed, finding herself exhausted by the effort. She has missed several classes and an appointment with her advisor, and she has not left the apartment. She has also not showered, dressed in anything other than sweats, or made herself a meal. From time to time, she eats a few spoonfuls of peanut butter or drinks a glass of (now sour) milk.

Ms. McLain has a large extended family, all of whom live on the West Coast. Her father died when she was 13 years old, being a victim of a single-car accident. At the time, there was a suspicion that he had committed suicide, but Ms. McLain's mother was adamant that this was not true. Ms. McLain's three siblings are all older and married. When she was living in California, she frequently saw her siblings and babysat for their children. She talks weekly with her mother via Skype, but she did not answer her mother's most recent Skype call. She did not answer the phone for several days, and when she finally did speak with her mother, she was tearful and uncommunicative.

Her friends have become concerned, and several of them have called or stopped by. She tells each of them that she is "fine" but otherwise refuses to say much.

THOUGHT QUESTIONS

1. Do you think that Ms. McLain has a mental disorder? If so, make a list of the factors in the description here that lead to that conclusion.
2. What problems, if any, do you see with Ms. McLain's daily activities? Again, make a list of the factors that contribute to this conclusion.
3. In what way do your two lists differ? In what ways are they the same?
4. Ms. McLain is a fifth-generation Irish American. Based on the limited information provided here, do you feel that her culture contributes to her current situation? What more would you need to know to make this judgment?
5. Would it make a difference to your assessment of the situation if Ms. McLain had previous similar episodes? Would it make a difference if this was the first/only time she'd experienced this type of episode?

Internet Resources

American Psychiatric Association DSM-5 Development homepage
http://www.dsm5.org/Pages/Default.aspx
Want to know more about how DSM-5 was developed? This site is the portal for information about the process as a whole and provides reports of the various working groups and research data that informed the process.

Centers for Disease Control and Prevention

http://www.cdc.gov/mentalhealth/

This link is for the homepage of the U.S. Centers for Disease Control and Prevention's Mental Health information. The site includes a wealth of information about mental disorders, their symptoms, prevalence, and treatment, as well as links to other resources. Much of the material is written for a lay audience.

National Institute of Mental Health

http://www.nimh.nih.gov/index.shtml

This is another Federal government site that includes a great deal of helpful information about mental health and mental disorders generally, as well as specific diagnostic groups.

National Institute of Mental Health Research Domain Criteria

http://www.nimh.nih.gov/research-priorities/rdoc/index.shtml

The Research Domain Criteria project of the National Institute of Mental Health is mentioned in Chapter 1. This site provides additional information about the project's activities.

References

American Psychiatric Association. (1952). *Diagnostic and statistical manual of mental disorders*. Washington, DC: Author.

American Psychiatric Association. (1968). *Diagnostic and statistical manual of mental* disorders (2nd ed.). Washington, DC: Author.

American Psychiatric Association. (1980). *Diagnostic and statistical manual of mental disorders* (3rd ed.). Washington, DC: Author.

American Psychiatric Association. (1987). *Diagnostic and statistical manual of mental disorders* (3rd ed., revised). Washington, DC: Author.

American Psychiatric Association. (1994). *Diagnostic and statistical manual of mental disorders* (4th ed.). Washington, DC: Author.

American Psychiatric Association. (2000). *Diagnostic and statistical manual of mental disorders* (4th ed., text revision). Washington, DC: Author.

American Psychiatric Association. (2012a). *DSM: History of the manual*. Retrieved from http://www.psychiatry.org/practice/dsm/dsm-history-of-the-manual.

American Psychiatric Association. (2012b). *DSM-5 overview: The future manual*. Retrieved from http://www.dsm5.org/about/Pages/DSMVOverview.aspx.

American Psychiatric Association. (2012c). *Frequently asked questions*. Retrieved from http://www.dsm5.org/about/Pages/faq.aspx.

American Psychiatric Association. (2012d). *Working group members*. Retrieved from http://www.dsm5.org/MeetUs/Pages/WorkGroupMembers.aspx.

American Psychiatric Association. (2013). *Diagnostic and statistical manual of mental disorders* (5th ed.). Washington, DC: Author.

APA Presidential Task Force on Evidence-Based Practice. (2006). Evidence-based practice in psychology. *American Psychologist, 61*(4), 271-285.

Arnett, J.J. (2008). The neglected 95%: Why American psychology needs to become less American. *American Psychologist, 63*, 602-614.

Belluck, P., & Carey, B. (2013, May 6). Psychiatry's guide is out of touch with science, experts say. *New York Times*. Retrieved from http://www.nytimes.com/2013/05/07/health/psychiatrys-new-guide-falls-short-experts-say.html?pagewanted=all&_r=0.

Blacker, D., & Tsuang, M.T. (1999). Classification and DSM-IV. In A. M. Nicholi (Ed.), *The Harvard guide to psychiatry* (3rd ed., pp. 65-73). Cambridge, MA: Harvard University Press.

Bonder, B., & Martin, L. (2013). *Culture in clinical care: Strategies for Competence* (2nd ed.). Thorofare, NJ: SLACK Incorporated.

Borckardt, J.J., Nash, M.R., Murphy, M.D., Moore, M., Shaw, D., & O'Neil, P. (2008). Clinical practice as natural laboratory for psychotherapy research: A guide to case-based time-series analysis. *American Psychologist, 63*, 77-95.

Boyd, J.H., Burke, J.D., Grundberg, E., Holzer, C.E., & Rae, D.S. (1984). Exclusion criteria of DSM-III: A study of co-occurrence of hierarchy-free syndromes. *Archives of General Psychiatry, 41,* 983-989.

Brauser, D. (2012, December 3). *Experts react to DSM-5 approval.* Retrieved from http://www.medscape.com/viewarticle/775526.

Brooks, D. (2013, May 27). Heroes of uncertainty. *New York Times.* Retrieved from http://www.nytimes.com/2013/05/28/opinion/brooks-heroes-of-uncertainty.html?_r=0.

Brown, A.S. (2011). The environment and susceptibility to schizophrenia. *Progress in Neurobiology, 93*(1), 23-58.

Caplan, P.J. (1991). How do they decide who is normal? The bizarre, but true, tale of the DSM process. *Canadian Psychology, 32,* 162-170.

Carey, B. (2008, December 17). Psychiatrists revise the book of human troubles. *New York Times.* Retrieved from http://www.nytimes.com/2008/12/18/health/18psych.html?pagewanted=1&_r=0.

Clay, R.A. (2013, April). The next DSM. *Monitor on Psychology,* 26-27.

Crocker, L. (2013, April 11). DSM-V: Hoarding, binge eating & more new mental-disorder diagnoses. *The Daily Beast.* Retrieved from http://www.thedailybeast.com/articles/2013/04/11/dsm-v-hoarding-binge-eating-more-new-mental-disorder-diagnoses.html.

DeAngelis, T. (1991). DSM being revised, but problems remain. *American Psychological Association Monitor, 22,* 12-13.

DeAngelis, T. (2013). The genetic dawn of mental illness. *Monitor on Psychology, 44*(3), 27-28.

Deibler, M.W. (2013, May 17). The DSM-5 is not crazy. *Slate.* Retrieved from http://www.slate.com/articles/health_and_science/medical_examiner/2013/05/defense_of_the_dsm_5_new_diagnoses_for_picking_bingeing_and_tantrums.html.

deJong, J.T. (2012). DSM-5 and culture [Abstract]. *Tijdschrift voor psychiatrie, 54*(9), 807-818.

Fabrega, H. (1992). Diagnosis interminable: Toward a culturally sensitive DSM-IV. *Journal of Nervous and Mental Disease, 180,* 5-7.

Friedman, R.A. (2013, May 20). The book stops here. *New York Times.* Retrieved from http://www.nytimes.com/2013/05/21/health/the-dsm-5-as-a-guide-not-a-bible.html.

Frances, A.J., First, M.B., Widiger, T.A., Miele, G.M., Tilly, S.M., Davis, W.W., & Pincus, H. (1991). An A to Z guide to DSM-IV conundrums. *Journal of Abnormal Psychology, 100,* 407-412.

Frey, B.B., Daaleman, T.P., & Peyton, V. (2005). Measuring a dimension of spirituality for health research: Validity of the Spirituality Index of Well-Being. *Research on Aging, 27,* 556-577.

Greenberg, G. (2013). *Book of woe: The DSM and the unmaking of psychiatry.* New York, NY: Blue Rider Press.

Horsfall, J. (2001). Gender and mental illness: An Australian overview. *Issues in Mental Health Nursing, 22,* 421-438.

Hwang, W.C., Myers, H.F., Abe-Kim, J., & Ting, J.Y. (2008). A conceptual paradigm for understanding culture's impact on mental health; the cultural influences on mental health (CIMH) model. *Clinical Psychology Review, 28,* 211-227.

Johnson, S.B. (2013). Increasing psychology's role in health research and health care. *American Psychologist, 68*(5), 311-321.

Kendall, R.E. (1991). Relationship between the DSM-IV and the ICD-10. *Journal of Abnormal Psychology, 100,* 297-301.

Kendler, K., Kupfer, D., Narrow, W., Phillips, K., & Fawcett, J. (2009). *Guidelines for making changes to DSM-V.* Retrieved from http://www.dsm5.org/ProgressReports/Documents/Guidelines-for-Making-Changes-to-DSM_1.pdf.

Klerman, G.L. (1988). Classification and DSM-III-R. In A.M. Nicholi (Ed.), *The new Harvard guide to psychiatry* (pp. 70-87). Cambridge, MA: Belknap Press.

Kupfer, D.J., First, M.B., & Regier, D.A. (2002). *A research agenda for DSM-V.* Washington, DC: American Psychiatric Press.

Maser, J.D., Kaelber, C., & Weise, R.E. (1991). International use and attitudes toward DSM-III and DSM-III-R: Growing consensus in psychiatric classification. *Journal of Abnormal Psychology, 100,* 271-279.

Mellsop, G., Varghese, F., Joshua, S., & Hicks, A. (1982). The reliability of Axis II of DSM-III. *The American Journal of Psychiatry, 139,* 1360-1361.

Mezzich, J.E., & Berganza, C.E. (2005). Purposes and models of diagnostic systems. *Psychopathology, 38,* 162-165.

Millon, T. (2004). *Masters of the mind: Exploring the story of mental illness from ancient times to the new millennium.* New York, NY: John Wiley & Sons.

Morey, L., & Ochoa, F. (1989). An investigation of adherence to diagnostic criteria: Clinical diagnosis of the DSM-III personality disorders. *Journal of Personality Disorders, 3,* 180-192.

Moriyama, I.M., Loy, R.M., & Robb-Smith, A.H.T. (2011). *History of the statistical classification of diseases and causes of death.* Rosenberg, H.M. & Hoyert, D.L. (Eds.). Hyattsville, MD: National Center for Health Statistics. Retrieved from http://www.cdc.gov/nchs/data/misc/classification_diseases2011.pdf.

National Institutes of Health. (2010). *PROMIS*. Retrieved from http://www.nihpromis.org/default#3.

National Institute of Mental Health. (n.d.). *Research domain criteria (RDoC)*. Retrieved from http://www.nimh.nih.gov/research-priorities/rdoc/index.shtml.

Painter, K. (2012). Evidence-based practices in community mental health: Outcome evaluation. *Journal of Behavioral Health Services & Research, 39*(4), 434-444.

Perkins, R., & Repper, J. (1998). *Dilemmas in community mental health practice*. Abingdon, England: Radcliffe Medical Press.

Phillips, J. (2011). DSM is a many-dimensioned thing. *Psychiatric Times*. Retrieved from http://www.psychiatrictimes.com/dsm-5-0/dsm-many-dimensioned-thing.

PLOS Medicine Editors. (2013). The paradox of mental health: Over-treatment and under-recognition. *PLOS Medicine*. doi:10.1371/journal.pmed.1001456.

Rogers, D.A. (2001, March 1). When, oh when, will psychology lay its own behavioral tracks without relying on psychiatry? *The National Psychologist*. Retrieved from http://nationalpsychologist.com/page/7?s=free+free.

Rosenberg, R.S. (2013, April 12). Abnormal is the new normal: Why will half of the U.S. population have a diagnosable mental disorder? *Slate*. Retrieved from http://www.slate.com/articles/health_and_science/medical_examiner/2013/04/diagnostic_and_statistical_manual_fifth_edition_why_will_half_the_u_s_population.html.

Spitzer, R.L., Endicott, J., & Robins, R.C. (1975). Research diagnostic criteria (RDC). *Psychopharmacology Bulletin, 11*, 22-24.

Spitzer, R.L., Forman, J.B.W., & Nee, J. (1979). DSM-III field trials I: Initial interrater diagnostic reliability. *The American Journal of Psychiatry, 136*, 818-820.

Stetka, B.S., & Correll, C.U. (2013). *A guide to DSM-5*. http://www.medscape.com/viewarticle/803884.

Szasz, T. (1974). *The myth of mental illness* (2nd ed.). New York, NY: Harper & Row.

Takayanagi, Y., Spira, A.P., Roth, K.B., Gallo, J.J., Eaton, W.W., & Mojtabai, R. (2014). Accuracy of reports of lifetime mental and physical disorders: Results from the Baltimore Epidemiological Catchment Area Study. *JAMA Psychiatry, 71*(3), 273-280. doi:10.1001/jamapsychiatry.2013.3579.

Taylor, R.R., & Jason, L.A. (1998). Comparing the DIS with the SCID: Chronic fatigue syndrome and psychiatric comorbidity. *Psychology and Health, 13*, 1087-1104.

Walker, M.T. (2006). The social construction of mental illness and its implications for the recovery model. *International Journal of Psychosocial Rehabilitation, 10*(1), 71-87.

Weisz, J.R., Jensen-Doss, A., & Hawley, K.M. (2006). Evidence-based youth psychotherapies versus usual care: A meta-analysis of direct comparisons. *American Psychologist, 61*, 671-689.

Widiger, T.A., Frances, A.J., Pincus, H.A., & Davis, W.W. (1990). DSM-IV literature reviews: Rationale, process, and limitations. *Journal of Psychopathology and Behavioral Assessment, 12*, 189-202.

Wilding, C., May, E., & Muir-Cochrane, E. (2005). Experience of spirituality, mental illness and occupation: A life-sustaining phenomenon. *Australian Occupational Therapy Journal, 52*, 2-9.

Williams, J.B.W. (1985). The multiaxial system of DSM-III: Where did it come from and where should it go? *Archives of General Psychiatry, 42*, 181-186.

Williams, J.B.W. (1988). Psychiatric classification. In J.A. Talbott, R.E. Hales, & S.C. Yudofsky (Eds.), *The American Psychiatric Press textbook of psychiatry* (pp. 201-223). Washington, DC: American Psychiatric Press.

World Health Organization. (1992). *International classification of diseases* (10th ed.). Geneva, Switzerland: Author.

World Health Organization. (2001). *International classification of functioning, disability, and health*. Geneva, Switzerland: Author.

Zimmerman, M., Jampala, C., Sierles, F.S., & Taylor, M.A. (1991). DSM-IV: A nosology sold before its time? *The American Journal of Psychiatry, 148*, 463-467.

DSM-5 and
Occupational Therapy

Learning Outcomes

By the end of this chapter, readers will be able to:
- Define the disease model of psychiatric diagnosis
- Discuss how the American Psychiatric Association's (APA) *Diagnostic and Statistical Manual of Mental Disorders* (DSM) and the World Health Organization's (WHO) *International Classification of Diseases* (ICD) have developed in parallel
- Describe the need for the WHO's *International Classification of Functioning, Disability and Health* (ICF)
- Discuss the ways in which occupational therapy categorization of psychosocial dysfunction differs from psychiatric diagnosis
- Describe how the ICF supports the views of occupational therapy about psychosocial dysfunction
- Identify the main points of several occupational therapy frames of reference for mental health
- Describe the six areas of focus for occupational therapy, as described in the *Occupational Therapy Practice Framework, Third Edition*
- Identify and discuss trends in mental health that have direct impact on the practice of occupational therapy

Bonder B.
Psychopathology and Function, Fifth Edition (pp 21-46).
© 2015 SLACK Incorporated.

KEY WORDS

- Disease model
- Occupational science
- Function
- Model of human occupation
- Allen cognitive disability model
- Person-environment occupational performance model

- Rehabilitation model
- Occupational adaptation model
- Selection, optimization, compensation model
- Kawa model
- Interpersonal relationship model
- Diagnostic overshadowing

CASE VIGNETTE

Andre Jackson is a 50-year-old homeless man and a veteran of Desert Storm. He entered the military immediately after graduating high school and had a military career of 12 years. After sustaining severe burns while in Iraq, he was treated at the Veterans Administration Hospital in his California hometown and was then discharged, both from the hospital and the military. Since that time, he has lived on the streets, working infrequently as a laborer. He receives a small disability pension. Mr. Jackson also occasionally stays in one of the local homeless shelters. He is an unpopular resident there because of his severe nightmares, from which he awakes screaming. He also has frequent temper outbursts that result in fights with other residents in the shelter. He dislikes staying in the shelter because they do not permit alcoholic beverages and because they insist that he shower before using one of the cots.

THOUGHT QUESTIONS

1. Do you think that Mr. Jackson has a mental disorder?
2. If so, what are the behaviors that led you to this conclusion?
3. If not, what do you think might account for his behavior?
4. What kinds of difficulties with daily activities are most important in Mr. Jackson's current situation? What thoughts do you have about interventions that might help Mr. Jackson to function more effectively?

Occupational therapy "diagnoses" differs substantially from medical and psychological diagnoses. The domain of occupational therapy is "achieving health, well-being, and participation in life through engagement in occupation" (American Occupational Therapy Association [AOTA], 2014, p. S4). This means that the focus of assessment, goal setting, and intervention is on the daily activities that clients must accomplish and those they want to accomplish.

This chapter examines the theoretical bases of psychological and occupational therapy conceptualizations of disorders, the impact of those conceptualizations on the diagnosis and beliefs about treatment, and the possibilities for interaction between the two systems. This chapter provides a general overview only, and readers are encouraged to refer to the texts that deal with psychosocial considerations in occupational therapy. Greater detail about assessment and about intervention is included in Chapters 22 and 23, respectively. You may also refer to the resource list at the end of this chapter.

To understand how occupational therapy fits in the mental health system, as well as how psychiatric disorders can affect care more generally, some discussion of the differing views of dysfunction is a necessary starting point.

Psychiatric Theories of Mental Disorders

What constitutes psychiatric disturbance is not fixed or absolute. Porter (1987) noted that "what is mental and what is physical, what is mad and what is bad, are not fixed points but culture relative" (p. 10). Ideas have changed throughout the centuries about what mental illness is and what interventions are appropriate. At some points in history, deviant or unusual behavior was accepted in the community, whereas at other times, individuals with these behaviors were institutionalized and kept out of sight. Treatment philosophies have shifted from so-called rational to moral to medical, and expectations about outcomes have shifted from optimistic to pessimistic and back again. All of these views have been influenced by and have influenced ideas about the origins and treatments of mental disorders.

Some theorists have speculated that deviance emerges from early childhood experiences (the analytic view; Freud, 1901) or innate personality (personality theory; Duggan et al., 2003), whereas others suspect that the problem is from faulty learning (behavioral theory; Skinner, 1953) or a skewed set of interpretations about events (cognitive theories; Rachman, 1997). Other theories emphasize neurobiological explanations or interactional models (Frager & Fadiman, 1998). As noted in Chapter 1, Szasz (1974) felt that psychiatric disorder did not exist, but instead was a reflection of the lack of acceptance of behavior that was outside of cultural norms, which is a view that has been reiterated by others over the years (cf. Small & Barnhill, 1998). Some theories (e.g., analytic) focus almost exclusively on internal processes and feelings, whereas others (e.g., cognitive) focus on thought processes; still others (e.g., behavioral) focus largely on observable behaviors.

In the last half of the 20th century, the definition of mental illness has shifted "from a diagnosis-focused to a person-focused definition of mental illnesses, and from an 'absence of disease' model to one that stresses positive psychological function for mental health" (Manderscheid et al., 2010, p. 1). This has been accompanied by a broader understanding that mental health contributes to overall health and well-being, which is reflective of a general shift in medicine from curing disease to prevention and health promotion.

As a result of a number of trends in health care—increased biological research, particularly genetic research; the move to evidence-based practice (EBP); and shifts in reimbursement trends—the *Diagnostic and Statistical Manual of Mental Disorders, Fifth Edition* (DSM-5; APA, 2013a) has moved away from an atheoretical stance toward a system that is more "etiologically based" (Aboraya, 2010); that is, developed on the basis of the underlying cause of a given disorder. This stance continues a shift in diagnosis toward a biologically based understanding of mental disorder. It implies that there are specific syndromes or conditions that constitute discrete and distinguishable entities identified on the basis of a constellation of symptoms, including psychological characteristics, behaviors, and physical findings. As shown in Chapter 1, this shift has led to considerable controversy about whether the DSM is too biologically based or not enough.

The **disease model** that categorizes mental disorders as illnesses rather than behavioral problems has long presented dilemmas in mental health care (Antonosky, 1972). Not all psychological theories fit neatly into the medical model. For example, behaviorists focus on mental disorders as being characterized by problematic behaviors, and their interventions focus on remediating those behaviors. Cognitive therapists conceptualize mental disorders as patterns of thought that lead to negative emotions and behaviors, and thus attempt to help clients alter the ways in which they view the world and their own situations. Neither of these approaches focuses on curing disease in the usual medical sense. The disease model has been criticized as being driven by particular segments of the research endeavor, notably psycho-pharmacological research (Healy, 2002). Another concern is that diagnosis and symptoms are not good predictors of functional skills, such as work performance and social skills (Tsang, Lam, Ng, & Leung, 2000). Perhaps most telling, Aboraya (2010) noted, "It is true that we are far from knowing the etiology of most mental disorders" (p. 34). Even so, the importance of the medical model to psychiatry continues to be evident in the centrality of the DSM diagnostic structure.

It is important to remember that the DSM-5 is not only biologically based, but culturally based as well (Alarcón, 2009). Although the DSM-5 includes an appendix listing various mental disorders described by other cultures, many feel that the diagnostic system itself continues to be strongly focused on Western beliefs and values about the causes and manifestations of psychological distress. Other explanatory models, including possession by spirits or imbalance of various elements of the self or of the self with nature, are not considered in the Western-based structure of diagnoses. However, large populations, both outside and within the United States, hold beliefs that are inconsistent with the DSM diagnostic system.

There are a number of reasons why diagnosis is important, as described in Chapter 1. Mezzich and Berganza (2005) identified the main purposes of diagnostic systems as (a) understanding a case, (b) planning effective clinical care, and (c) intervening to promote public health. They further noted that such systems must convey information. Decisions of third-party payers are simplified by attaching a label to a set of symptoms, and outcomes can then be evaluated based on change in that set of symptoms. Common understanding of categories is also vital in promoting research that will enhance understanding and—hopefully—treatment of specific disorders. The process of developing the DSM-5 (APA, 2013b) has "generated a wealth of knowledge about the prevalence and distribution of mental disorders worldwide, the physiology of the brain, and the lifelong influences of genes and environment on a person's health and behavior" (para. 1). For these reasons, it is unlikely that the diagnostic system will disappear at any time in the near future, in spite of the many criticisms noted in Chapter 1.

Psychiatrists acknowledge that diagnosis is only loosely related to function. Individuals who are diagnosed as schizophrenic may present with widely varying functional abilities; for instance, some may be able to hold jobs, whereas others may require the constant attention of an inpatient psychiatric facility. It is also true that individuals diagnosed with a particular disorder may vary on other emotional and behavioral attributes (APA, 2013a). In addition, there is acknowledgment that when the "disease" has been ameliorated, residual dysfunction in daily life may remain to be addressed (Warner, 2009). For example, individuals with schizophrenia often develop the disorder in mid-to-late adolescence. Medication and behavioral interventions may help these individuals to manage the positive symptoms of the disorder (e.g., hallucinations and delusions), but they may fail to learn many of the important life skills that are essential elements of normal adolescent development. When their positive symptoms have diminished, a set of functional deficits with regard to basic life tasks, such as work and leisure, remains.

The medical community has recognized the limitations of the traditional diagnostic structure. One attempt to deal with these limitations has been the development of the *International Classification of Functioning, Disability, and Health* (ICF; World Health Organization [WHO], 2001). This classification system is based on factors of the individual, including body functions and structures; the interface between the individual and the environment; activities; participation; and factors in the environment that support or restrict function and context. This system, like the DSM and the *International Classification of Diseases* (ICD), allows for alphanumeric categorization so that a score can be assigned that indicates what kind of dysfunction exists (for example, body function is assigned a "b"), and how severe the problem is (denoted with a 0 to 4 rating).

The ICF provides a description of function and disability that is separate from—but may be related to—biological disorder. Its creators indicate that it includes the following four major purposes:

1. "To provide a scientific basis for understanding and studying health and health-related states, outcomes, and determinates

2. To establish a common language for describing health and health-related states in order to improve communication between different users, such as health care workers, researchers, policy-makers, and the public, including people with disabilities

3. To permit comparison of data across countries, health care disciplines, services, and time

4. To provide a systematic coding scheme for health information systems" (WHO, 2001, p. 5)

This classification system is much closer to the view promoted by occupational therapy and recognizes that disease and dysfunction are not synonymous. However, the ICF conceptualization of function has limitations as related to occupational therapy (Hemmingsson & Jonsson, 2005). One concern is regarding the ICF's emphasis on observable behavior, which excludes the individual's subjective experience. In addition, the ICF's conceptualization of the environment and the environmental impact on function is relatively one-dimensional. As demonstrated later in this chapter, the *Occupational Therapy Practice Framework: Domain and Process* (AOTA, 2014) is a more useful and comprehensive guide for occupational therapists for the understanding of function. Nevertheless, the ICF is clear evidence that occupational therapy is not alone in recognizing function as a construct separate from disease or illness.

Like the DSM, the ICF was developed through a lengthy process that included research; consensus meetings of researchers, care providers, consumers, and policy makers; and public comment in locations around the world. The ICF was an attempt to be truly international and, therefore, cross-cultural in scope. This effort at cross-cultural awareness is an important attribute of the classification system as it relates to mental health and psychosocial dysfunction.

The emphasis on function in the ICF (WHO, 2001) is helpful for occupational therapists, for whom function is the primary concern. It has helped to bring occupational therapy into the mainstream in international health circles, as others increasingly recognize function as being vital to definitions of health and quality of life.

As discussed in Chapter 1, culture clearly influences perceptions of mental health. Although the DSM-5 (APA, 2013a) has expanded its treatment of culture, the primary categories reflect largely Western, possibly even U.S., beliefs. For example, premenstrual dysphoric disorder—described almost exclusively in industrialized countries and particularly in the United States—is included as a formal diagnosis, whereas *pribloqtoa*, *susto*, *nervios*, and *amok*, which are culturally mediated conditions from Inuit, Hispanic, and Malaysian cultures, are listed only in the appendix. An example of the kinds of challenges faced by the APA in addressing culture is the discussion of diagnostic criteria for posttraumatic stress disorder (Phillips & Phillips, 2010). There is evidence that the diagnostic framework does not adequately capture the kinds of situations encountered in some non-Western cultures where ongoing civil war and cultural beliefs about expressions of stress differ greatly from anything encountered in the United States. Given the increasingly diverse character of the United States, the existing classification system works poorly across cultures (Bonder & Martin, 2013). The DSM-5 (APA, 2013a) attempted a more robust acknowledgement of cultural factors than previous editions of the DSM, but there is still considerable work to be done to genuinely incorporate culture into the diagnostic structure.

Occupational Therapy View of Mental Disorder

Occupational therapy has its roots in mental health. Bream (2013) recounts work by numerous early thinkers in the field of occupational therapy who believed that "the greatest value of occupational therapy would be its impact on the mental health arena" (p. CE-1). There certainly is evidence that this belief is an accurate one, although the number and proportion of occupational therapists working in settings exclusively focusing on mental health is not large.

Originating during World War I in response to the horrors of that conflict,

> the first occupational therapy aides went to La Fauche, France, to serve at Base Hospital 117 near the front lines. Their assignment was to provide treatment to enable physically sound men suffering from war neurosis to return to duty as quickly as possible. (Low, 1992, p. 38)

War neurosis is now recognized as posttraumatic stress disorder (which is discussed in detail in Chapter 9). The therapists emphasized hands-on activities in a workshop environment, providing the soldiers with opportunities for creativity, which was a way to express emotional concerns through activity and to forget what they had recently been through. According to Low (1992), "Their work exemplified the value of activities as therapy" (p. 43).

The founders of occupational therapy included the psychiatrist Dr. Adolf Meyer, whose philosophy focused on interaction with the environment to balance the individual, natural rhythms that positively affect well-being and in spheres of occupation (Reitz, 1992). Occupational therapy was founded on humanistic principles during the Progressive Era in the United States—a time when the mental hygiene movement and the arts-and-crafts movement also emerged. Although the profession has at times strayed from those early values, the past several decades have seen renewed emphasis on occupation as contributing not only to physical function but to mental well-being as well. Turpin (2007) cited a presentation by Coleman in 2005 that focused on a need to "recover our belief in holism rather than responding to government and organizational pressures to see people as diagnoses and symptoms" (p. 469).

One factor that has encouraged efforts focused on recovering the fundamental beliefs of occupational therapy has been the establishment of **occupational science**, which is a discipline dedicated to the study and understanding of occupation (Zemke & Clark, 1996). Occupational science was "formally created in the last decades of the twentieth century by occupational therapists to study people as occupational beings" (Wilcock, 2005, p. 7). Occupational scientists are interested in understanding how occupational therapists "ignite our clients' intense engagement in a world of productivity and activity" (Wilcock, 2005, p. xiv). In enhancing this understanding, occupational scientists attempt to explain how occupation and well-being (physical, psychosocial, and spiritual) interact.

The practical implication of this is that although physicians (including psychiatrists) focus on disease, occupational therapists focus on **function** (i.e., the ability of individuals to accomplish their daily occupations; AOTA, 2014) and performance. It is quite possible for an individual to have a disease that results in no functional deficit, or at least one that does not require intervention. For example, an individual who has a head cold has a disease, but he or she may carry on with normal activities (Rogers, 1982).

On the other hand, some individuals who have no diagnosable disease—either physical or psychological—have deficits in occupational performance. For example, children from socioeconomically deprived backgrounds may have difficulty adapting to expectations in a school setting, and adults from isolated rural settings might show performance deficits when they move to the city to take factory jobs. These do not constitute diseases in the medical sense, but occupational therapists would be concerned about remediating performance deficits. Failure to address those deficits could certainly contribute to depression or anxiety in such individuals.

The idea that deficits in occupational performance contribute to poor quality of life and well-being is a consistent tenet of occupational therapy, regardless of the theoretical orientation of the therapist. Thus, individuals who adhere to Kielhofner's **model of human occupation** (MOHO; Kielhofner, 2002), which is a general systems model; the **Allen cognitive disabilities model** (Allen, 1985), which is a neurobiological model; or the **Person-Environment Occupational Performance** (PEOP) model (Christiansen & Baum, 1997) would all focus on function as the central concern of assessment and intervention. However, the specific problems identified on the basis of these theories would differ. In the case of the MOHO, a deficit might be identified in personal volition (i.e., interests and motivation to accomplish activities). The cognitive approach suggests the cognitive level (i.e., problem solving, the ability to acquire new information) as a source of difficulty in accomplishing activities. The PEOP model might lead to identification of a poor fit between environmental demand and individual skills. Likewise, the interventions suggested by the models would vary because the problems identified differed. However, the long-term goal of each is to enhance performance of everyday occupations.

The *Occupational Therapy Practice Framework: Domain and Process* (AOTA, 2014), which is the guiding document for practice developed by the AOTA Commission on Practice, focuses on the profession's "core belief in the positive relationship between occupation and health and its view of people as occupational beings" (p. S3). To address this overarching belief, therapists emphasize the following:

- Occupations
- Client factors
- Performance skills
- Performance patterns
- Context and environment
- Activity demands

Like the DSM and the ICF, the Practice Framework is a work in progress. It is derived from an earlier document, the Uniform Terminology Checklist (AOTA, 1994). The first version of the Practice Framework (AOTA, 2002) was developed through a lengthy process of literature review and discussion. The second edition was published in 2008 and represented a refinement of the first, rather than a wholesale revision. Likewise, the third edition (AOTA, 2014) refined and revised the conceptual system.

Gutman, Mortera, Hinojosa, and Kramer (2007) noted that:

> the Framework was developed as a document that could (1) describe the profession's philosophical assumptions, (2) define the profession's domain of concern, (3) offer direction for evaluation and intervention, and (4) help external audiences to better understand the profession's unique contributions to health care. (p. 119)

The Practice Framework attempts to use carefully defined and clear terminology to communicate the central values and practices of occupational therapy.

Table 2-1 summarizes the areas included in the current conceptualization of the domain of occupational therapy. Note that all of these areas are focused on performance, not on the labeling of deficits. Note also that the majority of areas encapsulate performance that is dependent on interrelationships among client factors (values, beliefs, spirituality, body functions, body structures), activity demands, and performance skills. This focus means that psychological,

TABLE 2-1

OCCUPATIONAL THERAPY DOMAIN

AREA OF OCCUPATION	CLIENT FACTORS	PERFORMANCE SKILLS	PERFORMANCE PATTERNS	CONTEXT AND ENVIRONMENT	ACTIVITY DEMANDS
ADL	Values, beliefs, and spirituality	Sensory perceptual skills	Habits	Cultural	Objects used and their properties
IADL	Body functions	Motor and praxis skills	Routines	Personal	Space demands
Rest and sleep	Body structures	Emotional	Roles	Physical	Social demands
Education		Cognitive skills	Rituals	Social	Sequencing and timing
Work		Communication and social skills	Temporal	Required actions	
Play				Virtual	Required body functions
Leisure					Required body structures
Social participation					

Republished with permission of American Occupational Therapy Association from Occupational therapy practice framework: Domain and process (2nd ed.). *American Journal of Occupational Therapy, 62*, 625-683, 2008; permission conveyed through Copyright Clearance Center, Inc.

cognitive, neuromuscular, and other skills must be in concert to ensure well-being—a view rather different from the view promoted in the DSM, which largely focuses on psychosocial and cognitive factors. As with the DSM and ICD, it can be assumed that new versions of the *Practice Framework* will emerge as new developments emerge in occupational therapy.

Domain of Occupational Therapy

Occupational therapy assumes that "people are shaped by what they have done, by their daily patterns of occupation" (Zemke & Clark, 1996, p. vii). The relevant questions for therapy relate to the kinds of choices that individuals make about their daily occupations, how those choices contribute to their sense of well-being, and how occupational therapists therapists and certified occupational therapy assistants (COTA) can structure interventions that facilitate participation in the activities that promote meaning and well-being.

Because, unlike physicians, occupational therapists focus on what it is that the clients need and want to do, their theoretical models for wellness differ as well. Occupational therapists develop interventions based on a set of theoretical beliefs about human performance and its enhancement.

Models That Assist in Understanding Behavior

Among these models are several that were noted previously—the Allen Cognitive Disabilities Model (Allen, 1985), the MOHO (Kielhofner, 2002), and the PEOP model (Christiansen & Baum, 1997). Allen's (1985) model suggests that individuals with mental disorders function at particular levels of cognitive ability that may or may not be modifiable; in cases where the individual's ability may not change, more supportive environments or activity changes can support function. The MOHO is a general systems model that addresses interactions among abilities, volition, and the environment. The PEOP, also a systems model, describes an interaction among individual characteristics, the environment, and occupations. Others models include the **rehabilitation model** (Anthony, 1979) and the **occupational adaptation model** (Schkade & Schultz, 1992; Schultz & Schkade, 1992). The **selection, optimization, and compensation model** (Baltes & Baltes, 1990), developed with an emphasis on older adults, is less focused on how disorders develop but is more focused on strategies for intervening. Newer models can be helpful in framing awareness of factors that receive additional emphasis as our understanding of occupation increases. For example, the growing interest in cultural factors in occupation is reflected in the **Kawa model** (Iwama, 2006). The Kawa model reduces the centrality of Western philosophy in understanding occupation, noting that concepts such as individualism and independence may not resonate in other cultures. Instead, the Kawa model's focus is on cultural relevance and safety. The theory emphasizes a water metaphor (*kawa* means water in Japanese), along with the importance of placing the individual in context. Another more recently developed model is the **interpersonal relationship model** (Taylor, 2008). This model emphasizes the importance of the therapeutic relationship in effective occupational therapy intervention and addresses strategies for balancing a focus on activity, with a focus on relationships.

Each model suggests a way of thinking about occupational function and dysfunction, including the sources of problems and the strategies for intervening. Effective therapy involves theory-based intervention that incorporates the model or a combination of models best validated by research as a means of framing assessment and intervention. Table 2-2 provides a brief summary of the beliefs of some of the best known conceptualizations of factors associated with occupational performance. Although this is not an exhaustive list, it indicates some of the theories in common use that offer descriptions of occupation in ways that can structure therapists' approaches.

Theories of Occupational Therapy Practice in Mental Health

It is important to note that almost all of the previous models include consideration of the client's cultural background, which is a key factor as identified in the *Practice Framework's* (AOTA, 2014) discussion of environment and contexts. The client's needs and wants will vary, depending not only on personal and environmental considerations but also on the cultural values and beliefs that are part of the individual's experience. These beliefs and values are vital when considering therapeutic interactions, and they can affect both major concerns (e.g., identification of treatment goals) and smaller concerns (e.g., choice of a specific activity to address those goals). Therapists must ensure that they gather and incorporate cultural considerations in all parts of the therapeutic process.

TABLE 2-2			
SOME THEORIES RELEVANT FOR OCCUPATIONAL THERAPY IN MENTAL HEALTH			
THEORY	*BELIEFS ABOUT DYSFUNCTION*	*INTERVENTION*	*OUTCOME*
Model of human occupation (Kielhofner, 2002)	Maladaptive cycles, feedback Does not meet needs for exploration and mastery Poorly developed or disordered volitional, habituation subsystems	Assessment: Evaluation of subsystems, environment, and feedback Intervention: Age-appropriate occupation	Adaptive cycles, age-appropriate systems
Rehabilitation model (Anthony, 1979)	Psychiatric disability Deficits in skilled performance	Assessment: Present and needed skills Intervention: Step organized program includes physical fitness and vocational activities	Increased repertoire of skilled behavior: physical, emotional, and intellectual Increased personal satisfaction and/or abilities Improved match between environment, occupation, and person
Person-environment-occupation performance model (Christiansen & Baum, 1997)	Deficits in person abilities Poor match between person, environment, and occupation Excessive occupational/environmental demands	Assessment: Individual skills, wishes and environmental, occupational demands Intervention: Enhancement of individual skills, clarification of personal goals, and modification of environment or occupation	Increased personal satisfaction and/or abilities Improved match between environment, occupation, and person
Occupational adaptation model (Schkade & Schultz, 1992; Schultz & Schkade, 1992)	Ineffective adaptive response Ineffective occupational response	Assessment: Information about occupational role expectations, person systems, and occupational adaptation Intervention: Focus on enhanced occupational adaptation	Effective adaptive response Effective occupational response
			(continued)

TABLE 2-2 (CONTINUED)			
SOME THEORIES RELEVANT FOR OCCUPATIONAL THERAPY IN MENTAL HEALTH			
THEORY	*BELIEFS ABOUT DYSFUNCTION*	*INTERVENTION*	*OUTCOME*
Kawa model (Iwama, 2006)	Culture and environment influence meaning and contribute to the definition of what constitutes undesirable states of being Context can enable and disable people	Assessment: Appreciate client in context Intervention: Focus on client goals in context. Find sources of life energy	Enable greater life flow
Intentional relationship model (Taylor, 2008)	Focus is on the importance of and strategies for building therapeutic relationships to address client concerns	Assessment: Focus on client preferences for structure of therapy sessions, client's perceptions about therapy sessions Intervention: Effective use of the self is critical to positive outcomes. Client defines a successful relationship. Activities and relationships must be balanced in intervention	Positive therapeutic relationships that facilitate positive outcomes of intervention
Selection, optimization, and compensation (Baltes & Baltes, 1990)	The process of human development from childhood into old age and age-related change in adaptive capacity, with a continuous interplay between growth and decline Individuals maximize the positive and minimize the negative by selection, optimization, and compensation (NOTE: This theory originated in the field of gerontology.)	Assessment: What activities does the individual want to do (select)? How can ability be maximized (optimize)? What new activities can fill gaps (compensate)? Intervention: Support optimization of abilities, implement new, compensating activities as needed.	Satisfying constellation of meaningful activities

Figure 2-1. An occupational therapist may evaluate the skills needed to undertake a specific job. (©2014 Shutterstock.com.)

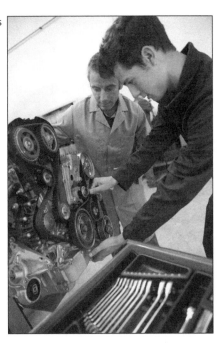

As is true in psychiatry and other mental health care professions, two primary factors influence treatment planning and intervention. The first of these is the diagnostic system that structures understanding of the individual's challenges and needs. The second is the theoretical framework that guides understanding of effective strategies for addressing those challenges and needs. Concepts related to the occupational therapy evaluation and interventions to address psychosocial well-being and disorder are discussed in greater detail in Chapters 22 and 23. Occupational therapists generally focus on the enhancement of client abilities in performance areas, skills, and patterns. The ultimate goal of occupational therapy, unlike medicine or psychology, is effective function in meaningful occupation. For example, as shown in Figure 2-1, occupational therapy would focus on an individual's ability to manage the cognitive, sensory–motor, and social aspects of a job. The belief of occupational therapists and COTAs is that a balance of occupation in all performance areas promotes the best possible quality of life for the individual (Meyer, 1922/1977).

A psychiatrist might interact with a client and note depressed mood and lethargy and say, "Here is someone who has a persistent depressive disorder. Let us treat the client with antidepressant medication and with verbal therapy to allow him to express his feelings." The occupational therapist might interact with the same client and note a general lack of interest and investment in activities. The occupational therapist might sum up the situation very differently and think, "Here is someone who has a pervasive sense of failure and no clear goals in life. Let us help him participate in activities that will affirm his strengths and encourage him to identify some goals that will give his life meaning." The two approaches are clearly different. In the best possible situation, they are complementary, each providing the client with something that will enhance his or her satisfaction with life, as well as his or her ability to contribute to society.

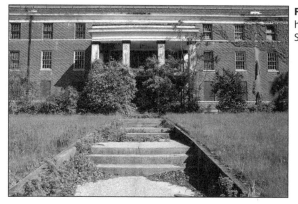

Figure 2-2. The old-style state psychiatric hospital has largely disappeared. (©2014 Shutterstock.com.)

Trends Affecting Mental Health Care in Occupational Therapy

Occupational therapy, like mental health care in general, must respond to an array of societal and political pressures and changes. Among those that have had the most impact on the delivery of occupational therapy services are the following:

- Changes in the service delivery systems for mental health, including sources of funding for care
- Changes in public policy and reimbursement structures
- Growing awareness of the common features of conditions conceptualized as "physical" and those conceptualized as "psychological"
- Increasing population diversity, coupled with growing appreciation of cultural difference in conceptualizations of health and disease
- A trend toward increased interdisciplinary intervention
- Increasing demands for accountability

Changes in Service Delivery and Sources of Funding for Care

Occupational therapy in mental health had its roots in the moral treatment movement of the late 19th and early 20th centuries (Christiansen & Haertl, 2014). This movement focused on humane care for individuals with mental disorders. These individuals were often housed in large psychiatric hospitals located in rural areas that were thought to promote calm and serenity (Figure 2-2). It was not unusual for individuals to spend decades in these institutions. Occupational therapists emphasized vocational activities, which were consistent with rural life (e.g., gardening, tending animals), and avocational activities, which were enjoyable and low stress (e.g., arts and crafts).

However, in the mid-twentieth century, in part as a result of improved medical (i.e., drug) treatment of mental disorders, there was a growing movement to return clients to the community. The Community Mental Health Center Act of 1963 (Rochefort, 1984) speeded the movement away from inpatient treatment (Griswold, 1999). Large state psychiatric hospitals were emptied, as a trend toward reintegration in the community spread. The idea that separating troubled individuals from their familiar environments, families, and friends was damaging to their recovery represented a significant shift in views about care. Occupational therapy was focused on assisting clients to develop the instrumental activities of daily living, which would enable them to cope with independent life in the community, as many had not managed money, shopped, or cooked in years.

Unfortunately, although well-intended and, in some instances, helpful, the Community Mental Health Center Act led to an array of new problems (Scharfstein, 2000). Some individuals did not have families to which to return, some individuals needed more intensive care than could be provided by community mental health centers, and funding was cut in times when the economy was slow, thus reducing services even more.

Nevertheless, long-term inpatient psychiatric care became increasingly rare. Over time, hospital stays decreased so that currently most consist of no more than a few days, and much of the care is provided in outpatient settings (Salinsky & Loftis, 2007). There has been an increase in hospitalization rates for adolescents and young adults in the past decade (Blader, 2011), but levels remain much lower than in the early 1960s and length of stay is usually very brief. A stay of several weeks or months is quite rare, except for some intensive substance abuse treatment programs.

Although community mental health centers still exist, their role in the treatment of mental disorders has greatly diminished. The system of care in mental health has become increasingly fragmented (Rosenberg, 2009), with services being offered in a multitude of forms and settings, and include the following:

- Inpatient psychiatric hospitals for short-term stays for individuals who represent an imminent danger to themselves or others (Horsfall, Cleary, & Hunt, 2010)
- Community mental health centers for short- to moderate-term outpatient psychotherapy (Auxier, Farley, & Seifert, 2011)
- Day treatment centers for individuals with serious mental disorders (Skalko, Williams, Snethen, & Cooper, 2008)
- Nursing homes and group homes for individuals needing long-term residential support (Felce et al., 2008; Molinari, Hedgecock, Branch, Brown, & Hyer, 2009)
- Primary care settings (e.g., through family practice offices) for brief consultation and medication (Madge, Foreman, & Baksh, 2008)
- Private pay psychotherapy services for individual or group therapy (Chen & Rizzo, 2010)
- Home health care for medication monitoring and management (Lichtenstein, 2012)
- Schools, either therapeutic or mainstream, for children with neurodevelopmental disorders (Kutcher & Wei, 2012)
- Psychiatric emergency rooms to manage individuals with acute, severe psychological symptoms (Simakhodskaya, Haddad, Quintero, & Malavade, 2009)

Occupational therapists and COTAs have a clear role in many of these settings, especially in community settings (Scaffa, Pizzi, & Chromiak, 2010), and there are numerous accounts of community-based intervention programs. For example, Bazyk (2011) described approaches to promotion of mental health in K-12 schools. An occupational therapist consulting with the teacher might help to design strategies that would support emotional expression, self-control, self-esteem, and emotional regulation. A number of studies confirm the value of both primary and tertiary prevention efforts in community-based settings to reduce bullying and aggression among school children (Bugenatl, Corpuz, & Schwartz, 2012). Prevention efforts can also support employment for individuals with developmental disabilities (Siporin & Lysack, 2004; Wuang, Wang, Huang, & Su, 2009) or individuals with severe mental illness (Chan, Tsang, & Li, 2009). An obvious dilemma is that the range of settings can contribute to fragmentation of care, which is a particular problem when a condition is either chronic or recurring (Hurst, 2013). Individuals with mental disorders often have poor problem solving, difficulty with follow-through, and trust issues that make such fragmentation particularly challenging.

Evidence of the effectiveness of community-based occupational therapy interventions has increased in the past two decades (Clark et al., 2001; Herzberg & Petrenchik, 2010; Holm, Santangelo, Fromuth, Brown, & Walter, 2000; Scaffa et al., 2010), providing important support for their value. As discussed later in this chapter, the integration of services presents a significant challenge in providing effective community-based care (Burson & Simpatico, 2002). Therefore, therapists must inform themselves about available services and mechanisms for ensuring that their clients receive appropriate referral. Awareness of and collaboration with other disciplines is vital for effective intervention in community settings.

Changes in Public Policy and Reimbursement Structures

Historically, paying for mental health services has been a challenge. Currently, primary sources of funding include Medicare and Medicaid; Social Security (through Social Security Disability); the Veteran's Administration; state or local government support for public hospitals, offices for support of children with developmental disabilities and vocational rehabilitation; and private insurance (Landsvek, Burns, Stambaugh, & Reutz, 2006; Substance Abuse and Mental Health Services Administration, 2011). The fact that there are so many different systems involved in the payment structure, as well as the limitations imposed by each, inevitably means that some individuals do not have the coverage needed. Those who do have coverage may find it to be limited, disjointed, and inadequate.

Two major pieces of relatively recent legislation have led to some progress in addressing this issue. The passage of the Affordable Care Act of 2010 (ACA; U.S. Department of Health and Human Services, 2014) was an effort to address the problem faced by the 17% of the U.S. population without health insurance coverage in 2010 (O'Hara & Caswell, 2012). Many of those individuals were the working poor—people at high risk for a wide variety of physical and psychological difficulties. The ACA reflects numerous compromises but falls well short of the kind of universal coverage that has long been discussed in this country (and exists in every other Western society). Nevertheless, its provisions increase the number of individuals who will have some form of health care. Because these provisions are being phased in over 10 years, it is too early to know the extent to which the law will actually reduce the number of uninsured individuals.

The ACA includes provisions that have the potential to improve mental health services (Stoffel, 2013). The ACA requires coverage of an array of problems, including serious mental illness and substance abuse. It provides chronic care management and care coordination, as well as opportunities for wellness and prevention programs. In particular, it focuses on recovery-oriented outcomes. Each of these provisions represents an opportunity for occupational therapists, whose long-standing interest in mental health care offers particular expertise for contribution.

From the perspective of mental health care, another bill has been equally important. The Mental Health Parity and Addiction Equity Act of 2008 (U.S. Department of Labor, 2012) requires insurers to cover mental health care in the same way that other kinds of medical care are covered. Prior to the passage of this bill, many insurance policies simply did not cover mental health services and many that did imposed stringent limitations on the dollar amounts, number of sessions, and conditions included.

In spite of the passage of these two bills, coverage remains incomplete. For example, Graham (2013) noted that the Mental Health Parity Bill left many issues unresolved, including the scope of coverage (a particular concern for occupational therapy), strategies for medical management, and lack of enforcement. The situation is particularly challenging for occupational therapy, which has not been incorporated into required coverage (Pitts et al., 2005).

Growing Awareness of the Common Features of Conditions Conceptualized as Physical and Those Conceptualized as Psychological

The distinctions between physical and psychological disorders are always arbitrary to some extent. Regardless of your practice setting, you will encounter individuals with both kinds of disorders; in fact, research suggests that there is no clear line between them (Kendall, 2001).

People with physical illnesses often benefit greatly from psychological interventions (Needham & Hill, 2010; Piazza, Charles, Sliwinski, Mogle, & Almeida, 2012). The impact of disorders such as arthritis, cancer, and heart disease can be reduced by paying attention to the anxiety and depression that may accompany them (Ali, Rollman, & Berger, 2010; Brothers, Yang, Strunk, & Andersen, 2011). Stress reduction is associated with lower rates of chronic disease (Piazza et al., 2012), as is intervention to reduce loneliness (Hawkley, Thisted, Masi, & Cacioppo, 2010). When chronic diseases occur, such as diabetes, psychological intervention can improve outcomes (Lewin et al., 2010).

At the same time, as discussed in other chapters of this book, there is increasing recognition that psychiatric disorders may have physical (genetic, autoimmune, and other) causes. Research on the etiology of autism is now focusing on genetics and chromosomal irregularities (Butler, Youngs, Roberts, & Hellings, 2012), as it is clearly a disorder associated with neurological function. Schizophrenia is believed to be caused by a combination of genetic factors and alterations in brain chemistry (Walsh et al., 2008).

Some disorders, such as Alzheimer's, fit within both the physical and psychological diagnostic systems. Multiple sclerosis, Parkinson's disease, and many other neurological disorders frequently manifest with psychological symptoms such as dementia, emotional lability, and depression. In fact, a chapter of the DSM-5 (APA, 2013a) addresses this specific issue and labels the cluster of neurocognitive disorders.

An important consideration in addressing the needs of individuals with mental disorders is **diagnostic overshadowing** (Thornicroft, Rose, & Kassam, 2007). This construct describes the fact that individuals with diagnosed mental disorders may have difficulty getting the medical care they need for other conditions due to the tendency of health care providers to dismiss their physical complaints. Yet, individuals with bipolar disorder can also develop cardiovascular problems and need treatment for physical conditions just as much as individuals with cardiovascular problems may need treatment for the depression that often accompanies the physical diagnosis. It is essential that health care professionals—including occupational therapists—recognize and avoid the potential to overlook real physical health issues in individuals with mental disorders.

It seems likely that as research continues, the line between the physical and the psychological will blur further. It is also the case that while working with clients whose disorders are categorized largely as physical, it is important to recognize that they may benefit from interventions that support their emotional, cognitive, and social needs as well. One strategy for managing this integration is the development of interdisciplinary teams in integrated care settings (Weiss, 2013). These integrated care settings involve a variety of providers across the range of behavioral and physical health needs in a single facility to reduce fragmentation and improve outcomes.

Increasing Population Diversity Coupled With Growing Appreciation of Cultural Difference in Conceptualizations of Health and Disease

As we have already seen, therapists must be aware of the cultural considerations related to mental disorders (Morales & Norcross, 2010). A growing body of research demonstrates the value of multiculturalism in working with ethnic minority clients. As is explicit in the DSM-5 (APA, 2013a), culture influences diagnosis and treatment, including not only the labels for the problem and the conceptualizations about etiology and prognosis but also treatment expectations, cooperation with recommended intervention, family involvement, and perceptions about side effects (Bonder & Martin, 2013; Flaskerud, 2000). Understanding cultural beliefs can also provide helpful interventions that may not be part of Western psychological tradition. Such treatments include acupuncture (Wu, Yeung, Schnyer, Wang, & Mischoulon, 2012), *tai chi* and *quigong* (Abbott & Lavretsky, 2013), as well as various herbal and spiritual remedies (Meisenhelder & Chandler, 2000). Incorporation of these kinds of beliefs into treatment can have a positive impact on outcomes.

In addition, cultural sensitivity as applied to typical Western interventions, such as cognitive behavioral therapy, can enhance outcomes of those approaches (Hayes, 2009). The essential factors in framing an intervention strategy include ensuring that assessment is reflective of cultural beliefs, identifying culturally mediated strengths and resources, and understanding the environmental factors, such as racism and discrimination, that contribute to an individual's problems. For occupational therapists, this means working with clients to identify culturally-relevant activities that are meaningful and motivating to the individual in the context of his or her beliefs and environment. Occupational therapists may find that incorporating activities such as *tai chi* and meditation into their interventions can be valuable in some situations, and there are many similar examples of non-Western activities that may be the focus of treatment with clients from a variety of backgrounds.

Interdisciplinary Intervention

Interdisciplinary care in mental health is an important strategy for working with clients needing mental health services (AOTA, 2011) and is one that presents challenges to effective care (Fortune & Fitzgerald, 2009). As therapists increasingly work in quarter- or half-way houses, community centers, sheltered living facilities, schools, and clients' homes, there is much "role blurring" among disciplines (Brown, Crawford, & Darongkamas, 2000). In addition to occupational therapists, the client may be treated by a psychiatric nurse; social worker; psychologist; art, music, dance, or recreation therapist; vocational counselor; and psychiatrist, and it may be difficult to maintain effective interaction among these various team members. In addition, it is important for all of these disciplines to recognize and value the professional scopes of practice of those with whom they collaborate (Kessler, 2014).

The nurse is primarily responsible for nursing care, medical management, and, in inpatient settings, for promoting the therapeutic milieu (Foster, 2001). A category of nurse practitioners exists that specifically focuses on psychiatric practice, and these nurses may also provide psychotherapy (National Panel for Psychiatric-Mental Health NP Competencies, 2003). Social workers deal with family issues and with discharge planning. Some social workers provide individual or group psychotherapy. Psychologists typically complete psychological assessments and, in some settings, provide individual and group psychotherapy (American Psychological Association, 2013). Art, music, and dance therapists offer opportunities for expression through nonverbal means, using the expressive arts as their media. Vocational counselors and job coaches focus on work-related skills and abilities, whereas recreation therapists focus on leisure abilities and interests. The psychiatrist provides medical care and prescribes medications, including psychotropic medications.

Occupational therapists focus on the assessment and remediation of performance of work, leisure, and self-care, as well as the underlying skills required to accomplish these activities. Their holistic view of activity helps them to integrate the perspectives of art, music, and dance, as well as those of recreation therapists, vocational counselors, and other members of the treatment team. They emphasize body functions and structures, motor skills, process skills, and communication/interaction skills, as well as the habits, routines, and roles required for optimal engagement in occupation (AOTA, 2014). To accomplish these interventions, occupational therapists often rely on the expertise of certified occupational therapy assistants who are effective at implementing treatment and making careful, thoughtful observations that contribute to refinement of intervention over time.

Ideally, the various mental health professionals work together to provide the best care for the client (Kessler, 2014). However, roles sometimes overlap and because cost containment has become an issue, efforts have been made to reduce the number of different therapists involved with each client. Occupational therapists have a broad perspective and can focus on issues that are vital to the client; they also have an obligation to recognize their limitations and call on others as appropriate.

Increasing Demands for Accountability

There is a growing demand for accountability and the demonstration that care is effective and worth reimbursement (Kazdin, 2011; Stepney & Rostila, 2011). The need for EBP—which, as discussed, has affected the development of the DSM—is particularly vital in health care because it attempts to control costs. If occupational therapists expect to continue to be included in this system, they must document their value (Gutman, 2011). Occupational therapists have an obligation to review the current literature and practice standards, which is a challenge in this era of information overload. One strategy for staying current is to regularly check search engines such as CINAHL and PsychInfo, which are available through most university libraries. Many excellent websites also provide current and regularly updated information about mental health care. The AOTA has designed several strategies for encouraging systematic literature reviews and for posting evidence-based reviews to inform clinicians. Several of these resources are listed at the end of this chapter. Therapists should visit these or similar sites on a regular basis to ensure that they are aware of the emerging scientific progress and practice trends.

Unfortunately, in the occupational therapy literature, there is a relative scarcity of research about mental health (Lloyd et al., 2010). This presents significant challenges for the profession as practitioners attempt to implement best practices. Another challenge for therapists is the need to ensure that use of EBP does not overshadow the views and values of the individual receiving treatment (Kazdin, 2011). Occupational therapists must be cautious about ignoring individual needs that are not described in the literature.

It is also important to be aware of other limitations of EBP (Hinojosa, 2013). Research can identify what is best for the average individual, but the average individual exists only as an artifact. Particularly in mental health, personal, social, environmental, and experiential factors interact to create unique situations that may require unique solutions. Another concern is that some forms of intervention are more difficult to study than others. In the upcoming chapters, psychopharmacology and CBT are frequently mentioned as effective treatments. This may be because they actually are most effective, but it also may be because they are more readily quantified and studied. Although there is considerable evidence for the effectiveness of psychodynamic psychotherapy (Shedler, 2010) and other forms of psychotherapeutic intervention (Barth et al., 2013), the volume of information is substantially less than for CBT and medication. Thus, although EBP can be helpful in guiding intervention, it is not without its drawbacks.

To make the best use of research evidence, practitioners should be prepared to evaluate the quality and meaning of research findings. Hodson and Craig (2010) recommended reflecting on the following five questions about a given research study:

1. What are the benefits and harms of the intervention?

2. Are there variations in the relative treatment effect?

3. Does the treatment effect vary with different baseline risk?

4. What are the predicted reductions in symptoms or risk for individuals?

5. Do the benefits of the intervention outweigh the harms? (p. 277)

Reminding oneself that these questions are relevant in determining how to view research results is a helpful way to recall that research varies in quality and relevance. Not every research finding is applicable to every client with a particular problem. Nevertheless, it is important to recognize that research can be essential in ensuring that clients receive the best care.

All of these trends make for a complex situation in which occupational therapy services are provided. Therapists must understand the system, the beliefs and values of their clients, and the beliefs and values of other professionals.

The chapters that follow describe the diagnostic categories in the DSM-5 (APA, 2013a), including diagnostic criteria, etiology, symptoms, and prognosis. They then describe the functional consequences of each disorder and its typical treatment. The disorders most likely to require occupational therapy services are emphasized, whereas others are described briefly. In reading these chapters, you will see that individuals with a variety of disorders may benefit from similar occupational therapy interventions because performance-related factors move across medical diagnoses.

Following the diagnosis-specific chapters, three chapters focus on aspects of intervention that directly affect the occupational therapy process in working with clients with mental disorders. Chapter 21 provides an overview of psychopharmacology, with an emphasis on what therapists need to know. Chapter 22 considers general approaches to the occupational therapy evaluation in psychosocial settings, and Chapter 23 addresses occupational therapy interventions. Although the individual diagnosis chapters provide information about evaluation and treatment that is directly linked to the conditions being described, occupational therapy approaches move across multiple psychiatric diagnoses. It is this reality that provides the most emphatic evidence of the differences among mental health disciplines. These differences relate to the central goal of occupational therapy, which is improved occupational performance.

Suggested Readings

Bruce, M.A., & Borg, B. (2002). *Psychosocial frames of reference: Core for occupation-based practice* (3rd ed.). Thorofare, NJ: SLACK Incorporated.

Cole, M.B., & Tufano, R. (2008). *Applied theories in occupational therapy: A practical approach.* Thorofare, NJ: SLACK Incorporated.

Scaffa, M., Reitz, S., & Pizzi, M. (2010). *Occupational therapy in the promotion of health and wellness.* Philadelphia, PA: F.A. Davis.

Sladyk, K., Jacobs, K., & MacRae, N. (2009). *Occupational therapy essentials for clinical competence.* Thorofare, NJ: SLACK Incorporated.

CASE STUDY

Al Dekmajian is a 50-year-old small business owner who lives in a suburban ranch home with his wife of 20 years and their two high school-aged sons. Mr. Dekmajian and his brother have a business that sells used comic books and sports cards, which has just expanded to its third location in a city in the Pacific Northwest. He met his wife when she applied for a clerk position in one of the stores. She still helps out occasionally, but she mostly stays home with their sons.

Although the business has been quite successful for several decades, opening a store at the third location has been stressful for the whole family. Mr. Dekmajian has been working very long hours, typically leaving the house around 9 o'clock in the morning and not returning until 11 or 12 o'clock at night. For a few months, he seemed exhausted when he returned, but lately he has been somewhat agitated and fidgety when he gets home.

In addition, Mr. Dekmajian's relationship with his brother has deteriorated significantly. They have shared responsibilities for more than two decades, but recently Mr. Dekmajian and his brother have had several screaming matches and they no longer speak to each other.

Mr. Dekmajian's wife describes him as generally cheerful and hard-working, but he has always had a temper. Although he has never struck her, she has been fearful on occasion and generally tries not to be around him when he is angry. However, over the past 2 years, these temper outbursts have become more frequent. On the most recent occasion, 1 week ago, he began throwing household items, breaking several plates, a vase, and a chair. She is aware that Mr. Dekmajian has used cocaine in the past because they used together on several occasions when they were dating. Although he denies current use of cocaine, she recognizes his behavior as similar to what she witnessed when they were dating.

THOUGHT QUESTIONS

1. What behaviors or emotions in this description suggest a mental disorder?
2. What functional consequences are resulting from Mr. Dekmajian's behaviors? That is, what occupational performance areas seem problematic?
3. How do you think Mr. Dekmajian's behavior might affect his wife and sons? What impact might his behavior have on their ability to accomplish needed and desired occupations?
4. Chapter 2 began with a case vignette about a 50-year-old man with issues related to anger. What is different about the two cases in this chapter? What are the common elements? In what ways might your thinking about the occupational performance of these two individuals be the same? Different?

Internet Resources

American Occupational Therapy Association
http://www.aota.org

The professional association for occupational therapists. A variety of publications about mental health, including position papers and practice guidelines, can be found at this site. Press releases, special interest group reports, advocacy initiatives, and other information are also included here.

American Psychiatric Association

http://www.psych.org

Medical research, including new information about diagnosis, laboratory testing, medication, and other treatments, can be found at this site.

American Psychological Association

http://www.apa.org

A good source of information about psychotherapeutic interventions.

MedMark, Psychiatry

http://www.medmark.org/psy/psychi2.htm

An excellent search engine for a wide array of topics, including various diagnoses, diagnostic testing, medication, and other intervention strategies. Includes a comprehensive list of other sources, including many appropriate for consumers.

National Alliance for the Mentally Ill

http://www.nami.org

This is the best known consumer organization on mental health and includes excellent information from the perspective of individuals with mental health problems. Includes educational, research, and advocacy information and is appropriate for both professionals and consumers.

National Library of Medicine

http://www.nlm.nih.gov

The National Library of Medicine houses both search engines and original documents. It is a comprehensive source for research literature and information about ongoing research and policy initiatives.

National Institute of Mental Health

http://www.nimh.nih.gov

The main body of funding research in mental health, this organization provides links to other sources, information about current research, and information about funding opportunities.

PsycPORT.com

http://www.psycport.com

Produced by the American Psychological Association, this website includes current news reports and press releases.

Internet Resources for Evidence-Based Practice

American Occupational Therapy Association, Evidence-Based Practice

http://www.aota.org/ebp

General resources and links to several practice areas.

American Occupational Therapy Association, Evidence-Based Practice

http://www.aota.org/Practice/Mental-Health/Evidence-based.aspx

Includes journal articles and critical appraisals specific to mental-health focused evidence.

ClinicalTrials.gov

An excellent resource for evidence about various mental health questions. This site is searchable by topic.

Cochrane Collaboration
http://www.cochrane.org
An excellent source for reviews of evidence included in a searchable database.

OT Seeker
http://www.otseeker.com
One of several occupational therapy-focused sources for research evidence.

PubMed
http://www.ncbi.nlm.nih.gov/sites/entrez?db+pubmed
The National Library of Medicine's searchable database, with thousands of abstracts and hundreds of full-text articles. Not specifically focused on integrating evidence, but a good mechanism for finding original research.

References

Abbott, R., & Lavretsky, H. (2013). Tai chi and quigong for the treatment and prevention of mental disorders. *Psychiatric Clinics of North America, 36*(1), 109-119.

Aboraya, A. (2010). Scientific forum on the Diagnostic and Statistical Manual of Mental Disorders, Fifth Edition (DSM-V)—An invitation. *Psychiatry, 7*(11), 32-36.

Alarcón, R.D. (2009). Culture, cultural factors and psychiatric diagnosis: Review and projections. *World Psychiatry, 8*(3), 131-139.

Ali, A.L., Rollman, B.L., & Berger, C.S. (2010). Comorbid mental health symptoms and heart diseases: Can health care and mental health care professionals collaboratively improve the assessment and management? *Health & Social Work, 35*(1), 27-38.

Allen, C. (1985). *Occupational therapy for psychiatric diseases: Measurement and management of cognitive disabilities.* Boston, MA: Little, Brown & Co.

American Occupational Therapy Association. (1994). Uniform terminology—third edition: Application to practice. *American Journal of Occupational Therapy, 48,* 1055-1059.

American Occupational Therapy Association. (2002). Occupational therapy practice framework: Domain & process. *American Journal of Occupational Therapy, 56*(6), 609-639.

American Occupational Therapy Association. (2008). Occupational therapy practice framework: Domain & process (2nd ed.). *American Journal of Occupational Therapy, 62,* 625-683.

American Occupational Therapy Association. (2011). *Fact sheet: Occupational therapy's role in mental health recovery.* Retrieved from http://www.aota.org/-/media/Corporate/Files/AboutOT/Professionals/WhatIsOT/MH/Facts/Mental%20Health%20Recovery.pdf.

American Occupational Therapy Association. (2014). Occupational therapy practice framework: Domain & process (3rd ed.). *American Journal of Occupational Therapy, 68*(Suppl. 1), S1-S48.

American Psychiatric Association. (2013a). *Diagnostic and statistical manual of mental disorders* (5th ed.). Washington, DC: Author.

American Psychiatric Association. (2013b). *Research background.* Retrieved from http://www.dsm5.org/Research/Pages/Default.aspx.

American Psychological Association. (2013). *Role of psychologists in addressing the mental and behavioral health concerns of the 21st century.* Retrieved from http://www.apa.org/about/gr/issues/health-care/role.aspx.

Anthony, W.A. (1979). *The principles of psychiatric rehabilitation.* Amherst, MA: Human Resource Development Press.

Antonosky, A. (1972). Breakdown: A needed fourth step in the conceptual armamentarium of modern medicine. *Social Science & Medicine, 6,* 537-544.

Auxier, A., Farley, T., & Seifert, K. (2011). Establishing an integrated care practice in a community health center. *Professional Psychology: Practice and Research, 42*(5), 391-397.

Baltes, P.B., & Baltes, M.M. (1990). Psychological perspectives on successful aging: The model of selective optimization with compensation. In P.B. Baltes & M.M. Baltes (Eds.), *Successful aging: Perspectives from the behavioral sciences* (pp. 1-34). New York, NY: Cambridge University Press.

Barth, J., Munder, T., Gerger, H., Nüesch, E., Trelle, S., Znoi, H., . . . Cuiipers, P. (2013). Comparative efficacy of seven psychotherapeutic interventions for patients with depression: A network meta-analysis. *PLoS Medicine, 10*(5), e1001454. doi:10.1371/journal.pmed.1001454.

Bazyk, S. (2011). *Mental health promotion, prevention, and intervention with children and youth: A guiding framework for occupational therapy.* Rockville, MD: American Occupational Therapy Association.

Blader, J.C. (2011). Acute inpatient care for psychiatric disorders in the United States, 1996 through 2007. *Archives of General Psychiatry, 68*(12), 1276-1283.

Bonder, B., & Martin, L. (2013). *Culture in clinical care: Strategies for competence* (2nd ed.). Thorofare, NJ: SLACK Incorporated.

Bream, S. (2013). The history of occupational therapy in adolescent mental health practice. *OT Practice, 18*(5), CE1-CE8.

Brothers, B.M., Yang, H.C., Strunk, D.R., & Andersen, B.L. (2011). Cancer patients with major depressive disorder: Testing a biobehavioral/cognitive behavior intervention. *Journal of Consulting and Clinical Psychology, 79,* 253-260.

Brown, B., Crawford, P., & Darongkamas, J. (2000). Blurred roles and permeable boundaries: The experience of multidisciplinary working in community mental health. *Health & Social Care in the Community, 8*(6), 425-435.

Bugenatl, D.B., Corpuz, R., & Schwartz, A. (2012). Preventing children's aggression: Outcomes of an early intervention. *Developmental Psychology, 48,* 1443-1439.

Burson, K., & Simpatico, T. (2002). Integrating service systems for people with psychiatric disabilities. *OT Practice,* 22-29.

Butler, M.G., Youngs, E.L., Roberts, J.L., & Hellings, J.A. (2012). Assessment and treatment in autism spectrum disorders: A focus on genetics and psychiatry. *Autism Research and Treatment, 2012,* 242537. doi:10.1155/2012/242537.

Chan, A.S.M., Tsang, H.W.H., & Li, S.M.Y. (2009). Case report of integrated supported employment for a person with severe mental illness. *American Journal of Occupational Therapy, 63,* 238-244.

Chen, J., & Rizzo, J. (2010). Racial and ethnic disparities in use of psychotherapy: Evidence from U.S. National survey data. *Psychiatric Services, 61*(4), 364-372.

Christiansen, C., & Baum, C. (1997). Person-environment occupational performance: A conceptual model for practice. In C. Christiansen & C. Baum (Eds.), *Occupational therapy: Enabling function and well-being* (2nd ed., pp. 46-70). Thorofare, NJ: SLACK Incorporated.

Christiansen, C., & Haertl, K. (2014). A contextual history of occupational therapy. In B.A.B. Schell, G. Gillen, & M.E. Scaffa (Eds.). *Willard & Spackman's occupational therapy* (12th ed., pp. 9-34). New York, NY: Wolters Kluwer/Lippincott Williams & Wilkins.

Clark, F., Azen, S.P., Carlson, M., Mandel, D., LaBree, L., Hay, J., . . . Lipson, L. (2001). Embedding health-promoting changes into the daily lives of independent-living older adults: Long-term follow-up of occupational therapy intervention. *Journal of Gerontology: Psychological Sciences, 56B,* P60-P63.

Duggan, C., Milton, J., Egan, V., McCarthy, L., Palmer, B., & Lee, A. (2003). Theories of general personality and mental disorder. *British Journal of Psychiatry, 182,* S19-S23.

Felce, D., Perry, J., Romeo, R., Robertson, J., Meek, A., Emerson, E., & Knapp, M. (2008). Outcomes and costs of community living: Semi-independent living and fully staffed group homes. *American Journal on Mental Retardation, 113*(2), 87-101.

Flaskerud, J.H. (2000). Ethnicity, culture, and neuropsychiatry. *Issues in Mental Health Nursing, 21,* 5-29.

Fortune, T., & Fitzgerald, M.H. (2009). The challenge of interdisciplinary collaboration in acute psychiatry: Impacts on the occupational milieu. *Australian Occupational Therapy Journal, 56*(2), 81-88.

Foster, S. (2001). *Role of the mental health nurse.* Eastbourne, England: Nelson Thomas.

Frager, R., & Fadiman, J. (1998). *Personality and personal growth* (4th ed.). New York, NY: Longman.

Freud, S. (1901/2003). *The psychopathology of everyday life.* New York, NY: Dover Publications.

Graham, J. (2013, March 11). Since 2008, insurers have been required by law to cover mental health—Why many still don't. *The Atlantic.* Retrieved from http://www.theatlantic.com/health/archive/2013/03/since-2008-insurers-have-been-required-by-law-to-cover-mental-health-why-many-still-dont/273562/.

Griswold, L.A.S. (1999). Community-based practice arenas. In M.E. Neistadt & E.B. Crepeau (Eds.), *Willard and Spackman's occupational therapy* (9th ed., pp. 810-815). Philadelphia, PA: Lippincott, Williams, Wilkins.

Gutman, S.A. (2011). Effectiveness of occupational therapy services in mental health practice. *American Journal of Occupational Therapy, 65*(3), 235-237.

Gutman, S.A., Mortera, M.H., Hinojosa, J., & Kramer, P. (2007). Revision of the occupational therapy practice framework. *American Journal of Occupational Therapy, 61,* 119-125.

Hawkley, L.C., Thisted, R.A., Masi, C.M., & Cacioppo, J.T. (2010). Loneliness predicts increased blood pressure: 5-year cross-lagged analyses in middle-aged and older adults. *Psychology and Aging, 25,* 132-141.

Hayes, P.A. (2009). Integrating evidence-based practice, cognitive-behavior therapy, and multicultural therapy: Ten steps for culturally competent practice. *Professional Psychology: Research and Practice, 40,* 354-360.

Healy, D. (2002). *The creation of psychopharmacology.* Cambridge, MA: Harvard University Press.

Hemmingsson, H., & Jonsson, H. (2005). The issue is—An occupational perspective on the concept of participation in the international classification of functioning, disability and health—Some critical remarks. *American Journal of Occupational Therapy, 59,* 569-576.

Herzberg, G., & Petrenchik, T.M. (2010). Health promotion for individuals and families who are homeless. In M.Scaffa, M. Reitz, & M. Pizzi (Eds.). *Occupational therapy in the promotion of health and wellness* (pp. 434-453). Philadelphia, PA: F.A. Davis.

Hinojosa, J. (2013). The evidence-based paradox. *American Journal of Occupational Therapy, 67,* e18-e23.

Hodson, E.M., & Craig, J.C. (2010). How to apply results from randomized trials and systematic reviews to individual patient care. *Nephrology, 15,* 277-280.

Holm, M.B., Santangelo, M.A., Fromuth, D.J., Brown, S.O., & Walter, H. (2000). Effectiveness of everyday occupations for changing client behaviors in a community living arrangement. *American Journal of Occupational Therapy, 54,* 361-371.

Horsfall, J., Cleary, M., & Hunt, G.E. (2010). Acute inpatient units in a comprehensive (integrated) mental health system: A review of the literature. *Issues in Mental Health Nursing, 31,* 273-278.

Hurst, M. (2013). Integrated care: Why did healthcare fragment in the first place and why should we integrate? Health homes, integrated care and the future of community psychiatry. Paper presented at: *11th Annual All-Ohio Institute on Community Psychiatry*, March 1-2, 2013.

Iwama, M.K. (2006). *The Kawa model: Culturally relevant occupational therapy.* Toronto, Ontario, Canada: Churchill Livingstone Elsevier.

Kazdin, A.E. (2011). Evidence-based treatment research: Advances, limitations, and next steps. *American Psychologist, 66*(8), 685-698.

Kendall, R.E. (2001). The distinction between mental and physical illness. *British Journal of Psychiatry, 178,* 490-493.

Kessler, J.F. (2014). Professionalism, communication, and teamwork. In B.A.B. Schell, G. Gillen, & M.E. Scaffa (Eds.). *Willard and Spackman's occupational therapy* (12th ed., pp. 452-465). New York, NY: Wolters Kluwer/Lippincott Williams & Wilkins.

Kielhofner, G. (Ed.). (2002). *Model of human occupation* (3rd ed.). Baltimore, MD: Lippincott, Williams & Wilkins.

Kutcher, S., & Wei, Y. (2012). Mental health and the school environment: Secondary schools, promotion and pathways to care. *Current Opinion in Psychiatry, 25*(4), 311-316.

Landsvek, J.A., Burns, B.J., Stambaugh, L.F., & Reutz, J.A. (2006). *Mental health care for children and adolescents in foster care: A review of research literature.* Casey Family Programs. Retrieved from http://www.casey.org/Resources/Publications/pdf/MentalHealthCareChildren.pdf.

Lewin, A.B., Storch, E.A., Williams, L.B., Duke, D.C., Silverstein, J.H., & Geffken, G.R. (2010). Brief report: Normative data on a structured interview for diabetes adherence in childhood. *Journal of Pediatric Psychology, 35,* 177-182.

Lichtenstein, D. (2012). Home- and community-based mental health services for youth: Is it working? *Brown University Child & Adolescent Behavior Letter, 28*(12), 1-7.

Lloyd, C., Williams, P.L., Simpson, A., Wright, D., Fortune, T., & Lal, S. (2010). Occupational therapy in the modern adult acute mental health setting: A review of current practice. *International Journal of Therapy & Rehabilitation, 17*(9), 483-493.

Low, J.F. (1992). The reconstruction aides. *American Journal of Occupational Therapy, 46,* 38-43.

Madge, N., Foreman, D., & Baksh, F. (2008). Starving in the midst of plenty? A study of training needs for child and adolescent mental health service delivery in primary care. *Child Psychology and Psychiatry, 13*(3), 463-478.

Manderscheid, R.W., Ryff, C.D., Freeman, E.J., McKnight-Eily, L.R., Dhingra, S., & Strine, T.W. (2010). Evolving definitions of mental illness and wellness. *Prevention of Chronic Disease, 7*(1), 1-6.

Meisenhelder, J.B., & Chandler, E.N. (2000). Faith, prayer, and health outcomes in elderly Native Americans. *Clinical Nursing Research, 9,* 191-203.

Meyer, A. (1922/1977). The philosophy of occupational therapy. *American Journal of Occupational Therapy, 31,* 639-642.

Mezzich, J.E., & Berganza, C.E. (2005). Purposes and models of diagnostic systems. *Psychopathology, 38*(4), 162-165.

Molinari, V., Hedgecock, D., Branch, L., Brown, L.M., & Hyer, K. (2009) Mental health services in nursing homes: A survey of nursing home administrative personnel. *Aging & Mental Health, 13*(3), 477-486.

Morales, E., & Norcross, J.C. (2010). Evidence-based practices with ethnic minorities: Strange bedfellows no more. *Journal of Clinical Psychology: In Session, 66,* 821-829.

National Panel for Psychiatric-Mental Health NP Competencies. (2003). *Psychiatric-mental health nurse practitioner competencies.* Retrieved from http://www.aacn.nche.edu/leading-initiatives/education-resources/PMHNP.pdf.

Needham, B., & Hill, T.D. (2010). Do gender differences in mental health contribute to gender differences in physical health? *Social Science & Medicine, 71*, 1472-1479.

O'Hara, B., & Caswell, K. (2012). *Health status, health insurance and medical services utilization: 2010.* Washington, DC: U.S. Census Bureau. Retrieved from http://www.census.gov/prod/2012pubs/p70-133.pdf.

Phillips, J., & Phillips, J. (2010, August 15). The cultural dimension in DSM-5: PTSD. *Psychiatric Times.* Retrieved from http://www.psychiatrictimes.com/dsm-5-0/cultural-dimension-dsm-5-ptsd.

Piazza, J.R., Charles, S.T., Sliwinski, M.J., Mogle, J., & Almeida, D.M. (2012). Affective reactivity to daily stressors and long-term risk of reporting a chronic physical health condition. *Annals of Behavioral Medicine, 45*, 110-120.

Pitts, D.B., Lamb, A., Ramsey, D., Learnard, L., Clark, F., Scheinholtz, M., . . . Nanoff, T. (2005). *Promotion of OT in mental health systems.* Retrieved from http://uspra.info/Education/Conference2011/HANDOUTS/OT_in_Mental_Health_Systems.pdf.

Porter, R. (1987). *A social history of madness.* New York, NY: Weidenfeld & Nicolson.

Rachman, S. (1997). The evolution of cognitive behaviour therapy. In D. Clark, C.G. Fairburn, & M.G. Gelder (Eds.). *Science and practice of cognitive behaviour therapy* (pp. 1-26). Oxford, England: Oxford University Press.

Reitz, S.M. (1992). A historical review of occupational therapy's role in preventive health and wellness. *American Journal of Occupational Therapy, 46*, 50-55.

Rochefort, D.A. (1984). Origins of the "third psychiatric revolution": The Community Mental Health Centers Act of 1963. *Journal of Health Politics, Policy and Law, 9*(1), 1-30.

Rogers, J.C. (1982). Order and disorder in medicine and occupational therapy. *American Journal of Occupational Therapy, 36*, 29-35.

Rosenberg, L. (2009). Mental health and addiction policy: What next? *Journal of Behavioral Health Services and Research, 36*(2), 127-128.

Salinsky, E., & Loftis, C.W. (2007, August 1). Shrinking inpatient psychiatric capacity: Cause for celebration or concern? *Issue Brief, no. 823.* Washington, DC: National Health Policy Forum.

Scaffa, M., Pizzi, M., & Chromiak, S.B. (2010). Promoting mental health and emotional well-being. In M.Scaffa, M. Reitz, & M. Pizzi (Eds.), *Occupational therapy in the promotion of health and wellness* (pp. 329-349). Philadelphia, PA: F.A. Davis.

Scharfstein, S. (2000). What ever happened to community mental health? *Psychiatric Services (Washington, DC), 15*(5), 616-620.

Schkade, J.K., & Schultz, S. (1992). Occupational adaptation: Toward a holistic approach for contemporary practice, part 1. *American Journal of Occupational Therapy, 46*, 829-838.

Schultz, S., & Schkade, J.K. (1992). Occupational adaptation: Toward a holistic approach for contemporary practice, part 2. *American Journal of Occupational Therapy, 46*, 917-926.

Shedler, J. (2010). The efficacy of psychodynamic psychotherapy. *American Psychologist, 65*(2), 98-109.

Simakhodskaya, Z., Haddad, F., Quintero, M., & Malavade, K. (2009). Innovative use of crisis intervention services with psychiatric emergency room patients. *Primary Psychiatry, 16*(9), 60-65.

Siporin, S., & Lysack, C. (2004). Quality of life and supported employment: A case study of three women with developmental disabilities. *American Journal of Occupational Therapy, 58*, 455-465.

Skalko, T., Williams, R., Snethen, G., & Cooper, N.L. (2008). ECU horizons day treatment program: A case report of collaboration between community mental health providers and an academic recreational therapy program. *Therapeutic Recreation Journal, 42*(2), 132-142.

Skinner, B.F (1953). *Science and human behavior.* New York, NY: MacMillan.

Small, R.F., & Barnhill, L.R. (Eds.). (1998). *Practicing in the new mental health marketplace: Ethical, legal, and moral issues.* Washington, DC: American Psychological Association.

Stepney, P., & Rostila, I. (2011). Towards an integrated model of practice evaluation balancing accountability, critical knowledge and developmental perspectives. *Health Sociology Review, 20*(2), 133-146.

Stoffel, V.C. (2013). Opportunities for occupational therapy behavioral health: A call to action. *American Journal of Occupational Therapy, 67*(2), 140-145.

Substance Abuse and Mental Health Services Administration, Center for Behavioral Health Statistics and Quality. (2011, July 7). *The NSDUH report: Sources of payment for mental health treatment for adults.* Rockville, MD: Author.

Szasz, T. (1974). *The myth of mental illness* (2nd ed.). New York, NY: Harper & Row.

Taylor, R.R. (2008). *The intentional relationship: Occupational therapy and the use of self.* Philadelphia, PA: F.A. Davis.

Thornicroft, G., Rose, D., & Kassam, A. (2007). Discrimination in health care against people with mental illness. *International Review of Psychiatry, 19*(2), 113-122.

Tsang, H., Lam, P., Ng, B., & Leung, O. (2000). Predictors of employment outcome for people with psychiatric disabilities: A review of the literature since the mid '80s. *Journal of Rehabilitation, 66*(2), 19-31.

Turpin, M. (2007). Recovery of our phenomenological knowledge in occupational therapy. *American Journal of Occupational Therapy, 61,* 469-473.

U.S. Department of Health and Human Services. (2014). *About the law.* Retrieved from http://www.hhs.gov/healthcare/rights/index.html.

U.S. Department of Labor. (2012). *2012 Report to Congress: Compliance with the Mental Health Parity and Addiction Equity Act of 2008.* Retrieved from http://www.dol.gov/ebsa/publications/mhpaeareporttocongress2012.html.

Walsh, T., McClellan, J. M., McCarthy, S. E., Addington, A. M., Pierce, S. B., Cooper, G. M., . . . Sebat, J. (2008). Rare structural variants disrupt multiple genes in neurodevelopmental pathways in schizophrenia. *Science, 320,* 539-543.

Warner, R. (2009). Recovery from schizophrenia and the recovery model. *Current Opinions in Psychiatry, 22*(4), 374-380.

Weiss, A.J. (2013). *Interdisciplinary teams in integrated care. Health homes, integrated care and the future of community psychiatry.* Paper presented at 11th Annual All-Ohio Institute on Community Psychiatry, March 1-2, 2013, Cleveland, OH.

Wilcock, A.A. (2005). 2004 CAOT conference keynote address: Occupational science: Bridging occupation and health. *Canadian Journal of Occupational Therapy, 72,* 5-12.

World Health Organization. (2001). *International classification of functioning, disability and health* (ICF). Geneva, Switzerland: Author.

Wu, J., Yeung, A.S., Schnyer, R., Wang, Y., & Mischoulon, D. (2012). Acupuncture for depression: A review of clinical applications. *Canadian Journal of Psychiatry, 57*(7), 397-405.

Wuang, Y., Wang, C., Huang, M., & Su, C. (2009). Prospective study of the effect of sensory integration, neurodevelopmental treatment, and perceptual–motor therapy on the sensorimotor performance in children with mild mental retardation. *American Journal of Occupational Therapy, 63,* 441-452.

Zemke, R., & Clark, R. (Eds.). (1996). *Occupational science: The evolving discipline.* Philadelphia, PA: F.A. Davis.

Neurodevelopmental Disorders

Learning Outcomes

By the end of this chapter, readers will be able to:
- Discuss the causes, symptoms, and typical interventions for neurodevelopmental disorders
- Discuss cultural factors in diagnosing neurodevelopmental disorders
- Discuss lifespan considerations of neurodevelopmental disorders
- Describe functional deficits that accompany neurodevelopmental disorders
- Describe interventions to prevent and/or remediate neurodevelopmental disorders
- Describe occupational therapy interventions for neurodevelopmental disorders

Bonder B.
Psychopathology and Function, Fifth Edition (pp 47-92).
© 2015 SLACK Incorporated.

KEY WORDS

- Dual diagnosis
- Intelligence quotient
- Habilitation
- Rehabilitation
- Sensory stimulation
- Social skills training
- Communication
- Speech
- Language
- Expressive
- Receptive
- Dyslexia
- Dyscalculia
- Tic
- Idiopathic

CASE VIGNETTE

In an inner-city elementary school, the teachers share concerns about classroom management. In their discussions, they discover that the kinds of problems with which they are dealing are consistent: children are inattentive, restless, and prone to frequent outbursts of temper. In addition, the children have difficulty interacting with each other and experience difficulty persisting in the tasks set for them. These factors result in chaos in many classrooms much of the time.

The teachers realize that the children come from difficult circumstances. Many are from single parent homes or are in the care of grandparents or other relatives. The parents do not seem particularly involved in their children's education, and they rarely show up for school open houses or parent–teacher conferences. Some of the parents have obvious substance abuse issues or other psychiatric disorders. Some of the children come to school in dirty or torn clothing, and many have difficulty affording school supplies.

Although the teachers are sympathetic to these problems and are committed to helping their students secure the best education possible, they are also frustrated. The teachers have limited time to manage individual behavioral problems, and their most frequent intervention is to send a difficult child to the principal's office.

An occupational therapist is present during one of the teachers' discussions and offers to assess the situation. The teachers are surprised because they think of the occupational therapist as someone to whom they should refer children with disabilities or poor handwriting. However, they are perfectly willing to accept any help they can get, and, although skeptical, they agree to have her visit their classrooms and make suggestions.

THOUGHT QUESTIONS

1. What explanations do you see for the problems facing the teachers?
2. Do you think the children have psychiatric disorders?
3. Why might an occupational therapist be involved in this circumstance?
4. What contribution might an occupational therapist make when a mental disorder has not been diagnosed?

NEURODEVELOPMENTAL DISORDERS

- Intellectual disabilities
  - Intellectual disability (intellectual development disorder)
  - Global developmental delay
- Communication disorders
  - Speech sound disorder
  - Childhood-onset fluency disorder (stuttering)
  - Social (pragmatic) communication disorder
- Autism spectrum disorder
- Attention-deficit/hyperactivity disorder
- Specific learning disorder
- Motor disorders
  - Developmental coordination disorder
  - Stereotypic movement disorder
- Tic disorders
  - Tourette's disorder
  - Persistent (chronic) motor or vocal tic disorder

Neurodevelopmental disorders are conditions that emerge early in life and are, in general, lifelong. In the previous *Diagnostic and Statistical Manual of Mental Disorders* (DSM), this cluster of disorders was called Disorders of Infancy, Childhood, and Adolescence (American Psychiatric Association [APA], 2000). However, because these disorders are thought to be lifelong, because there is treatment for some previously life-shortening conditions, such as Down syndrome, and because diagnostic criteria have become more explicit, it is increasingly common to see adults diagnosed with early-life onset mental disorders (e.g., autism [Morgan et al., 2002], intellectual disabilities [Hassiotis et al., 2008], and attention-deficit/hyperactivity disorder [ADHD; Kessler et al., 2006]). For this and other reasons, the fifth edition of the DSM (DSM-5) has relabeled this cluster of disorders. It was thought that Neurodevelopmental Disorders better captured both the etiology and the time of onset for this diagnostic group while acknowledging that the disorders persist into adulthood (APA, 2013).

Many of the diagnoses found in other categories of the DSM-5 (APA, 2013) and covered in later chapters (e.g., mood and anxiety disorders) may also occur in children or adolescents. The differences in manifestation that are sometimes seen in children will be discussed in the chapters that discuss adult-onset disorders.

Childhood and adolescence are characterized by numerous stresses, some of which may contribute to diagnosable psychiatric disorders (Hollenstein & Lougheed, 2013). Normal stressors include physical development and maturation, emphasis on education, and family tensions, among many others. Sexual, emotional, and/or physical abuse are surprisingly common experiences for children. Depression, suicidal ideation or action, substance abuse, adjustment disorders, and sexual acting-out may result. Some theorists suggest that these difficulties may be part of normal development, particularly during adolescence (Freud, 1958). This view is supported by those who feel that modern society presents more difficult dilemmas than what existed in earlier times (Newman & Newman, 2003), among these are parental divorce, early placement in day care, and availability of and peer pressure to use drugs and alcohol.

This view is not universal (Hollenstein & Lougheed, 2013), and some researchers have found adolescents to be largely well adjusted. Overall, the evidence is unclear, and debates rage on about the effects of divorce and other societal trends on the well-being of adolescents. These disputes await resolution through further research. However, there is no question that children and adolescents can experience an array of psychological difficulties.

The process of diagnosing children and adolescents must take into account what reflects normal behavior and what represents dysfunction severe enough to warrant labeling. The DSM-5 (APA, 2013) has attempted to provide very specific criteria about the symptoms required for diagnosis, but there remains an element of subjectivity. Some practitioners suggest that diagnosing the young is particularly challenging because psychiatric disorders still carry a social stigma that may affect the future development of the child.

As with all psychiatric diagnoses, those of childhood and adolescence may occur independently or in conjunction with other problems. The concept of **dual diagnosis** is a frequent theme in the literature, referring to an individual who has two concurrent diagnoses (e.g., intellectual disability and depression; Dykens & Hodapp, 2001) or any number of simultaneous psychiatric disorders. By one estimate, 25% of individuals with intellectual disabilities also have some other psychiatric condition (Dykens & Hodapp, 2001), whereas other researchers place the figure at anywhere from 20% to 74% (Dosen & Day, 2001), with as many as 10% of these individuals reporting depression (Walker, Dosen, Buitelaar, & Janzing, 2011). Dual diagnosis complicates both the diagnostic process and treatment, requiring integration of treatment approaches. The issue of dual diagnosis is discussed in greater detail in Chapter 17.

The current chapter reviews the neurodevelopmental diagnoses in detail, as many are likely to be seen by occupational therapists. The major diagnoses in this category are listed in the box on p. 49. Table 3-1 provides information about prevalence of these disorders.

Intellectual Disabilities

The specific diagnostic criteria for intellectual disabilities (formerly known as mental retardation [APA, 2000]) focus on intellectual and functional deficits. Intellectual disabilities begin early in development and are distinct from the intellectual deficits that might accompany traumatic brain injury or cerebrovascular accident, which are conditions that can develop at any time in life (APA, 2013).

Measurement of intellectual capacity or **intelligence quotient** (IQ) is most often performed using standardized instruments, such as the Wechsler Intelligence Scale for Children (WISC; Wechsler, 2004). The WISC measures verbal IQ based on listening and answering examiner questions, measuring comprehension, vocabulary, and general information, and performance IQ is measured through timed problems that require manipulation of puzzles and blocks. The WISC is valid and reliable for children aged 6 years and older; there is also a preschool version that can be used with children aged 4 years. For younger children, several other instruments, including the Stanford-Binet (Roid, 2003) and the Kaufman Assessment Battery (Kaufman & Kaufman, 1983), are more appropriate. Intelligence testing has been criticized for its potential cultural bias and for the fact that it measures only two dimensions of a construct—intelligence—which is much more complex (Nisbett et al., 2012). It does not, for example, measure creativity or emotional and social intelligence. However, the diagnosis of intellectual disabilities often involves such testing, although the DSM-5 (APA, 2013) encourages the use of multiple methods of measurement.

Intellectual disability is one of the diagnoses in which function is specifically addressed (APA, 2013). By definition, individuals with intellectual disabilities struggle in most spheres of occupation. They may have difficulty with education, self-care, social interactions, and communication. In addition, they struggle with activities that require judgment (for example, they may be more gullible than most). Assessment of functional deficit is typically observational and based on comparison with developmental norms, such as by the Denver Developmental Milestones assessment test (Frankenberg & Dobbs, 1967). Such individuals may be disruptive, or sometimes, even aggressive, and they may be victims or perpetrators of

TABLE 3-1			
PREVALENCE OF NEURODEVELOPMENTAL DISORDERS			
DIAGNOSIS	*PREVALENCE (%)*	*GENDER RATIO (M:F)*	*SOURCE*
Intellectual disability	1; severe: 0.006%	1.6:1 (mild) 1.2:0.1 (severe)	APA, 2013
Language disorder		~2:1	Weindrich, Jennen-Steinmetz, Laucht, Esser, & Schmidt, 2000
Autism spectrum disorder	1	4:1	Autism and Developmental Disabilities Monitoring Network Surveillance Year 2006 Principal Investigators & Centers for Disease Control, 2009
ADHD	5 (children); 2.5 (adults)	2:1	Faraone, Sergeant, Gillberg, & Biederman, 2003
Specific learning disorder	5 to 15 (children); 4 (adults)	~2:1	APA, 2013
Developmental coordination disorder	5 to 6	Between 2:1 and 7:1	APA, 2013
Stereotypic movement disorder	3 to 4		APA, 2013
Tic disorder	Tic disorder	Between 2:1 and 4:1	APA, 2013

a variety of criminal activities, such as physical and sexual abuse. These behaviors lack the intent that may be found in an individual with a conduct disorder or an antisocial personality (described in Chapters 16 and 19, respectively), reflecting instead on an inability to fully understand social norms about behavior.

Intellectual disabilities are categorized as mild, moderate, severe, or profound (APA, 2013). Individuals with the mildest intellectual disabilities demonstrate slightly slowed development, immaturity, and modest difficulties in school environments. Moderate intellectual disabilities are reflected in slow progress in reading and other academic areas, difficulty in social situations, and some challenges in self-care. Severe intellectual disabilities lead to limited academic achievement, including, inability to read or manipulate numbers. Social and self-care abilities are compromised to the extent that considerable support from others is required. Individuals with profound intellectual disability typically require total care in all spheres. Although individuals with less severe conditions may be able to function in ordinary settings, individuals with profound disability may require institutional care.

It is important to remember that individuals with intellectual disabilities may also have other coexisting mental disorders, such as depression, and their difficulty with problem solving and lack of awareness of risk and danger, can lead to accidental injury (APA, 2013; Kozlowski, Matson, Sipes, Hattier, & Bamburg, 2011). Other common coexisting diagnoses are ADHD, bipolar disorders, autism spectrum disorder, impulse control disorder, and numerous others (Chaplin, 2009).

Care must be exercised when considering cultural factors in a diagnosis of intellectual disability (Fraine & McDade, 2009). For example, newly immigrated children may have language delays caused by the need to shift from one language to another. Children from agrarian backgrounds or those who have experienced significant trauma in refugee situations may have developmental delays, but these delays may be largely situational and may resolve as adjustment to a new situation moves forward.

Where the diagnosis of intellectual disability does not quite fit, but some characteristics are present, the individual may be diagnosed with global developmental delay or unspecified intellectual disability (also known as intellectual development disorder; APA, 2013). Global developmental delay is a diagnosis made for a child under the age of 5, when it is difficult to accurately assess intellectual capacity. When the child is old enough to participate in standardized testing, the diagnosis will be revisited. Unspecified intellectual disability is the diagnosis when an individual over the age of 5 cannot participate in intelligence testing because of some associated physical limitation or severe behavioral challenges. Severe hearing impairment, blindness, or some motor disabilities would be examples of these situations.

Intellectual disabilities are typically identified before the child reaches school age (APA, 2013), although in mild cases, it may be classroom behavior that leads to an eventual diagnosis. In cases where there is an identifiable genetic cause (e.g., trisomy 21 [Down syndrome]), there may be an associated physical presentation that supports the diagnosis. Most of the time, intellectual capacity is stable, but there are conditions (e.g., Rett syndrome, San Phillippo syndrome) where there may be either intermittent or progressive deterioration. In almost all circumstances, the condition is lifelong. Coexisting conditions, such as hearing impairments or epilepsy, may lead to lower functioning. In those cases, addressing the additional condition (prescribing hearing aids for hearing impairments or medication for epilepsy) may improve functional ability. Intellectual disability must be carefully distinguished from such disorders as autism, ADHD, specific learning disabilities, and schizophrenia. Intellectual disability can also be comorbid with these conditions if the individual meets the specific diagnostic criteria for more than one.

Etiology

Risk factors for intellectual disabilities are multifactorial and can be categorized based on cause or on time of onset (Schalock, 2011). Causes are biological (maternal illness, genetic disorders; Vorstman & Ophoff, 2013), educational (lack of educational opportunity, impoverished parenting), social (poverty, domestic violence), or behavioral (e.g., maternal alcohol use; O'Leary et al., 2013). Onset may occur during the prenatal period (e.g., maternal alcohol use or genetic flaw), perinatal (e.g., hypoxia during birth), or postnatal (e.g., lead exposure or child abuse).

In some cases, etiology is very clear, whereas in others it is less obvious. Some genetic disorders (e.g., trisomy 21, fragile X syndrome [Cornish, Turk, & Hagerman, 2008], Williams syndrome [Martens, Wilson, & Reutens, 2008]) cause intellectual disabilities, as do some prenatal problems such as fetal alcohol syndrome or maternal malnutrition (Chandrasena, Mukherjee, & Turk, 2009). A variety of physical problems during early childhood may also lead to intellectual disabilities, including low birth weight (Schendel & Bhasin, 2008); exposure to toxic substances (e.g., lead and mercury); diseases, such as meningitis; nutritional deficiencies (Moretti et al., 2008); and injury, especially head trauma. A strong association exists between epilepsy and intellectual disabilities, although whether this is a causative relationship is unclear (Besag, 2002).

Environmental factors may also contribute to intellectual disabilities (Ramey & Ramey, 1999; van der Schuit, Peeters, Segers, van Balkom, & Verhoeven, 2009). Parental deprivation

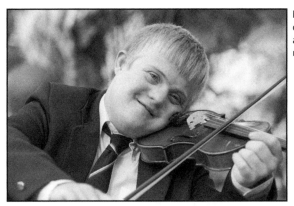

Figure 3-1. A young man with Down syndrome, a common cause of intellectual disability, enjoys a leisure occupation that is meaningful to him. (©2014 Shutterstock.com.)

or absence of adequate stimulation may lead to slowed development and low IQ. Early malnutrition is also a factor. Bijou (1992) identified several categories of causes of intellectual disability, including biomedical pathology, cultural–familial conditions, and restricted development. It is noteworthy also that many individuals with intellectual disabilities have accompanying psychiatric diagnoses.

Prognosis

Prognosis is dependent on both cause and intervention (Pratt & Gradanus, 2007). Intellectual capacity is typically stable across the lifespan, but thoughtful intervention that is focused on functional capacity can have significant impact on the individual's ability to participate in mainstream society.

Management of associated medical conditions is essential. A significant proportion of individuals with intellectual disabilities also have accompanying epilepsy (Leunissen et al., 2011). Treatment of the epilepsy with appropriate drugs can contribute to improved function, even in the absence of increased intelligence, as measured by standardized tests. Other physical disorders that can accompany Down syndrome, which is one of the many causes of intellectual disability, include ophthalmic disorders, hearing impairment, thyroid problems, orthopedic problems, cancer, obesity, and congenital heart disorders (Steingass, Chicoine, McGuire, & Roizen, 2011). Most individuals with Down syndrome have symptoms of Alzheimer's disease by age 40—a fact that indicates additional intervention may be required to address emerging functional deficits at that time.

In addition, as will be discussed in greater detail in this chapter, interventions that focus on specific behaviors can have a significant impact on functional ability. Thus, although it is unlikely that intellectual disability will be reversed, the functional disability can be addressed. It is also important to note that increasingly, individuals with intellectual disabilities can develop their strengths and effectively integrate into society and live meaningful and productive lives (Figure 3-1).

Implications for Function and Treatment

By definition, a diagnosis of intellectual disability means that the individual has limitations in function (APA, 2013). Those deficits are global, unlike some that are found in diagnostic categories based on a single occupation or skill (e.g., communication or motor skills disorders [described later]). This means that function will be affected in all areas. The degree to which function is impaired relates to the level of intellectual disability. An individual with a mild disability may be able to manage self-care, education, and vocational activities, although at a somewhat limited level and with the need for more intense education and training to acquire the needed skills, whereas an individual with profound intellectual disability may remain severely limited, regardless of intervention.

Functional decrements are related to the etiology of the intellectual disability (Dykens & Hodapp, 2001). For example, children with Prader-Willi syndrome show a high degree of food-seeking behavior, high rates of tantrums and impulsivity, and increased risk for the development of psychosis in adolescence. Williams syndrome is associated with deficits in visuospatial skills and face-processing deficits, hypersociability, and also with superior musical skill (Martens et al., 2008), a reminder that mental difficulties do not eliminate the potential for significant strengths.

In areas of occupation, individuals with intellectual disabilities are limited in performing activities of daily living (Kottorp, Bernspång, & Fisher, 2003), as well as being limited in instrumental activities of daily living, education, work, play, and leisure. Rest and sleep may or may not be affected, but social participation may be diminished (Verdonschot, de Witte, Reichrath, Buntinx, & Curfs, 2009), either because of skill deficits on the part of the individual or because of lack of opportunity. Some of these children find themselves being shunned by others, so their social lives are impoverished, even if they have the capacity to interact.

All skills are affected (Kottorp et al., 2003), including motor and praxis skills and cognitive skills in particular. Diminished body functions include significant impairment of all aspects of mental functions. Sensory functions, neuromuscular functions, and voice and speech functions may also be affected. The individual may be clumsy, have difficulty with speech, and show signs of sensory-integrative deficits (Gal, Dyck, & Passmore, 2010). Cardiovascular, skin, and other body functions may or may not be affected, depending on the specific cause of the intellectual disability. For example, some genetic conditions, such as trisomy 21 (Down syndrome) carry a high risk of cardiovascular flaws (Clur, Oude Rengerink, Ottenkamp, & Bilardo, 2011).

Because the characteristics of intellectual disabilities are largely behavioral, medical treatment—particularly medication—is useful only to address accompanying medical issues. For example, epilepsy may be treated with a variety of drugs, such as valproate and some of the benzodiazepines (Striano & Belcastro, 2013). Side effects must be carefully monitored, as they can impair cognitive function, but remediation of the seizure disorder can improve cognition. Antipsychotic medications are also sometimes used (Tsiouris, Kim, Brown, Pettinger, & Cohen, 2013; Unwin & Deb, 2011), although their efficacy is questionable when the condition is a straightforward intellectual disability, as opposed to a situation in which there is a comorbid diagnosis of schizophrenia or other psychosis. It is always important to monitor medications to make sure that side effects do not cause additional problems.

A child with intellectual disability is likely to have motor, social, cognitive, sensory, and psychological deficits, although he or she may have relatively less motor delay than cognitive delay or less social delay than motor delay. For example, some children who have an intellectual disability may be quite sociable, but they have difficulty with academic skills. Deficits are also roughly correlated with IQ, so that a child whose condition is labeled profound based on IQ test scores is likely to have severely impaired function in all areas (Dykens & Hodapp, 2001).

Self-injurious behavior is noted in a subset of these individuals, particularly those with severe developmental delay (Furniss & Biswas, 2012). Aggression has also been noted as a problem for some individuals with severe or profound intellectual disability (Pert & Jahoda, 2008). Not only can individuals who have intellectual disabilities be possible perpetrators of aggression, they are also more likely than others to be victimized. Deficits in emotional regulation skills—combined with difficulties in other skill areas—negatively affect performance patterns. Each of these problems requires particular attention in the assessment and intervention process.

The most common interventions are behavioral and educational. The Individuals with Disabilities Education Act (U.S. Department of Education, 2004) requires that children have access to education and the needed support services to enhance their learning. Thus, most schools have classroom aides, special education teachers, occupational therapists, and other service providers who can help to structure educational interventions that are likely to support learning in such individuals.

Education may extend to the family, both for purposes of prevention (e.g., educating pregnant women about the need for good nutrition) and for management of the child with an intellectual disability. This may reduce the stress that has been noted in families with children with intellectual disabilities (Hodapp, Ly, Fidler, & Ricci, 2001). Because intellectual disability occurs in young children, parents may well experience a period of grief, as well as longer term coping challenges as they strive to meet their child's unexpected needs.

Behavioral interventions focus on specific functional deficits. For example, many individuals with intellectual disabilities struggle with social interactions. Behavior modification that includes modeling, direct instruction, practice, and reinforcement of helpful behaviors can promote improved social skills (Benson & Valenti-Hein, 2001; Walton & Ingersoll, 2013). As another example, behavioral programs to support physical activity can contribute to health and improved quality of life (Lante, Walkley, Gamble, & Vassos, 2011).

Behavioral interventions can be valuable both for children and adults (Bielecki & Swender, 2004; Cohen, Heller, Alberto, & Fredrick, 2008). Enhanced social and vocational function can be promoted through a program that carefully outlines the steps involved in each task and then provides reinforcement as the individual accomplishes each step. Less attention has been paid to leisure and play, but there is every reason to believe that this also can be enhanced through behavioral and educational approaches (Lifter, 2000). Young adults with intellectual disabilities are likely to be concerned about the transition to adulthood, thus, a focus on specific work skills can be essential (Forte, Jahoda, & Dagnan, 2011).

Residential intervention may be necessary for some individuals (Embregts, 2009). In residential treatment facilities, interaction with staff can lead to more independent functioning. Increasingly, however, efforts are being made to maintain individuals with intellectual disabilities in the community (Neely-Barnes, Marcenko, & Weber, 2008). The client's preferences for both location of service and types of services are an increasing focus as well, where the individual is able to make such choices. In addition, the needs of families are important, as their lives are also affected by the individual's condition (Faust & Scior, 2008).

Implications for Occupational Therapy

As discussed in Chapter 2, the *Occupational Therapy Practice Framework, Third Edition* (American Occupational Therapy Association [AOTA], 2014) emphasizes the ability of individuals to participate in meaningful occupations and to perform needed daily tasks. Occupations for children includes play, socialization, education, and mastery of self-care skills. In general, children with intellectual disabilities mirror their nondelayed peers, but they are slower to master developmental tasks. Children with intellectual disabilities might show preference for certain kinds of play (e.g., rough and tumble play) for a longer period of time than nondelayed children (Case-Smith & Kuhaneck, 2008).

An understanding of the precise nature of function of the individual child is vital, as there is a broad range of functional ability among children identified as having intellectual disabilities (Dolva, Coster, & Lilja, 2004). In 5-year-old children with Down syndrome who were evaluated with the Pediatric Evaluation of Disability Inventory, some areas of function had score ranges of 20 points or more, demonstrating the wide range of ability that can accompany a specific diagnostic group.

For individuals who are delayed, the goal of treatment is most often **habilitation** (enabling) instead of **rehabilitation**, which supports reinstituting or improving function, because they must acquire skills they never had, rather than regain those lost. Because function varies from individual to individual and is based on both sociocultural and biological factors (Dosen & Day, 2001), it is important to understand the cause of the delay in the individual, as well as his or her own particular strengths.

In general, goals of occupational therapy focus on facilitating maximal performance. This requires careful evaluation of both deficits and strengths in all potential occupations (AOTA, 2014). Individuals with intellectual disabilities often wish to perform the same activities as their peers and are able to accomplish many developmental milestones, albeit more slowly than others. A young person with an intellectual disability may, for example, enjoy repetitive tasks, making him or her well suited for work that others might prefer to avoid.

At the same time, realistic appraisal is necessary. It is essential to understand what constitutes the starting point for a particular individual and that the duration of the learning process for a particular skill may place limits on his or her eventual achievement. Physical well-being in terms of body functions and body structures must be attended to (Kreuger, van Exel, & Nieboer, 2008) in concert with focus on occupations and skills, such as social and communication skills.

Occupational therapy interventions focused on addressing functional deficits in individuals with intellectual disabilities can be of great value (Drysdale, Casey, & Porter-Armstrong, 2008; Hällgren & Kottorp, 2005; Kåhlin & Haglund, 2009; Wuang, Ho, & Su, 2013). It is most helpful to focus intervention on occupations, skills, and performance patterns. Strategies to address contexts can also be of value in minimizing the functional deficits caused by excessive environmental demands. In many instances, specific interventions—such as the Children's Friendship Training program (Chandrasena et al., 2009), which promotes social skills and interactions—can be beneficial.

Skills require specific intervention. Motor, language, cognitive, and sensory processing skills are typically delayed. Accomplishment of play, self-care, and academic work may be limited in the absence of adequate skill level. However, some therapists have suggested that sensory integration may help to remediate these problems (May-Benson & Koomar, 2010; Pizzamiglio et al., 2008). In addition, neurodevelopmental treatment and perceptual motor therapy may enhance sensorimotor skills (Wuang, Wang, Huan, & Su, 2009). Neurodevelopmental treatment focuses on muscle tone; stability and mobility, whereas perceptual motor intervention is focused on providing a range of structured activities that provide sensory and motor practice. For individuals who are profoundly delayed, early intervention may need to focus on swallowing, in preparation for eating, and on movement to facilitate self-care activities like dressing.

A wide array of interventions in the home and in the community can address occupations. A home program may focus on activities of daily living (ADL), instrumental activities of daily living (IADL), leisure, and play through parent education and mentoring, as well as through direct practice for the child (Hällgren & Kottorp, 2005; Wuang et al., 2013). Community-based interventions can enhance community skills, as well as education and work abilities (Drysdale et al., 2008; Kåhlin & Haglund, 2009). Such programs can emphasize concrete, step-by-step learning of ADL, IADL, and work-related activities. It is vital to incorporate the family into the intervention because the disorder can have significant impact on family occupations, as well as individual occupations (Sachs & Nasser, 2009).

Occupations that are of initial concern include self-care and play. Play is developmentally important for all children (Lifter, 2000). Limitations in play may restrict later academic ability, social interaction, and language. Play training and play intervention, emphasizing provision of opportunities for participation, prompting, and encouraging these behaviors, can have an impact beyond that occupation. Self-care may focus on such activities as dressing skills. In one school, children aged 6 to 10 years spent several weeks playing "Simon Says," pointing to body parts on dolls, doing the "Hokey-Pokey" ("you put your left foot in…"), and so on. Two months later, the children were ready to begin putting legs into pant legs and arms into sleeves. It should be noted that **sensory stimulation** is a component of these activities and may also have a therapeutic benefit. Sensory stimulation involves providing a variety of patterned forms of sensory input that includes tactile, visual, auditory, and other inputs.

It is also important for these children to identify play activities at which they can succeed. Many have siblings they would like to emulate, but Little League may be beyond them unless leagues are specially organized to meet their needs. Not only must the individual identify leisure interests, but he or she must also have the mobility skills to get to those activities. For elementary school-aged children, this might focus on bike riding. Later, training and practice in the use of public transportation may be of value.

As these children age, vocational training and training in independent living skills, including **social skills training** (Hughes et al., 2011) and sex education, become increasingly important. Social skills training is a strategy for teaching specific social conventions, such as greetings, responses to others' greetings, conversational strategies, and departures, allowing for role play with feedback and repeated practice. Although individuals who are delayed may desire to engage in the same activities as their peers who are not delayed, they tend to conceptualize at a concrete level. Because many will live independently or in semisheltered environments, they need to understand the accompanying responsibilities. For example, one young woman expressed a wish for a baby until she sat through an independent living group while a baby doll cried in the background. Another young man planned to go to the movies every day until he was shown a realistic example of financial planning when the therapist had him put his pay from the sheltered workshop in piles to represent rent, food costs, transportation, and so on. For both individuals, the intervention served as a reality check about their skills. This kind of parenting and independent living education, combined with a focus on vocational issues, is increasingly important as more individuals with intellectual disabilities acquire these roles (Rose, Perks, Fidan, & Hurst, 2010).

Although the research evidence is insufficient to make a clear recommendation, some research supports the value of aerobic exercise as a way to improve physical and psychosocial health for individuals with developmental delay (Andriolo, El Dib, Ramos, Atallah, & Silva, 2010). Because exercise has demonstrated benefit for others, there is certainly no reason to doubt its effectiveness with these individuals, and, at minimum, it will improve general health status.

Individuals with intellectual disabilities most often prefer to integrate as much as possible into the world around them. Jahoda, Kemp, Riddell, and Banks (2007) undertook a review of the literature of feelings about work. They found that the greatest quality of life was reported by individuals with intellectual disabilities who were able to work in competitive employment, compared with those in sheltered work or who were unemployed. Their review also found that IQ was correlated with work and type of work; thus, not all individuals were capable of competitive employment. Therapists can focus on efforts to assist individuals to secure employment in the least sheltered setting they can manage and on assisting employers to structure the workplace effectively.

Technological devices can provide some assistance (Hoppestad, 2013) as a means of structuring the environment to reduce demand. Devices must be carefully evaluated, and training should be provided until the individual is comfortable with their use. It is important to choose wisely because some devices add to rather than reduce complexity of tasks.

As can be inferred from this discussion, treatment may occur in a variety of sites, including the home, a special school, a regular school, an institution, a sheltered workshop, or a supervised living facility. Increasingly, as a result of legislative emphasis on allowing every child access to the least restrictive environment, service is being provided in regular schools.

Communication Disorders

Communication disorders are characterized by deficits in **communication**, methods for conveying meaning among individuals, including **speech** (the production of sound) and **language** (form, function, and use of spoken symbols), to produce behaviors that allow interaction with others (APA, 2013).

The main features of communication disorders are difficulties acquiring and using language due to either incomprehension or production of language (APA, 2013). These problems are apparent in both **expressive** (ability to produce meaningful sounds) and **receptive** (ability to understand others' communication) language. Vocabulary and grammar are typically limited. and this, in turn, limits ability to interact. Communication challenges, in turn, limit participation in other activities, including socialization and education. As is true for most of the neurodevelopmental disorders, the diagnosis is not made unless the deficits deviate significantly from normal expectations.

Often, a family history of language disorders exists (APA, 2013). The child may be shy or reticent and have more difficulty communicating outside of familiar settings (e.g., away from home).

In some situations, the diagnosis of a language disorder does not precisely fit the situation. Related diagnoses include speech sound disorder, childhood-onset fluency disorder (stuttering), social (pragmatic) communication disorder, and unspecified communication disorder (APA, 2013). An "unspecified" category exists for every DSM diagnosis used for conditions that meet some but not all the characteristics of the main diagnostic group. The disorders must be distinguished from intellectual disability, autism, schizophrenia, and depression, and they may coexist with any of these disorders.

Etiology

The typical expectation about development of language is single-word production at approximately age 1 year and sentence production at approximately age 2 years, with comprehension emerging prior to expression (Nicholls, Eadie, & Reilly, 2011). However, there is considerable variability in development, in that delay until the age of 2 years in single-word use is not unheard of among children who acquire normal language use by the time they begin school. In addition, language acquisition may be delayed in bilingual households because of the need to process additional information and master a larger numbers of sounds.

As an example of these normal variations, consider the situation of a mother who brought her 3-year-old son to the family physician, expressing concern that the child had not yet spoken a recognizable word. The physician asked a series of questions that revealed the child was the youngest of four children; the other three of whom were quite verbal and very solicitous of the child. Also in the household were both parents, two grandparents, and a nanny. The physician suggested that perhaps the child simply had no need to speak, since his needs and wants were anticipated by the others in the household. Sure enough, that autumn when the three older siblings headed off to school full time, the child began speaking in complete sentences.

Stuttering has a significant genetic component (Nippold, Packman, Hammer, Scheffner, & Finn, 2012). Other causes of delay in language acquisition are hearing or other sensory impairments, intellectual disability, and some neurological disorders, such as epilepsy or autism (APA, 2013).

Prognosis

A language disorder that is diagnosed before age 4 is likely to be uncertain and unstable (APA, 2013) because there are broad variations in language acquisition. After age 4, differences between the individual and peers will be both more evident and more stable over time, typically persisting into adulthood. Roughly three quarters of children who stutter will eventually develop normal speech, assuming they receive appropriate therapy (Nippold et al., 2012). Speech sound disorder can be effectively treated through speech therapy and is unlikely to be lifelong unless it is accompanied by a language disorder.

Receptive impairments have a poorer prognosis than expressive impairments (APA, 2013). Early intervention seems to have a positive impact (Bernhardt & Major, 2005), with some individuals achieving normal language over time.

Implications for Function and Treatment

Various communication disorders impair social, educational, and—depending on the content of the job—vocational occupations (Adams et al., 2012; Hollo, 2012). The main performance skill affected is, obviously, communication. Performance patterns, expressed through roles, habits, and rituals, are affected only to the extent that the individual's communication deficits interfere with desired roles and patterns. For example, one young man exhibited childhood-onset fluency disorder (stuttering), evident since age 2. He struggled to produce single words and, on occasion, took as long as 5 minutes to complete a single sentence. He was able to reduce the frequency and severity of his stuttering over years of intensive speech therapy. However, he was never able to eliminate the problem. He had to deal with an array of social issues throughout his schooling, particularly bullying from some of the other students. He also struggled with oral presentations during his K-12 education. However, he was quite bright and likeable, and he developed a small group of loyal friends who shielded him from the students who were less accepting. Although his teachers continued to insist that he give the same oral presentations in class as other students—arguing that he needed to acquire this skill to be successful in the workplace—they allowed him additional time in the presentations and were somewhat more generous in their grading. In fact, over time, his presentation skills did improve. Ultimately, he chose a career as a medical technologist—a vocation that did not require extensive oral communication. He was quite successful, ultimately rising to supervisor of the department in a large teaching hospital. He married and had three children—one of whom also had childhood-onset fluency disorder.

As this example shows, treatment can be effective, although language deficits may persist (Adams et al., 2012). Unless there is a clear accompanying medical condition, medication is unlikely to be a part of treatment for language disorders. On the other hand, speech–language therapy with a behavioral focus, as well as behavioral strategies for management of accompanying anxiety, can be quite helpful (Smith-Lock, Leitao, Lambert, & Nickels, 2013). Individually structured intervention in the context of the classroom setting is likely to be helpful. Involving families in treatment can also be of value (Roberts, Kaiser, Oetting, & Hadley, 2012). Interventions are delivered in a variety of ways: to individuals, groups, and to whole classrooms (Roulstone, Wren, Bakopoulou, & Lindsay, 2012).

In planning an intervention, it is important to distinguish between children who have only a specific language deficit and those who have autism, ADHD, or social anxiety. The most helpful interventions include speech therapy and cognitive behavioral approaches to the accompanying anxiety and distress.

Implications for Occupational Therapy

Occupational therapists working with children with communication disorders may focus at the level of skill or occupations. In working on communication skills, there is some evidence for the value of sensory integration interventions (Roberts, King-Thomas, & Boccia, 2007). Occupational therapists can effectively collaborate with speech–language pathologists by providing safe environments in which the child can practice communication skills that are the focus of speech therapy. The occupational therapist can also help the child to identify social and leisure activities that deemphasize verbal communication to enhance the child's self-esteem and sense of self-confidence.

Autism Spectrum Disorder

Autism spectrum disorder is one of the diagnostic groupings that has been most altered in DSM-5, with considerable associated controversy (Stetka & Volkmar, 2012). Among the changes is the deletion of Asperger's syndrome, a DSM-IV diagnosis (APA, 2000), which was conceptualized as a less severe form of autism. Instead, the DSM-5 (APA, 2013) places autism along a spectrum, with Asperger's syndrome subsumed as a point on that continuum. Asperger's is now categorized as mild autism.

The most significant features of autism spectrum disorder are severe deficits in communication and social interaction, along with repetitive, patterned, and unproductive behaviors (APA, 2013). These features are often accompanied by significant emotional and behavioral difficulties, as the individual may be anxious, agitated, or withdrawn in situations that require social interaction (Georgiades, et al., 2011).

The difficulties with social interaction are more than shyness or withdrawal and are characterized by avoidance or peculiar behavior (Bishop, Gahagan, & Lord, 2007). As an example, a child with autism disorder may show no interest in what peers are doing even when sitting right next to them, may vigorously resist giving up an object of focus (sharing a toy for example), and may ignore direct efforts of other children to start a conversation. Obviously, it is important to evaluate such behavior, compared with what is normal for the child's age and culture. Many 2-year-old children are unwilling to share toys, but by age 3 or so, parallel or small-group play is typical. The child with autism will show no signs of making this developmental shift. Further, the ferocity of the refusal to participate with others is striking.

The same can be said of the repetitive behavior features of autism. Although young children often have somewhat patterned behaviors ("step on a crack, break your mother's back") and many appreciate routine in their lives, the child with autism may be absolutely insistent on such patterns and have significant emotional outbursts if these patterns are disrupted (APA, 2013).

The diagnosis of autism is typically made relatively early in life, often before age 2 (Shumway et al., 2011). However, in less severe cases, the diagnosis may be made later because the interaction and behavior patterns are not clearly distinct from those of other children until expectations for behavior have become more complex. In some cases, there is apparent normal development followed by deterioration, which is reported by parents to occur at approximately age 2 (Kalb, Law, Landa, & Law, 2010). This pattern of deterioration is puzzling to parents, and it has contributed to a belief held by some that autism is caused by childhood vaccination, particularly the measles/mumps/rubella vaccine (Richler et al., 2006). Although this belief has no scientific support—and has been repeatedly refuted by well-designed research studies—some parents continue to refuse to allow their children to be vaccinated.

Autism is not associated with deterioration over time. The occasional reports of deterioration in function may actually reflect the child's inability to reach more challenging developmental milestones. Typically the symptoms are stable, although function may improve in adolescence and adulthood as the individual develops compensatory skills (Anderson, Maye, & Lord, 2011; APA, 2013).

It is possible to specify severity as one of the following (APA, 2013):

- "Level 3 Requiring very substantial support
- Level 2 Requiring substantial support
- Level 1 Requiring support" (p. 52)

At level 3, severe communication and behavioral deficits occur so that the individual may have little intelligible speech and may demonstrate severe distress when any changes to the environment or alterations of a very patterned, restricted behavioral profile occur. On the other hand, at level 1, deficits in communication cause noticeable impairment, but individuals may be able to speak in complete sentences and interact with others, although those interactions may be stilted or odd. They may be relatively inflexible and have difficulty switching tasks, organizing, or problem solving. However, individuals with level 1 deficits may be able to function, with some difficulty, in normal educational and vocational settings.

Autism may coexist with ADHD (van Steijn et al., 2012), social anxiety (White, Bray, & Ollendick, 2012), schizophrenia (Gadow, 2012), and mood disorders (Simonoff et al., 2012). It must also be distinguished from these disorders when a diagnosis is made.

Etiology

The etiology of autism is increasingly well understood. At one point, it was considered a problem of inadequate parenting, believed to be associated with maternal coldness, absence, or rejection (Weininger, 1993). This idea has been discredited, and current hypotheses center on the possibility of some sort of neurological dysfunction, possibly of genetic origin (APA, 2013). Brain abnormalities have been found in the cerebellum, limbic system, and cortex of these individuals, and there is evidence of defective lateralization (Townsend et al., 2001). There are reports that children with autism have more brain cells and heavier brains, compared with other children (Courchesne et al., 2011). In addition, neurochemical abnormalities have been found, with suspicion focused on the role of dopamine agonists. There is speculation that maternal nutrition or hormonal status affect in utero development of the fetus (Lyall, Pauls, Santangelo, Spiegelman, & Ascherio, 2011). The most recent report on the etiology of autism indicates that there are patches of cortical disorganization of neurons in the prefrontal and temporal cortex in children with autism (Stoner et al., 2014).

A great deal of research interest has focused on genetic causes for the brain and biochemical changes that seem to be associated with autism (Abel et al., 2013; McPartland, Coffman, & Pelphrey, 2011). The strongest evidence points to a genetic source of the disorder (Johnson, Giarelli, Lewis, & Rice, 2013). Family studies reveal a risk of 60% for monozygotic twins. In addition, there is a 90% risk for some degree of social and behavioral problems in the second twin, even in the absence of an autism spectrum disorder.

Prognosis

In general, the prognosis is poor for individuals with autism (Lord et al., 2006; Shumway et al., 2011). In one study, almost 90% of the participants—all individuals with autism— had been receiving disability income 30 years after initial diagnosis (Mordre et al., 2012). Individuals with higher IQ, with special skills and interests, and who receive effective educational interventions are less likely to need disability income later in life. Another study found two main risk factors (symptom severity and speech ability) and two main protective factors (communication skill and person-related cognition), but even taking these into account, children with autism showed relatively little change over the course of 3 years (Darrou et al., 2010). The prognosis is particularly poor for individuals with a dual diagnosis of intellectual disability and autism (Bryson, Bradley, Thompson, & Wainwright, 2008).

Long-term consequences include increased stress for families of adolescents and adults with autism because of the additional responsibilities for care of these individuals.

Implications for Function and Treatment

Autism is one of the many mental disorders in which impaired function in daily activities is a diagnostic criterion. Function can be significantly affected in social settings (Patterson, Smith, & Jelen, 2010). Individuals with autism typically experience moderate to severe difficulty with ADL, IADL, education, work, leisure, and play (Jung & Sainato, 2013). Family occupations are affected as well as parents alter their choices about what family activities to undertake, how they prepare for those activities, and what the experiences mean to them and to the child (Bagby, Dickie, & Baranek, 2012).

Individuals with autism can show extreme impairments in communication and social skills, as well as in most functional areas (APA, 2013). These impairments may be characterized by peculiarities in function or by absence of engagement in expected occupations. For example, an individual with autism may be able to speak but may put words together in ways that are not meaningful to others. Similarly, he or she may be able to perform specific fine motor tasks but is unable to put them together into a meaningful sequence to accomplish a specific task.

The deficits in function can be quite severe, sometimes precluding most forms of normal goal-oriented occupation. Individuals with autism are often unable to perform ADL and IADL, have disturbed patterns of play, and may be unable to study and, later, work. Communication skills are particularly poor (Christensen-Sandfort & Whinnery, 2013). Half of the individuals with autism never develop speech and most fail to use speech in a functional way. Social participation is severely impaired (Teitt, Eastman, O'Donnell, & Deitz, 2010), with decreased imitation and social response. Sensory and self-regulatory symptoms are associated with more severe autism and accompanying greater dysfunction (Silva & Schalock, 2012). For example, autonomic and behavioral responses to auditory stimuli are heightened in these individuals (Chang et al., 2012).

Habits and patterns can be excessively rigid. Some individuals with autism find novel stimuli unpleasant and resist any change in environment (DeGrace, 2004). This can present challenges for family members because the individual's difficulty with change can constrain the function of the entire family, and going out to eat or to a movie may be very challenging with such a child.

Individuals with autism may have areas of unusually good function, such as excellent rote memory, visual/spatial skills, or attention to detail (Bennett & Heaton, 2012). These abilities may be associated with selective attention to particular features of the surroundings that other children might not notice.

This selective attention may be accompanied by stereotypic interactions with objects, such as spinning them or placing them in particular patterns. Individuals with autism typically display excessively routinized and unproductive patterns of behavior. Their stereotypic movements and verbalizations are quite entrenched, but they do not contribute to functional outcomes. All of these functional issues fall along a continuum, with individuals whose disorder is at the milder end of the spectrum having fewer and less severe deficits than those with the most severe disorders.

Because the etiology of autism is as yet unclear, treatment is not well-established. A wide array of treatments has been attempted, including both psychosocial and biological strategies. All these treatments focus on the behavioral manifestations of the condition rather than on cure, something that requires a better understanding of the underlying biological factors associated with the disorder.

Behavioral interventions are widely recommended (Reichow, Barton, Boyd, & Hume 2012), with a focus on developing speech, increasing behaviors such as ADL skills, and decreasing undesirable behaviors such as peculiar movements. More and more children with autism spectrum disorder—particularly those with less severe conditions—are in community settings, such as public schools, and are often in special classes. However, many programs are still provided at special schools or inpatient settings, as they are usually designed to provide high levels of patterned input throughout the day (Bryant & Battles, 2006).

Behavior modification and cognitive behavioral approaches have been utilized for specific deficits (Patterson et al., 2010; White, Ollendick, Scahill, Oswald, & Albano, 2009). There is consensus that intensive intervention, involving roughly 25 hours per week, is needed (Maglione et al., 2012). Low impact intervention is less successful (Eldevik, Eikeseth, Jahr, & Smith, 2006). Applied behavior analysis is considered a best practice in some areas and involves careful assessment of specific behaviors, accompanied by detailed plans for intervention based on behavior modification principles. Depending on the severity of the condition, it may be necessary to focus initially on very small units of behavior (e.g., making eye contact or picking up a new toy). At the less severe end of the spectrum, behavioral therapy can minimize social and behavioral deficits. For example, adults with level 1 autism may be able to avoid repetitive movement while in public situations and may be able to learn to interact with others fairly effectively. Speech therapy can address some of the typical communication deficits (Adams et al., 2012).

A number of comprehensive programs that incorporate a constellation of environmental and behavioral strategies have been reported and appear to be at least modestly beneficial. One such program is the Treatment and Education of Autistic and Related Communication-Handicapped Children (Mesibov & Shea, 2010). This program includes structure of the environment, visual supports for function, a focus on the child's special interests, and meaningful, child-initiated communication. Its focus on the child's interests makes this program particularly relevant for consideration by occupational therapists.

Early intervention is important (Rogers, 2001). Early intervention can provide families with a sense of relief that their concerns are being taken seriously and can help ensure that appropriate treatment strategies are identified. Because of their unique sets of strengths and weaknesses, tailored early intervention can help children with autism learn most effectively. It is possible that early intervention may be associated with better outcomes, although the research on this issue is equivocal.

Biological intervention focuses on drug treatment to ameliorate symptoms such as anxiety and hyperactivity. Nontraditional antipsychotic medications, such as risperidone, seem to be effective in managing aggressive behavior (West & Waldrop, 2006). An array of psychopharmacological agents may be provided to individuals with autism (Sung, Fung, & Cai, 2010) to address specific behavioral or emotional concerns, such as anxiety, explosive behavior, self-injurious behavior, sleep problems, and so on. There is no medication that addresses the core symptoms of the disorder.

Vitamins (Ferraro, 2001) and special diets (Santhanam & Kendler, 2012) are other biological interventions that have been attempted. Removing gluten and casein from an individual's diet has been proposed as a mechanism to reduce symptoms, but much of the diet-based research has been performed in an uncontrolled fashion or with small samples.

It should be noted that over the years a wide array of interventions of questionable value has been advocated (Ferraro, 2001). One largely discredited, but still popular intervention, is avoidance of sugar and artificial dyes in the diet. There is no good research to document the effectiveness of this approach. Although it is understandable that parents wish to find a cure, an important role for the therapist is to help them understand the limits of these kinds of recommendations and to help them avoid a sense of guilt if they do not or cannot devote the kind of time and attention required to provide these interventions.

Implications for Occupational Therapy

Because children with autism may be severely impaired, observation must often be substituted for formal evaluation, and treatment goals must be sensitive to the probability that change will occur in very small steps. Interestingly, evaluation for adaptive function seems to be particularly important to ensure diagnostic accuracy (Tomanik, Pearson, Loveland, Lane, & Shaw, 2007). Occupational therapy has a significant role in ensuring that children diagnosed with autism actually fit the criteria.

Case-Smith and Arbesman (2008) identified six main clusters of strategies used most often by occupational therapists working with children with autism. These strategies include the following:

1. Sensory integration
2. Relationship-based approaches
3. Developmental skills approaches
4. Sensory-cognitive approaches
5. Parent-focused intervention
6. Behavioral interventions

There is some limited evidence about the value of music therapy (Gold, Wigram, & Elefant, 2006), as well as motor-based role-playing for children with level 1 autism (Gutman, Raphael-Greenfield, & Rao, 2012). Comprehensive intervention that takes advantage of many of these strategies is the most effective (Tomchek, LaVesser, & Watling, 2010).

Alternative mechanisms, such as *qigong* massage, may improve social and language skills (Silva, Schalock, Ayres, Bunse, & Budden, 2009). Additional research will be needed to confirm these findings, and caution must be exercised as some children with autism would find touch distressing. Yoga has also been shown to increase acceptable behavior in the classroom (Koenig, Buckley-Reen, & Garg, 2012).

Behavioral and sensory integration interventions seem to be the treatments most frequently described in occupational therapy (Case-Smith & Arbesman, 2008; Pfeiffer, Koenig, Kinnealey, Sheppard, & Henderson, 2011; Schaaf, Hunt, & Benevides, 2012). In general, treatment focus is on basic self-care and communication. Motivation and attention are also key issues. Behavioral techniques may be helpful in both enhancing attention and in training children with autism to perform sequences of activities related to self-care. It is important to point out that some researchers have found that sensory integration is less effective than behavior modification in ameliorating behavioral problems (Devlin, Healy, Leader, & Hughes, 2011).

One area of controversy is the value of mainstreaming for children with autism (Humphrey, 2008). Although there are those who argue that children with autism are excessively disruptive to other students, there is evidence that their inclusion improves some of their behavioral symptoms. At the same time, their inclusion provides benefits for other children in the class by challenging stereotypes and promoting peer understanding.

Environmental modification in the classroom may support function of children with autism and have the added benefit of helping other children who are excessively sensitive to sensory input (e.g., children with ADHD; Kinnealey et al., 2012). Alternative seating using therapy balls has been shown to increase in-seat behavior (Bagatell, Mirigliani, Patterson, Reyes, & Test, 2010). Although this specific intervention may not work with every child, it is an example of a simple strategy that may have substantial benefits for some children.

It is likely that occupational therapy is best provided in the context of multidisciplinary intervention (Aldred, Pollard, Phillips, & Adams, 2001; Jordan, 2001), particularly because it is not clear which of the many educational, behavioral, environmental, and biological treatments are most effective (Gabriels, Hill, Pierce, Rogers, & Wehner, 2001).

A number of new technologies seem helpful in working with children with autism. Computer-assisted communication can be of considerable benefit. For children with autism, predictability and routine are important, and computers can provide highly structured instruction that is, nonetheless, individualized. Assistive technologies are also being developed to provide prompts during social interaction and other structured input to facilitate occupations.

Keyboarding to encourage self-expression also seems helpful (Giese, 2008), perhaps because it allows the child to convey his or her ideas without the need to interact directly with another human being. Augmentative communication strategies are particularly valuable because of the severe communication deficits that characterize the disorder (Shane, 2006). Other technologies are being developed to provide social prompts and other input to compensate for the child's difficulty with sorting and interpreting sensory input (Tartaro & Cassell, 2006).

Two other important considerations for occupational therapy intervention are the inclusion of families (Bendixen et al., 2011; Dunn, Cox, Foster, Mische-Lawson, & Tanquary, 2012; Foster, Dunn, & Lawson, 2013) and the importance of facilitating the transition from adolescence into the adult world.

Families are profoundly affected by the needs of a child with autism. Understanding the disorder, learning management mechanisms, and learning how to recognize the strengths of the child can help to reduce caregiver stress and improve both the child's and the family's functioning.

One of the major stressors for the individual with autism and the family is the transition to adult life (Crabtree, 2011). Individuals with autism, insofar as they can, need to explore and enter the world of work (Waite, 2013). They need to learn community mobility (Precin, Otto, Popalzai, & Samuel, 2012) and other ADL and IADL skills that will allow them to live in the least restrictive, most satisfying environment. For some individuals at the less severe end of the autism spectrum, a focus on social behaviors can ease the transition (Gutman et al., 2012). However, in some instances, the goal of the transition must be to find a suitable supported environment for the young adult. For example, one family, whose young adult son with autism struggled to find a way to make a living, have a social life, and become independent from his parents, ultimately located a farm in a nearby rural community that housed adults with autism, providing supported living and a work environment to which the young man could contribute.

Finally, as is true regardless of the disorder under consideration, a focus on an individual's strengths is essential (Kotler & Koenig, 2012). One example of an individual with autism who has forged a meaningful and satisfying life is Temple Grandin (Grandin & Panek, 2013). Dr. Grandin described a childhood during which she struggled to manage her sensory processing difficulties and her daily activities. She ultimately earned a doctor of philosophy degree, focused her attention on a love of animals, and worked to make the slaughter of animals for food a more humane process. She now advocates for access to opportunity for individuals with autism. Although Dr. Grandin's life story is well known, there are many other successful individuals who have found ways to compensate for the challenges of their symptoms and to capitalize on their unique strengths. Dr. Grandin's life demonstrates that individuals with autism have unique contributions to make to the world around them, and helping them to reach their potential can make a difference to their families and communities, as well as to their own lives.

Attention-Deficit/Hyperactivity Disorder

Attention-deficit/hyperactivity disorder (ADHD) is characterized by inattention, hyperactivity, and impulsivity (APA, 2013). The inattention is reflected in difficulty with arousal control, visual and auditory sensory processing, and distractibility. This results in difficulty completing tasks and maintaining focus, compounded by excessive attention to irrelevant stimuli. The hyperactivity component is characterized by age-inappropriate difficulty sitting still. The child may squirm, run around, talk incessantly, and fidget. Impulsivity is demonstrated by recklessness, impetuosity, and disinhibition. All these behaviors result in difficulty with tasks of daily living and in poor classroom performance.

In addition to the criteria listed, the diagnosis should specify whether there is a combined presentation that includes both inattention and hyperactivity-impulsivity for the past 6 months, or whether the presentation includes predominantly inattentive presentation or predominantly hyperactive–impulsive presentation. It is also important to specify whether the condition is in partial remission (fewer than the full criteria during the past 6 months) and whether it is mild, moderate, or severe.

Most often, ADHD is identified during the early school years when behavioral expectations for attention and focus increase (Cherkasova, Sulla, Dalena, Pondé, & Hechtman, 2013). There is a trend toward earlier diagnosis, as well as diagnosis during adulthood, but school performance during primary school years is still the main trigger to diagnosis. One of the challenges in diagnosis is that adult tolerance for impulsive behavior varies. A child might be diagnosed before entering school if the parents are sensitive to the child's level of energy and activity, whereas the same behaviors might not be diagnosed in a child whose parents and teachers expect and tolerate higher levels of activity. Nevertheless, some children struggle with the most basic expectations of the school setting and express their frustration in acting out behavior (Figure 3-2).

Conditions that may be comorbid with ADHD include conduct and oppositional defiant disorder, specific learning disorders, mood and anxiety disorders, Tourette syndrome, obsessive-compulsive disorder, and autism spectrum disorder (Chu, 2003). The presence of one of these additional conditions influences prognosis.

Etiology

It is fairly well established that ADHD is a neurological condition that almost certainly has a genetic component. Findings include evidence of reduced cerebral blood flow, decreased right frontal lobe size, changes in the caudate nucleus and cerebellum, poorly regulated levels of dopamine, and abnormal electroencephalogram patterns (Chu, 2003). It seems probable that the environment has a role in the production of behaviors typifying ADHD. This helps to explain why some children with ADHD can be quite attentive and functional in some settings, for example, when playing video games, whereas very distractible and impulsive in others, such as at a swimming pool or skating rink.

Among other contributing factors that have been hypothesized, the idea of a dietary influence has been largely discredited (Bradley & Golden, 2001). Hypoxia during birth, maternal

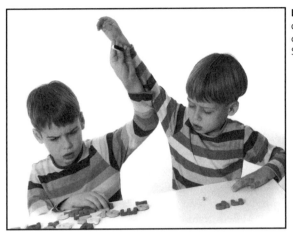

Figure 3-2. Children with ADHD may have difficulty managing their frustration in classroom and social situations. (©2014 Shutterstock.com.)

smoking, low birth weight, and other environmental factors do seem to be associated with ADHD.

Prognosis

Only about half of children with ADHD remain symptomatic in adulthood (APA, 2013). This means that the prognosis is a reasonably good one. Factors that influence the outcome include the severity of symptoms, presence of comorbid conditions, family situation, intelligence, socioeconomic status, and treatment (Chu, 2003).

The severity of symptoms affects not only the likelihood of an initial diagnosis but also the long-term outcome. Roughly 60% to 80% of preschool children diagnosed with ADHD will retain the diagnosis in primary school (Cherkasova et al., 2013). The severity of the impulsive and hyperactive behavior will also influence the extent to which the child can ultimately manage school and work occupations.

A potential negative consequence of ADHD is the possibility that the child will become depressed or develop low self-esteem as a result of the social disapproval or academic difficulties that often accompany the disorder (Faraone & Doyle, 2001). Understandably, the prognosis is less favorable if ADHD is accompanied by intellectual disability or some other behavioral disorder, such as conduct disorder or substance abuse (Lynskey & Hall, 2001).

Implications for Function and Treatment

Children with ADHD are able to function in many areas. They are usually able to perform age-appropriate ADL and IADL, play, and interact with peers. Generally speaking, social participation and education are most impaired. Peers and adults may find the excessive activity and difficulty concentrating annoying and avoid or chastise the child. In some instances, poor impulse control leads the child to behave in a socially inappropriate or antisocial fashion, again leading to disapproval and even legal difficulties. These children may have difficulty in peer relationships persisting into adolescence (Vilardo, DuPaul, Kern, & Hojnoski, 2013).

Developmental stages alter the ways in which ADHD is expressed (Anastopoulos, Klinger, & Temple, 2001). In toddlers, it can manifest as impatience to gain desired objects. In preschool children, inattentiveness may be noted as these children move rapidly from one activity to another. Often, it is entry into kindergarten that brings first recognition of the problem, as school introduces the requirement that children sit still and attend for increasing time periods. However, the fact that the inattentiveness and hyperactivity may vary with the situation can be challenging, as parents may perceive that nothing is wrong, whereas teachers are reporting misbehavior in school (Lench, Levine, & Whalen, 2013). In other instances, hyperactivity is clear in the home environment as well. One parent reported that her son routinely ran out into the street while playing, with total disregard for traffic. She indicated that he could sit still for only a few minutes while watching TV or listening to her read. This example may not be typical of all children with ADHD, as some can focus well on particular kinds of activities (e.g., watching TV), whereas other activities generate significant hyperactivity (particularly in school).

Poor concentration and impulse control are notable, as are deficits in executive function (Barnett, Maruff, & Vance, 2009; Graziano, McNamara, Geffken, & Reid, 2013). In addition, these children may have sensory overresponsivity and/or anxiety (Reynolds & Lane, 2009). These present significant problems in the academic sphere. Not only is learning impaired, but teachers find these children difficult to manage, thus compounding the students' learning problems. They often do poorly in school and then become anxious about their performance, exacerbating their learning difficulties. Other activities that require concentration or attention may be difficult or impossible for these children, limiting the play and leisure activities in which they are able to participate. Because of their inattention, they have difficulty establishing effective performance patterns.

In adolescence, individuals with ADHD may engage in a variety of risky behaviors associated with driving, drug use, and sexual behavior (Hosain, Berenson, Tennen, Bauer, & Wu, 2012; White & Buehler, 2012). Individuals with ADHD may be less sensitive to punishment than others (Humphreys & Lee, 2011). Social interactions can be affected at any age, but this dilemma is particularly pronounced in adolescence (Glass, Flory, & Hankin, 2012).

Medication is often part of the treatment for ADHD, with methylphenidate, atomoxetine, and dexamphetamine all being recommended (Didoni, Sequi, Panei, & Bonati, 2011). Studies have shown that these medications increase children's on-task behavior and improve academic work. Use of medication is somewhat controversial, as the side effects can be problematic, and they may not be helpful for every child with ADHD (Sroufe, 2012). In addition, because their use is now widespread, and because diagnosis is somewhat imprecise, there is a belief that some children are being medicated simply for being children. Studies of medication in adults with ADHD support their use, with reports of reduced symptoms, improved function, and generally low rates of side effects (Bitter, Angyalosi, & Czobor, 2012; Prasad et al., 2013).

Many psychological and behavioral treatments are also used to reduce the symptoms of ADHD. These include behavior therapy, psychotherapy, family therapy, social skills training, parent training, and school-based educational interventions (Frank-Briggs, 2011). These interventions appear to be helpful in many situations, and are more acceptable to families that are uncomfortable with medication. In some situations, the two categories of intervention are used in concert. Behavioral approaches attempt to reinforce efforts to concentrate and control hyperactivity (Döpfner & Rothenberger, 2007).

Environmental strategies include design of low-stimulus environments in which distractions are kept to a minimum. Teacher and parent education can be helpful in providing these individuals with management strategies. Cognitive-behavioral therapy and social skills training are of value with older children (Barkley, 2004). Peer coaching is among the other interventions reported as being helpful to address social dysfunction (Vilardo et al., 2013). It seems likely that a combination of psychosocial and pharmacological interventions is most helpful, although there are calls for reducing the role of medication and increasing the role of other interventions (Pelham, 2002).

A challenge in successful intervention for children with ADHD is ensuring effective parental collaboration (Dreyer, O'Laughlin, Moore, & Milam, 2010). Caregivers can be stressed and exhausted by expectations of their support of school-based and environmental interventions. Although parents often prefer behavioral interventions, these require time and effort, which may be in short supply in the home.

Implications for Occupational Therapy Intervention

As the name of the ADHD disorder implies, attention is an important factor when work-ing with these children. It is helpful to provide treatment in the setting where problems occur, thus school-based interventions are desirable (AOTA, 2014). Occupational therapy may be helpful in the specific environmental structuring needed to minimize distraction and may help the child focus on the task at hand. Occupational therapy may also provide patterned, sequenced sensory input to attempt to help the child better organize his or her reactions to the environment. Ideally, this input is provided through play or other meaningful occupations.

Many specific interventions have been reported in the research literature. For example, a cognitive–functional intervention promoted significant improvement in executive function and improved cognitive strategies supporting occupations (Hahn-Markowitz, Manor, & Maeir, 2011). The intervention involved 10 hour-long sessions in the child's home, each of which focused on a specific occupational goal (e.g., organizing his or her backpack, playing with a friend for 15 minutes without arguing). The parents were instructed in strategies for reinforcing successful accomplishment of each goal. Another intervention reported using the simple addition of a stability ball to seat children with ADHD (Fedewa & Erwin, 2011). Children seated in this way showed increased attention and decreased hyperactivity.

Self-regulated strategy development can assist elementary and middle school-aged children with ADHD (Lienemann & Reid, 2008). Self-esteem is an important issue. Identification of activities these children do well can be enormously helpful in convincing them that they do have strengths, despite repeated scolding from exasperated adults.

Often, the occupational therapist teaches parents (Chu & Reynolds, 2007) and teachers to manage difficult behaviors. Assisting them in optimally structuring the learning or home environment, breaking tasks into chunks, or providing deep touch to help the child gain con-trol, may help the adult to cope better and the child to function better.

Early intervention is particularly valuable. One program for preschool-aged children and their families demonstrated long-term value over 18 months (Jones, Daley, Hutchings, Bywater, & Eames, 2008). Of course, because ADHD is so often undiagnosed until the child reaches school age, it may be difficult to implement early-intervention programming.

At the same time, it is important to remember that functional deficits can persist into adulthood. Occupational therapists can assist such adults to develop strategies for coping with the performance challenges posed by short attention span and poor executive functioning (Gutman & Szczepanski, 2005).

Specific Learning Disorder

The specific learning disorder focuses on a particular area of function: the ability to learn in academic settings. The diagnostic criteria make it possible to be specific about the exact nature of the difficulty (APA, 2013). Therefore, for impairment in reading, it is possible to indicate whether the problem is with word reading accuracy, reading rate or fluency, or read-ing comprehension as the problem area. These difficulties are sometimes labeled **dyslexia**. For difficulty in writing, it is possible to specify spelling, grammar and punctuation, or clar-ity and organization. Impairment in mathematics can be noted as difficulty with number sense, memorization of arithmetic facts, difficulty with calculation, and difficulty with math reasoning. These difficulties are sometimes called **dyscalculia**. It is also possible to specify whether the problem is mild, moderate, or severe.

The most evident and important diagnostic feature is difficulty learning as a result of specific skill deficits (APA, 2013). These deficits reflect ability noticeably and measurably below that of peers or what is expected at a particular age. Most of the time, these difficulties are evident early in primary school, although in cases where the difficulty is mild they may not be evident until the challenge of the material to be learned increases. For example, a child with impairment in math reasoning may manage to acquire the skills needed for basic math calculation, but struggle when reasoning involved in geometry or algebra becomes necessary. A further feature is the specificity of the difficulty. Unlike intellectual development disorder—where the learning deficits are global—a child with a specific learning disorder may, for example, be able to manage reading and writing without difficulty, while struggling with math. It is important to be aware that a child with one learning disorder may well have several; therefore, a comprehensive evaluation is warranted (Landerl & Moll, 2010).

Specific learning disorder is almost always diagnosed in elementary school (Warnke, 1999), although—particularly when the difficulty is in math reasoning—it may not be apparent until middle school, when mathematical concepts are taught at a more complex level. Specific learning disorder is often concomitant with fine motor difficulties. Symptoms that may be recognized in preschool can include lack of interest in playing rhyming games and other word games, difficulty recognizing letters or numbers, and difficulty breaking words into their parts. The disorder occurs across cultures, with slight variations, depending on the kind of language (e.g., alphabetic versus nonalphabetic) and the requirements within that culture for the ability in question (APA, 2013). Children with this disorder may also have comorbid ADHD, communication disorders, developmental coordination disorder, autism spectrum disorder, or other mental disorders (APA, 2013).

Etiology

Specific learning disorders may be the result of inadequate neurons or inadequate neural connections in particular regions of the brain (Gordon, 2004). Prematurity and very low birth weight are associated with specific learning disorder (APA, 2013). It appears that genetic factors may also contribute, although etiology is not well established. Most literature supports a biological/neurological component (Grigorenko, 2001; Keogh, 2002), whereas family studies indicate a genetic factor (Plomin, 2001). Family studies also suggest that prevalence of learning disorders is higher in children whose parents have a history of substance abuse (Martin, Romig, & Kirisci, 2000). It is unclear whether this finding is related to prenatal exposure to drugs or environmental factors during development.

Prognosis

With appropriate intervention, students may be able to find strategies for managing their deficits, although in many cases, the particular skill continues to require substantial effort. One clear recommendation for treatment is to identify the problem early. Children who show delay in language development, have speech or coordination difficulties, or who have an unusually short attention span can be identified as young as 2.5 years of age and should be evaluated for possible learning disabilities (American Academy of Pediatrics Subcommittee on Attention-Deficit/Hyperactivity Disorder, 2011). According to the American Academy of Pediatrics (2011), intervention to promote gross motor development, practice with speech, shape recognition, and other skills—begun at a very early age—can reap considerable benefits. Technology offers new strategies for intervention. A computer-based program that targets auditory temporal processing and language skills improved reading and language function for middle-school children with learning disabilities (Given, Wasserman, Chari, Beattie, & Eden, 2008).

Some children grow out of their learning difficulties over time. For these children, specific learning disorder may represent a developmental lag, rather than a chronic disorder. Some researchers believe that learning disorders are developmental variants, rather than true psychiatric disorders (Gilger & Kaplan, 2001; Keogh, 2002). If this is true, it might be expected that some of these children would catch up developmentally. For other children, learning disorders have long-term negative consequences. Approximately 5% of people with learning disorders are unresponsive to treatment, and these individuals may represent those with true disorder, as opposed to developmental variants (Keogh, 2002).

Learning disorders may well persist (Shalev, Auerbach, Manor, & Gross-Tsur, 2000), although many individuals acquire management strategies. Without adequate intervention, school failure and subsequent occupational failure may occur (Geary, 2011; Rimrodt & Lipkin, 2011). In addition, greater severity of the disability, as well as coexisting conditions such as ADHD, are predictive of poorer outcomes (APA, 2013). It is also important to recognize that learning disabilities can coexist with other conditions (Capozzi et al., 2008). Among the most common comorbidities is ADHD (Capano, Minden, Chen, Schachar, & Ickowicz, 2008). Another challenging condition is the coexistence of self-injurious behavior (Lovell, 2008). In each of these cases, intervention must include attention to both the learning disability and to the coexisting condition.

Implications for Function and Treatment

Function is impaired in specific areas of academic performance, which is defined by the nature of the learning disability. It is not entirely clear whether the dysfunction is at the level of occupation or skill. In all probability, skills are deficient and contribute to difficulties in performance.

Treatment must begin with careful evaluation to determine the exact nature of the child's difficulty (Bowers & Bailey, 2001). Following assessment, plans can be made to remediate the deficits, often through occupational therapy. Therapy may emphasize the development of motor and praxis skills through gross and fine motor activities and communication and social skills through direct training. In addition, teachers can develop instructional plans that make use of the alternate pathways available to the child. For example, some children find mnemonic devices helpful (Wolgemuth, Cobb, & Alwell, 2008). A child with auditory learning difficulties may be able to make use of visual substitutes and vice versa. These adaptive mechanisms can be helpful, but they must be individualized. For example, one child with a disorder of written expression had great difficulty writing, but she was able to express herself eloquently by using the computer when writing.

Individualized educational strategies can be helpful in addressing difficulties with language in both reading and written expression (Berninger & O'Malley, 2011), and accompanying emotional difficulties are best treated with psychotherapy (Vedi & Bernard, 2012). Evidence exists that music education can be helpful in improving reading skills (Cogo-Moreira et al., 2012).

For dyscalculia, strategies identified as being effective include repeated practice, segmentation of subject matter, small interactive groups, and use of cues in strategy learning (Kaufmann & von Aster, 2012). From time to time, psychotherapy and medication may be helpful in managing the accompanying anxiety or frustration that arises from difficulty learning.

Implications for Occupational Therapy Intervention

Occupational therapy plays a major role in addressing learning disorders (cf., Case-Smith, Richardson, Schultz, Humphry, & Rogers, 2005; Parham & Fazio, 2007). Treatment of children with learning disorders is the primary role for therapists in school systems. Screening is particularly important because parents and teachers may not recognize the indicators of the problem. Informing parents and teachers about signs of learning disorders can be quite valuable.

In addition, occupational therapists can assist teachers and parents in managing the difficulties with learning and in providing direct treatment to the child. Sensory integration is among the interventions that appear to be of value (Bundy, Lane, Fisher, & Murray, 2002). Students also benefit from neuropsychological interventions, cognitive training, accommodation, and compensation (Bowers & Bailey, 2001). One particularly important issue is the transferability of skill from academic to vocational settings as individuals reach adolescence. It is clear that demands of the workplace differ from those of academic settings and that skills and accommodations learned in school may not be adequate for the new challenges (Bowers & Bailey, 2001).

Motor Disorders

Several motor disorders exist and include the following:
- Developmental coordination disorder
- Stereotypic movement disorder
- Tic disorder

In general, these disorders are all characterized by motor deficits or dysfunctions that interfere with normal performance.

Developmental Coordination Disorder

Developmental coordination disorder is characterized by delayed and inadequate development of age-appropriate motor skills. This diagnosis is usually made on the basis of observation of an informant (parent, teacher) over time. The child displays delays in achieving expected motor milestones, such as sitting, walking, and manipulating objects (Wilson, Ruddock, Smits-Engelsman, Polatajko, & Blank, 2013). To make a diagnosis, it is important to note that the child must have had the opportunity to acquire a specific skill. For example, although children between the ages of 6 and 10 typically learn to ride a bicycle, the diagnosis of developmental coordination disorder could not be made if a child cannot ride a bike because he or she never had the opportunity to learn to do so.

The disorder is most often recognized in early childhood when the individual does not achieve developmental milestones (APA, 2013) and then continues through adolescence and adulthood as the individual strives to learn new motor activities, such as building models, handwriting, playing softball, driving, and using tools.

Developmental coordination disorder must be distinguished from motor impairments due to other medical conditions, such as cerebral palsy, intellectual disability, ADHD, autism spectrum disorder, and a medical condition called joint hypermobility syndrome (APA, 2013). This disorder occurs frequently with specific learning disorder, autism spectrum disorder, and ADHD, as well as disruptive and emotional behavior problems (APA, 2013).

Because the central concern is on motor function in this and other motor disorders, fewer cultural factors exist than with disorders that more directly affect communication, social interaction, or education.

Etiology

Low birth weight is one factor (Zwicker et al., 2013) that is associated with developmental coordination disorder. In addition, prenatal exposure to alcohol, genetic factors, and neurological dysfunction of unspecified origin has also been implicated (APA, 2013).

Prognosis

As with learning disorders, some children simply grow out of their difficulties, particularly if they are provided with opportunities for physical practice and perceptual motor training (Barnhart, Davenport, Epps, & Nordquist, 2003). However, for many children, the difficulties persist into adulthood. Although the characteristics of the developmental coordination disorder can contribute to various functional difficulties, in general they are less disabling than those of many other mental disorders.

Implications for Function and Treatment

Motor disorders are characterized by poor performance on a wide array of motor tasks (Asonitou, Koutsouki, Kourtessis, & Charitou, 2012; Wilson et al., 2013). Children with developmental coordination disorder do worse on all motor performance than do peers without the disorder. In addition, the condition often occurs with specific learning disorders—particularly focused on language skills—leading to significant challenges in school settings (Adi-Japha, Strulovich-Schwartz, & Julius, 2011).

Deficits at the skill level contribute to difficulties in several occupations. Beyond having difficulty with educational performance, affected individuals may have peer problems as well (Wagner, Bös, Jascenoka, Jekauc, & Peterman, 2012). These may be a result of the clumsiness that causes children with motor disorders to struggle in sports, as well as with academic tasks such as writing, which require motor control. Boys with developmental coordination disorder are less likely than their peers to participate in sports activities, and they are more likely to report loneliness (Poulsen, Ziviani, Cuskelly, & Smith, 2007). Among the long-term negative consequences of this constellation of difficulties is the emergence of other mental disorders, especially anxiety and depression (Emck, Bosscher, van Wieringen, Doreleijers, & Beek, 2012).

For all of these reasons, early intervention is essential (Wilson et al., 2013). There is compelling evidence that occupational and physical therapy are among the most helpful strategies (Smits-Engelsman et al., 2013). The emphasis of intervention is on motor practice and compensatory strategies.

Implications for Occupational Therapy

Occupational therapists are directly involved in the treatment of developmental coordination disorder. In addition to screening, assessment, and consultation with teachers and parents, therapists provide direct treatment (Smits-Engelsman et al., 2013). Play that encourages gross motor activity has the potential to strengthen muscles and provide sensory input that may enhance motor and praxis skills. Perceptual motor training has been shown to be helpful, as have task-oriented occupational therapy interventions that emphasize specific practice of skills. There is also evidence that this set of strategies can improve coordination, successful pursuit of occupations, and quality of life (Kaiser, 2013).

Stereotypic Movement Disorder

As distinct from developmental coordination disorder, in which motor performance is slow or ineffective, stereotypic movement disorder is characterized by excessive and nonfunctional movement. The condition may be mild, moderate, or severe (APA, 2013). The specifiers also allow clinicians to note situations in which the individual engages in self-injurious behavior and can be associated with a medical or genetic condition or environmental factor.

The most significant feature of stereotypic movement disorder is the presence of motor behaviors that are repetitive and apparently purposeless (APA, 2013). Often, the individual will have a particular patterned behavior that is repeated over and over, such as twirling of the hair, rocking, or flapping the hands. Some of these movements, such as eye-poking, may be self-injurious, although self-injury is not a required feature of the diagnosis.

The stereotypic movement disorder is most often noted within the first 2 years of life, and the mean age of diagnosis is 6 (Freeman, Soltanifar, & Baer, 2010). Symptoms must be differentiated from ADHD, autism spectrum disorder, tic disorders, obsessive-compulsive disorders, and other neurological or medical conditions (APA, 2013).

Etiology

One significant risk factor of stereotypic movement disorder is the presence of another condition, such as blindness, a genetic disorder (e.g., Rett syndrome), or autism (Freeman et al., 2010). In children who do not have another condition, the disorder often resolves.

Tic Disorders

Three tic disorders are included in the motor disorder category of the DSM-5 (APA, 2013): Tourette's disorder, persistent (chronic) motor or vocal tic disorder, and provisional tic disorder. A **tic** is a "sudden, rapid, recurrent, nonrhythmic motor movement or vocalization" (APA, 2013, p. 81).

Etiology

The etiology of tic disorders is unclear (Shprecher & Kurlan, 2009). Speculation exists that they may be genetic, but the other leading cause is **idiopathic** (i.e., unknown).

Prognosis

The prognosis for tic disorders is relatively good (Ludolph, Roessner, Münchau, & Müller-Vahl, 2012; Roessner, Hoekstra, & Rothenberger, 2011). One third of children with tic disorders become completely free of tics as adults, and another third are much improved. Less than 20% of people with these diagnoses still have significant tics as adults.

Implications for Function and Treatment

The main concern with regard to tic disorders is the impact on the child's social interactions (Lin, Lai, & Gau, 2012). Children with tic disorders may be perceived as odd and can become stigmatized as a result.

Motor skills and occupations requiring motor skills (leisure sports participation, for example) can be affected (Bo & Lee, 2013; Wilson et al., 2013).

Intervention strategies include motor practice, anxiety management skill development, and contextual strategies to minimize triggers for the tics (Ludolph et al., 2012; Smits-Engelsman et al., 2013). Cognitive behavioral therapy has been demonstrated to be effective, either in combination with medication or on its own (O'Connor et al., 2009). Because it is probable that the child will outgrow the tic disorder, supportive interventions to help with academic, leisure, and social activities and to support the child's self-esteem are valuable.

Implications for Occupational Therapy

Occupational therapy interventions focus largely on the development of gross motor skills through meaningful activities (Kaiser, 2013). In addition, carefully designed behavioral interventions focused on developing new habits and relaxation and function-based strategies for managing environmental triggers and social interactions can enhance engagement in occupations (Rowe, Yuen, & Dure, 2013). Attention to relevant occupations, including handwriting practice to support educational efforts and practice that contributes to participation in sports, can have a positive impact on the child's quality of life. Opportunities to capitalize on strengths also have a positive impact by improving peer standing and building self-esteem. Table 3-2 summarizes the diagnostic criteria and functional consequences of the disorders described in this chapter.

Cultural Considerations

Culture affects both a diagnosis and treatment. For example, parental views of their children's activity can affect the probability that a child is diagnosed with ADHD (Starr, 2007). Characteristics of several Hispanic groups, which place high value on interactive learning for young children, lead to greater probability of diagnosis because of the greater potential for the child's behavior to affect others. In other groups, particularly those with agrarian traditions and lower expectations for formal education, ADHD may be diagnosed less frequently. General mistrust of the medical system seems to be associated with greater skepticism about the use of medications to treat ADHD among African-Americans.

As another example, motor disorders may be identified differently, depending on the culture (e.g., in some children, a motor disorder may be noted when he or she tries to learn to play soccer, whereas in other cultures, children may not play organized sports), but the impact of the disorder is similar, regardless of culture.

Cultural background must be considered in designing an intervention. For example, in Japan, there is not yet a strong self-help culture, although there is a growing trend in this direction (Tsuda, 2006). Family members of individuals with intellectual disability who are recent immigrants from Japan might be less aggressive in seeking services for their children, requiring professionals to be more energetic in both advocating for the child and teaching the family how to pursue such advocacy activities.

Although early intervention is clearly important, cultural factors can mediate against the condition being identified and the treatment begun (Wilder, Dyches, Obiakor, & Algozzine, 2004). In some cultures, there is reluctance to identify the problem or there is limited understanding of behaviors that Western health care providers might identify as being characteristic of a mental disorder. The behavior may carry sufficient stigma so that families are reluctant to bring it to the attention of health care providers (cf., Baker, 2013). In other cultures (e.g., Latino), the presence of a child with a disability is perceived as placing a special obligation on the parents to provide care, resulting in reluctance to seek outside help.

Table 3-2		
Neurodevelopmental Disorders		
Disorder	*Diagnostic Criteria (APA, 2013)*	*Implications for Function*
Intellectual disabilities	Deficits in intellectual functioning, emerging during the developmental period, that include problem solving, planning, abstract reasoning, academic learning, and other intellectual functioning Test scores of two standard deviations below the mean are considered reflective of intellectual disability Deficits in adaptive functioning that limit activities of daily life, social participation and independent living	Deficits in all occupations. Roles may not be affected Habits and routines may be difficult to establish Deficits in cognitive skills and process and communication skills likely; motor skills may or may not be affected Range from mild to severe
Communication disorders	Difficulty in acquiring and using language, including spoken, written, and sign language, with ability are below those expected for age. Accompanying functional limitations Not caused by a hearing impairment, another medical explanation, or intellectual disability	School and social occupations likely to be affected; other performance areas may be unaffected Habits and routines unaffected in most instances Social and communication skills affected Other skills may be unaffected
Speech sound disorder	Difficulty producing sounds, not resulting from medical condition, that limits effective communication Onset is during early development	School and social occupations likely to be affected; other performance areas may be unaffected Habits and routines unaffected in most instances Social and communication skills affected Other skills may be unaffected
		(continued)

TABLE 3-2 (CONTINUED)

NEURODEVELOPMENTAL DISORDERS

DISORDER	DIAGNOSTIC CRITERIA (APA, 2013)	IMPLICATIONS FOR FUNCTION
Childhood-onset fluency disorder (stuttering)	Difficulty with normal language that may include: • Sound or syllable repetition • Broken words • Blocking (audible or silent) • Circumlocutions to avoid difficult words • Physical tension during speech • Other difficulty producing words Begins in early development and causes anxiety and limits participation in social, educational, and vocational activities Not the result of a medical condition	School and social occupations likely to be affected; other performance areas may be unaffected Habits and routines unaffected in most instances Social and communication skills affected Other skills may be unaffected
Social (pragmatic) communication disorder	Difficulty in the social use of communication that causes functional problems, and that may include: • Difficulty with social communication like greeting and sharing information • Difficulty matching communication to the context • Difficulty following conversational rules like turn-taking and acknowledging understanding Onset in early development	School and social occupations likely to be affected; other performance areas may be unaffected Habits and routines unaffected in most instances Social and communication skills affected Other skills may be unaffected
Autism spectrum disorder	Deficits in social interaction and communication including: • Limited social-emotional reciprocity • Inadequate nonverbal communication • Difficulty establishing and understanding relationships	All occupations may show mild to severe deficits May exhibit excessively (but unproductively) patterned behavior Deficits in process skills pronounced, and motor skills likely to be affected Social, communication, sensory skills all likely to be affected

(continued)

TABLE 3-2 (CONTINUED)

NEURODEVELOPMENTAL DISORDERS

DISORDER	DIAGNOSTIC CRITERIA (APA, 2013)	IMPLICATIONS FOR FUNCTION
Autism spectrum disorder (continued)	Restricted, repetitive patterns of behavior that result in dysfunction, and might include: • Stereotyped movement, speech, or use of objects • Inflexible adherence to routines or ritualized patterns of behavior • Distress at small changes or transitions • Restricted interests with abnormal intensity • Unusual response to sensory input Symptoms present in early development, although possibly not be fully apparent until social demands make them obvious	Motor performance may not be goal directed
Attention-deficit/ hyperactivity disorder (ADHD)	Persistent inattention that interferes with development in social, academic, and occupational spheres, with or without hyperactivity Typically includes: • Inattention • Hyperactivity and impulsivity Some symptoms before age 12 and in two or more settings	Affects education, work, and social occupations in particular May also affect play, leisure, and ADL/IADL Habits and routines impaired; roles are not typically affected Motor skills not impaired, process skills affected, manifested by impulsivity and poor control. Communication minimally affected
Specific learning disorder	Six months or more of difficulty learning that interferes with academic performance, and can be seen as: • Inaccurate, slow, or difficulty in word reading and/or understanding what is read • Difficulty with spelling and/or written expression • Difficulty with mathematical reasoning and number concepts	Education is the occupation most affected. Other occupations likely to be unaffected Cognitive and sensory processing skills affected. Other skill areas likely to be unimpaired

(continued)

TABLE 3-2 (CONTINUED)		
NEURODEVELOPMENTAL DISORDERS		
DISORDER	DIAGNOSTIC CRITERIA (APA, 2013)	IMPLICATIONS FOR FUNCTION
Specific learning disorder (continued)	Beginning during school years but may be more apparent as academic demands increase	Habits, patterns roles impaired particularly in expectations of formal educational settings; otherwise probably unimpaired
Motor Disorders		
Developmental coordination disorder	Beginning early in development, acquisition and skill in coordinated motor activity is below what is expected for the individual's age and opportunities to learn motor skills Deficits interfere with function	Most occupations unaffected except insofar as motor skills are required Most skills unaffected except for motor skills Habits, roles, patterns unaffected except those for which motor skills are central
Stereotypic movement disorder	Beginning early in development, repetitive and purposeless motor behavior that interferes with activities and may result in self-injury	Most occupations unaffected except insofar as motor skills are required Most skills unaffected except for motor skills Habits, roles, patterns unaffected except those for which motor skills are central

Tic disorders	*Tourette's disorder*
	  Multiple motor and one or more vocal tics have occurred at some time during the disorder and persist for at least 1 year
	Persistent (Chronic) Motor or Vocal Tic disorder
	  Multiple motor or vocal tics but not both that persist for at least 1 year but do not meet criteria for Tourette's disorder
	Provisional Tic disorder
	  Single or multiple motor and/or vocal tics present for less than 1 year when criteria for other tic disorders are not met
	
	All tic disorders have onset before age 18
		Most occupations unaffected except insofar as motor skills are required
		
		Social occupations may be affected
		
		Most skills unaffected except for motor skills
		
		Habits, roles, patterns unaffected except those for which motor skills are central

Lifespan Considerations

As has been described throughout the previous sections, many neurodevelopmental disorders are stable across the lifespan. This fact, plus the reality that medical management has improved, means that many more individuals with neurodevelopmental disorders are living into adulthood and into later life (Sinai, Bohnen, & Strydom, 2012; Torr & Davis, 2007). For individuals with intellectual disability, there are growing numbers of opportunities for independent or semi-independent living in group homes, as well as vocational opportunities—especially for those with mild to moderate intellectual limitations. For example, one grocery store chain in a large urban area has a policy of hiring young adults with intellectual disabilities as baggers. Other businesses are, likewise, finding it worthwhile to hire such individuals. Nevertheless, families are concerned as their children with intellectual disabilities "age out" of the services that are provided to children (Dyke, Bourke, Llewellyn, & Leonard, 2013); thus, the parents confront the probability that their children will survive them and that they will need to identify other support options.

Individuals with trisomy 21 are likely to develop early-onset Alzheimer's disease (Sokol, Maloney, Long, Ray, & Lahiri, 2011). Although the reasons for this are poorly understood, researchers are exploring the possible molecular and genetic commonalities. For these individuals, a long period of relative stability of function may deteriorate quickly with the onset of symptomatic Alzheimer's disease.

In comparison, the outlook is different for children with communication disorders. Although some language disorders continue throughout life, many children improve, particularly those who receive treatment. These disorders are more persistent in individuals with receptive language disorder, with implications for decreased vocational and social functioning (Clegg, Hollis, Mawhood, & Rutter, 2005).

Individuals with level 2 and level 3 autism show continued signs of the disorder throughout life. As is true for individuals with intellectual disabilities, families tend to be the primary caregivers and coordinators of services. As such children reach age 21—the point at which children's services typically end—concerns about living arrangements, financial support, and vocational activities become pronounced.

There are an increasing number of services for adults with autism, including group homes and sheltered employment (Autism Speaks, 2013). However, too often, these services require the financial resources that many families simply do not have.

Adults with autism, again depending on the severity of the condition, can participate in daily activities, including work and leisure occupations (Haertl, Callahan, Markovics, & Sheppard, 2013). For example, one young man was able to complete a college degree in accounting. He obtained a job with the Internal Revenue Service and married a young woman who also had an autism spectrum disorder. Although their relationship appeared to others to be a bit distant, both expressed great satisfaction with their lives.

Unlike intellectual disability (particularly when it is moderate to severe) or autism spectrum disorder (again, when it is moderate to severe), the impact of ADHD can be somewhat less pervasive. However, when ADHD is severe, does not respond well to medication and other interventions, and persists into adolescence, it can affect function into adulthood (Burke, 2013). Adults with ADHD may struggle in work settings, although they may manage other spheres of life more effectively (Hirshman, 2013).

The other disorders described in this chapter, including specific learning disorder and tic disorders, have variable courses that may or may not affect adult functioning. Certainly, it is important to continue treatment across the lifespan to evaluate function and to address the limitations of adults who may have continuing challenges as a result of a neurodevelopmental disorder.

CASE STUDY

Ethan Langston is a 17-year-old boy living in an affluent suburb of a large East Coast city. His father is a research biologist at a high-profile state university. His mother worked as a teacher until Ethan was 3 years old.

When Ethan was 2 years old, his parents noticed that he had a number of peculiar motor habits; he would sit for long periods of time waving a hand in front of his eyes and was unresponsive to his surroundings. He also rocked forward and backward most of the time when he was seated. His speech was infrequent and somewhat garbled, and he was physically awkward. All of these observations were in marked contrast to Ethan's older brother, who was a very verbal and well-coordinated child.

Dr. and Mrs. Langston were somewhat concerned about Ethan; however, Mrs. Langston's mother often reminded them that children develop differently, and she urged that they have patience. When the Langstons attempted to have Ethan attend preschool, he displayed a whole new set of problem behaviors. He would scream every time Mrs. Langston brought him into the classroom, and his teacher reported that he screamed frequently during the day. He did not interact with the other children and became enraged when they attempted to take a toy he was using, regularly striking the other children. When Ethan was not screaming or focused on a toy, he would rock back and forth for hours. Within a month, the school officials indicated they would not be able to manage his behavior.

The Langstons took Ethan to a neurologist who, following an extensive evaluation, indicated that Ethan had an autism spectrum disorder and referred the family to a child psychiatrist. He recommended that they find a therapeutic program for Ethan to help reduce his problem behaviors and get him ready for school placement.

The psychiatrist referred the family to a local program for children with autism spectrum disorder that offered preschool and elementary school in a therapeutic setting. The family decided against enrolling Ethan, as Mrs. Langston and her mother were convinced that he just needed a bit of special attention and could learn to manage in a regular school. Until Ethan reached the age of 5, Mrs. Langston worked with him every day, implementing an exercise program, reading to him, and creating a low-stress, low-stimulation environment. She sought information about autism and its treatment and began to advocate for Ethan with the local school so that he could be supported in a regular schoolroom, provided he had an aide and an Individualized Education Program.

Ethan's school years were marked by challenges. He acquired reading and math skills slowly and had frequent temper outbursts. His interaction with other children was inappropriate, as he was not able to share toys, he never made eye contact with others, and his verbalizations were repetitive and not always understandable. As a result, the other students generally avoided him. He became obsessed with watching sports on television and would decompensate whenever his favorite team lost, stalking up and down the sidewalk in front of his house shouting and throwing things. As a result, when he was in high school, the neighbors called the police on several occasions.

Now that Ethan is 17 years old and in his last year of high school, his parents are concerned about what comes next.

(continued)

CASE STUDY (CONTINUED)

THOUGHT QUESTIONS

1. What aspects of Ethan's functioning do you think are particularly problematic?
2. Why do you think the family might have insisted that Ethan attend a regular school?
3. What do you think are likely to be the family's current concerns about Ethan's future? What more do you need to know about the family occupations?
4. What additional information would you want to gather to understand Ethan's occupational profile? How might that added information help you to decide on a plan of action?

Internet Resources

American Association on Intellectual and Developmental Disabilities
http://aaidd.org/
A self-help organization for individuals and families, providing a great deal of information and helpful links to other resources.

The Arc
http://www.thearc.org/page.aspx?pid=2444
A self-help organization for individuals with intellectual disabilities and their families. This organization provides numerous publications and links.

Autism Now
http://autismnow.org/
A national self-help organization providing not only information and resources focused on understanding autism, but other developmental disabilities as well.

Autism Speaks
http://www.autismspeaks.org/family-services/resource-library
The resource library at this site is exceptionally well-organized and rich.

Canadian Centre on Substance Abuse
http://www.ccsa.ca
This organization is included here specifically for its resources for addressing fetal alcohol syndrome.

Higashida, Y. (2013). *The reason I jump.* **New York, NY: Random House.**
This book was written by a 13-year-old Japanese boy with severe autism spectrum disorder. It is a clear and moving description of his perceptions about the world and about his condition, and it offers exceptionally valuable insights for therapists, parents, and anyone else who wants to understand the world of autism.

National Center for Learning Disabilities
http://www.ncld.org/
Focused primarily on assisting parents of children with learning disabilities.

References

Abel, K.M., Dalman, C., Svensson, A.C., Susser, E., Dal, H., Idring, S., . . . Magnusson, C. (2013). Deviance in fetal growth and risk of autism spectrum disorder. *American Journal of Psychiatry, 170*(4), 391-398.

Adams, C., Lockton, E., Freed, J., Faile, J., Earl, G., McBean, K., . . . Law, J. (2012). The Social Communication Intervention Project: A randomized controlled trial of the effectiveness of speech and language therapy for school-age children who have pragmatic and social communication problems with or without autism spectrum disorder. *International Journal of Language & Communication Disorders, 47*(3), 233-244.

Adi-Japha, E., Strulovich-Schwartz, O., & Julius, M. (2011). Delayed motor skill acquisition in kindergarten children with language impairment. *Research in Developmental Disabilities, 32*(6), 2963-2971.

Aldred, C., Pollard, C., Phillips, R., & Adams, C. (2001). Multidisciplinary social communication intervention for children with autism and pervasive developmental disorder: The Child's Talk Project. *Educational and Child Psychology, 18*(2), 76-87.

American Academy of Pediatrics Subcommittee on Attention-Deficit/Hyperactivity Disorder, Steering Committee on Quality Improvement and Management. (2011). American Academy of Pediatrics clinical practice guideline: ADHD: Clinical practice guideline for the diagnosis, evaluation, and treatment of attention-deficit/hyperactivity disorder in children and adolescents. *Pediatrics, 128*(5), 1007-1022.

American Occupational Therapy Association. (2014) Occupational therapy practice framework: Domain & process (3rd ed.). *American Journal of Occupational Therapy, 68*(Suppl 1), S1-S48.

American Psychiatric Association. (2000). *Diagnostic and statistical manual of mental disorders* (4th ed., text revision). Washington, DC: Author.

American Psychiatric Association. (APA; 2013). *Diagnostic and statistical manual of mental disorders* (5th ed.). Washington, DC: Author.

Anastopoulos, A.D., Klinger, E.E., & Temple, E.P. (2001). Treating children and adolescents with attention-deficit/hyperactivity disorder. In J.N. Hughes, A.M. LaGreca, & J.C. Close (Eds.), *Handbook of psychological services for children and adolescents* (pp. 245-266). Oxford, England: Oxford University Press.

Anderson, D.K., Maye, M.P., & Lord, C. (2011). Changes in maladaptive behaviors from midchildhood to young adulthood in autism spectrum disorder. *American Journal on Intellectual & Developmental Disabilities, 116*(5), 381-397.

Andriolo, R.G., El Dib, R.P., Ramos, L., Atallah, A.N., & da Silva, E.M.K. (2010). Aerobic exercise training programmes for improving physical and psychosocial health in adults with Down syndrome. The *Cochrane Database of Systematic Reviews*. doi:10.1002/14651858.CD005176.pub4

Asonitou, K., Koutsouki, D., Kourtessis, T., & Charitou, S. (2012). Motor and cognitive performance differences between children with and without developmental coordination disorder (DCD). *Research in Developmental Disabilities, 33*(4), 996-1005.

Autism and Developmental Disabilities Monitoring Network Surveillance Year 2006 Principal Investigators, & Centers for Disease Control and Prevention (CDC). (2009). Prevalence of autism spectrum disorders— Autism and Developmental Disabilities Monitoring Network, United States, 2006. *Morbidity and Mortality Weekly Report Surveillance Summaries, 58*(10), 1-20.

Autism Speaks. (2013). *Adults with autism: What services and programs are available at twenty-two?* Retrieved from http://www.autismspeaks.org/family-services/community-connections/adults-autism-what-services-and-programs-are-available-twenty-two.

Bagatell, N., Mirigliani, G., Patterson, C., Reyes, Y, & Test, L. (2010). Effectiveness of ball chairs on classroom participation in children with autism spectrum disorders. *American Journal of Occupational Therapy, 64*, 895-903.

Bagby, M.S., Dickie, V.A., & Baranek, G.T. (2012). How sensory experiences of children with and without autism affect family occupations. *American Journal of Occupational Therapy, 66*(1), 78-86.

Baker, A. (2013, June 30). Working to combat the stigma of autism. *New York Times*. Retrieved from http://mobile.nytimes.com/2013/07/01/nyregion/in-queens-an-effort-to-combat-autisms-stigma-among-korean-americans.html?tbm=nws&pagewanted=all&.

Barkley, R.A. (2004). Adolescents with attention-deficit/hyperactivity disorder: An overview of empirically based treatments. *Journal of Psychiatric Practice, 10*(1), 39-56.

Barnett, R., Maruff, P., & Vance, A. (2009). Neurocognitive function in attention-deficit-hyperactivity disorder with and without comorbid disruptive behaviour disorders. *Australian & New Zealand Journal of Psychiatry, 43*(8), 722-730.

Barnhart, R.C., Davenport, M.J., Epps, S.B., & Nordquist, V.M. (2003). Developmental coordination disorder. *Physical Therapy, 83*, 722-731.

Bendixen, R.M., Elder, J.H., Donaldson, S., Kairalla, J.A., Valcante, G., & Ferdig, R.E. (2011). Effects of a father-based in-home intervention on perceived stress and family dynamics in parents of children with autism. *American Journal of Occupational Therapy, 65*, 679-687.

Bennett, E., & Heaton, E. (2012). Is talent in autism spectrum disorders associated with a specific cognitive and behavioural phenotype? *Journal of Autism & Developmental Disorders, 42*(12), 2739-2753.

Benson, B.A., & Valenti-Hein, D.C. (2001). Cognitive and social learning treatment. In A. Dosen & K. Day (Eds.), *Treating mental illness and behavior disorders in children and adults with mental retardation* (pp. 101-118). Washington, DC: American Psychiatric Press.

Bernhardt, B., & Major, E. (2005). Speech, language and literacy skills 3 years later: A follow-up study of early phonological and metaphonological intervention. *International Journal of Language & Communication Disorders, 40*(1), 1-27.

Berninger, V.W., & O'Malley May, M. (2011). Evidence-based diagnosis and treatment for specific learning disabilities involving impairments in written and/or oral language. *Journal of Learning Disabilities, 44*(2), 167-183.

Besag, F.M. (2002). Childhood epilepsy in relation to mental handicap and behavioural disorders. *Journal of Child Psychology and Psychiatry, and Allied Disciplines, 43*, 103-131.

Bielecki, J., & Swender, S.L. (2004). The assessment of social functioning in individuals with mental retardation: A review. *Behavior Modification, 28*, 694-708.

Bijou, S.W. (1992). Concepts of mental retardation. *The Psychological Record, 42*, 305-322.

Bishop, S., Gahagan, S., & Lord, C. (2007). Re-examining the core features of autism: A comparison of autism spectrum disorder and fetal alcohol spectrum disorder. *Journal of Child Psychology & Psychiatry, 48*(11), 1111-1121.

Bitter, I., Angyalosi, A., & Czobor, P. (2012). Pharmacological treatment of adult ADHD. *Current Opinion in Psychiatry, 25*(6), 529-534.

Bo, J., & Lee, C. (2013). Motor skill learning in children with developmental coordination disorder. *Research in Developmental Disabilities, 34*(6), 2047-2055.

Bowers, T.G., & Bailey, M.D. (2001). Specific learning disorders: Neuropsychological aspects of psychoeducational remediation. *Innovations in Clinical Practice: A Source Book, 19*, 49-61.

Bradley, J.D.D., & Golden, C.J. (2001). Biological contributions to the presentation and understanding of attention-deficit/hyperactivity disorder: A review. *Child Psychology Review, 21*, 907-929.

Bryant, S., & Battles, C. (2006). When school is home: Looking at a residential placement for children with autism. *Exceptional Parent, 36*(4), 20-23.

Bryson, S.E., Bradley, E.A., Thompson, A., & Wainwright, A. (2008). Prevalence of autism among adolescents with intellectual disabilities. *Canadian Journal of Psychiatry, 53*, 449-451.

Bundy, A.C., Lane, S.J., Fisher, A.G., & Murray, E.A. (2002). *Sensory integration theory and practice* (2nd ed.). Philadelphia, PA: F.A. Davis.

Burke, M.G. (2013). Adolescent ADHD has major negative effect on adult functioning. *Contemporary Pediatrics, 30*(3), 8-10.

Capano, L., Minden, D., Chen, S.X., Schachar, R.J., & Ickowicz, A. (2008). Mathematical learning disorder in school-age children with attention-deficit hyperactivity disorder. *Canadian Journal of Psychiatry, 53*, 392-399.

Capozzi, F., Casini, M.P., Romani, M., Gennaro, L., Nicolais, G., & Solano, L. (2008). Psychiatric comorbidity in learning disorder: Analysis of family variables. *Child Psychiatry and Human Development, 39*, 101-110.

Case-Smith, J., & Arbesman, M. (2008). Evidence-based review of interventions for autism used in or of relevance to occupational therapy. *American Journal of Occupational Therapy, 62*(4), 416-429.

Case-Smith, J., & Kuhaneck, H.M. (2008). Play preferences of typically developing children and children with developmental delays between ages 3 and 7 years. *OTJR: Occupation, Participation and Health, 28*, 19-29.

Case-Smith, J., Richardson, P., Schultz, W., Humphry, R., & Rogers, J. (2005). *Occupational therapy for children* (5th ed.). St. Louis, MO: Mosby.

Chandrasena, A.N., Mukherjee, R.A.S., & Turk, J. (2009). Fetal alcohol spectrum disorders: An overview of interventions for affected individuals. *Child and Adolescent Mental Health, 14*, 162-167.

Chang, M.C., Parham, L.D., Blanche, E.I., Schell, A., Chou, C., Dawson, M., & Clark, F. (2012). Autonomic and behavioral responses of children with autism to auditory stimuli. *American Journal of Occupational Therapy, 66*, 567-576.

Chaplin, R. (2009). Annotation. New research into general psychiatric services for adults with intellectual disability and mental illness. *Journal of Intellectual Disability Research, 53*(Part 3), 189-199.

Cherkasova, M., Sulla, E.M., Dalena, K.L., Pondé, M.P., & Hechtman, L. (2013). Developmental course of attention deficit hyperactivity disorder and its predictors. *Journal of the Canadian Academy of Child & Adolescent Psychiatry, 22*(1), 47-54.

Christensen-Sandfort, R.J., & Whinnery, S.B. (2013). Impact of milieu teaching on communication skills of young children with autism spectrum disorder. *Topics in Early Childhood Special Education, 32(4),* 211-222.

Chu, S. (2003). Attention deficit hyperactivity disorder (ADHD) part one: A review of the literature. *International Journal of Therapy & Rehabilitation, 10(5),* 218-227.

Chu, S., & Reynolds, S. (2007). Occupational therapy for children with attention deficit hyperactivity disorder (ADHD), part 2: A multicentre evaluation of an assessment and treatment package. *British Journal of Occupational Therapy, 70(10),* 439-448.

Clegg, J., Hollis, C., Mawhood, L., & Rutter, M. (2005). Developmental language disorders—a follow-up in later adult life. Cognitive, language and psychosocial outcomes. *Journal of Child Psychology & Psychiatry, 46(2),* 128-149.

Clur, S.A., Oude Rengerink, K., Ottenkamp, J., & Bilardo, C.M. (2011). Cardiac function in trisomy 21 fetuses. *Ultrasound in Obstetrics & Gynecology, 37(2),* 163-171.

Cogo-Moreira, H., Andriolo, R.B., Yazigi, L., Ploubis, G.B. Brandão de vila, C.R., & Mari, J.J. (2012). Music education for improving reading skills in children and adolescents with dyslexia. *Cochrane Database of Systematic Reviews, 8,* CD009133.

Cohen, E.T., Heller, K.W., Alberto, P., & Fredrick, L.D. (2008). Using a three-step decoding strategy with constant time delay to teach word reading to students with mild and moderate mental retardation. *Focus on Autism and Other Developmental Disabilities, 23,* 67-78.

Cornish, K., Turk, J., & Hagerman, R. (2008). The fragile X continuum: New advances and perspectives. *Journal of Intellectual Disability Research, 52,* 469-482.

Courchesne, E., Mouton, P.R., Calhoun, M.E., Semendeferi, K., Ahrens-Barbeau, C., Hallet, M.J., . . . Pierce, K.(2011). Neuron number and size in prefrontal cortex of children with autism. *Journal of the American Medical Association, 306(18),* 2001-2010.

Crabtree, L. (2011, July 4). Autism is lifelong: Community integration of adults on the autism spectrum. *OT Practice,* 8-12.

Darrou, C., Pry, R., Pernon, E., Michelon, C., Aussilloux, C., & Baghdadli, A. (2010). Outcome of young children with autism. *Autism: The International Journal of Research & Practice, 14(6),* 663-677.

DeGrace, B.W. (2004). The everyday occupation of families with children with autism. *American Journal of Occupational Therapy, 56,* 543-550.

Devlin, S., Healy, O., Leader, G., & Hughes, B. (2011). Comparison of behavioral intervention and sensory-integration therapy in the treatment of challenging behavior. *Journal of Autism & Developmental Disorders, 41(10),* 1303-1320.

Didoni, A., Sequi, M., Panei, P., & Bonati, M. (2011). One-year prospective follow-up of pharmacological treatment in children with attention-deficit/hyperactivity disorder. *European Journal of Clinical Pharmacology, 67(10),* 1061-1067.

Dolva, A., Coster, W., & Lilja, M. (2004). Functional performance in children with Down syndrome. *American Journal of Occupational Therapy, 58,* 621-629.

Döpfner, M., & Rothenberger, A. (2007). Behavior therapy in tic-disorders with co-existing ADHD. *European Child & Adolescent Psychiatry, 16*(Suppl. 1) I/89-I/99.

Dosen, A., & Day, K. (2001). Epidemiology, etiology, and presentation of mental illness and behavior disorders in persons with mental retardation. In A. Dosen & K. Day (Eds.), *Treating mental illness and behavior disorders in children and adults with mental retardation* (pp. 3-24). Washington, DC: American Psychiatric Press.

Dreyer, A.S., O'Laughlin, L., Moore, J., & Milam, Z. (2010) Parental adherence to clinical recommendations in ADHD evaluation clinic. *Journal of Clinical Psychology, 66,* 1101-1120.

Drysdale, J., Casey, J., & Porter-Armstrong, A. (2008). Effectiveness of training on the community skills of children with intellectual disabilities. *Scandinavian Journal of Occupational Therapy, 15(4),* 247-255.

Dunn, W., Cox, J., Foster, L., Mische-Lawson, L., & Tanquary, J. (2012). Impact of a contextual intervention on child participation and parent competence among children with autism spectrum disorders: A pretest-posttest repeated-measures design. *American Journal of Occupational Therapy, 55(5),* 520-528.

Dyke, P., Bourke, J., Llewellyn, G., & Leonard, H. (2013). The experiences of mothers of young adults with an intellectual disability transitioning from secondary school to adult life. *Journal of Intellectual & Developmental Disability, 38(2),* 149-162.

Dykens, E.M., & Hodapp, R.M. (2001). Research in mental retardation: Toward an etiologic approach. *Journal of Child Psychology and Psychiatry, and Allied Disciplines, 42,* 49-71.

Eldevik, S., Eikeseth, S., Jahr, E., & Smith, T. (2006). Effects of low-intensity behavioral treatment for children with autism and mental retardation. *Journal of Autism & Developmental Disorders, 36(2),* 211-224.

Embregts, P.J. (2009). Residential treatment following outpatient treatment for children with mild to borderline intellectual disabilities: A study of child and family characteristics. *Research in Developmental Disabilities, 30(5),* 1062-1067.

Emck, C., Bosscher, R.J., van Wieringen, P.C.W., Doreleijers, T., & Beek, P.J. (2012). Psychiatric symptoms in children with gross motor problems. *Adapted Physical Activity Quarterly, 29*(2), 161-178.

Faraone, S.V., & Doyle, A.E. (2001). The nature and heritability of attention-deficit/hyperactivity disorder. *Child and Adolescent Psychiatric Clinics of North America, 10*, 299-316.

Faraone, S.V., Sergeant, J., Gillberg, C., & Biederman, J. (2003). The worldwide prevalence of ADHD: Is it an American condition? *World Psychiatry, 2*(2), 104-113.

Faust, H., & Scior, K. (2008). Mental health problems in young people with intellectual disabilities: The impact on parents. *Journal of Applied Research in Intellectual Disabilities, 5*, 414-424.

Fedewa, A.L., & Erwin, H.E. (2011). Stability balls and students with attention and hyperactivity concerns: Implications for on-task and in-seat behavior. *American Journal of Occupational Therapy, 65*, 393-399.

Ferraro, F.R. (2001). Survey of treatments for childhood autism. *Psychology and Education, 38*(2), 29-41.

Forte, M., Jahoda, A., & Dagnan, D. (2011). An anxious time? Exploring the nature of worries experienced by young people with a mild to moderate intellectual disability as they make the transition to adulthood. *British Journal of Clinical Psychology, 50*(4), 398-411.

Foster, L., Dunn, W., & Lawson, L. (2013). Coaching mothers of children with autism: A qualitative study for occupational therapy practice. *Physical & Occupational Therapy in Pediatrics, 33*(2), 253-263.

Fraine, N., & McDade, R. (2009). Reducing bias in psychometric assessment of culturally and linguistically diverse students from refugee backgrounds in Australian schools: A process approach. *Australian Psychologist, 44*(1), 16-26.

Frank-Briggs, A.I. (2011). Attention deficit hyperactivity disorder (ADHD). *Journal of Pediatric Neurology, 9*(3), 291-298.

Frankenburg, W.K., & Dobbs, J.B. (1967). The Denver developmental screening test. *Journal of Pediatrics, 71*(2), 181-191.

Freeman, R.D., Soltanifar, A., & Baer, S. (2010). Stereotypic movement disorder: Easily missed. *Developmental Medicine & Child Neurology, 52*(8), 733-738.

Freud, A. (1958). Adolescence. *Psychoanalytic Study of Children, 13*, 255-278.

Furniss, F., & Biswas, A.B. (2012). Recent research on aetiology, development and phenomenology of self-injurious behaviour in people with intellectual disabilities: A systematic review and implications for treatment. *Journal of Intellectual Disability Research, 56*(5), 453-475.

Gabriels, R.L., Hill, D.E., Pierce, R.A., Rogers, S.J., & Wehner, B. (2001). Predictors of treatment outcome in young children with autism. *Autism, 5*, 407-429.

Gadow, K.D. (2012). Schizophrenia spectrum and attention-deficit/hyperactivity disorder symptoms in autism spectrum disorder and controls. *Journal of the American Academy of Child & Adolescent Psychiatry, 51*(10), 1076-1084.

Gal, E., Dyck, M.J., & Passmore, A. (2010). Relationships between stereotyped movements and sensory processing disorders in children with and without developmental or sensory disorders. *American Journal of Occupational Therapy, 64*, 453-461.

Geary, D.C. (2011). Consequences, characteristics, and causes of mathematical learning disabilities and persistent low achievement in mathematics. *Journal of Developmental & Behavioral Pediatrics, 32*(3), 250-263.

Georgiades, S., Szatmari, P., Duku, E., Zwaigenbaum, L., Bryson, S., Roberts, W., . . . Pathways in ASD Study Team. (2011). Phenotypic overlap between core diagnostic features and emotional/behavioral problems in preschool children with autism spectrum disorder. *Journal of Autism & Developmental Disorders, 41*(10), 1321-1329.

Giese, T. (2008, September 22). The art of written expression through keyboarding. *OT Practice, 13*(17), 17-21.

Gilger, J.W., & Kaplan, B.J. (2001). Atypical brain development: A conceptual framework for understanding developmental learning disabilities. *Developmental Neuropsychology, 20*, 465-481.

Given, B.K., Wasserman, J.D., Chari, S.A., Beattie, K., & Eden, G.F. (2008). A randomized controlled study of computer-based intervention in middle school struggling readers. *Brain Language, 106*(2), 83-97.

Glass, K., Flory, K., & Hankin, B.L. (2012). Symptoms of ADHD and close friendships in adolescence. *Journal of Attention Disorders, 16*(5), 406-417.

Gold, C., Wigram, T., & Elefant, C. (2006). Music therapy for autistic spectrum disorder. *Cochrane Database of Systematic Reviews, 2*, CD004381.pub2. doi:10.1002/14651858

Gordon, N. (2004). The "medical" investigation of specific learning disorders. *Journal of Pediatric Neurology, 2*(1), 3-8.

Grandin, T., & Panek, R. (2013). *The autistic brain: Thinking across the spectrum*. New York, NY: Houghton Mifflin Harcourt.

Graziano, P.A., McNamara, J.P. Geffken, G.R., & Reid, A.M. (2013). Differentiating co-occurring behavior problems in children with ADHD: Patterns of emotional reactivity and executive functioning. *Journal of Attention Disorders, 17*(3), 249-260.

Grigorenko, E.L. (2001). Developmental dyslexia: An update on genes, brains, and environments. *Journal of Child Psychology and Psychiatry, and Allied Disciplines, 42*, 91-125.

Gutman, S.A., Raphel-Greenfield, E.I., & Rao, A.K. (2012). Effect of a motor-based role-play intervention on the social behaviors of adolescents with high-functioning autism: Multiple-baseline single-subject design. *American Journal of Occupational Therapy, 66*(5), 529-537.

Gutman, S.A., & Szczepanski, M., (2005). Adults with attention deficit hyperactivity disorder: Implications for occupational therapy intervention. *Occupational Therapy in Mental Health, 21*(2), 13-38.

Haertl, K., Callahan, D., Markovics, J., & Sheppard, S.S. (2013). Perspectives of adults living with autism spectrum disorder: Psychosocial and occupational implications. *Occupational Therapy in Mental Health, 29*(1), 27-41.

Hahn-Markowitz, J., Manor, I. & Maeir, A. (2011). Effectiveness of cognitive-functional (cog-fun) intervention with children with attention deficit hyperactivity disorder: A pilot study. *American Journal of Occupational Therapy, 65*, 384-392.

Hällgren, M., & Kottorp, A. (2005). Effects of occupational therapy intervention on activities of daily living and awareness of disability in persons with intellectual disabilities. *Australian Occupational Therapy Journal, 52*(4), 350-359.

Hassiotis, A., Strydom, A., Hall, I., Ali, A., Lawrence-Smith, G., Meltzer, H., . . . Bebbington, P. (2008). Psychiatric morbidity and social functioning among adults with borderline intelligence living in private households. *Journal of Intellectual Disability Research, 52*, 95-106.

Hirshman, J.L. (2013). ADHD in adults. Health homes, integrated care and the future of community psychiatry. Paper presented at: *11th All-Ohio Institute on Community Psychiatry.* March 1-2, 2013. Cleveland, OH.

Hodapp, R.M., Ly, T.M., Fidler, D.J., & Ricci, L.A. (2001). Less stress, more rewarding: Parenting children with Down syndrome. *Parenting Science and Practice, 1*, 317-337.

Hollenstein, T., & Lougheed, J.P. (2013). Beyond storm and stress: Typicality, transactions, timing, and temperament to account for adolescent change. *American Psychologist, 68*(6), 444-454.

Hollo, A. (2012). Language and behavior disorders in school-age children: Comorbidity and communication in the classroom. *Perspectives on School-Based Issues, 13*(4), 111-119.

Hoppestad, B.S. (2013). Current perspective regarding adults with intellectual and developmental disabilities accessing computer technology. *Disability & Rehabilitation: Assistive Technology, 8*(3), 190-194.

Hosain, G.M.M., Berenson, A.B., Tennen, H., Bauer, L.O., & Wu, Z.H. (2012). Attention deficit hyperactivity symptoms and risky sexual behavior in young adult women. *Journal of Women's Health, 21*(4), 463-468.

Hughes, C., Golas, M., Cosgriff, J., Brigham, N., Edwards, C., & Cashen, K. (2011). Effects of a social skills intervention among high school students with intellectual disabilities and autism and their general education peers. *Research & Practice for Persons with Severe Disabilities, 36*(1/2), 46-61.

Humphrey, N. (2008). Including pupils with autistic spectrum disorders in mainstream schools. *Support for Learning, 23*, 41-47.

Humphreys, K., & Lee, S. (2011). Risk taking and sensitivity to punishment in children with ADHD, ODD, ADHD+ODD, and controls. *Journal of Psychopathology & Behavioral Assessment, 33*(3), 299-307.

Jahoda, A., Kemp, J., Riddell, S., & Banks, P. (2007). Feelings about work: A review of the socio-emotional impact of supported employment on people with intellectual disabilities. *Journal of Applied Research in Intellectual Disabilities, 21*, 1-18.

Johnson, N.L., Giarelli, E., Lewis, C., & Rice, C.E. (2013). Genomics and autism spectrum disorder. *Journal of Nursing Scholarship, 45*(1), 69-78.

Jones, K., Daley, D., Hutchings, J., Bywater, T., & Eames, C. (2008). Efficacy of the Incredible Years Programme as an early intervention for children with conduct problems and ADHD: Long-term follow-up. *Child: Care, Health and Development, 34*, 380-390.

Jordan, R. (2001). Multidisciplinary work for children with autism. *Educational and Child Psychology, 18*(2), 5-14.

Jung, S., & Sainato, D.M. (2013). Teaching play skills to young children with autism. *Journal of Intellectual & Developmental Disability, 38*(1), 74-90.

Kåhlin, I., & Haglund, L. (2009). Psychosocial strengths and challenges related to work among persons with intellectual disabilities. *Occupational Therapy in Mental Health, 25*(2), 151-163.

Kaiser, M. (2013). Children with developmental coordination disorder: The effects of combined intervention on motor coordination, occupational performance, and quality of life. *Journal of Occupational Therapy, Schools & Early Intervention, 6*(1), 44-53.

Kalb, L.G., Law, J.K., Landa, R., & Law, P.A. (2010). Onset patterns prior to 36 months in autism spectrum disorders. *Journal of Autism & Developmental Disorders, 40*(11), 1389-1402.

Kaufman, A.S., & Kaufman, N.L. (1983). *Kaufman assessment battery for children.* Circle Pines, MN: American Guidance Service.

Kaufmann, L., & von Aster, M. (2012). The diagnosis and management of dyscalculia. *Deutsches Aerzteblatt International, 109*(45), 767-778.

Keogh, B.K. (2002). Research on reading and reading problems: Findings, limitations, and future directions. In K.G. Butler & E.R. Silliman (Eds.), *Speaking, reading, and writing in children with language learning disabilities: New paradigms in research and practice* (pp. 27-44). Mahwah, NJ: Erlbaum Associates.

Kessler, R.C., Adler, L., Barkley, R., Biederman, J., Conners, C.K., Demler, O., . . . Zavlavsky, A.M. (2006). The prevalence and correlates of adult ADHD in the United States: Results from the National comorbidity survey replication. *Evidence Based Mental Health, 9*(4), 116-121.

Kinnealey, M., Pfeiffer, B., Miller, J., Roan, C., Shoener, R., & Ellner, M.L. (2012). Effect of classroom modification on attention and engagement of students with autism or dyspraxia. *American Journal of Occupational Therapy, 66*, 511-519.

Koenig, K.P., Buckley-Reen, A., & Garg, S. (2012). Efficacy of Get Ready to Learn Yoga program among children with autism spectrum disorders: A pretest-posttest control group design. *American Journal of Occupational Therapy, 66*, 538-546.

Kotler, P.D., & Koenig, K.P. (2012). Authentic partnerships with adults with autism: Shifting the focus to strengths. *OT Practice, 17*(2), 6-9.

Kottorp, A., Bernspång, B., & Fisher, A.G. (2003). Activities of daily living in persons with intellectual disability: Strengths and limitations in specific motor and process skills. *Australian Occupational Therapy Journal, 50*(4), 195-204.

Kozlowski, A.M., Matson, J.L., Sipes, M., Hattier, M.A., & Bamburg, J.W. (2011). The relationship between psychopathology symptom clusters and the presence of comorbid psychopathology in individuals with severe to profound intellectual disability. *Research in Developmental Disabilities, 32*(5), 1610-1604.

Kreuger, L., van Exel, J., & Nieboer, A. (2008). Needs of persons with severe intellectual disabilities: A Q-methodological study of clients with severe behavioural disorders and severe intellectual disabilities. *Journal of Applied Research in Intellectual Disabilities, 21*, 466-476.

Landerl, K., & Moll., K. (2010). Comorbidity of learning disorders: Prevalence and familial transmission. *Journal of Child Psychology and Psychiatry, 51*, 287-294.

Lante, K.A., Walkley, J.W., Gamble, M., & Vassos, M.V. (2011). An initial evaluation of a long-term, sustainable, integrated community-based physical activity program for adults with intellectual disability. *Journal of Intellectual & Developmental Disability, 36*(3), 197-206.

Lench, H.C., Levine, L.J., & Whalen, C.K. (2013). Exasperating or exceptional? Parents' interpretations of their child's ADHD behavior. *Journal of Attention Disorders, 17*(2), 141-151.

Leunissen, C.L., de la Parra, N.M., Tan, I.Y., Rentmeester, T.W., Vader, C.I., Veendrick-Meekes, M.J., & Aldenkamp, A.P. (2011). Antiepileptic drugs with mood stabilizing properties and their relation with psychotropic drug use in institutionalized epilepsy patients with intellectual disability. *Research in Developmental Disabilities, 32*(6), 2660-2668.

Lienemann, T.O., & Reid, R. (2008). Using self-regulated strategy development to improve expository writing with students with attention deficit hyperactivity disorder. *Exceptional Children, 74*, 471-486.

Lifter, K. (2000). Linking assessment to intervention for children with developmental disabilities or at-risk for developmental delay: The Developmental Play Assessment (DPA) instrument. In K. Gitlin-Weiner, A. Sandgrund, & C.E. Schaefer (Eds.), *Play diagnosis and assessment* (2nd ed., pp. 228-261). New York, NY: Wiley.

Lin, Y.J., Lai, M.C., & Gau, S.S. (2012). Youths with ADHD with and without tic disorders: Comorbid psychopathology, executive function and social adjustment. *Research in Developmental Disabilities, 33*(3), 951-963.

Lord, C., Risi, S., DiLavore, P.S., Shulman, C., Thurm, A., & Pickles, A. (2006). Autism from 2 to 9 years of age. *Archives of General Psychiatry, 63*, 694-670.

Lovell, A. (2008). Learning disability against itself: The self-injury/self-harm conundrum. *British Journal of Learning Disabilities, 36*, 109-121.

Ludolph, A.G., Roessner, V., Münchau, A., & Müller-Vahl, K. (2012). Tourette syndrome and other tic disorders in childhood, adolescence and adulthood. *Deutsches Ärzteblatt International, 109*(48), 821-828.

Lyall, K., Pauls, D., Santangelo, S., Spiegelman, D., & Ascherio, A. (2011). Maternal early life factors associated with hormone levels and the risk of having a child with an autism spectrum disorder in the Nurses Health Study II. *Journal of Autism & Developmental Disorders, 41*(5), 618-627.

Lynskey, M.T., & Hall, W. (2001). Attention deficit hyperactivity disorder and substance use disorders: Is there a causal link? *Addiction, 96*, 815-822.

Maglione, M.A., Gans, D., Das, L., Timbie, J., Kasari, C., & Technical Expert Panel, HRSA Autism Intervention Research—Behavioral (AIR-B) Network. (2012). Nonmedical interventions for children with ASD: Recommended guidelines and further research needs. *Pediatrics. 130*(Suppl. 2), S169-S178.

Martens, M.A., Wilson, S.J., & Reutens, D.C. (2008). Research review: Williams syndrome: A critical review of the cognitive, behavioral, and neuroanatomical phenotype. *Journal of Child Psychology and Psychiatry, 49,* 576-608.

Martin, C.S., Romig, C.J., & Kirisci, L. (2000). DSM-IV learning disorders in 10- to 12-year-old boys with and without a parental history of substance use disorders. *Preventive Science, 1,* 107-113.

May-Benson, T.A., & Koomar, J.A. (2010). Systematic review of the research evidence examining the effectiveness of interventions using a sensory integrative approach for children. *American Journal of Occupational Therapy, 64,* 403-414.

McPartland, J.C., Coffman, M., & Pelphrey, K.A. (2011). Recent advances in understanding the neural bases of autism spectrum disorder. *Current Opinion in Pediatrics, 23*(6), 628-632.

Mesibov, G.B., & Shea, V. (2010). The TEACCH program in the era of evidence-based practice. *Journal of Autism and Developmental Disorders, 40,* 570-579.

Mordre, M., Groholt, B., Knudsen, A., Sponheim, E., Mykletun, A., & Myhre, A. (2012). Is long-term prognosis for pervasive developmental disorder not otherwise specified different from prognosis for autistic disorder? Findings from a 30-Year follow-up study. *Journal of Autism & Developmental Disorders, 42*(6), 920-928.

Moretti, P., Peters, S.U., Gaudio, D., Sahoo, T., Hyland, K., Bottiglieri, T., . . . Scaglia, F. (2008). Brief report: Autistic symptoms, developmental regression, mental retardation, epilepsy, and dyskinesias in CNS folate deficiency. *Journal of Autism and Developmental Disorders, 38,* 1170-1177.

Morgan, C.N., Roy, M., Nasr, A., Chance, P., Hand, M., Mlele, T., & Roy, A. 2002). A community survey establishing the prevalence rate of autistic disorder in adults with learning disability. *Psychiatric Bulletin, 26,* 127-130.

Neely-Barnes, S., Marcenko, M., & Weber, L. (2008). Does choice influence quality of life for people with mild intellectual disabilities? *Intellectual and Developmental Disabilities, 46*(1), 12-26.

Newman, B.M., & Newman, P.R. (2003). *Development through life: A psychosocial approach* (8th ed.). Belmont, CA: Wadsworth/Thomson Learning.

Nicholls, R.J., Eadie, P.A., & Reilly, S. (2011). Monolingual versus multilingual acquisition of English morphology: What can we expect at age 3? *International Journal of Language & Communication Disorders, 46*(4), 449-463.

Nippold, M.A., Packman, A., Hammer, C., Scheffner, C., & Finn, P. (2012). Managing stuttering beyond the preschool years. *Language, Speech & Hearing Services in Schools, 43*(3), 338-343.

Nisbett, R.E., Aronson, J., Blair, C., Dickens, W., Flynn, J., Halpern, D.F., & Turkheimer, E. (2012). Intelligence: New findings and theoretical developments. *American Psychologist, 67*(2), 130-159.

O'Connor, K.P., Laverdure, A., Taillon, A., Stip, E., Borgeat, F., & Lavoie, M. (2009). Cognitive behavioral management of Tourette's syndrome and chronic tic disorder in medicated and unmedicated samples. *Behavior Research and Therapy, 47,* 1090-1095.

O'Leary, C., Leonard, H., Bourke, J., D'Antoine, H., Bartu, A., & Bower, C. (2013). Intellectual disability: Population-based estimates of the proportion attributable to maternal alcohol use disorder during pregnancy. *Developmental Medicine & Child Neurology, 55*(3), 271-277.

Parham, L.D., & Fazio, L.S. (2007). *Play in occupational therapy for children* (2nd ed.). Philadelphia, PA: Elsevier.

Patterson, S.Y., Smith, V., & Jelen, M. (2010). Behavioural intervention practices for stereotypic and repetitive behaviour in individuals with autism spectrum disorder: A systematic review. *Developmental Medicine & Child Neurology, 52*(4), 318-327.

Pelham, W.E. (2002). Psychosocial interventions for ADHD. In P.S. Jensen & J.R. Cooper (Eds.), *Attention deficit hyperactivity disorder: State of the science • best practices* (pp. 12-1-12-24). Kingston, NJ: Civic Research Institute.

Pert, C., & Jahoda, A. (2008). Social goals and conflict strategies of individuals with mild to moderate intellectual disabilities who present problems of aggression. *Journal of Intellectual Disability Research, 52*(Part 5), 393-403.

Pfeiffer, B.A., Koenig, K., KInnealey, M., Sheppard, M., & Henderson, L. (2011). Effectiveness of sensory integration interventions in children with autism spectrum disorders: A pilot study. *American Journal of Occupational Therapy, 65,* 76-85.

Pizzamiglio, M.R., Nasti, M., Piccardi, L., Zotti, A., Vitturini, C., Spitoni, G., . . . Morelli, D. (2008). Sensorymotor rehabilitation in Rett syndrome. *Focus on Autism and Other Developmental Disabilities, 23,* 49-62.

Plomin, R. (2001). Genetic factors contributing to learning and language delays and disabilities. *Child and Adolescent Psychiatric Clinics of North America, 10,* 259-277.

Poulsen, A.A., Ziviani, J.M., Cuskelly, M., & Smith, R. (2007). Boys with developmental coordination disorder: Loneliness and team sports participation. *American Journal of Occupational Therapy, 61,* 451-462.

Prasad, V., Brogan, E., Mulvaney, C., Grainge, M., Stanton, W., & Sayal, K. (2013). How effective are drug treatments for children with ADHD at improving on-task behaviour and academic achievement in the school classroom? A systematic review and meta-analysis. *European Child & Adolescent Psychiatry, 22*(4), 203-216.

Pratt, H.D., & Gradanus, D.E. (2007). Intellectual disability (mental retardation) in children and adolescents. *Primary Care, 34*(2), 375-386.

Precin, P., Otto, M., Popalzai, K., & Samuel, M. (2012). The role for occupational therapists in community mobility training for people with autism spectrum disorders. *Occupational Therapy in Mental Health, 28*(2), 129-146.

Ramey, S.L., & Ramey, C.T. (1999). Early experience and early intervention for children "at risk" for developmental delay and mental retardation. *Mental Retardation and Developmental Disabilities Research Reviews, 5*, 1-10.

Reichow, B., Barton, E.E., Boyd, B.A. & Hume, K. (2012). Early intensive behavioral intervention (EIBI) for young children with autism spectrum disorders (ASD). *Cochrane Database of Systematic Reviews, 10*, CD009260.

Reynolds, S., & Lane, S.J. (2009). Sensory overresponsivity and anxiety in children with ADHD. *American Journal of Occupational Therapy, 63*, 433-440.

Richler, J., Luyster, R., Risi, S., Hsu, W., Dawson, G., Bernier, R., . . . Lord, C. (2006). Is there a 'regressive phenotype' of autism spectrum disorder associated with the measles-mumps-rubella vaccine? A CPEA study. *Journal of Autism & Developmental Disorders, 36*(3), 299-316.

Rimrodt, S.L., & Lipkin, P.H. (2011). Learning disabilities and school failure. *Pediatrics in Review, 32*(8), 315-324.

Roberts, J.E., King-Thomas, L., & Boccia, M.L. (2007). Behavioral indexes of the efficacy of sensory integration therapy. *American Journal of Occupational Therapy, 61*(5), 555-562.

Roberts, M.Y., Kaiser, A.P., Oetting, J., & Hadley, P. (2012). Assessing the effects of a parent-implemented language intervention for children with language impairments using empirical benchmarks: A pilot study. *Journal of Speech, Language & Hearing Research, 55*(6), 1655-1670.

Roessner, V., Hoekstra, P., Rothenberger, A. (2011). Tourette's disorder and other tic disorders in DSM-5: A comment. *European Child & Adolescent Psychiatry, 20*(2), 71-74.

Rogers, S. (2001). Diagnosis of autism before the age of 3. *International Review of Research in Mental Retardation, 23*, 1-31.

Roid, G.H. (2003). *Stanford-Binet intelligence scales* (5th ed.). Itasca, IL: Riverside.

Rose, J., Perks, J., Fidan, M., & Hurst, M. (2010). Assessing motivation for work in people with developmental disabilities. *Journal of Intellectual Disabilities, 14*(2), 147-155.

Roulstone, S., Wren, Y., Bakopoulou, I., & Lindsay, G. (2012). Interventions for children with speech, language and communication needs: An exploration of current practice. *Child Language Teaching & Therapy, 28*(3), 325-341.

Rowe, J., Yuen, H.K., & Dure, L.S. (2013). Comprehensive behavioral intervention to improve occupational performance in children with Tourette disorder. *American Journal of Occupational Therapy, 67*, 194-200.

Sachs, D., & Nasser, K. (2009). Facilitating family occupations: Family member perceptions of a specialized environment for children with mental retardation. *American Journal of Occupational Therapy, 63*, 453-462.

Santhanam, B., & Kendler, B. (2012). Nutritional factors in autism: An overview of nutritional factors in the etiology and management of autism. *Integrative Medicine: A Clinician's Journal, 11*(1), 46-49.

Schaaf, R.C., Hunt, J., & Benevides, T. (2012). Occupational therapy using sensory integration to improve participation of a child with autism: A case report. *American Journal of Occupational Therapy, 66*(5), 547-555.

Schalock, R.L. (2011). The evolving understanding of the construct of intellectual disability. *Journal of Intellectual & Developmental Disability, 36*(4), 223-233.

Schendel, D., & Bhasin, T.K. (2008). Birth weight and gestational age characteristics of children with autism, including a comparison with other developmental disabilities. *Pediatrics, 121*, 1155-1164.

Shalev, R., Auerbach, J., Manor, O., & Gross-Tsur, V. (2000). Developmental dyscalculia: Prevalence and prognosis. *European Child & Adolescent Psychiatry, 9*(Suppl. 2), 558-564.

Shane, H.C. (2006). Using visual scene displays to improve communication instruction in persons with autism spectrum disorders. *Perspectives on Augmentative and Alternative Communication, 15*, 7-13.

Shprecher, D., & Kurlan, R. (2009). The management of tics. *Movement Disorders, 24*(1), 15-24.

Shumway, S., Thurm, A., Swedo, S., Deprey, L., Barnett, L., Amaral, D., . . . Ozonoff, S. (2011). Brief report: Symptom onset patterns and functional outcomes in young children with autism spectrum disorders. *Journal of Autism & Developmental Disorders, 41*(12), 1727-1732.

Silva, L.M.T., & Schalock, M. (2012). Sense and self-regulation checklist, a measure of comorbid autism symptoms: Initial psychometric evidence. *American Journal of Occupational Therapy, 66*, 177-186.

Silva, L.M.T., Schalock, M., Ayers, R., Bunse, C., & Budden, S. (2009). Quigong massage treatment for sensory and self-regulation problems in young children with autism: A randomized controlled trial. *American Journal of Occupational Therapy, 63*, 423-432.

Simonoff, E., Jones, C.R.G., Pickles, A., Happé, F., Baird, G., & Charman, T. (2012). Severe mood problems in adolescents with autism spectrum disorder. *Journal of Child Psychology & Psychiatry, 53*(11), 1157-1166.

Sinai, A., Bohnen, I., & Strydom, A. (2012). Older adults with intellectual disability. *Current Opinion in Psychiatry, 25*(5), 359-364.

Smith-Lock, K.M., Leitao, S., Lambert, L., & Nickels, L. (2013). Effective intervention for expressive grammar in children with specific language impairment. *International Journal of Language & Communication Disorders, 48*(3), 265-282.

Smits-Engelsman, B.C., Blank, R., van der Kaay, A.C., Mosterd-van der Meijs, R., Vlugt-van den Brand, E., .. . Wilson, P.H. (2013). Efficacy of interventions to improve motor performance in children with developmental coordination disorder: A combined systematic review and meta-analysis. *Developmental Medicine & Child Neurology, 55*(3), 229-237.

Sokol, D.K., Maloney, B., Long, J.M., Ray, B., & Lahiri, D.K. (2011). Autism, Alzheimer disease, and fragile X: APP, FMRP, and mGluR5 are molecular links. *Neurology, 76*(15), 1344-1352.

Sroufe, L.A. (2012, January 28). Ritalin gone wrong. *New York Times.* Retrieved from http://www.papsyblog.org/2012/02/ritalin-gone-wrong.html.

Steingass, K.J., Chicoine, B., McGuire, D., & Roizen, N.J. (2011). Developmental disabilities grown up: Down syndrome. *Journal of Developmental & Behavioral Pediatrics, 7,* 548-558.

Stoner, R., Chow, M.L., Boyle, M.P., Sunkin, S.M., Mouton, P.R., Roy, S., . . . Courchesne, E. (2014). Patches of disorganization in the neocortex of children with autism. *New England Journal of Medicine, 370,* 1209-1219.

Starr, H.L. (2007). The impact of culture on ADHD. *Contemporary Pediatrics, 2*(12), 38-40, 42, 45-50.

Stetka, B., & Volkmar, F. (2012, July 10). Two major concerns in autism. *Medscape Psychiatry.* Retrieved from http://www.medscape.com/viewarticle/766687_3.

Striano, P., & Belcastro, V. (2013). Treating myoclonic epilepsy in children: State-of-the-art. *Expert Opinion on Pharmacotherapy, 14*(10), 1355-1361.

Sung, M., Fung, D.S.S., & Cai, Y. (2010). Pharmacological management in children and adolescents with pervasive developmental disorder. *Australian and New Zealand Journal of Psychiatry, 44,* 410-428.

Tartaro, A., & Cassell, J. (2006). Using virtual peer technology as an intervention for children with autism. In J. Lazar (Ed.), *Towards universal usability: Designing computer interfaces for diverse user populations* (pp. 231-262). New York, NY: John Wiley & Sons.

Teitt, A., Eastman, M., O'Donnell, S., & Deitz, J. (2010). Skills for life: Promoting social participation in preteens and teens with autism spectrum disorder. *Developmental Disabilities Special Interest Section Quarterly, 33*(3), 1-4.

Tomanik, S.S., Pearson, D.A., Loveland, K.A., Lane, D.M., & Shaw, J.B. (2007). Improving the reliability of autism diagnoses: The utility of adaptive behavior. *Journal of Autism and Developmental Disorders, 37,* 921-928.

Tomchek, S., LaVesser, P., & Watling, R. (2010). The scope of occupational therapy services for individuals with an autism spectrum disorder across the life course. *American Journal of Occupational Therapy, 64*(Suppl.), S125-S136.

Torr, J., & Davis, R. (2007). Ageing and mental health problems in people with intellectual disability. *Current Opinion in Psychiatry, 20*(5), 467-471.

Townsend, J., Westerfield, M., Leaver, E., Makeig, S., Jung, T., Pierce, K., . . . Courchesne, E. (2001). Event-related brain response abnormalities in autism: Evidence for impaired cerebello-frontal spatial attention networks. *Cognitive Brain Research, 11,* 127-145.

Tsiouris, J., Kim, S., Brown, W., Pettinger, J., & Cohen, I. (2013). Prevalence of psychotropic drug use in adults with intellectual disability: Positive and negative findings from a large scale study. *Journal of Autism & Developmental Disorders, 43*(3), 719-731.

Tsuda, E. (2006). Japanese culture and the philosophy of self-advocacy: The importance of interdependence in community living. *British Journal of Learning Disabilities, 34,* 151-156.

Unwin, G.L., & Deb, S. (2011). Efficacy of atypical antipsychotic medication in the management of behaviour problems in children with intellectual disabilities and borderline intelligence: A systematic review. *Research in Developmental Disabilities, 32*(6), 2121-2133.

U.S. Department of Education (2004). *Building the Legacy: IDEA 2004.* Retrieved from http://idea.ed.gov/.

van der Schuit, M., Peeters, M., Segers, E., van Balkom, H., & Verhoeven, L. (2009). Home literacy environment of pre-school children with intellectual disabilities. *Journal of Intellectual Disability Research, 53*(Part 12), 1024-1037.

van Steijn, D.J., Richards, J.S., Oerlemans, A.M., de Ruiter, S.W., van Aken, M.A.G., Franke, B., . . . Nanda, N.J. (2012). The co-occurrence of autism spectrum disorder and attention-deficit/hyperactivity disorder symptoms in parents of children with ASD or ASD with ADHD. *Journal of Child Psychology & Psychiatry, 53*(9), 954-963.

Vedi, K., & Bernard, S. (2012). The mental health needs of children and adolescents with learning disabilities. *Current Opinion in Psychiatry, 25*(5), 353-358.

Verdonschot, M.M.L., de Witte, L.P., Reichrath, E., Buntinx, W.H.E., & Curfs, L.M.G. (2009). Community participation of people with an intellectual disability: A review of empirical findings. *Journal of Intellectual Disability Research*, *53*(Part 4), 303-318.

Vilardo, B.A., DuPaul, G, Kern, L., & Hojnoski, R.L. (2013). Cross-age peer coaching: Enhancing the peer interactions of children exhibiting symptoms of ADHD. *Child & Family Behavior Therapy*, *35*(1), 63-81.

Vorstman, J.A., & Ophoff, R.A. (2013). Genetic causes of developmental disorders. *Current Opinion in Neurology, 26*(2), 128-136.

Wagner, M.O., Bös, K., Jascenoka, J., Jekauc, D., & Peterman, F. (2012). Peer problems mediate the relationship between developmental coordination disorder and behavioral problems in school-aged children. *Research in Developmental Disabilities, 33*(6), 2072-2079.

Waite, A. (2013). Workin' on it: Helping adults with autism ease into the work world. *OT Practice, 18*(2), 9-13.

Walker, J.C., Dosen, A., Buitelaar, J.K., & Janzing, J.G.E. (2011). Depression in Down syndrome: A review of the literature. *Research in Developmental Disabilities, 32*, 1432-1440.

Walton, K., & Ingersoll, B. (2013). Improving social skills in adolescents and adults with autism and severe to profound intellectual disability: A review of the literature. *Journal of Autism & Developmental Disorders, 43*(3), 594-615.

Warnke, A. (1999). Reading and spelling disorders: Clinical features and causes. *European Child & Adolescent Psychiatry, 8*(Suppl. 3), III/2-III/12.

Wechsler, D. (2004). *The Wechsler intelligence scale for children* (4th ed.). London, England: Pearson Assessment.

Weindrich, D., Jennen-Steinmetz, C., Laucht, M., Esser, G., & Schmidt, M.H. (2000). Epidemiology and prognosis of specific disorders of language and scholastic skills. *European Child & Adolescent Psychiatry, 9*(3), 186-194.

Weininger, O. (1993). Attachment, affective contact, and autism. *Psychoanalytic Inquiry, 13*, 49-62.

West, L., & Waldrop, J. (2006). Risperidone use in the treatment of behavioral symptoms in children with autism. *Pediatric Nursing, 32*(6), 545-551.

White, J., & Buehler, C. (2012). Adolescent sexual victimization, ADHD symptoms, and risky sexual behavior. *Journal of Family Violence, 27*(2), 123-132.

White, S., Bray, B., & Ollendick, T. (2012). Examining shared and unique aspects of social anxiety disorder and autism spectrum disorder using factor analysis. *Journal of Autism & Developmental Disorders, 42*(5), 874-884.

White, S.W., Ollendick, T., Scahill, L., Oswald, D., & Albano, A.M. (2009). Preliminary efficacy of a cognitive-behavioral treatment program for anxious youth with autism spectrum disorders. *Journal of Autism & Developmental Disorders, 39*(12), 1652-1662.

Wilder, L.K., Dyches, T.T., Obiakor, F.E., & Algozzine, B. (2004). Focus on autism and other developmental disabilities. *Journal of Autism and Developmental Disorders, 19*, 105-113.

Wilson, P.H., Ruddock, S., Smits-Engelsman, B., Polatajko, H., & Blank, R. (2013). Understanding performance deficits in developmental coordination disorder: A meta-analysis of recent research. *Developmental Medicine & Child Neurology, 55*(3), 217-228.

Wolgemuth, J.R., Cobb, R.B., & Alwell, M. (2008). The effects of mnemonic interventions on academic outcomes for youth with disabilities: A systematic review. *Learning Disabilities Research and Practice, 23*, 1-10.

Wuang, Y., Wang, C., Huang, M., & Su, C. (2009). Prospective study of the effect of sensory integration, neurodevelopmental treatment, and perceptual-motor therapy on the sensorimotor performance in children with mild mental retardation. *American Journal of Occupational Therapy, 63*, 441-452.

Wuang, Y.P., Ho, G.S., & Su, C.Y. (2013). Occupational therapy home program for children with intellectual disabilities: A randomized, controlled trial. *Research in Developmental Disabilities, 34*(1), 528-537.

Zwicker, J.G., Yoon, S.W., Mackay, M., Petrie-Thomas, J., Rogers, M., & Synnes, A.R. (2013). Perinatal and neonatal predictors of developmental coordination disorder in very low birthweight children. *Archives of Disease in Childhood, 98*(2), 118-122.

Schizophrenia Spectrum and Other Psychotic Disorders

Learning Outcomes

By the end of this chapter, readers will be able to:

- Describe the symptoms of schizophrenia and other psychotic disorders
- Differentiate among various psychotic disorders
- Identify the causes of the psychotic disorders
- Discuss the prevalence of psychotic disorders
- Describe treatment strategies for psychotic disorders
- Discuss the occupational perspective of psychotic disorders, including specific intervention considerations

Bonder B.
Psychopathology and Function, Fifth Edition (pp 93-117).
© 2015 SLACK Incorporated.

KEY WORDS

- Positive symptoms
- Hallucinations
- Delusions
- Negative symptoms
- Flat affect
- Anhedonia
- Avolition
- Prodromal

- Residual
- Loose association
- Waxy rigidity
- Tardive dyskinesia
- Catatonia ·
- Catalepsy
- Echolalia
- Echopraxia

CASE VIGNETTE

Dr. Enid Mitchell is a 43-year-old pharmacist who has come to a local community mental health center where she is well known. She has been unemployed for the past 3 years and lives with her mother. During this time, she has been repeatedly hospitalized for fatigue, feelings of extreme anger, and difficulty experiencing emotion. Although she indicates she does not feel depressed or euphoric and does not have hallucinations or delusions, she tells the therapists she feels strongly that people are out to get her, and she demonstrates considerable difficulty concentrating to respond to the therapist's questions. She alternately expresses guilt about various aspects of her life and expresses accusations that others are interfering with her ability to succeed. She is in constant motion during the conversation with the therapist and repeatedly indicates she needs to get back to her "projects."

Dr. Mitchell's most recent hospitalization occurred when she was picked up by the police. She had been found standing outside a neighbor's house in a snow storm—dressed only in pajamas—screaming that "they" were poisoning her. She told the police, on the way to the psychiatric emergency department, that she had not been able to sleep for days and felt unable to stop moving. She indicated that she was in the midst of several important projects in her home, and that she needed to get back right away to start several more.

During her hospitalization, she received several medications that seemed to help her become calmer. She was seen by an occupational therapist, who tried to help her manage her behavior so she could go back to work; however, these efforts were unsuccessful.

THOUGHT QUESTIONS

1. Do you believe that Dr. Mitchell has a mental disorder?
2. If so, what behaviors, thoughts, or other symptoms do you identify that suggest this view?
3. Of the symptoms you identified, which might cause Dr. Mitchell problems in her work as a pharmacist?

SCHIZOPHRENIA SPECTRUM AND OTHER PSYCHOTIC DISORDERS

- Schizotypal (personality) disorder
- Delusional disorder
- Brief psychotic disorder
- Schizophreniform disorder
- Schizophrenia

- Schizoaffective disorder
- Substance or medication-induced psychotic disorder
- Catatonia

Psychotic disorders are among the most disabling psychiatric conditions. Of the psychotic disorders, schizophrenia is the best known, serving as the prototypical mental illness in various media representations. These media portrayals tend to be somewhat misleading, and often cast the individual with schizophrenia as a violent criminal. Although psychotic disorders are, in fact, associated with rates of violence somewhat higher than of the general population, much of this increase is attributable to higher rates of comorbid substance abuse (Fazel, Gulati, Linsell, Geddes, & Grann, 2009). This finding suggests that it is essential to distinguish between the symptoms of psychosis and the symptoms of substance abuse and to treat each appropriately.

The fifth edition of the *Diagnostic and Statistical Manual of Mental Disorders* (DSM-5; American Psychiatric Association [APA], 2013) identifies the characteristics that must be present for the diagnosis to be made, including a minimum duration and a specific constellation of symptoms that must include at least some **positive symptoms** of psychosis: **hallucinations** (i.e., distorted sensory experiences, such as hearing voices that are not evident to others), **delusions** (i.e., firmly held, fixed beliefs that are not held by others, such as a belief that one is being pursued by the Federal Bureau of Investigation, when it is inconsistent with reality), disorganized thinking; or some combination of these. Note that the term *positive* refers to the fact that a symptom is present and does not imply that it is good. In fact, hallucinations and delusions are typically quite frightening. One young man noted that when he looked into the mirror, he saw his own face with fire burning in his eye sockets (Figure 4-1).

Schizophrenia also includes **negative symptoms,** such as **flat affect** (lack of emotional expression and response) and **anhedonia** (lack of experience of pleasure). These negative symptoms, which reflect the absence of expected emotion and behavior, can persist long after positive symptoms, delusions, or hallucinations have been reduced. These symptoms have a major impact on function over the long term.

There are a number of significant changes in the most recent diagnostic criteria, compared with previous editions of the DSM (APA, 2013; Tandon, 2013). Among these changes is a stronger requirement for the presence of positive symptoms and a dimensional diagnostic system that permits rating each of eight symptoms on a scale of severity from 1 (least severe) to 4 (most severe). Perhaps the most significant change is the deletion of subcategories of schizophrenia, such as paranoid type, disorganized type, and undifferentiated schizophrenia. The only subcategory that remains is catatonia, which is now described as a symptom, rather than a separate form of schizophrenia. Catatonia will be described in detail in this chapter.

As you review the diagnoses in this group, keep in mind that personality disorders are listed in two areas of this book. Each disorder is mentioned in the chapter describing the spectrum that most closely parallels the symptoms (i.e., schizotypal personality disorder is listed among the psychotic disorders in this chapter). The disorders also appear in a separate

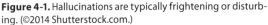

Figure 4-1. Hallucinations are typically frightening or disturbing. (©2014 Shutterstock.com.)

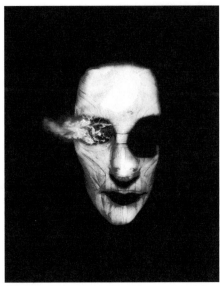

chapter that includes all the personality disorders, and they will be discussed in detail in that chapter; therefore, details about schizotypal disorder will be also provided in Chapter 19. Prevalence of the various psychotic disorders is shown in Table 4-1.

Remember also that each diagnostic cluster offers an opportunity to diagnose the condition with labels such as "other" or "due to a medical condition." These labels allow the clinician to make it clear that the client's symptoms do not fully conform to those required for a more definitive diagnosis. They also allow the clinician to identify conditions that are the result of a medical illness. For example, schizophrenia-like symptoms may be seen in some individuals with multiple sclerosis (Sarısoy, Terzi, Gümüş & Pazvantoğlu, 2013), traumatic brain injury (Schwarzbold et al., 2008), and other medical conditions. In such cases, the diagnosis would be psychotic disorder due to another medical condition (APA, 2013).

Delusional Disorder

The primary feature of delusional disorder is the presence of one or more delusions for at least 1 month (APA, 2013). Other criteria include the absence of all the symptoms required for a diagnosis of schizophrenia; the absence of functional or behavioral peculiarities, except for those related to the delusions; delusions that last longer than any symptoms of depression or mania; and symptoms that cannot be attributed to substance abuse or a medical condition. The delusions may encompass any content, with the most prominent being the following:

- Erotomanic, in which the individual believes that he or she is loved by someone else, usually a prominent figure whom the individual does not actually know
- Grandiose, in which the individual believes he or she has some special, great characteristic
- Jealous, in which the individual is convinced that a spouse or lover is unfaithful
- Somatic, in which the individual believes that he or she has some gross physical problem
- Persecutory, in which the individual believes that he or she is being conspired against (this is the most common)

TABLE 4-1			
PREVALENCE OF SCHIZOPHRENIA SPECTRUM AND OTHER PSYCHOTIC DISORDERS			
DIAGNOSIS	*PREVALENCE*	*GENDER RATIO (M:F)*	*SOURCE*
Delusional disorder	0.02%	1:1	APA, 2013
Brief psychotic disorder	9% (first-onset psychosis)	1:1	APA, 2013
Schizophreniform disorder	0.03% to 0.07%	1:1	APA, 2013
Schizophrenia	4% (lifetime)	1:1	Saha, Chant, Welham, & McGrath, 2005
Schizoaffective disorder	0.03%	Slightly more prevalent in women	APA, 2013
Catatonia	35% of those with schizophrenia have this symptom		APA, 2013

The disorder most often occurs in middle or later life, and it is more common in first-generation immigrants, although it is not clear why this might be the case. One possibility is that individuals with hearing impairment or whose English is not good may misunderstand what is occurring around them, which may cause them to believe they are being persecuted. In addition, neurocognitive changes have been identified in individuals with delusional disorder (Abdel-Hamid & Brüne, 2008).

The course of delusional disorder is variable, although it is most often chronic, with exacerbations and remissions. Impairment of vocational, avocational, and self-care occupations is rare, whereas social impairment is frequent and often severe. Client outcome appears best when somatic delusions are most evident and worse in cases of which erotomanic or paranoid content is prevalent (Bourgeois, Khan, & Hilty, 2013). Treatment includes antipsychotic medications, which appear to have limited benefits, psychotherapy, and cognitive behavioral therapy.

As indicated in the diagnostic criteria, function is—on the whole—unimpaired, except as related to the delusion. It is important to distinguish delusional disorder from obsessive-compulsive disorders, delirium, schizophrenia, and mood disorders. It is also important for the clinician to understand the cultural and religious beliefs (e.g., belief in possession by spirits) that could be misconstrued as delusional.

The next two disorders to be described are psychotic disorders, which are similar to schizophrenia, but of shorter duration. These are brief psychotic disorders, a label that is used for a psychosis of 1 month or less, and schizophreniform disorder, a duration of which is 1 to 6 months. The descriptions of these disorders are provided herein. Because the implications for function, treatment, and occupational therapy are similar, the two disorders are presented together.

Brief Psychotic Disorder

The diagnostic criteria for brief psychotic disorder include one or more of the symptoms associated with psychosis (APA, 2013): delusions, hallucinations, disorganized speech, or disorganized behavior lasting more than 1 day but less than 1 month. The disorder is diagnosed only if it is not associated with a medical condition. The criteria allow for specification about the presence or absence of stressors, as well as whether onset is postpartum.

The brief psychotic disorder most often emerges in adolescence or early adulthood and may be a precursor to a more chronic psychotic disorder. It must be differentiated from other medical conditions, substance abuse-related disorders, mood disorders, other psychotic disorders, and personality disorders.

Etiology

A number of theories exist about the etiology of brief psychotic disorder. All of the possible causes of schizophrenia described herein may apply (remember, brief psychotic disorder is often a precursor of schizophrenia). In addition, inflammation has been implicated (Suvisaari & Mantere, 2013). In some instances, brief psychotic disorder is directly related to substance abuse (Shah, Vu, Thomas, Hartman, & Sharma, 2013).

Prognosis

The prognosis for brief psychotic disorder is variable (Correll et al., 2008). It is a precursor to full schizophrenia in approximately 9% of all cases of schizophrenia. However, in other cases, the disorder remits completely within the 1 month time frame that characterizes the diagnosis. If the psychosis is a result of substance use, removing the substance often resolves the psychotic symptoms.

Schizophreniform Disorder

Schizophreniform disorder includes the same symptoms as schizophrenia, but with a shorter duration—between 1 and 6 months—at which point, a diagnosis of schizophrenia would be appropriate. Thus, the main distinction of schizophreniform disorder is duration, and an individual with a diagnosis of schizophreniform disorder might improve, or might, at the end of 6 months, have the schizophreniform disorder diagnosis changed to schizophrenia.

The etiology of schizophreniform disorder is thought to be the same as for brief psychotic disorder and schizophrenia, and the prognosis outcome ranges from a probable recovery if the symptoms remain confined to those comparable with brief psychotic disorder and a more dire outcome if symptoms progress to schizophrenia.

Implications for Function and Treatment

During the period in which psychotic symptoms are present, function is severely impaired, just as it is in schizophrenia (Carrión et al., 2011; Zanelli et al., 2010). Cognition is particularly impaired, with resultant deterioration of social and vocational roles.

Treatment is typically pharmacological in nature, using some of the many antipsychotic medications, such as chlorpromazine, that are now available (Ehlis et al., 2005). Although the most recently developed antipsychotic medications are more effective than previous generations and less likely to cause severe side effects, significant challenges still exist in taking these medications (Stetka & Correll, 2014). Because of the potential side effects of antipsychotic medications and the fundamental symptoms of the various psychotic disorders, maintaining effective medication strategies can be difficult (Berger et al., 2012). See Chapter 21 for details about antipsychotic medications.

Implications for Occupational Therapy

Occupational therapy has several important roles in the management of brief psychotic disorder and schizophreniform disorder. The occupational therapist may be called on to monitor the effectiveness of medications as they are introduced. Therapy can focus on minimizing the damage to occupational status that results from a period of severe disorder. However, as demonstrated in the case of Dr. Mitchell in this chapter's vignette, therapy efforts are not always successful.

On the other hand, occupational therapy can make a significant difference in the long-term functional impact of shorter-term psychotic disorders. For example, an interior designer for a large architectural firm became increasingly paranoid and disorganized over a period of 6 weeks. She came to the office looking disheveled, was increasingly unable to complete her work, and was found one day in her office pacing, muttering, and throwing objects. She would not let anyone in the office and screamed, "They're all out to get me." Her supervisor called emergency medical services, and she was taken to a local emergency department. The emergency department admitted the interior designer to a psychiatric unit for observation. During that time, she was placed on an antipsychotic medication and gradually became calmer. Within 1 week, she was able to return home with support from a home health nurse. However, her employer was reluctant to allow her to return to work. The home health nurse asked an occupational therapist for a consultation and, in concert with the client, they mapped a plan for her to reenter the workplace gradually. With the client's permission, her employer was also consulted, and a strategy was designed that involved her returning to work on a part-time basis and being assigned to low-stress projects. Over the next 6 months, the woman made a complete recovery and returned to her premorbid functional status.

Schizophrenia

Schizophrenia is diagnosed on the basis of presence of two or more of the major signs of psychosis for a significant portion of at least 1 month (APA, 2013). At least one symptom must include delusions, hallucinations, or disorganized speech. The second may be another one of the three symptoms, disorganized or catatonic behavior, or negative symptoms such as diminished emotional expression or **avolition** (i.e., the absence of motivation and energy).

Unlike the psychotic disorders described earlier in this chapter, schizophrenia is explicitly associated with dysfunction in at least one major functional area (e.g., work, interpersonal relationships, or self-care). In children, this dysfunction is marked by failure to acquire the function at all. Later in life, it is marked by deterioration in function. Although delusional disorder, brief psychotic disorder and schizophreniform disorder all often lead to functional deficits, the presence of these disorders are not specific diagnostic criteria as they are for schizophrenia.

Signs of disturbance must persist for at least 6 months, although symptoms may be less pronounced in **prodromal** periods, those that lead up to major psychosis, or **residual** periods, which is the time when psychotic symptoms lessen after a major episode. Specifiers allow for indication of whether it is a first episode or one of multiple episodes, whether it is in partial or full remission, or whether it is continuous. The condition must be distinguished from mood disorders, other psychotic disorders, obsessive–compulsive disorder, posttraumatic stress disorder, and autism. Relatively high comorbidity exists with substance-related disorders and anxiety disorders.

Schizophrenia is most notably a disorder of thought and perception. Delusions occur frequently in schizophrenia, the most common being delusions of persecution, fear that one is being followed or will be harmed by others; delusions of reference, the belief that one is being talked about by others; or delusions of grandeur (i.e., the belief that one possesses special powers, abilities, or gifts). Loosening of associations, incoherence, or excessively concrete or abstract thought is also characteristic. Someone with **loose associations**—a thought and conversational style marked by odd departures from the topic—might answer a question about the weather by launching into a discussion of weather patterns in outer space. An excessively concrete response might be that there are two rain drops on the window of a red car outside, whereas an excessively abstract answer might be that weather describes the meaning of life.

Perception and affect are also disturbed. Hallucinations are typical. Auditory hallucinations (i.e., hearing voices) are most common (Moritz & Larøi, 2008), although any sense may be involved. The individual may smell peculiar smells and interpret this as being poisonous gas in the room or he or she may see strange figures when looking at his or her own face in the mirror. Affect is either flat or inappropriate. Some individuals with schizophrenia are totally expressionless, whereas others may have bizarre smiles, laugh inappropriately, and so on.

Peculiar psychomotor behavior may be present. Odd mannerisms, grimacing, hyperactivity, or **waxy rigidity** may be observed. Individuals with waxy rigidity may sit for hours at a time without moving and will retain whatever position they are placed in. For example, if the therapist moves the individual's hand in front of his or her face, the individual will hold it there, motionless.

The sense of self is also impaired. The individual may have difficulty discriminating between self and others or between self and the environment. Age of onset is typically adolescence or early adulthood (Tandon, Keshavan, & Nasrallah, 2008), although there are often precursors (e.g., odd behavior or affect) or even onset in childhood.

Negative symptoms are present in approximately one third of all individuals with schizophrenia (Mäkinen, Miettunen, Isohanni, & Koponen, 2008). These symptoms are particularly problematic with regard to long-term outcomes and function. As a result, quality of life can be severely impacted between active phases of the disorder. Medication is less effective in treating negative symptoms of the disorder.

Schizophrenia can be comorbid with depression, bipolar disorder, a personality disorder, and/or substance abuse. It must be differentiated particularly from bipolar disorder, although there is some commonality of symptoms with many other mental disorders.

Etiology

A variety of theories exist about the emergence of schizophrenia. A family pattern can be demonstrated, even when the individual is not raised by the biological family (DeVylder & Lukens, 2013; Tandon et al., 2008). The risk for first-degree relatives of an individual with schizophrenia is 10 times higher than in the general population, and a child whose parents both have schizophrenia has a 50% risk of developing the disorder (Stetka & Correll, 2014).

This familial pattern has led to considerable research about the possibility of a genetic cause for schizophrenia (Dempster, Vian, Pidsley, & Mill, 2013; Desbonnet, Waddington, & O'Tuathaigh, 2009; Lin & Mitchell, 2008). There now is little doubt that genes contribute to the condition, although the specific gene or genes remain to be identified.

Genes alone are not sufficient to cause the emergence of the disease (Brown, 2012; Demjaha, MacCabe, & Murray, 2012), and not all individuals who are genetically predisposed develop schizophrenia, even identical twins. Some theorists suggest that environmental factors (Prasad et al., 2010), including a variety of psychosocial stressors, such as maladjusted family relationships, contribute as well. This vulnerability model (Harvey, 2001) suggests that multiple factors, both biological and psychosocial, must be present for the disorder to emerge. Stress has been examined as an etiologic factor, and although it seems unlikely that it causes schizophrenia, it appears to be a factor of exacerbations (Bentall & Fernyhough, 2008). Poor parenting and family dysfunction may play a role in the emergence of the disorder in individuals with a predisposition, but poor parenting alone is insufficient to cause schizophrenia (Wan, Abel, & Green, 2008; Wan, Warren, Salmon, & Abel, 2008). However, childhood trauma of various types clearly contributes (Thompson et al., 2009).

Other possible factors being studied include traumatic brain injury as a predisposing factor (Kim, 2008) and the possibility that schizophrenia is a syndrome that reflects accelerated aging (Kirkpatrick, Messias, Harvey, Fernandez-Egea, & Bowie, 2008). A variety of studies have examined the role of biochemical changes, neurological factors, and other physical agents in the emergence of the disorder (Basar & Güntekin, 2008; Geyer & Vollenweider, 2008). Exposure to infection in utero has also been hypothesized as a contributing factor (Brown & Susser, 2002), as has the relationship between schizophrenia and other physical diseases. For example, individuals with comorbid schizophrenia and diabetes show greater cognitive impairment than others (Takayanagi, Cascella, Sawa, & Eaton, 2012), leading to speculation that there are some common etiological features. In summary, it appears that schizophrenia has multiple, probably interacting, causes (Stetka & Correll, 2014).

The diagnosis of schizophrenia is more common in lower socioeconomic groups, but this may be an outcome of the disease, rather than a predisposing factor. Because schizophrenia is marked by functional decline, the individual may have difficulty holding a job and, therefore, experience downward socioeconomic mobility. Poor premorbid functioning, particularly social functioning (Tarbox & Poque-Geile, 2008) and emotional processing (Phillips & Seidman, 2008), characterizes individuals who ultimately develop schizophrenia. Risk of developing schizophrenia is also higher in recent immigrants to the United States (Weiser et al., 2008). However, it is not clear whether this is a consequence of the stresses of immigration or bias or lack of understanding on the part of health care professionals.

The wide range of factors currently being investigated reflects the fact that much remains to be learned about the causes of schizophrenia, in spite of the intense research interest in the disorder.

Prognosis

Schizophrenia has been thought to have a poor prognosis, although review of the literature suggests there is variability (Emsley, Chiliza, & Schoeman, 2008) and some evidence indicates that client outcomes may not be as poor as previously thought (Whitty et al., 2008). Improved medication options may account for some of the outcome differences, although it is possible that methodological issues in studying the prognosis of schizophrenia may have contributed to excessive pessimism. Strong evidence exists that discontinuation of medication is a significant predictor of relapse (Leucht et al., 2012).

Several factors of the specific manifestations of schizophrenia predict better or worse outcomes. Individuals with higher levels of negative symptoms and greater cognitive dysfunction have worse functional outcomes (Versterager et al., 2012). Higher levels of education and brief duration of untreated psychosis also predict better outcomes (Whitty et al., 2008).

The specifics of onset and the course of the disorder affect function and outcomes. Individuals who experience early onset, with significant premorbid symptoms, typically have a more problematic course (Nordt, Müller, Rössler, & Lauber, 2007). For example, a young adult who was isolated and lethargic as a teenager, had few friends, and did poorly in school might later manifest symptoms of schizophrenia, continue to have few friends, and find employment difficult, even during the residual phase. In contrast, an individual who held a job, had a social circle, and who developed schizophrenia in his or her late 20s would be likely to do much better during residual periods.

Suicide occurs in approximately 10% to 13% of individuals with schizophrenia (Skodlar, Tomori, & Parnas, 2008). The subject of suicide and suicide prevention will be covered in more detail in Chapter 6. Schizophrenia is also associated with a higher risk for various other physical ailments, including cardiovascular disease, which leads to high rates of early mortality (Schultz, North, & Shields, 2007).

Implications for Function and Treatment

Schizophrenic symptoms occur in three predictable phases (Yee et al., 2010). The first is a prodromal phase in which function begins to deteriorate. The individual withdraws from friends and family. Work, self-care, and avocational activities suffer. The individual may stop bathing, begin to have trouble relating to people at work or school, and spend most free time staring in a mirror or just sitting.

The active phase is characterized by delusions and hallucinations, thought disorder, and other psychotic symptoms. This phase may occur spontaneously or as a result of stress. The residual phase symptoms often are similar to those of the prodromal phase. During this phase, functional level continues to be below the highest level ever achieved. Most individuals continue to have flat affect, peculiar behavior, and functional difficulties between active phases. They usually have few friends or interests, ignore self-care, and may have problems concentrating well enough to work.

Symptoms of schizophrenia vary from individual to individual, and the specific cluster of symptoms determines how function will be affected. For example, apathy (a negative symptom) is associated with substantial functional deficits as a consequence of the demotivation that defines it (Konstantakopoulos et al., 2011). On the other hand, hallucinations may affect function less, particularly because hallucinations can be more readily managed with medication.

For some individuals, function during the prodromal and residual phases may be minimally affected. This is particularly true where supportive treatment, such as outpatient counseling, is available. Individuals who can identify the environments in which demand and stress are relatively low may do well, and they may maintain or regain reasonable measures of social and self-care function. In addition, if a supportive work environment with low levels of stress and an understanding supervisor can be found, individuals with schizophrenia may be able to hold jobs, particularly during the residual phase (Baksheev, Allott, Jackson, McGorry, & Killackey, 2012). Among the many challenges to vocational recovery is the potential for discrimination; this can pose problems in social interactions during recovery as well (Üçok, Karadayi, Emiroğlu, & Sartorius, 2013).

Occupations are likely to be affected during the acute phases of the disorder. Individuals with active psychotic symptoms are likely to have difficulty with work, social interaction, self-care, and leisure occupations. These deficits are almost certainly a consequence of the limitations in skill areas. Visual processing is typically impaired (Perez, Shafer, & Cadenhead, 2012), as is emotional identification (Tremeau & Antonius, 2012). Communication skills, emotional regulation, and visual–motor perception are affected as well (Szöke et al., 2008). In addition, processing speed and working memory are impaired, with severity of these impairments mirroring the severity of other schizophrenic symptoms (Su, Tsai, Su, Tang, & Tsai, 2011). These deficits are, in turn, associated with body structure/body function issues, including, changes in brain structure and activity (Onitsuka et al., 2006).

This multiplicity of problems at numerous levels of function has significant implications for treatment. Because of the varied impact of the disorder, treatment must be provided through a combination of modalities. Psychotropic medications are clearly effective (Hasan et al., 2012). The older antipsychotic medications, referred to as "typical" or "conventional," are most effective in reducing the positive symptoms of the disorder, possibly minimizing the number of exacerbations and lengthening the intervals between active periods. However, these medications do little to ameliorate the negative symptoms and tend to have problematic side effects. Newer, "atypical" medications have fewer side effects and show promise in treating negative symptoms.

One challenge in implementing drug treatment is poor cooperation with medication schedules (Jónsdóttir et al., 2013). Because of the unpleasant side effects, individuals often decide to stop taking the medications (McCann, Clark, & Lu, 2009). Short-term side effects can include dry mouth, sleepiness, and tremors. Longer term side effects include **tardive dyskinesia**, a permanent condition that damages voluntary movement. Tardive dyskinesia is a serious medication side effect that is described in greater detail in Chapter 21, in addition to other helpful and problematic effects of these medications.

Not only are the side effects unpleasant, it can be struggle for an individual with a psychotic disorder to remember the medication schedules (Glazer & Byerly, 2008). Medication reminders, using technological devices, have had mixed success to date. Thus, although psychopharmacological treatment has shown considerable improvement, it continues to be problematic, particularly over long periods of time (Busch, Lehman, Goldman, & Frank, 2009).

There is growing attention to strategies to tailor medication to the specifics of the subtype of schizophrenia (Farooq, Agid, Foussais, & Remington, 2013). Such approaches recommend identifying biological markers, developing a mechanism for clinical staging, and carefully monitoring responses to treatment to refine the specifics of pharmacological interventions.

A variety of other biological treatments have been attempted, including neurogenesis (Eisch et al., 2008) and transcranial magnetic stimulation (Prikryl & Prikrylova, 2013). However, no sufficient data exist to determine whether these treatments have had an impact.

Cognitive interventions are used frequently, based on the theory that schizophrenia is a cognitive disorder (Demily & Franck, 2008; Sivec & Montesano, 2012). Cognitive training has been shown to have a positive impact (Kurtz, Wexler, Fujimoto, Shagan, & Seltzer, 2008; Maples & Velligan, 2008), although evidence is incomplete about whether this translates into improved function (Kontis, Reeder, Landau, & Wykes, 2013).

Clear evidence exists that biological treatments are most effective when they are combined with psychosocial interventions, especially cognitive–behavioral therapy (Rathod, Phiri, & Kingdon, 2010), environmental and social therapies (Beebe, 2002), and life skills training (Tungpunkom & Nicol, 2008).

Environmental supports in the community can enable individuals to live outside hospital settings in spite of continuing functional deficits (Velligan et al., 2010). These include ongoing therapy, medication, and social support that is provided by community mental health centers. Some individuals with schizophrenia do well in sheltered environments, such as group homes and sheltered workshops. Halfway houses in which individuals can live while reintegrating into the community may ease the transition from inpatient care to the community.

During the active period of the disorder, individuals with schizophrenia often require hospitalization. Although drug treatment is initiated, the individual may also be placed in a therapeutic milieu or in a behavioral program. Brief hospital stays may be beneficial, particularly if community follow-up is available. Cognitive behavioral therapy may be initiated during hospitalization and continued when the client is discharged (Rector & Beck, 2012).

Many types of psychotherapy—individual and group—have been attempted with clients diagnosed with schizophrenia, with varying degrees of success. However, reasonable evidence of success exists to support personal therapy, cognitive behavioral therapy, and cognitive enhancement therapy (Brus, Novakovic, & Friedberg, 2012), but less evidence exists about the value of psychodynamic psychotherapy, although given the limitations of antipsychotic medications, there is reason to consider this intervention. A variety of art and body-based group therapies are cost effective in reducing negative symptoms (Priebe et al., 2013). Behavioral therapy may focus on cognition, including executive function, which has been implicated as a major factor in the cognitive deficits shown by individuals with schizophrenia (Kluwe-Schiavon, Sanvicente-Vieira, Kristensen, & Grassi-Oliveira, 2013).

In addition, family therapy is often used, both to assist the family in dealing with the problem of schizophrenia and to remediate psychosocial stressors related to family interaction (Smerud & Rosenfarb, 2011). Family psychoeducation, in particular, seems to be valuable in this regard.

Physical health is a serious concern in an individual with schizophrenia, in part because of the side effects of long-term use of antipsychotic medications. Weight control can be a problem (Lowe & Lubos, 2008), as can cardiovascular disease. Individuals with schizophrenia tend to be physically inactive, thus they are at higher risk for health problems to occur that accompany lack of exercise (Jerome et al., 2009; Millar, 2008). Close monitoring of physical health is essential (Llorca, 2008). Some researchers explored the impact of complementary strategies, such as acupuncture, for both maintaining physical health and ameliorating the symptoms of psychosis (Samuels, Gropp, Singer, & Oberbaum, 2008).

Perhaps most important, individuals with chronic psychiatric conditions, such as schizophrenia, need to find meaning and purpose in life, but this is no small challenge (Kuperberg, 2008; Pitkänen, Hätönen, Kuosmanen, & Väimäki, 2009; Tali, Rachel, Adiel, & Marc, 2009). As discussed later in this chapter, helping the individual to find such meaning and purpose can be an important contribution of occupational therapy and may explain why body therapies (Priebe et al., 2013) are effective.

Implications for Occupational Therapy

Similar to many other organic mental disorders, schizophrenia affects a broad array of occupations and skills (Lipskaya, Jarus, & Kotler, 2011; Urlic & Lentin, 2010), as well as performance patterns. Not only does the disorder affect function (among other occupations and skills), the medication prescribed for treatment may impair body functions and complicate management. Because of this, occupational therapy intervention must be comprehensive, with particular emphasis on occupational engagement (Bejerholm & Eklund, 2007). Motor and praxis, sensory perceptual, cognitive, and communication and social skills must be assessed, and history and current status of self-care, leisure, and work must be considered.

Occupations may be enhanced through activities and instrumental activities of daily living training (Hamera & Brown, 2000). Vocational assessment and work skills training are also part of the intervention, particularly as individuals prepare for discharge into community settings. Work as an activity is clearly important for an intervention and for an outcome (Bond & Drake, 2008; Liu, Hollis, Warren, & Williamson, 2007; Lysaker, Davis, Bryson, & Bell, 2009). An important strategy for therapists to consider is matching job demands to the skills of the individual (Kopelowicz, Liberman, Wallace, Aguirre, & Mintz, 2006).

Strengths as well as weaknesses should be assessed. There is a tendency to ignore strengths when dealing with someone who has a disorder with a poor prognosis; however, important assets that often exist can be built upon. For example, one client was quite artistic and creative. As his schizophrenia improved, he was able to find work as a greeting card artist for a company noted for somewhat "off the wall" cards.

Another young woman with a long history of psychosis simply decided one day that the other clients on her ward at the state hospital were depressing and that she did not want to be like them anymore. Her recovery was long and arduous, but she eventually returned to school and became an effective psychotherapist. Her case demonstrates, among other things, the importance of motivation as a crucial asset (McCann, 2002).

Motivating clients with schizophrenia is no easy matter, as many not only experience the lethargy that is symptomatic of the disorder but they become quite discouraged. Frequently, careful probing is necessary to uncover the activities that have meaning for the person and the ways in which they can be therapeutic. For the woman described in the last paragraph, school was that activity. She wanted to understand as much as possible about her own condition. Those individuals who have reasonable levels of self-esteem and persistence do better overall (Eklund & Bejerholm, 2007), and there is now evidence that interventions that promote positive recovery attitudes and hope can make a significant difference in outcomes of care (Kukla, Salyers, & Lysaker, 2013).

Remediating an individual's skill deficits through education and behavioral or sensorimotor approaches is vital. The woman described previously had few social skills. She had to learn to make eye contact and to engage in social interaction before she could consider going to school. More global "life skills" training (Mairs & Bradshaw, 2004)—with emphasis on role development (Schindler & Baldwin, 2005)—may have value. Improvements in cognition, functional competence, and real-world behavior have been observed as a result of life skills training (Bowie, McGurk, Mausbach, Patterson, & Harvey, 2012). Occupational therapists should make sure that the individual can function in a variety of settings. Not only must occupations and skills be remediated, but self-esteem must be addressed. Functional deficits often lead to negative self-assessment and poor quality of life (Laliberte-Rudman, Yu, Scott, & Pajouhandeh , 2000).

Clients with schizophrenia have indicated that the meaning of quality of life was based on activity, social interaction, time, disclosure, "being normal," finances, and management of their illness. Managing time (Minato & Zemke, 2004), connecting and belonging, and making choices and maintaining control were themes related to these seven factors. Spirituality is also an important consideration to ensure that the individual finds meaning (Smith & Suto, 2012). Too often, quality of life is overlooked in considering treatment (Laliberte-Rudman et al., 2000).

Work is an important focus of intervention (Cook, 2009; Evans, 2006; Liu et al., 2007). Leisure is also a concern because individuals with schizophrenia may find that unstructured time is hard to manage. One woman, whose only leisure activity was watching television, had frequent exacerbations of her hallucinations as she came to believe that the television was talking directly to her and telling her that she was an evil person.

Differing occupational therapy theories suggest differing occupational therapy interventions. Therapists who subscribe to the cognitive model (Allen, 1985) emphasize identification of a specified cognitive level and intervene by adapting tasks and environment to fit the appropriate level if the client's ability is assessed to be too poor to allow improvement. Those therapists who subscribe to the model of human occupation (Kielhofner, 2002) will instead emphasize both skills and volition, and will attempt to assist the client in enhancing the skills while also identifying meaningful occupations that are reflected in volition. The differences among theories are discussed briefly in Chapter 2 of this text; however, it is beyond the scope of this book to deal with the subject in detail. Therapists should inform themselves about differing theories and the research that supports and refutes each. Although much research remains to be performed to validate specific theories, mounting evidence exists that occupational therapy contributes significantly to positive outcomes in addressing the problems of individuals with schizophrenia (cf., Bejerholm, 2010; Waghorn, Lloyd, & Clune, 2009).

When working with individuals with schizophrenia, occupational therapists may have an important role in educating family and employers as well. Advocacy efforts on behalf of the individual may be vital to the long-term success of the intervention and, over time, may help to change the social attitudes that stigmatize such individuals.

Schizoaffective Disorder

The diagnosis of schizoaffective disorder is made when symptoms of schizophrenia are present, with at least one period of illness during which there is a major episode of depression or mania (see Chapters 5 and 6 for more information about these mood disorders). Delusions or hallucinations must be present for 2 or more weeks, without a major mood episode at some point during the illness, although the mood episodes must be present for the majority of the duration of the illness.

Specifiers are used to clarify whether the mood symptoms are bipolar or depressive, whether there is coexisting catatonia, and/or whether it is a first episode (e.g., acute, in partial remission, or in full remission) or a multiple episode disorder (e.g., acute, in partial remission, or in full remission). The severity of the condition can be rated on a 5-point scale. The disorder must be differentiated from other psychotic disorders, mood disorders, and substance-related disorders. It is frequently comorbid, with substance-related disorders.

Etiology

As is true for many of the psychotic and mood disorders, a strong genetic component is evident as an etiological factor for schizoaffective disorder, although the specific genetic factors are not clear (Coryell, 2008). Among the added risk factors for schizoaffective disorder are loss of a parent—especially as a result of suicide—advanced parental age at birth, urban residence, and preterm birth (Laursen, Munk-Olsen, Nordentoft, & Mortensen, 2007).

Prognosis

The course of schizoaffective disorder is typically of a chronic nature, but the prognosis is better than that of schizophrenia and worse than that of a mood disorder (Horan, Blanchard, Clark, & Green, 2008). Because it has become increasingly clear that psychotic and mood disorders share common etiological features, it has also become clear that they share features relative to course and outcome.

Implications for Function and Treatment

Unlike schizophrenia—for which functional impairment is a diagnostic criterion—in schizoaffective disorder there may or may not be functional deficits. However, as this disorder bridges the psychotic and mood disorders, it is reasonable to expect that at least some functional deficits will be present. In particular, cognitive ability, especially visual–spatial and visual–motor coordination are affected, although not as severely as in schizophrenia (Stip, et al., 2005).

Implications for Occupational Therapy

Occupational therapy assessment should consider the factors that are relevant in both schizophrenia and the mood disorders. The thought disorders that characterize psychosis and the affective impairments that characterize bipolar and depressive disorders may all be manifested in schizoaffective disorder, leading to deficits in self-care, leisure, work, and social occupations.

Not a great deal of research exists in occupational therapy that is specifically focused on intervention for individuals with schizoaffective disorder. However, there have been suggestions that cognitive interventions may be effective (Waltermire, Walton, Steese, Riley, & Robertson, 2010). Reintegration of an individual into the community is an important emphasis for occupational therapists (Kopelowicz, Wallace, & Zarate, 1998). This is a good reminder for occupational therapists that the focus is on functional needs, rather than on the specifics of psychiatric diagnosis. It is the functional manifestations of schizoaffective disorder—or any other mental disorder—that guide the occupational therapist's assessment and intervention.

Substance and Medication-Induced Psychotic Disorders

As indicated in the previous descriptions, substance-related disorders are common comorbid conditions of psychotic disorders. The DSM-5 (APA, 2013) includes a specific category for substance-induced disorders in most of its diagnostic categories. The most common substances associated with psychosis are alcohol, cannabis, phencyclidine and other hallucinogens, inhalants, sedative and hypnotics, and cocaine. Between 7% and 25% of individuals presenting with psychosis have a substance-induced condition.

The severity and persistence of substance-induced psychosis vary considerably. In some instances, psychosis lasts well after the substance has been removed. During acute episodes, function is most often severely affected, although removal of the substance may improve function. Individuals with substance-induced psychosis are frequently seen in emergency departments. Remember, too, that there is a correlation between comorbid substance abuse and psychosis in terms of risk of violence (Berger et al., 2012).

Catatonia

In previous versions of the DSM, catatonia was considered a form of schizophrenia, along with paranoid and disorganized types. However, in the new version, **catatonia** is listed as a symptom that is associated with many other mental disorders, including depression and bipolar disorder. It is included in the DSM-5 (APA, 2013) as a specifier, rather than as a distinct condition, and is characterized by the presence of three or more of the following:

- Stupor (absence of psychomotor activity, failure to interact with the environment)
- **Catalepsy** (passive induction of a posture against gravity, such as an arm held in front of the face for long periods of time)
- Waxy flexibility (resistance to being positioned by the therapist)
- Mutism (absence of verbal response in the absence of aphasia)
- Negativism (opposition or failure to respond to instructions or stimuli)
- Posturing (spontaneous, active maintenance of a posture against gravity)
- Mannerism (odd caricature of normal actions)
- Stereotypy (repetitive, frequent, nongoal-directed movement)
- Agitation
- Grimacing
- **Echolalia** (mimicking others' speech)
- **Echopraxia** (mimicking others' movements)

When these symptoms are present, the major diagnosis—for example, schizophrenia, autism, or other mental disorder—is listed first, with the catatonia included to further define the nature of the disorder. The presence of catatonia negatively impacts function and prognosis. Table 4-2 provides a summary of diagnostic criteria and functional consequences of the psychotic disorders.

	Table 4-2	
Diagnostic Criteria and Functional Impact: Schizophrenia and Other Psychotic Disorders		
Disorder	*Diagnostic Criteria (APA, 2013)*	*Implications for Function*
Delusional disorder	One or more delusions for at least 1 month, without meeting criteria for schizophrenia Minimal functional or behavioral deficits Delusions more pronounced than any symptoms of depression or mania	Minimal impact on function
Brief psychotic disorder	More than a day but less than 1 month of one or more symptoms of psychosis: • Delusions • Hallucinations • Disorganized behavior • Disorganized speech	Deficits in occupations, performance skills, patterns Body systems/body functions likely to be affected at least briefly Most likely impact is on cognition and emotional regulation skills
Schizophreniform disorder	Same symptoms as schizophrenia Duration between 1 and 6 months	Deficits in occupations, performance skills, patterns Body systems/body functions are likely to be affected at least briefly Most likely impact is on cognition and emotional regulation skills
Schizophrenia	Two or more signs of psychosis for a period of at least the majority of 1 month At least one of the following: • Delusions • Hallucinations • Disorganized speech	Deficits in all occupations Habits, routines, and roles are either not established or impaired during exacerbations
		(continued)

TABLE 4-2 (CONTINUED)		
DIAGNOSTIC CRITERIA AND FUNCTIONAL IMPACT: SCHIZOPHRENIA AND OTHER PSYCHOTIC DISORDERS		
DISORDER	DIAGNOSTIC CRITERIA (APA, 2013)	IMPLICATIONS FOR FUNCTION
Schizophrenia (continued)	May also include • Catatonic behavior • Negative symptoms (diminished emotional expression, avolition, low energy) Significant dysfunction	Process skills and communication significantly affected, as are social, emotional regulation, and cognitive skills Motor skills may be intact (or may be affected by medication)
Schizoaffective disorder	Same symptoms as schizophrenia At least one major episode of depression or mania At some point, delusions or hallucinations for two or more weeks without a major mood episode, but mood episodes present much of the time	Similar to schizophrenia with particular deficits in emotional regulation, volition
Catatonia	A specifier rather than a distinct disorder Three or more symptoms, that may include (among others): • Absence of psychomotor activity, failure to interact with environment • Catalepsy • Waxy flexibility • Mutism • Failure to respond to instruction or stimuli • Repetitive non-goal-directed movement • Agitation • Echolalia or echopraxia	Similar to schizophrenia, with particular deficits in motor, cognitive, and emotional regulation skills

Cultural Considerations

The diagnostic criteria for psychotic disorders assume a particular set of cultural values and beliefs, and it is now well established that these values and beliefs are not consistently held across cultures. For example, there are those who firmly believe in spirits and spirit healing (Seeman, 2010). Visions and other sensory experiences that might be considered hallucinations in Western cultures can be part of important religious and life stage events in other cultures (Van Gennep, 2010). For example, in some Latino cultures, religious beliefs affect interpretation of events, and it would be an error to interpret reports that an individual is hearing the voice of God as a pathological delusion (Loue & Sajatovic, 2008).

Culture is defined by the symbols, values, and behaviors it promotes. "Cultural meanings attributed to schizophrenia are very often embedded in conflicts between 'tradition' and modernity, for example, between witchcraft and medicine, between client advocacy groups and psychiatric orthodoxy, or between competing religious groups or sects" (Jenkins & Barrett, 2004, p. 6). The subjective nature of interpretations of experience require that caution be exercised in attributing mental disorder to experiences or beliefs that make sense in the context of the particular individual's culture.

Another cultural consideration relates to the health disparities that are prevalent in the United States. Consistent evidence exists of the overdiagnosis of schizophrenia among African Americans (Barnes, 2008). This overdiagnosis leads to inaccurate and ineffective treatment and to stigma that can affect many aspects of daily life.

Lifespan Considerations

Although individuals with schizophrenia undergo exacerbations and remissions, functional deficits tend to persist (van Os & Kapur, 2009). Many individuals who have been diagnosed with one of the psychotic disorders continue to require treatment and support throughout life. Treatment typically involves antipsychotic medication, as well as a variety of therapeutic and social supports. One challenge of the long-term use of antipsychotic medications is they can lead to significant side effects, which, themselves, increase functional deficits.

The fact that onset of schizophrenia often occurs in adolescence or young adulthood means that individuals may miss important developmental accomplishments in education, work, leisure, and social participation. For example, occupational therapy may be the only discipline to consider and provide sex education for adolescents and young adults with schizophrenia (Penna & Sheehy, 2000). Because individuals often develop schizophrenia at a time when most young people are developing their social and sexual relationships, this occupation may be significantly impaired. Sexual behavior is important to self-esteem and identity. Attention to this and other developmental milestones can greatly enhance quality of life.

Older adults with schizophrenia have typically endured an extended illness, dating back to their early lives. By the time they reach later life, the neurological components of the disorder may be prominent, and the individual may have significantly lowered energy and motivation. In addition, he or she may have significant and permanent deficits that are associated with long-term antipsychotic medication use. Acute episodes of hallucinations and delusions may have diminished, but the individual may have sustained continual negative symptoms. Efforts to build an occupational life that enhances quality of life are central to therapeutic interventions. As is true in many cases where illness causes occupational deficits, the occupational therapist may be the primary clinician focused on the importance of daily occupations to satisfaction with life.

CASE STUDY

Arthur White is a 32-year-old man who was diagnosed with schizophrenia at age 18. Prior to that time, he had been an awkward and asocial child and teenager whose parents described him as "odd." However, he managed to finish high school and begin college. He dropped out of college during his first semester. At the same time, he began to ignore his personal hygiene, avoid people, and mutter to himself. He indicated at that time that he heard voices telling him that he was a new god.

He was treated by a psychiatrist with antipsychotic medications and had a good initial response. He became more interactive and reported that the voices stopped. Nevertheless, he was not able to return to college, and he took a job as a clerk at a video store. Since that time, his work history has been spotty, and he has had at least three exacerbations of his condition. During each of these episodes, he stopped caring for his personal hygiene, began pacing and muttering, and withdrew from any social contact.

Currently, Mr. White lives at home with his parents. However, they are both in their late 70s and are deeply concerned about his future. He has been unable to hold a job for more than a few months at a time, and he frequently stops taking his medication. He is 5 feet 9 inches tall, weighs 260 pounds, and smokes heavily. He has no friends and spends most of his time playing video games.

Mr. White's psychiatrist has long been concerned about his status and referred him for a third time to occupational therapy. After failing to follow up previously, Mr. White decides (with considerable urging from his parents) to make an appointment.

Mr. White and the therapist discuss his daily activities. The therapist—aware that activities have unique meanings both from an individual and a cultural perspective (Asaba, 2008)—explores Mr. White's feelings about his daily activities. The therapist also explores the meanings of his hallucinations, aware that these may provide some insight about his feelings about his disorder and its place in his life (Moore, 2007).

Together, they determine that Mr. White is not uncomfortable with his current situation, but he recognizes that his parents are concerned. He, too, feels some anxiety about what will happen if they can no longer care for him. Mr. White decides that he might like to try some kind of part-time employment as a step toward self-sufficiency, and he and the therapist carefully consider what that might mean in terms of his self-care, occupational patterns, and social interactions. They make a step-by-step plan, including various self-checks that Mr. White can use to assess his own progress, and they arrange for a follow-up appointment in 1 month, at which time he can report on his progress and they can modify the plan.

THOUGHT QUESTIONS

1. Describe Mr. White's positive and negative symptoms.
2. What developmental accomplishments is Mr. White likely to have missed?
3. What might you expect in terms of Mr. White's relationship with his parents? How would this differ from the typical adult child and parents relationship?
4. How might you investigate options with regard to Mr. White's living situation, to help address his parents' concerns?
5. What might be some strategies for addressing Mr. White's occupational profile beyond his interest in work?
6. What other occupations must Mr. White address to become more independent?

Internet Resources

MayoClinic.com

http://www.mayoclinic.com/health/schizophrenia/DS00196

The Mayo Clinic provides an overview of information about schizophrenia and an assortment of links to additional information. Its message is a positive one, which suggests that individuals with schizophrenia can lead productive lives with good quality.

MedlinePlus

http://www.nlm.nih.gov/medlineplus/schi zophrenia.html

The National Library of Medicine provides access to professional literature and the most current research on schizophrenia (and other psychiatric disorders).

National Alliance for Mental Illness (NAMI)

http://www.nami.org/Template.cfm?Section=By_Illness&Template=/TaggedPage/TaggedPageDisplay.cfm&TPLID=54&ContentID=23036

NAMI is a well-known and well-regarded self-help organization for individuals with psychiatric disorders. The website provides a wealth of information for individuals and their families and for health care professionals who want to advocate for their clients.

National Institute of Mental Health

http://www.nimh.nih.gov/health/topics/schizophrenia/index.shtml

This National Institute of Mental Health provides definitions, resources, and links to additional information. This website is helpful for both health care professionals and consumers.

Northeast Ohio Medical University Best Practice in Schizophrenia Treatment (BeST) Center

http://www.neomed.edu/academics/bestcenter

This website provides an array of reports and resources that are focused on evidence-based intervention for the treatment of schizophrenia.

References

Abdel-Hamid, M., & Brüne, M. (2008). Neuropsychological aspects of delusional disorder. *Current Psychiatry Reports, 10,* 229-234.

Allen, C. (1985). *Occupational therapy for psychiatric diseases: Measurement and management of cognitive disorders.* Boston, MA: Little, Brown & Co.

American Psychiatric Association (2013). *Diagnostic and statistical manual of mental disorders* (5th ed.). Washington, DC: Author.

Asaba, E. (2008). Hashi-ire: Where occupation, chopsticks, and mental health intersect. *Journal of Occupational Science, 15*(2), 74-79.

Baksheev, G.N., Allott, K., Jackson, H.J., McGorry, P.D., & Killackey, E. (2012). Predictors of vocational recovery among young people with first-episode psychosis: Findings from a randomized controlled trial. *Psychiatric Rehabilitation Journal, 35,* 421-427.

Barnes, A. (2008). Race and hospital diagnosis of schizophrenia and mood disorders. *Social Work, 53*(1), 77-83.

Basar, E., & Güntekin, B. (2008). A review of brain oscillations in cognitive disorders and the role of neurotransmitters. *Brain Research, 1235,* 172-193.

Beebe, L.H. (2002). Problems in community living identified by people with schizophrenia. *Journal of Psychosocial Nursing and Mental Health Services, 40*(2), 34-38, 52-53.

Bejerholm, U. (2010). Relationships between occupational engagement and status of and satisfaction with sociodemographic factors in a group of people with schizophrenia. *Scandinavian Journal of Occupational Therapy, 17*(3), 244-254.

Bejerholm, U., & Eklund, M. (2007). Occupational engagement in persons with schizophrenia: Relationships to self-related variables, psychopathology, and quality of life. *American Journal of Occupational Therapy, 61*, 21-32.

Bentall, R.P., & Fernyhough, C. (2008). Social predictors of psychotic experiences: Specificity and psychological mechanisms. *Schizophrenia Bulletin, 34*, 1012-1020.

Berger, A., Edelsberg, J., Sanders, K.N., Alvir, J.M.J., Mychaskiw, M.A., & Oster, G. (2012). Medication adherence and utilization in patients with schizophrenia or bipolar disorder receiving aripiprazole, quetiapine, or ziprasidone at hospital discharge: A retrospective cohort study. *BMC Psychiatry, 12*(99). doi:10.1186/1471-244X-12-99

Bond, G.R., & Drake, R.E. (2008). Predictors of competitive employment among patients with schizophrenia. *Current Opinion in Psychiatry, 21*, 362-369.

Bourgeois, J.A., Khan, R.A., & Hilty, D.M. (2013). Delusional disorder. *Medscape.* Retrieved from http://emedicine.medscape.com/article/292991-overview#a11.

Bowie, C.R., McGurk, S.R., Mausbach, B., Patterson, T.L., & Harvey, P.D. (2012). Combined cognitive remediation and functional skills training for schizophrenia: Effects on cognition, functional competence, and real-world behavior. *American Journal of Psychiatry, 169*(7), 710-718.

Brown, A.S. (2012). Epidemiologic studies of exposure to prenatal infection and risk of schizophrenia and autism. *Developmental Neurobiology, 72*(10), 1272-1276.

Brown, A.S., & Susser, E.S. (2002). In utero infection and adult schizophrenia. *Mental Retardation and Developmental Disability Research Reviews, 8*, 51-57.

Brus, M., Novakovic, M., & Friedberg, A., (2012). Psychotherapy for schizophrenia: A review of modalities and their evidence base. *Psychodynamic Psychiatry, 40*(4), 609-616.

Busch, A.B., Lehman, A.F., Goldman, H., & Frank, R.G. (2009). Changes over time and disparities in schizophrenia treatment quality. *Medical Care, 47*, 199-207.

Carrión, R.E., Goldberg, T.E., McLaughlin, D., Auther, A.M., Correll, C.U., & Cornblatt, B.A. (2011). Impact of neurocognition on social and role functioning in individuals at clinical high risk for psychosis. *American Journal of Psychiatry, 168*(8), 806-813.

Cook, S. (2009). Occupational therapy for people with psychotic conditions in community settings: A pilot randomized controlled trial. *Clinical Rehabilitation, 23*, 40-52.

Correll, C.U., Smith, C.W., Auther, A.M., McLaughlin, D., Shah, M., Foley, C., . . . Cornblatt, B.A. (2008). Predictors of remission, schizophrenia, and bipolar disorder in adolescents with brief psychotic disorder or psychotic disorder not otherwise specified considered at very high risk for schizophrenia. *Journal of Child and Adolescent Psychopharmacology, 18*(5), 475-490.

Coryell, W. (2008). Schizoaffective and schizophreniform disorders. In S.H. Fatemi & P.J. Clayton (Eds.), *The medical basis of psychiatry* (3rd ed., pp. 109-123). Totowa, NJ: Humana.

Demily, C., & Franck, N. (2008). Cognitive remediation: A promising tool for the treatment of schizophrenia. *Expert Review of Neurotherapeutics, 8*, 1029-1036.

Demjaha, A., MacCabe, J.H., & Murray, R.M. (2012). How genes and environmental factors determine the different neurodevelopmental trajectories of schizophrenia and bipolar disorder. *Schizophrenia Bulletin, 38*(2), 209-214.

Dempster, E., Vian, A.J., Pidsley, R., & Mill, J. (2013). Epigenetic studies of schizophrenia: Progress, predicaments, and promises for the future. *Schizophrenia Bulletin, 39*(1), 11-16.

Desbonnet, L., Waddington, J.L., & O'Tuathaigh, C.M. (2009). Mutant models for genes associated with schizophrenia. *Biochemical Society Transactions, 37*, 308-312.

DeVylder, J.E., & Lukens, E.P. (2013). Family history of schizophrenia as a risk factor for axis I psychiatric conditions. *Journal of Psychiatric Research, 47*(2), 181-187.

Ehlis, A.Z., Herrmann, J., Ringel, M.J., Jacob, T., Fallgatter, C., & Andreas J. (2005). Beneficial effect of atypical antipsychotics on prefrontal brain function in acute psychotic disorders. *European Archives of Psychiatry and Clinical Neuroscience, 255*(5), 299-307.

Eisch, A.J., Cameron, H.A., Encinas, J.M., Meltzer, L.A., Ming, G.L., & Overstreet-Wadiche, L.S. (2008). Adult neurogenesis, mental health, and mental illness: Hope or hype? *The Journal of Neuroscience, 28*, 11785-11791.

Eklund, M., & Bejerholm, U. (2007). Temperament, character, and self-esteem in relation to occupational performance in individuals with schizophrenia. *OTJR: Occupation, Participation, and Health, 27*, 52-69.

Emsley, R., Chiliza, B., & Schoeman, R. (2008). Predictors of long term outcome in schizophrenia. *Current Opinion in Psychiatry, 21*, 173-177.

Evans, H. (2006). Vocational rehabilitation for people with a diagnosis of schizophrenia: What evidence should be considered by occupational therapists? *Mental Health Occupational Therapy, 11*(1), 11-17.

Farooq, S., Agid, O., Foussias, G., & Remington, G. (2013). Using treatment response to subtype schizophrenia: Proposal for a new paradigm in classification. *Schizophrenia Bulletin, 39*(6), 1169-1172.

Fazel, S., Gulati, G., Linsell, L., Geddes, J.R., & Grann, M. (2009). Schizophrenia and violence: Systematic review and meta-analysis. *PLoS Medicine, 6*(8), e1000120. Retrieved from http://www.plosmedicine.org/article/info%3Adoi%2F10.1371%2Fjournal.pmed.1000120.

Geyer, M.A., & Vollenweider, F.X. (2008). Serotonin research: Contributions to understanding psychosis. *Trends in Pharmacological Sciences, 29*, 445-453.

Glazer, W.M., & Byerly, M.J. (2008). Tactics and technologies to manage nonadherence in patients with schizophrenia. *Current Psychiatry Reports, 10*, 359-369.

Hamera, E., & Brown, C.E. (2000). Developing a context-based performance measure for persons with schizophrenia: The test of grocery shopping skills. *American Journal of Occupational Therapy, 54*, 20-25.

Harvey, P.D. (2001). Vulnerability to schizophrenia in adulthood. In R.E. Ingram & J.M. Price (Eds.), *Vulnerability to psychopathology: Risk across the lifespan* (pp. 355-381). New York, NY: Guilford.

Hasan, A.F., Wobrock, P., Lieberman, T., Glenthoj, J., Gattaz, B., Thibaut, W.F., . . . The WFSBP Task Force on Treatment Guidelines for Schizophrenia. (2012). World Federation of Societies of Biological Psychiatry (WFSBP) guidelines for biological treatment of schizophrenia, part 1: Update 2012 on the acute treatment of schizophrenia and the management of treatment resistance. *World Journal of Biological Psychiatry, 13*(5), 318-378.

Horan, W.P., Blanchard, J.J., Clark, L.A., & Green, M.F. (2008). Affective traits in schizophrenia and schizotypy. *Schizophrenia Bulletin, 34*, 856-874.

Jenkins, J.H., & Barrett, R.J. (2004). Introduction. In J.H. Jenkins & R.J. Barrett (Eds.), *Schizophrenia, culture, and subjectivity: The edge of experience* (pp. 1-11). Cambridge, England: Cambridge University Press.

Jerome, G.J., Young, D.R., Dalcin, A., Charleston, J., Anthony, C., Hayes, J., . . . Daumit, G.L. (2009). Physical activity levels of persons with mental illness attending psychiatric rehabilitation programs. *Schizophrenia Research, 108*, 252-257.

Jónsdóttir, H., Opjordsmoen, S., Birkenaes, A. B., Simonsen, C., Engh, J. A., Ringen, P. A., . . . Andreassen, O.A. (2013). Predictors of medication adherence in patients with schizophrenia and bipolar disorder. *Acta Psychiatrica Scandinavica, 127*(1), 23-33.

Kielhofner, G. (Ed.). (2002). *A model of human occupation: Theory and application* (3rd ed.). Philadelphia, PA: Lippincott Williams & Wilkins.

Kim, E. (2008). Does traumatic brain injury predispose individuals to develop schizophrenia? *Current Opinion in Psychiatric Research, 21*, 286-289.

Kirkpatrick, B., Messias, E., Harvey, P.D., Fernandez-Egea, E., & Bowie, C.R. (2008). Is schizophrenia a syndrome of accelerated aging? *Schizophrenia Bulletin, 34*, 1024-1032.

Kluwe-Schiavon, B., Sanvicente-Vieira, B., Kristensen, C.H., & Grassi-Oliveira, R. (2013). Executive functions rehabilitation for schizophrenia: A critical systematic review. *Journal of Psychiatric Research, 47*(1), 91-104.

Konstantakopoulos, G., Ploumpidis, D., Oulis, P., Patrikelis, P., Soumani , A., Papadimitriou, G.N., & Politis, A.M. (2011). Apathy, cognitive deficits and functional impairment in schizophrenia. *Schizophrenia Research, 133*(1-3), 193-198.

Kontis, D.H., Reeder, V., Landau, C., & Wykes, T. (2013). Effects of age and cognitive reserve on cognitive remediation therapy outcome in patients with schizophrenia. *American Journal of Geriatric Psychiatry, 21*(3), 218-230.

Kopelowicz, A., Liberman, R.P., Wallace, C.J., Aguirre, F., & Mintz, J. (2006). Differential performance of job skills in schizophrenia: An experimental analysis. *Journal of Rehabilitation, 72*, 31-39.

Kopelowicz, A., Wallace, C.J., & Zarate, R. (1998). Teaching psychiatric inpatients to re-enter the community: A brief method of improving the continuity of care. *Psychiatric Services, 49*(10), 1313-1316.

Kukla, M., Salyers, M.P., & Lysaker, P.H. (2013). Levels of patient activation among adults with schizophrenia: Associations with hope, symptoms, medication adherence, and recovery attitudes. *Journal of Nervous & Mental Disease, 201*(4), 339-344.

Kuperberg, G.R. (2008). Building meaning in schizophrenia. *Clinical EEG and Neuroscience, 39*, 99-102.

Kurtz, M.M., Wexler, B.E., Fujimoto, M., Shagan, D.S., & Seltzer, J.C. (2008). Symptoms versus neurocognition as predictors of change in life skills in schizophrenia after outpatient rehabilitation. *Schizophrenia Research, 102*, 303-311.

Laliberte-Rudman, D., Yu, B., Scott, E., & Pajouhandeh, P. (2000). Exploration of the perspectives of persons with schizophrenia regarding quality of life. *American Journal of Occupational Therapy, 54*, 137-147.

Laursen, T.M., Munk-Olsen, T., Nordentoft, M., & Mortensen, P.B. (2007). A comparison of selected risk factors for unipolar depressive disorder, bipolar affective disorder, schizoaffective disorder, and schizophrenia from a Danish population-based cohort. *Journal of Clinical Psychiatry, 68*(11), 1673-1681.

Leucht, S., Tardy, M., Komossa, K., Heres, S., Kissling, W., Salanti, G., & Davis, J.M. (2012). Antipsychotic drugs versus placebo for relapse prevention in schizophrenia: A systematic review and meta-analysis. *Lancet, 379*(9831), 2063-2071.

Lin, P.I., & Mitchell, B.D. (2008). Approaches for unraveling the joint genetic determinants of schizophrenia and bipolar disorder. *Schizophrenia Bulletin, 34,* 791-797.

Lipskaya, L., Jarus, T., & Kotler, M. (2011). Influence of cognition and symptoms of schizophrenia on IADL performance. *Scandinavian Journal of Occupational Therapy, 18*(3), 180-187.

Liu, K.W.D., Hollis, V., Warren, S., & Williamson, D.L. (2007). Supported-employment program processes and outcomes: Experiences of people with schizophrenia. *American Journal of Occupational Therapy, 61,* 543-554.

Llorca, P.M. (2008). Monitoring patients to improve physical health and treatment outcome. *European Neuropsychopharmacology, 18*(Suppl. 3), S140-S145.

Loue, S., & Sajatovic, M. (2008). Auditory and visual hallucinations in a sample of severely mentally ill Puerto Rican women: An examination of the cultural context. *Mental Health, Religion and Culture, 11,* 597-608.

Lowe, T., & Lubos, E. (2008). Effectiveness of weight management interventions for people with serious mental illness who receive treatment with atypical antipsychotic medications. A literature review. *Journal of Psychiatric and Mental Health Nursing, 15,* 857-863.

Lysaker, P.H., Davis, L.W., Bryson, G.J., & Bell, M.D. (2009). Effectiveness of cognitive behavioral therapy on work outcomes in vocational rehabilitation for participants with schizophrenia spectrum disorders. *Schizophrenia Research, 107,* 186-191.

Mairs, H., & Bradshaw, T. (2004). Life skills training in schizophrenia. *British Journal of Occupational Therapy, 67,* 217-224.

Mäkinen, J., Miettunen, J., Isohanni, M., & Koponen, H. (2008). Negative symptoms in schizophrenia: A review. *Nordic Journal of Psychiatry, 62,* 334-341.

Maples, N.J., & Velligan, D.I. (2008). Cognitive adaptation training: Establishing environmental supports to bypass cognitive deficits and improve functional outcomes. *American Journal of Psychiatric Rehabilitation, 11*(2), 164-180.

McCann, T.V. (2002). Uncovering hope with clients who have psychotic illness. *Journal of Holistic Nursing, 20*(1), 81-99.

McCann, T.V., Clark, E., & Lu, S. (2009). Subjective side effects of antipsychotics and medication adherence in people with schizophrenia. *Journal of Advanced Nursing, 65,* 534-543.

Millar, H. (2008). Management of physical health in schizophrenia: A stepping stone to treatment success. *European Neuropsychopharmacology, 18*(Suppl. 2), S121-S128.

Minato, M., & Zemke, R. (2004). Time use of people with schizophrenia living in the community. *Occupational Therapy International, 11,* 177-191.

Moore, M. (2007). 'Can there be value in madness?' *Mental Health Occupational Therapy, 12*(3), 86-88.

Moritz, S., & Larøi, F. (2008). Differences and similarities in the sensory and cognitive signatures of voice-hearing, intrusions and thoughts. *Schizophrenia Research, 102,* 96-107.

Nordt, C., Müller, B., Rössler, W., & Lauber, C. (2007). Predictors and course of vocational status, income, and quality of life in people with severe mental illness: A naturalistic study. *Social Science & Medicine, 65*(7), 1420-1429.

Onitsuka, T., Niznikiewicz, M.A., Spence, K.M., Frumin, M., Kuroki, N., Lucia, L.C., . . . McCarley, R.W. (2006). Functional and structural deficits in brain regions subserving face perception in schizophrenia. *American Journal of Psychiatry, 163*(3), 455-462.

Penna, S., & Sheehy, K. (2000). Sex education and schizophrenia: Should occupational therapists offer sex education to people with schizophrenia? *Scandinavian Journal of Occupational Therapy, 7,* 126-131.

Perez, V.B., Shafer, K.M., & Cadenhead, K.S. (2012). Visual information processing dysfunction across the developmental course of early psychosis. *Psychological Medicine, 42*(10), 2167-2179.

Phillips, L.K., & Seidman, L.J. (2008). Emotion processing in persons at risk for schizophrenia. *Schizophrenia Bulletin, 34,* 888-903.

Pitkänen, A., Hätönen, H., Kuosmanen, L., & Väimäki, J. (2009). Individual quality of life of people with severe mental disorders. *Journal of Psychiatric and Mental Health Nursing, 16,* 3-9.

Prasad, K.M., Talkowski, M.E., Chowdari, K.V. ,McClain, L., Yolken, R.H., & Nimgaonkar, V.L. (2010). Candidate genes and their interactions with other genetic/environmental risk factors in the etiology of schizophrenia. *Brain Research Bulletin, 83*(3-4), 86-92.

Priebe, S.S., Reininghaus, M., Wykes, U., Bentall, T., Lauber, R., McCrone, C., . . . Eldridge, S. (2013). Effectiveness and cost-effectiveness of body psychotherapy in the treatment of negative symptoms of schizophrenia–A multi-centre randomised controlled trial. *BMC Psychiatry, 13,* 26-33

Prikryl, R.K., & Prikrylova, H. (2013). Can repetitive transcranial magnetic stimulation be considered effective treatment option for negative symptoms of schizophrenia? *The Journal of ECT, 29*(1), 67-74.

Rathod, S., Phiri, P., & Kingdon, D. (2010). Cognitive behavioral therapy for schizophrenia. *Psychiatric Clinics of North America, 33*(3), 527-536.

Rector, N.A., & Beck, A.T. (2012). Cognitive behavioral therapy for schizophrenia: An empirical review. *Journal of Nervous & Mental Disease, 200*(10), 832-839.

Saha, S., Chant, D., Welham, J., & McGrath, J. (2005). A systematic review of the prevalence of schizophrenia. *PLoS Medicine, 2*(5), e141. doi:10.1371/journal.pmed.0020141

Samuels, N., Gropp, C., Singer, S.R., & Oberbaum, M. (2008). Acupuncture of psychiatric illness: A literature review. *Behavior Medicine, 34*(Summer), 55-62.

Sarisoy, G., Terzi, M., Gümüs, K., & Pazvantoğlu, O. (2013). Psychiatric symptoms in patients with multiple sclerosis. *General Hospital Psychiatry, 35*(2), 134-140.

Schindler, V.P., & Baldwin, S.A.M. (2005). Role development: Application to community-based clients. *Israel Journal of Occupational Therapy, 14*(1), E3-E18.

Schultz, S.H., North, S.W., & Shields, C.G. (2007). Schizophrenia: A review. *American Family Physician, 75*, 1821-1829.

Schwarzbold, M., Diaz, A., Martins, E.T., Rufino, A., Amante, L.N., Thais, M.E., . . . Walz, R. (2008). Psychiatric disorders and traumatic brain injury. *Neuropsychiatric Disease Treatment, 4*(4), 797-816.

Seeman, M.V. (2010). Raves, psychosis, and spirit healing. *Transcultural Psychiatry, 47*(3), 491-501.

Shah, U.R., Vu, C., Thomas, R., Hartman, D.W., & Sharma, T.R. (2013). Alcohol-induced psychotic disorder in a 42-year-old female patient. *Journal of the American Academy of Physician Assistants (JAAPA), 26*(2), 30, 32, 36.

Sivec, H.J., & Montesano, V.L. (2012). Cognitive behavioral therapy for psychosis in clinical practice. *Psychotherapy, 49*(2), 258-270.

Skodlar, B., Tomori, M., & Parnas, J. (2008). Subjective experience and suicidal ideation in schizophrenia. *Comprehensive Psychiatry, 49*, 482-488.

Smerud, P.E., & Rosenfarb, I.S. (2011). The therapeutic alliance and family psychoeducation in the treatment of schizophrenia: An exploratory prospective change process study. *Couple and Family Psychology: Research and Practice, 1*, 85-91.

Smith, S., & Suto, M.J. (2012). Religious and/or spiritual practices: Extending spiritual freedom to people with schizophrenia. *Canadian Journal of Occupational Therapy, 79*(2), 77-85.

Stetka, B.S., & Correll, C.U. (2014, January 16). 7 advances in schizophrenia. *Medscape.* Retrieved from http://www.medscape.com/viewarticle/819068.

Stip, E., Sepehry, A.A., Prouteau, A., Briand, C., Nocole, L. Lalonde, P., & Lesage, A. (2005). Cognitive discernible factors between schizophrenia and schizoaffective disorder. *Brain & Cognition, 59*(3), 292-295.

Su, C., Tsai, P., Su, W., Tang, T., & Tsai, A.Y. (2011). Cognitive profile difference between Allen cognitive levels 4 and 5 in schizophrenia. *American Journal of Occupational Therapy, 65*, 453-461.

Suvisaari, J., & Mantere, O. (2013). Inflammation theories in psychotic disorders: A critical review. *Infectious Disorders Drug Targets, 13*(1), 59-70.

Szöke, A., Trandafir, A., Dupont, M.E., Méary, A., Schürhoff, F., & Leboyer, M. (2008). Longitudinal studies of cognition in schizophrenia: Meta-analysis. *The British Journal of Psychiatry, 192*, 248-257.

Takayanagi, Y., Cascella, N.G., Sawa, A., & Eaton, W.W. (2012). Diabetes is associated with lower global cognitive function in schizophrenia. *Schizophrenia Research, 142*(1-3), 183-187.

Tali, S., Rachel, L.W., Adiel, D., & Marc, G. (2009). The meaning in life for hospitalized patients with schizophrenia. *Journal of Nervous & Mental Disease, 197*, 133-135.

Tandon, R. (2013, May 6). From DSM-5: Four important changes in the diagnosis of schizophrenia. *Psychiatry Weekly, 8*(10). Retrieved from http://www.psychweekly.com/aspx/article/articledetail.aspx?articleid=1567.

Tandon, R., Keshavan, M.S., & Nasrallah, H.A. (2008). Schizophrenia, "just the facts." What we know in 2008. 2. Epidemiology and etiology, *Schizophrenia Research, 102*, 1-18.

Tarbox, S.I., & Poque-Geile, M.F. (2008). Development of social functioning in preschizophrenia children and adolescents: A systematic review. *Psychological Bulletin, 134*, 561-583.

Thompson, J.L., Kelly, M., Kimhy, D., Harkavy-Friedman, J.M., Khan, S., Messinger, J.W., . . . Corcoran, C. (2009). Childhood trauma and prodromal symptoms among individuals at clinical high risk for psychosis. *Schizophrenia Research, 108*, 176-181.

Tremeau, F., & Antonius, D. (2012). Review: emotion identification deficits are associated with functional impairments in people with schizophrenia [Commentary]. *Evidence Based Mental Health, 15*(4), 106.

Tungpunkom, P., & Nicol, M. (2008). Life skills programmes for chronic mental illness. *Cochrane Database of Systematic Reviews*, Issue 2. Art. No.: CD000381. doi:10.1002/14651858.CD000381.pub.2

Ücok, A., Karadayi, G., Emiroğlu, B., & Sartorius, N. (2013). Anticipated discrimination is related to symptom severity, functionality, and quality of life in schizophrenia. *Psychiatry Research, 209*(3), 333-339. doi:10.1016/j.psychres.2013.02.022

Urlic, K., & Lentin, P. (2010). Exploration of the occupations of people with schizophrenia. *Australian Occupational Therapy Journal, 57*(5), 310-317.

Van Gennep, A. (2010). *The rites of passage.* London, England: Chapman & Hall.

van Os, J., & Kapur, S. (2009). Schizophrenia. *Lancet, 374*(9690), 635-645.

Velligan, D.I., Weiden, P.J., Sajatovic, M., Scott, J., Carpenter, D., Ross, R., & Docherty, J.P. (2010). Strategies for addressing adherence problems in patients with serious and persistent mental illness: Recommendations from the Expert Consensus Guidelines. *Journal of Psychiatric Practice, 16*(5), 306-324.

Versterager, L., Christensen, T., Olsen B.B., Krarup, G., Melau, M., Forchhammer, H.B., & Nordentoft, M. (2012). Cognitive and clinical predictors of functional capacity in patients with first episode schizophrenia. *Schizophrenia Research, 141*(2-3), 251-256.

Waghorn, G., Lloyd, C., & Clune, A. (2009). Reviewing the theory and practice of occupational therapy in mental health rehabilitation. *British Journal of Occupational Therapy, 72*(7), 314-323.

Wan, M.W., Abel, K.M., & Green, J. (2008). The transmission of risk to children from mothers with schizophrenia: A developmental psychopathology model. *Clinical Psychology Review, 28*, 613-637.

Wan, M.W., Warren, K., Salmon, M.P., & Abel, K.M. (2008). Patterns of maternal responding in postpartum mothers with schizophrenia. *Infant Behavior and Development, 31*, 532-538.

Waltermire, D., Walton, L., Steese, B., Riley, J. & Robertson, A. (2010). Assessing sensory characteristics of the work environment for adults with schizophrenia or schizoaffective disorder. *OT Practice, 15*(7), 12-5, 16-7.

Weiser, M., Werbeloff, N., Vishna, T., Yoffe, R., Lubin, G., Shmushkevitch, M., & Davidson, M. (2008). Elaboration on immigration and risk for schizophrenia. *Psychological Medicine, 38*, 1113-1119.

Whitty, P., Clarke, M., McTigue, O., Browne, S., Kamali, M., Kinsella, A., . . . O'Callaghan, E. (2008). Predictors of outcome in first-episode schizophrenia over the first 4 years of illness. *Psychological Medicine, 38*(8), 1141-1146.

Yee, C.M., Mathis, K.I., Sun, J.C., Sholty, G.L., Lang, P.J., Bachman, P., . . . Nuechterlein, K.H. (2010). Integrity of emotional and motivational states during the prodromal, first-episode, and chronic phases of schizophrenia. *Journal of Abnormal Psychology, 119*(1), 71-82.

Zanelli, J., Reichenberg, A., Morgan, K., Fearon, P., Kravariti, E., Dazzan, P., . . . Murray, R.M. (2010). Specific and generalized neuropsychological deficits: A comparison of patients with various first-episode psychosis presentations. *American Journal of Psychiatry, 167*(1), 78-85.

Bipolar and Related Disorders

Learning Outcomes

By the end of this chapter, readers will be able to:
- Describe the symptoms of bipolar and other related disorders
- Identify the causes of bipolar disorders
- Discuss the prevalence of bipolar disorders
- Describe treatment strategies for bipolar disorders
- Discuss the occupational perspective on bipolar disorders, including specific intervention consideration

Bonder B.
Psychopathology and Function, Fifth Edition (pp 119-134).
© 2015 SLACK Incorporated.

KEY WORDS

- Manic episode
- Hypomanic episode
- Major depressive episode
- Insomnia

- Hypersomnia
- Flight of ideas
- Rapid cycling

CASE VIGNETTE

George Gonzales is a 34-year-old insurance salesman who has been in the insurance line of work for 10 years. He was initially quite successful, but approximately 4 years ago, he experienced a period during which he felt sad and anxious. For a period of roughly 1 month, he experienced insomnia, poor appetite, and anhedonia, and his work suffered. He has never recovered to his previous level of productivity.

Mr. Gonzales is a third-generation Mexican American, and his large extended family was quite supportive during his initial illness. His *abuela* (grandmother) recommended an herbal supplement that he tried. The family also encouraged him to attend church to help him to resolve his difficulties (which they categorized as "*nervios*"—which translates as "nerves" and has components of anxiety and depression). However, none of these recommendations made any difference in his feelings of sadness, and he finally sought medical help.

His primary care physician prescribed a selective serotonin reuptake inhibitor (SSRI), and over a period of several weeks, he began to feel better. He discontinued the SSRI after 6 months, and he had no additional problems until 10 days ago.

At that time, he became quite dysfunctional, spending 1 week partying at night and shopping during the day. He began several home remodeling projects, each of which was abandoned within minutes, leaving the house in disarray. He emptied the joint savings account he shared with his wife, and he stopped eating, bathing, and shaving.

These symptoms have now been replaced by a repeat of the sadness, anxiety, and anhedonia he experienced 4 years ago. He is having difficulty getting out of bed, tearfully expresses remorse for the behavior of the past week, and indicates that he "just wants to die."

THOUGHT QUESTIONS

1. Do you believe Mr. Gonzales has a mental disorder?
2. If so, what behaviors, thoughts, or other symptoms do you identify as being problematic?
3. Of those symptoms, which might cause problems for Mr. Gonzales in his work?
4. What cultural factors do you believe might be important in this situation? How might you gather more information to respond more fully to this question?

BIPOLAR AND RELATED DISORDERS

- Bipolar I disorder
- Bipolar II disorder

- Cyclothymic disorder

Bipolar disorders are characterized by a disturbance of mood: excessive elation or some combination of periods of elation and excessive energy that are usually, although not always, interspersed with periods of depression and lethargy. Because mood impacts one's world view, these disorders tend to affect functional ability in a global fashion. The bipolar disorders most often fluctuate between mania and depression, although an individual who has a single manic episode may be diagnosed with bipolar I disorder.

The bipolar and related disorders section of the *Diagnostic and Statistical Manual of Mental Disorders* (DSM) has been significantly reconfigured in the newest version. In earlier editions, bipolar disorders were included in the same section as depression and other mood disorders; however, in the new framework for the fifth edition (DSM-5; American Psychiatric Association [APA], 2013), the bipolar disorders appear in a separate chapter. In addition, the DSM-5 notes that they have been placed "between the chapters on schizophrenia spectrum and other psychotic disorders and depressive disorders in recognition of their place as a bridge between the two diagnostic classes in terms of symptomatology, family history, and genetics" (p. 123). This description of the relationship among disorders represents a new conceptualization of a spectrum of diagnostic clusters based on expanded understanding of the underlying biological mechanisms of the various conditions (Smith, Barch, & Csernansky, 2009).

Bipolar disorders must be differentiated from major depressive disorder, anxiety disorders, attention-deficit/hyperactivity disorder (ADHD), and personality disorders. It is common for an individual who has been diagnosed with any of the disorders in this chapter to have a coexisting substance use disorder, and any of the disruptive disorders (e.g., ADHD, conduct disorder) and anxiety disorders are also common comorbid conditions.

This chapter will provide detailed coverage of bipolar I, bipolar II, and cyclothymic disorder, which are the most common presentations of the bipolar group. Etiology, prognosis, function, and treatment will be discussed together for bipolar I and bipolar II disorders, as they share many common features. Keep in mind that bipolar disorders—as is true for all other disorders—may be induced by substance use or some medical conditions and that some disorders in this group do not fit the typical symptom clusters; therefore, they would be considered as "other" or "unspecified." Table 5-1 shows the prevalence of the common bipolar disorders.

Bipolar I Disorder

As indicated earlier, the bipolar disorders have in common the presence of behaviors that are excessively energetic and active, to the point that function is altered or impaired. Bipolar I disorder is the most severe of the group, and its first criterion is that the individual had at least one **manic episode**. A manic episode includes a period of abnormal and persistent elevated, expansive, or irritable mood, combined with abnormal and persistently increased goal-directed activity or energy (APA, 2013). At the same time, the individual shows at least three other symptoms of mania: inflated self-esteem or grandiosity, decreased need for sleep, excessive talkativeness or pressure to speak, distractibility, or increased goal-directed activity or psychomotor agitation. The individual's activities may have the potential for adverse consequences (e.g., financial difficulties, legal difficulties, physical injury), and the symptoms impair function or require hospitalization.

Sometimes these symptoms are first seen following the treatment for depression, as was true for Mr. Gonzales, described in the case vignette. Assuming that the individual's symptoms meet the standards listed earlier, they would be considered as a manic episode, even when they appear to have resulted from the treatment of depression. At least one full manic

TABLE 5-1			
PREVALENCE OF BIPOLAR DISORDERS			
DIAGNOSIS	*PREVALENCE*	*GENDER RATIO (M:F)*	*SOURCE*
Bipolar I	0.6%	1.1:1	APA, 2013
Bipolar II	0.8% (United States); 0.3% (worldwide) 3% to 4%	Uncertain	APA, 2013; Merikangas & Lamers, 2012
Bipolar I and II combined	1% to 2%		Fagiolini et al., 2013
Cyclothymic disorder	0.4% to 1%	1:1 (probable, although women seek treatment more frequently than men)	APA, 2013

episode is required for a diagnosis of bipolar I disorder, and many individuals with bipolar I disorder have recurring episodes.

In addition to meeting the criteria for a manic episode, bipolar I disorder may include one or more **hypomanic episodes** before, after, or both before and after the manic episode. These hypomanic episodes differ from a manic episode in terms of duration (a minimum of 4 days, rather than 1 full week) and in terms of the functional consequences of the behavior, with manic episodes being the more severe manifestation of symptoms. To be diagnosed with a hypomanic episode, an individual must show abnormal and persistent elevated activity, three or more of the behavioral signs discussed previously, and a change in functioning from periods when the person is not symptomatic. However, a hypomanic episode is not sufficiently problematic to lead to deficits in social and work functioning or to require hospitalization. If psychotic symptoms are present, the condition is a manic episode, by definition, and would contribute to a diagnosis of bipolar I.

The individual may also have one or more **major depressive episodes** before, after, or both before and after the manic episode. To be diagnosed with a major depressive episode, the individual must show five symptoms that represent a change from prior function (APA, 2013). One of the symptoms present must be either depressed mood or anhedonia. The individual may also experience weight loss or loss of appetite, **insomnia** (difficulty sleeping), **hypersomnia** (excessive sleeping), fatigue or low energy, feelings of worthlessness or guilt, problems concentrating, and suicidal ideation or attempt. The symptoms must cause distress and functional impairment, and they must be distinguished from grief reaction following a loss.

Each manic episode is severe—usually with abrupt onset—and characterized by major changes in attitude, behavior, and cognition (Bhattacharya et al., 2011). For men, the most prominent symptoms are increased motor activity, psychosis, and grandiosity, whereas for women, emotional lability and moodiness are more prominent. The decreased need for sleep, talkativeness, **flight of ideas**, distractibility, increased activity, and excessive involvement in pleasurable activities with disregard for the consequences. Flight of ideas is characterized by rapid attention shifts from topic to topic, without logical connections. Typical behaviors for individuals experiencing a manic episode may include spending money wildly or involvement in inappropriate sexual activities. Functioning is impaired in all spheres, with marked deficits in occupational and social functioning. Hospitalization is often required.

Emotional lability can be seen, as the individual may be expansive and grandiose one minute and angry and hostile the next. Frequent rapid shifts from mania to depression occur, and, occasionally, the symptoms of the two appear together. Furthermore, the individual may be oblivious to his or her behavior and is totally unaware there is a problem.

Manic episodes may be preceded by a prodromal period during which early symptoms emerge. Insomnia, excessive energy, difficulty concentrating, and other manic symptoms may appear. The majority of individuals who experience manic episodes have prodromal symptoms (Brietzke et al., 2012).

In summary, a bipolar I diagnosis requires that the person has had at least one manic episode. Hypomanic and major depressive episodes may also occur, but the bipolar I diagnosis does not require the presence of either. Several ways exist in which the diagnosis is further described by the specifiers, including severity (mild, moderate, or severe), with psychotic features, in partial or full remission, and, if warranted, with a variety of possible accompanying conditions such as anxiety, mixed features, **rapid cycling** (i.e., quick change from mania to depression and back again), with seasonal pattern, and so on.

As with all mental disorder diagnoses, part of the diagnostic process is the exclusion of other possible disorders. If hallucinations and delusions are present, they must be accompanied by alterations in mood. Schizophrenia, other psychotic disorders, and organic factors— such as intoxication—must be ruled out. These disorders, particularly substance-related disorders, may also be comorbid. Although thought disorders may be present in individuals who experience manic episodes, mood alterations are the most prominent feature of the symptom constellation.

Bipolar II Disorder

Bipolar II disorder is characterized by at least one hypomanic episode, with at least one major depressive episode. As distinct from bipolar I disorder, the individual must not ever have had a manic episode, meaning that the disorder is somewhat less severe. The distinction is based on the extent of functional changes and the possible need for hospitalization. For a diagnosis of bipolar I disorder, severe functional deficits with potential need for hospitalization are required; however, for bipolar II, these deficits are explicitly excluded. The criteria for a hypomanic episode include (APA, 2013) a period of abnormally elevated or irritable mood, with abnormally increased activity or energy for most of several days. Mood and energy changes consist of at least three signs of mania, including grandiosity or inflated self-esteem, decreased need for sleep, talkativeness or pressured speech, flight of ideas, distractibility, and increase in goal-directed activity. These activities may have a high potential for adverse outcomes, and they represent a change from normal behavior. The symptoms are evident to others, but they are not severe enough to cause significant functional impairment or hospitalization.

The symptoms of a major depressive disorder are included in the discussion of bipolar I disorder. The symptoms are identical in the diagnostic criteria for bipolar II disorder. The criteria for bipolar II disorder include at least one hypomanic episode but no manic episode (APA, 2013). These symptoms cause significant distress or functional impairment (APA, 2013).

Specifiers can clarify whether the most recent episode was hypomania or depression, whether there are signs of anxiety, mixed features, rapid cycling (i.e., rapid shifts from depression to hypomania and back, with few periods during which the individual is relatively asymptomatic). Specifiers also exist for psychotic features, peripartum onset, and seasonal pattern. Severity can be noted as mild, moderate, or severe.

Most often, an individual with bipolar II disorder seeks help during a depressive episode (APA, 2013). The individual may find that the hypomanic episodes are less troubling, although family, friends, and coworkers typically find them quite problematic. In fact, one of the challenges in managing bipolar disorders is that the individual might actually enjoy the manic or hypomanic periods, in spite of the fact that these episodes can cause long-term negative consequences. The impulsivity that appears during the hypomanic episodes can be associated with substance abuse, sexual acting out, and other evidence of impulse control difficulty (Meade et al., 2012). The unpredictability of mood may also increase suicide risk as the individual shifts from excessive energy to depressed mood (Gonda et al., 2012). The lifetime risk of at least one suicide attempt is 33% among individuals with bipolar II disorder.

Bipolar II disorder is associated with other mental disorders, and approximately 60% of diagnosed individuals have three or more comorbid diagnoses (APA, 2013). These other disorders include substance abuse (37% of individuals) and anxiety (70% of individuals). When comorbid conditions exist, they are closely associated with the bipolar II circumstances; for example, anxiety is strongly associated with depressive episodes.

Etiology

Bipolar disorders most often emerge in adolescence or young adulthood, although a middle-adulthood age of onset is not uncommon (Coryell, Fiedorowicz, Leon, Endicott, & Keller, 2013). Two major patterns of onset are noted, one is characterized by early and repeated depression and the other is characterized by initial manic symptoms (Forty et al., 2009).

A clear familial pattern in bipolar disorder exists (Hankin, 2009). The risk for developing bipolar I disorder is between 40% and 70% in twin and family studies (Hauser & Correll, 2013). This finding—combined with the fact that psychotropic medications are effective—suggests a biological basis for the disorder. However, psychosocial factors also appear to be involved. It is vital to understand the underlying biology but also to be aware of the environmental, social, and personal factors, as well as the stressors that contribute to risk (Hauser & Correll, 2013). These factors could include complications during pregnancy and childbirth, season of birth, and stressful life events—although evidence is limited to support any of these as independent risk factors in the development of bipolar disorder.

Prognosis

Although single manic or depressive episodes may resolve relatively quickly, bipolar disorder is most often chronic (González-Pinto, Aldama, Mosquera, & González Gómez, 2007). In particular, early onset is predictive of a more difficult and chronic course (Coryell et al., 2013), as is a course that includes repeated periods of depression, in addition to early onset (Forty et al., 2009). Degree of cognitive impairment during an individual's first manic episode is associated with functional outcome but not with clinical outcome (Torres et al., 2011)—meaning that less cognitive dysfunction will not necessarily be associated with reduced manic symptoms or shorter episodes, but it does predict better resumption of function thereafter.

The prognosis for specific manic episodes is good (Bowden et al., 2003). The duration of episodes varies, although, if untreated, they may last for 1 month or more. Longer episodes, with cycling through depressive episodes, are associated with the need for hospitalization and require longer stays than those for most other disorders (Martin-Carrasco et al., 2012). Often, there is a pattern of recurring episodes, meaning that without maintenance treatment, it is probable that the individual will have manic episodes on a periodic basis. In some individuals, the episodes follow a particular pattern, perhaps appearing each spring (Cassidy & Carroll, 2002), whereas in others, their appearance may be unpredictable. In still others, there may be a single episode, with no recurrence. In approximately 13% of cases, manic episodes result

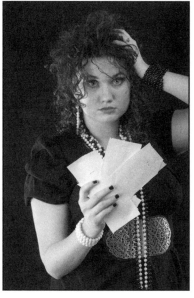

Figure 5-1. Individuals experiencing a manic episode may show poor control of their finances. (©2014 Shutterstock.com.)

in interaction with the criminal justice system (Christopher, McCabe, & Fisher 2012), and approximately half of individuals who experience one manic episode have repeated manic episodes (Yatham, Kauer-Sant'Anna, Bond, Lam, & Torres, 2009).

Implications for Function and Treatment

Function is severely impaired in bipolar I disorder, but it is somewhat less impaired in bipolar II disorder. Judgment is extremely poor, and individuals tend to engage in acting-out behaviors. For example, the individual may begin to gamble wildly, take drugs, abuse alcohol, argue with colleagues at work, or engage in promiscuous sexual activity or uncontrolled and excessive spending (Figure 5-1). Impulsiveness and grandiosity interfere with vocational and social activities, alienate coworkers and friends (Malhi, Bargh, Cahsman, Frye, & Gitlin, 2012), and decrease the individual's ability to complete tasks.

Changes in cognition and perception occur. Motor skill does not change, but hyperactivity is almost always present; in fact, a diagnosis of ADHD may be made in children when the actual problem is a bipolar disorder (Skirrow, Hosang, Farmer, & Ahserson, 2012). It appears that changes in central nervous system function contribute to the characteristic symptom constellation (Michalak, Murray, Young, & Lam, 2008). In particular, executive function is impaired, and the extent of this impairment is associated with the overall functional deficits (Lopera-Vaszuez, Bell, & López-Jaramillo, 2011). Individuals with bipolar disorders often lack insight, particularly during manic or hypomanic episodes (Yen et al., 2009), which makes it difficult to design interventions that the individual perceives as suitable. Individuals with bipolar disorders may be able to function reasonably normally between episodes, although some cognitive and neurological signs may persist. Bipolar disorders typically have a serious negative impact on quality of life (Michalak et al., 2008).

Depending on the frequency and duration of the manic periods, it is possible that individuals with bipolar disorders may hold jobs, have families, and carry on other activities during periods of remission. However, all of these functions are impaired during episodes and often result in loss of job and family disruption. In individuals who have reasonable levels of function between episodes, maintenance treatment with drugs, as well as family therapy to assist

Figure 5-2. During manic and hypomanic episodes, individuals may show poor judgment about their activities. (©2014 Shutterstock.com.)

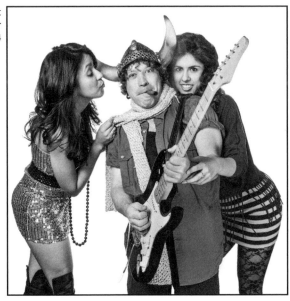

others to understand the disorder, may be effective. However, recent research suggests that at least some executive function and psychosocial impairment persists even when the disorder is in remission (Yen et al., 2009).

The primary treatment for bipolar disorders is medication, typically lithium (Pfennig, Bschor, Falkai, & Bauer, 2013). However, to prevent recurrence, medication must be continued in maintenance doses for long periods of time. Although lithium can be effective, it presents a set of problems related to the potential for toxicity from the drug and the possible unwillingness of the individual to follow the prescribed regimen. There is a significant subset of individuals for whom lithium is not effective, and research on alternatives is scarce (Sienaert, Lambrichts, Dols, & De Fruyt, 2013). It appears that a number of other drugs—including ketamine and risperidone—may be tried, and in cases where no psychopharmacological agent is beneficial, electroconvulsive therapy is occasionally implemented.

Group psychotherapy, family therapy, educational approaches, and behavioral interventions have all shown some effectiveness, particularly in combination with medication (Kauer-Sant'anna, Bond, Lam, & Yatham, 2009). Cognitive behavioral intervention has demonstrated value above and beyond psychoeducational approaches (Zaretzky, Lancer, Miller, Harris, & Parikh, 2008).

Because of the severity of manic episodes, hospitalization—often involuntary—is frequently warranted (Baker, 2001). While in manic episodes, individuals demonstrate extremely poor judgment and must often be protected from a tendency to engage in illegal or imprudent acts or to abuse drugs (Figure 5-2). Quick action is recommended to provide treatment for individuals during these episodes to prevent catastrophic consequences (Garlow, 2008).

When hospitalization is part of the treatment, it is usually brief. The primary objective is to protect the individual from harming himself or herself or others as a result of poor judgment and impulsivity. When medications have begun to ameliorate the symptoms, hospitalization is no longer necessary. However, individuals with bipolar disorder who need hospitalization typically have residual functional deficits (Dickerson et al., 2010).

Implications for Occupational Therapy

During acute episodes, an important role for the occupational therapist is to monitor behavior changes and provide a structured environment in which behavior can be managed. A typical manic client might breeze into the clinic to begin "building a castle," starting by nailing two boards together, then switch to "creating a new Mona Lisa," then switch to making a leather coat after the first stroke of paint is on the canvas, and so on. Helping the individual to focus and setting limits to contain manic impulses are important elements of initial interventions. Monitoring the signs of behavior change in daily activities as medication is introduced is an important contribution to making decisions about long-term treatment.

Between episodes, the occupational therapist may assist the individual in coping with the possibility of a chronic illness. The individual needs to learn the signs of an impending episode to know when to seek help. In addition, activity patterns may need to be examined to determine whether some stressful activities should be stopped or changed. If bipolar disorder onset was early in life, the assessment of skills and remediation of skill deficits may be needed, as skill acquisition can be impaired if manic episodes are frequent (Baker, 2001). Function in all occupations should be assessed to determine how stress can be managed and how quality of life can be maximized.

For most individuals who have manic episodes, occupations and skills are minimally impaired between episodes. However, behavior during episodes may have long-term consequences in terms of lost friends, family disputes, lost jobs, and financial difficulties. Self-esteem and self-concept are likely to be damaged by both the chronic nature of the disorder and the enormous fluctuations in personality that characterizes it (Baker, 2001). When an individual is sometimes withdrawn, sad, and lethargic and at other times is energetic and effervescent, it is difficult for him or her to form a clear picture of his or her abilities and desires. It is also difficult to feel good about one's function when it is so unstable.

Medication may help the individual to reach a more even keel, but it cannot repair the damage done to self-concept by these mood swings. The occupational therapist must help the individual identify strengths, weaknesses, likes, and dislikes through exposure to a wide range of activities. Psychoeducational approaches may assist in achieving these goals (González Isasi, Echeburúa, Liminana, & González-Pinto, 2012).

For some individuals, needed skills may have been lost or may never have been acquired. One young mother had fluctuated between feeling withdrawal from her two preschool children when she was not with them to extreme irritability when they were present. The mother needed training in parenting skills to resolve this issue and to begin repairing the damage done by her inconsistent and unpredictable behavior. This course is fairly typical of individuals with long-standing bipolar disorder, particularly those who have not had adequate diagnosis and treatment.

Clients need to learn how to avoid or manage these difficulties by altering their lifestyle, monitoring symptoms, and getting family members involved (Murray et al., 2011). One woman recognized that she would begin to have problems as soon as the lilacs bloomed each spring. Her husband learned to put away the credit cards then, and she learned to go see her physician immediately.

The education of family members, consultation with supervisors at work, and advocacy for the individual are all important aspects of effective occupational therapy intervention.

Cyclothymic Disorder

Cyclothymic disorder is a chronic disorder in which episodes of hypomania and depressed mood (but without a major depressive episode) are interspersed. Cyclothymic disorder is the least severe of the bipolar disorders and is characterized by multiple periods of hypomanic and depressive symptoms that are not serious enough to meet the criteria for hypomanic or depressive episodes (APA, 2013). Although less severe, the individual has symptoms most of the time over several years.

Cyclothymic disorder typically emerges during adolescence or early adulthood. It is frequently accompanied by substance abuse or sleep disorders.

Because cyclothymia is less severe than bipolar I or bipolar II disorder, functional capacity is less impaired. In fact, some individuals report that they are unusually productive during hypomanic episodes. Vocational function is affected during depressed periods. Social function is often impaired, as the wide, unpredictable mood swings may cause difficulty for those around the individual. Substance use may become a problem as the individual attempts to manage the depressed episodes or loses capacity for good judgment during hypomanic episodes. The fact that mood and behavioral swings are less severe than in individuals with bipolar I and bipolar II disorders sometimes means that diagnosis is delayed. Family members, employers, and others may find the individual quite difficult to deal with during periods of hypomanic or depressed mood, and they may be unaware that the individual is trying to cope with a mental disorder.

For example, one woman who had a cyclothymic disorder applied for a management position with a large bank. Her resume included a wide array of impressive accomplishments. During the interview process, the human resources specialist found it difficult to pin down the applicant's precise contributions to the various achievements she claimed. The applicant became annoyed when asked for details and stormed out of the office, saying that the bank did not deserve her. Needless to say, she did not get the job, but a series of similar encounters led to a period of depression, during which the woman finally sought help.

Strong evidence exists that individuals with cyclothymic disorder are at high risk for developing either bipolar I or bipolar II disorder (Alloy, Abramson, Urosevic, Nusslock, Jager-Hyman, 2010). In particular, elevated mid-frontal left cortical activity is associated with conversion to bipolar I or II (Nusslock et al., 2012).

Implications for Occupational Therapy

The principles discussed for the more severe disorders can be applied equally to cyclothymic disorder. Although the functional impact is less, cyclothymic disorder can be a frustrating problem because of its chronicity. In addition, because symptoms are less severe, it can more difficult to recognize periods during which the individual is worse. This alone can result in significant difficulties related to the depression and irritability that characterize the disorder. Thus, the individual may benefit from support in coping with chronic illness, as well as acquiring education and information and assistance in clarifying valued goals and activities.

Individuals who tend to have hypomanic symptoms often have difficulty with time management. They may be overcommitted and may create interpersonal friction by being unable to meet their commitments. Effective use of time and realistic self-appraisal are important goals for occupational therapy.

Cyclothymic disorder requires a combination of approaches, much like those suggested for bipolar disorder. Although the functional impairments are less extreme, their impact on self-esteem should not be minimized. Table 5-2 shows the symptoms and functional deficits of the most frequently diagnosed mood disorders.

TABLE 5-2

DIAGNOSTIC CRITERIA AND FUNCTIONAL DEFICITS: BIPOLAR AND RELATED DISORDERS

DISORDER	DIAGNOSTIC CRITERIA (APA, 2013)	IMPLICATIONS FOR FUNCTION
Bipolar I disorder	At least one manic episode: • Abnormal elevated or irritable mood with abnormal increased activity • Symptoms may include: • Grandiosity • Decreased need for sleep • Excessive talkativeness and/or pressured speech • Distractibility • Increased activity or psychomotor agitation • Involvement in activities with potential for bad consequences • Need for hospitalization, or psychotic signs May include one or more hypomanic episodes and/or one or more major depressive episodes Distress and dysfunction	Work, social, leisure occupations, habits, roles, and routines deteriorate during episodes Motor hyperactivity Process deficits Communication not severely affected Function tends to improve between episodes
Bipolar II disorder	At least one hypomanic episode lasting 4 or more days including (among others): • Elevated or irritable mood with abnormally increased activity and/or energy • Grandiosity • Decreased need for sleep • Flight of ideas • Distractibility • Excessive involvement in activities with a high probability of bad outcome • Change in function from normal behavior • Not severe enough to cause substantial functional impairment or a need for hospitalization (note that this is a distinguishing characteristic as opposed to the criteria for a manic episode) At least one major depressive episode and no manic episode	As above, but some-what less severe

(continued)

TABLE 5-2 (CONTINUED)		
DIAGNOSTIC CRITERIA AND FUNCTIONAL DEFICITS: BIPOLAR AND RELATED DISORDERS		
DISORDER	*DIAGNOSTIC CRITERIA (APA, 2013)*	*IMPLICATIONS FOR FUNCTION*
Cyclothymic disorder	At least 2 years with multiple periods of hypomanic symptoms that do not meet the criteria for a hypomanic episode and depressive symptoms that do not meet the criteria for a major depressive episode Symptoms are present at least half the time Does not meet the criteria for a manic, hypomanic, or major depressive episode	As above, but sufficiently less severe to allow for reasonable function most of the time

Cultural Considerations

Cultural factors may affect the timing of diagnosis following the onset of symptoms, the consequences for the individual in terms of access to and outcomes of care, and the outcomes for individuals with bipolar disorder who have other accompanying medical conditions (Warren, 2007). In the United States, some individuals from a variety of minority cultures are likely to experience longer delay until a diagnosis is made, partially because of perceptions about mental disorders. Symptoms and perceived etiology may also differ from culture to culture (Alarcón, 2009). In the case of bipolar disorder, the extent to which manic behavior is tolerated can vary, as can the acceptability of use of medication (short- or long-term). Another important issue is the extent to which the disorder carries a stigma in different cultures (Vázquez et al., 2011).

Lifespan Considerations

Early development of bipolar disorder is predictive of a more severe and chronic course that includes greater functional deficits and the possibility that psychopharmacological intervention will be less effective (Hauser & Correll, 2013). Between one-half and two-thirds of individuals diagnosed with bipolar I disorder develop the condition prior to age 18. Hauser and Correll (2013) speculated that early identification of such individuals, perhaps by recognizing prodromal symptoms, might improve treatment outcomes. Diagnosing bipolar disorder in children is complicated by the potential for overlap among symptoms with other disorders, such as ADHD (Fields & Fristad, 2009). The disorder is relatively rare in children, in spite of the fact that the number of children diagnosed with bipolar disorder has increased significantly over the past two decades.

Symptoms found in children may differ somewhat from those described in adults and usually reflect developmental stage. Anxiety, school refusal or school problems, and acting-out are all common. These children often have low self-esteem. School and social function are likely to be impaired. Irritability, aggressive behavior, anger outbursts, emotional hypersensitivity, and mood lability are particularly prominent during prodromal periods for children at high risk of developing one of the bipolar disorders (Hauser & Correll, 2013). Thus, intervention must be sensitive to the age and stage of the individual child. The question of medication for children is a difficult one. Lithium has substantial side effects and risks; therefore, alternative management strategies may be preferable if possible.

Older adults with bipolar disorder are at high risk of developing dementia (Aprahamian, Nunes, & Forlenza, 2013). This has significant implications for function, as either bipolar disorder by itself or dementia by itself contributes to functional deficits. The combination of the two can make dysfunction more severe and intervention more complex. Another complicating factor in the treatment of older adults is that the process of metabolizing medications changes and often results in a need to monitor and reconsider medication types and doses (Dolder, Depp, & Jeste, 2007).

Most often, an older adult with bipolar disorder has had the condition life long. For these individuals, depressive symptoms become more prevalent in later life (Coryell, Fiedorowicz, Solomon, & Endicott, 2009). Some individuals may develop the condition late in life, although this is relatively uncommon (Carlino, Stinnett, & Kim, 2013).

Internet Resources

Helpguide.org
http://www.helpguide.org/mental/bipolar_disorder_symptoms_treatment.htm
This is a self-help organization that provides information about many mental disorders. It has accessible language and is good for consumers.

National Alliance on Mental Illness
http://nami.org/Content/NavigationMenu/Mental_Illnesses/Bipolar1/Home_-_What_is_Bipolar_Disorder_.htm
A resource listed in many chapters, NAMI is an advocacy and self-help organization that provides consumer information. The site encourages individuals with mental disorders to advocate for themselves.

National Institute of Mental Health
http://www.nimh.nih.gov/health/publications/bipolar-disorder/index.shtml
A good summary of the bipolar disorders, with links to other sites and resources.

TeensHealth
http://kidshealth.org/teen/your_mind/mental_health/bipolar.html
Information focused on families with children and adolescents with mental disorders, including bipolar disorder.

CASE STUDY

Marvin Wright is a 60-year-old Black widower. He has four children ranging in age from 22 to 26. Two of his daughters live with him, one because she has a serious alcohol abuse problem, and the other to "take care of" him. Mr. Wright is aware that he has also been known to drink to excess, but he explains regularly to his daughter that unlike her, he can manage because he is unusually bright and capable. Although he is typically a loving father and grandfather, the younger generations are somewhat afraid of him because he has frequent tempter outbursts. Although he has never physically abused any of his children or grandchildren, they are anxious about the possibility.

Mr. Wright was a postal worker but lost his job following a major blow-up in which he accused his supervisor of failing to recognize his superior work ethic and his frequent innovations that are designed to speed mail delivery. The supervisor, who had been supportive because of Mr. Wright's usually engaging personality, had frequently given Mr. Wright written warnings about his excessive absence from work and for his verbal abuse of customers and coworkers.

Prior to the firing, the supervisor had insisted that Mr. Wright have an evaluation by the Employee Assistance Program offered through the post office. Mr. Wright resisted, but eventually went for evaluation. The counselor discovered that in addition to his drinking to excess, Mr. Wright was in serious financial difficulty. He had accumulated substantial debt financing his "inventions" and gambling. Mr. Wright burst into tears in the counselor's office, repeating that he was "a failure and a very bad person." The counselor referred Mr. Wright to a psychiatrist and strongly encouraged him to make an appointment in the near future. Mr. Wright went back to work, and subsequently had the encounter with his supervisor that resulted in his firing.

Mr. Wright went home and got directly into bed, where he stayed for the next 3 days. He was uninterested in eating, declined suggestions from his daughters that he get up to spend time with them, and did not bathe or dress.

After 3 days, Mr. Wright got out of bed, resumed his activities, and spent time looking at help-wanted ads. For several weeks, he tried unsuccessfully to find another job. He finally decided to see the psychiatrist to whom he had been referred.

The psychiatrist prescribed lithium, noting how important it is that Mr. Wright take the medication exactly as prescribed. He made a follow-up appointment, and he referred Mr. Wright to an occupational therapist.

An occupational profile interview with the occupational therapist revealed that Mr. Wright used to have a lot of valued occupations, but he currently has great difficulty focusing on any of them. He is either too distracted or too upset to participate in any of them. He is very worried about finding a new job, but he also fluctuates between feeling that he is too good for any employer and feeling that he is worthless.

THOUGHT QUESTIONS

1. What functional deficits are evident in Mr. Wright's current situation?
2. Of these deficits, which might be most critical to address first?
3. What are some factors in Mr. Wright's history that could help to structure a meaningful occupational profile?
4. What would be the highest priority in helping Mr. Wright regain a level of function that is supportive of his needs?

References

Alarcón, R.D. (2009). Culture, cultural factors and psychiatric diagnosis: Review and projections. *World Psychiatry, 8*(3), 131-139.

Alloy, L.B., Abramson, L.Y., Urosevic, S., Nusslock, R., & Jager-Hyman, S. (2010). Course of early-onset bipolar spectrum disorders during the college years: A behavioral approach system dysregulation perspective. In D.J. Miklowitz & D. Cicchetti (Eds.), *Understanding bipolar disorder: A developmental psychopathology perspective* (pp. 166-191). New York, NY: Guilford.

American Psychiatric Association. (2013). *Diagnostic and statistical manual of mental disorders* (5th ed.). Washington, DC: Author.

Aprahamian, I., Nunes, P.V., & Forlenza, O.V. (2013). Cognitive impairment and dementia in late-life bipolar disorder. *Current Opinion in Psychiatry, 26*(1), 120-123.

Baker, J.A. (2001). Bipolar disorders: An overview of the current literature. *Journal of Psychiatric and Mental Health Nursing, 5,* 437-441.

Bhattacharya, A., Khess, C.R.J., Munda, S.J., Bakhala, A.K., Praharaj, S. K., & Kumar, M. (2011). Sex difference in symptomatology of manic episode. *Comprehensive Psychiatry, 52*(3), 288-292.

Bowden, C.L., Calabrese, J.R., Sachs, G., Yatham, L.N., Asghar, L.A., Hompland, M., . . . Lamictal 606 Study Group. (2003). A placebo-controlled 18-month trial of lamotrigine and lithium maintenance treatment in recently manic or hypomanic patients with bipolar I disorder. *Archives of General Psychiatry, 60*(4), 392-400.

Brietzke, E., Mansur, R.B., Soczynska, J.K., Kapczinski, F., Bressan, R.A., & McIntyre, R.S. (2012). Towards a multifactorial approach for prediction of bipolar disorder in at risk populations. *Journal of Affective Disorders, 140*(1), 82-91.

Carlino, A.R., Stinnett, J.L., & Kim, D.R. (2013). New onset of bipolar disorder in late life. *Psychosomatics: Journal of Consultation Liaison Psychiatry, 54*(1), 94-97.

Cassidy, F., & Carroll, B.J. (2002). Seasonal variation of mixed and pure episodes of bipolar disorder. *Journal of Affect Disorders, 68,* 25-31.

Christopher, P.P., McCabe, P.J., & Fisher, W.H. (2012). Prevalence of involvement in the criminal justice system during severe mania and associated symptomatology. *Psychiatric Services, 63*(1), 33-39.

Coryell, W., Fiedorowicz, J., Leon, A.C., Endicott, J., & Keller, M.B. (2013). Age of onset and the prospectively observed course of illness in bipolar disorder. *Journal of Affective Disorders, 146*(1), 34-38.

Coryell, W., Fiedorowicz, J., Solomon, D., & Endicott, J. (2009). Age transitions in the course of bipolar I disorder. *Psychological Medicine, 39*(8), 1247-1252.

Dickerson, F., Origoni, A., Stallings, C., Khushalani, S., Dickinson, D., & Medoff, D. (2010). Occupational status and social adjustment six months after hospitalization early in the course of bipolar disorder: A prospective study. *Bipolar Disorders, 12*(1), 10-20.

Dolder, C.R., Depp, C.A., & Jeste, D.V. (2007). Biological treatments of bipolar disorder in later life. In M. Sajatovic & F.C. Blow (Eds.), *Bipolar disorder in later life* (pp. 71-93). Baltimore, MD: Johns Hopkins University Press.

Fagiolini, A., Forgione, R., Maccari, M., Cuomo, A., Morana, B., Dell'Osso, M.C., . . . Rossi, A. (2013). Prevalence, chronicity, burden and borders of bipolar disorder *Journal of Affective Disorders, 148*(2-3), 161-169.

Fields, B.W., & Fristad, M.A. (2009). Assessment of childhood bipolar disorder. *Clinical Psychology: Science and Practice, 16,* 166-181.

Forty, L., Jones, L., Jones, I., Smith, D.J., Caesar, S., Fraser, C., . . . Craddock, N. (2009). Polarity at illness onset in bipolar I disorder and clinical course of illness. *Bipolar Disorder, 11*(1), 82-88.

Garlow, S.J. (2008). Interventions for acute mood episodes in patients with bipolar disorder. *Journal of Clinical Psychiatry, 69*(2), e05.

Gonda, X., Pompili, M., Serafini, G., Montebovi, F., Campi, S., Dome, P., . . . Rihmer, Z. (2012). Suicidal behavior in bipolar disorder: Epidemiology, characteristics and major risk factors. *Journal of Affective Disorders, 143*(1-3), 16-26.

González Isasi, A., Echeburúa, E., Limiñana, J.M., & González-Pinto, A. (2012). Psychoeducation and cognitive-behavioral therapy for patients with refractory bipolar disorder: A 5-year controlled clinical trial. *European Psychiatry, 29*(3), 134-141. doi:10.1016/j.eurpsy.2012.11.002.

González-Pinto, A., Aldama, A., Mosquera, F., & González Gómez, C. (2007). Epidemiology, diagnosis and management of mixed mania. *CNS Drugs, 21,* 611-626.

Hankin, B.L. (2009). Etiology of bipolar disorder across the lifespan: Essential interplay with diagnosis, classification, and assessment. *Clinical Psychology: Science and Practice, 16*(2), 227-230.

Hauser, M., & Correll, C.U. (2013). The significance of at-risk or prodromal symptoms for bipolar I disorder in children and adolescents. *The Canadian Journal of Psychiatry/La Revue Canadienne de Psychiatrie, 58*(1), 22-31.

Kauer-Sant'anna, M., Bond, D.J., Lam, R.W., & Yatham, L.N. (2009). Functional outcomes in first-episode patients with bipolar disorder: A prospective study from the Systematic Treatment Organization Program for Early Mania project. *Comprehensive Psychiatry, 50*(1), 1-8.

Lopera-Vaszuez, J., Bell, V., & López-Jaramillo, C. (2011). What is the contribution of executive dysfunction to the cognitive profile of bipolar disorder? A well-controlled direct comparison study. *Revista Colombiana de Psiquiatría, 40*(Suppl. 1), 64S-75S.

Malhi, G.S., Bargh, D.M., Cahsman, E., Frye, M.A., & Gitlin, M.A. (2012). The clinical management of bipolar disorder complexity using a stratified model. *Bipolar Disorders, 14*(Suppl. 2), 66-89.

Martin-Carrasco, M., Gonzalez-Pinto, A., Gala, J.L., Ballesteros, J., Maurino, J., & Vieta, E. (2012). Number of prior episodes and the presence of depressive symptoms are associated with longer length of stay for patients with acute manic episodes. *Annals of General Psychiatry, 11.* Retrieved from http://www.annals-general-psychiatry.com/content/11/1/7.

Meade, C.S., Fitzmaurice, G.M., Sanchez, A.K., Griffin, M.L., McDonald, L.J., & Weiss, R.D. (2012). The relationship of manic episodes and drug abuse to sexual risk behavior in patients with co-occurring bipolar and substance use disorders: A 15-month prospective analysis. *AIDS and Behavior, 15*(8), 1829-1833.

Merikangas, K.R. & Lamers, F. (2012). The 'true' prevalence of bipolar II disorder. *Current Opinion in Psychiatry, 25*(1), 19-23.

Michalak, E.E., Murray, G., Young, A.H., & Lam, R.W. (2008). Burden of bipolar depression: Impact of disorder and medications on quality of life. *CNS Drugs, 22,* 389-406.

Murray, G., Suto, M., Hole, R., Hale, S., Amari, E., & Michalak, E.E. (2011). Self-management strategies used by 'high functioning' individuals with bipolar disorder: From research to clinical practice. *Clinical Psychology & Psychotherapy, 18*(2), 95-109.

Nusslock, R., Harmon-Jones, E., Alloy, L.B., Urosevic, S., Goldstein, K., & Abramson, L.Y. (2012). Elevated left mid-frontal cortical activity prospectively predicts conversion to bipolar I disorder. *Journal of Abnormal Psychology, 121*(3), 592-601.

Pfennig, A., Bschor, T., Falkai, P., & Bauer, M. (2013). The diagnosis and treatment of bipolar disorder. *Deutsches Ärzteblatt International, 110*(6), 92-100.

Sienaert, P., Lambrichts, L., Dols, A., & De Fruyt, J. (2013). Evidence-based treatment strategies for treatment-resistant bipolar depression: A systematic review. *Bipolar Disorders, 15*(1), 61-69.

Skirrow, C., Hosang, G.M., Farmer, A.E., & Ahserson, P. (2012). An update on the debated association between ADHD and bipolar disorder across the lifespan. *Journal of Affective Disorders, 141*(2-3), 143-159.

Smith, M.J., Barch, D.M., & Csernansky, J.G. (2009). Bridging the gap between schizophrenia and psychotic mood disorders: Relating neurocognitive deficits to psychopathology. *Schizophrenia Research, 107*(1), 69-75.

Torres, I.J., De Freitas, C.M., DeFreitas, V.G., Bond, D.J., Junz, M., Honer, W.G., . . . Yatham, L.N. (2011). Relationship between cognitive functioning and 6-month clinical and functional outcome in patients with first manic episode bipolar I disorder. *Psychological Medicine, 41*(5), 971-982.

Vázquez, G.H., Kapczinski, F., Magalhaes, P.V., Córdoba, R., Jaramillo, C., Rosa, A. R., . . . The Ibero-American Network on Bipolar Disorders (IAN-BD) Group. (2011). Stigma and functioning in patients with bipolar disorder. *Journal of Affective Disorders, 130*(1-2), 323-327.

Warren, B.J. (2007). Cultural aspects of bipolar disorder: Interpersonal meaning for clients and psychiatric nurses. *Journal of Psychosocial Nursing and Mental Health Services, 45*(7), 32-37.

Yatham, L.N., Kauer-Sant'Anna, M., Bond, D.J., Lam, R.W., & Torres, I. (2009). Course and outcome after the first manic episode in patients with bipolar disorder: Prospective 12-month data from the systematic treatment optimization program for early mania project. *Canadian Journal of Psychiatry, 54,* 105-112.

Yen, C., Cheng, C., Huang, C., Ko, C., Yen, J., Chang, Y., & Chen, C. (2009). Relationship between psychosocial adjustment and executive function in patients with bipolar disorder and schizophrenia in remission: The mediating and moderating effects of insight. *Bipolar Disorders, 11*(2), 190-197.

Zaretsky, A., Lancer, W., Miller, C., Harris, A., & Parikh, S.V. (2008). Is cognitive-behavioral therapy more effective than psychoeducation in bipolar disorder? *Canadian Journal of Psychiatry, 53,* 441-448.

Depressive Disorders

Learning Outcomes

By the end of this chapter, readers will be able to:
- Describe the symptoms of depressive disorders
- Differentiate among the depressive disorders on the basis of symptoms and onset
- Identify the causes of depressive disorders
- Describe treatment strategies for depressive disorders
- Discuss occupational therapy interventions for depressive disorders
- Discuss the prevalence and causes of suicidal ideation and suicide attempts
- Discuss strategies for screening for suicide risk
- Describe interventions to reduce suicide risk

Bonder B.
Psychopathology and Function, Fifth Edition (pp 135-157).
© 2015 SLACK Incorporated.

CASE VIGNETTE

Andrea McCardle is a 24-year-old administrative assistant for a nonprofit organization in a medium-sized city. She has a reputation as a hard worker, and her employer especially appreciates her consistent attendance. She is a slightly plump but attractive young woman who is described by friends as likeable and fun. She gets along well with her coworkers and frequently goes out with some of them after work for a drink. On weekends, she likes to go to movies, and she often visits her family who lives in a town approximately 2 hours away.

In the past month, Ms. McCardle has missed work on several occasions. Her productivity has been poor, and her supervisor has had to chastise her several times for making errors. She has refused to go out with her friends and has not been to see her family during that month. Twice in the past 2 weeks, a coworker has found her crying in the women's room. When the coworker has asked what is bothering her, she tries to hide her tears and simply says, "I'm fine." Her coworkers and family are all concerned about her.

THOUGHT QUESTIONS

1. Do you believe that Ms. McCardle has a mental disorder?
2. If so, what behaviors, thoughts, or other symptoms do you identify as being problematic?
3. Of those symptoms, which might cause Ms. McCardle's daily occupations to suffer?

DEPRESSIVE DISORDERS

- Disruptive mood dysregulation disorder
- Major depressive disorder, single and recurrent episodes
- Persistent depressive disorder (dysthymia)
- Premenstrual dysphoric disorder

As a group, depressive disorders are characterized by "sad, empty, or irritable mood" (American Psychiatric Association [APA], 2013). The symptoms in this cluster of disorders also include somatic and cognitive changes, which typically affect an individual's ability to function. As noted in Chapter 5, these disorders were grouped with the bipolar disorders in previous editions of the *Diagnostic and Statistical Manual of Mental Disorders* (DSM); however, their separation in the fifth edition (DSM-5) reflects the sense that bipolar disorders

TABLE 6-1			
PREVALENCE OF DEPRESSIVE DISORDERS			
DIAGNOSIS	*PREVALENCE*	*GENDER RATIO (M:F)*	*SOURCE*
Disruptive mood dysregulation disorder	Estimated at 2% to 5%	Unknown	APA, 2013
Major depressive disorder	7%	1:1.5 to 1:1.3	APA, 2013
Persistent depressive disorder (dysthymia)	3% to 6%		Sansone & Sansone, 2009
Premenstrual dys-phoric disorder	3.1% of menstruating women	Women only	Tschudin, Bertea, & Zemp, 2010

represents a mid-ground between schizophrenia and other psychoses and the depressive disorders in terms of severity and etiology.

Depressed mood is characteristic of all the disorders in this chapter. The distinctions among the disorders are severity, duration of episodes, degree of chronicity, and presumed etiology. As shown in Table 6-1, depressive disorders are very common.

Disruptive Mood Dysregulation Disorder

Disruptive mood dysregulation disorder is new to the DSM-5 (APA, 2013). It was included to reduce the overdiagnosis of bipolar disorders in children. However, it is one of the more controversial changes in this DSM revision, with critics suggesting that it will lead to a different kind of overdiagnosis. The contention of the critics is that its criteria are indistinguishable from the normal temper outbursts that are commonly found in children (Deibler, 2013). On the other hand, because of the potential stigma, significant concerns exist about diagnosing young children with bipolar disorder, about the possible overlap between bipolar and attention-deficit/hyperactivity disorder (ADHD) diagnoses, and other disorders perceived as severe and lifelong (Zepf & Holtmann, 2012).

According to the APA (2013), the criteria for disruptive mood dysregulation disorder include severe and repeated temper outbursts out of proportion to their circumstances and inappropriate for the individual's developmental stage. These outbursts occur three or more times per week, and the child has irritable mood during most of the time between outbursts. For a diagnosis to be made, this behavior pattern must have been present for most of the previous year, and occurs in at least two settings. The diagnosis is made for children between the ages of 6 and 18, although onset must be before age 10. These criteria reflect the behavior of a child who has very frequent and severe temper outbursts, with irritable behavior between episodes, and whose behavior does not meet the criteria for bipolar or depressive disorders. As discussed in Chapter 16, the disorder must also be distinguished from several of the disruptive, impulse control, and conduct disorders. In addition, manic, hypomanic, and depressive disorders must be ruled out, along with substance abuse.

Because disruptive mood dysregulation disorder is a new diagnosis, there is little firm evidence about etiology, prognosis, functional implications, and treatment. It seems that this will be a relatively frequent diagnosis in childhood, but it is less frequent in adults (Copeland, Angold, Costello, & Egger, 2013). It also appears that the disorder is comorbid with several other emotional and behavioral disorders, perhaps as much as 32% to 92% of the time (Copeland et al., 2013). Initial research suggests that these children have higher than normal rates of social impairments and school difficulties, they use social and psychological services more frequently, and they live in poverty more frequently than other children.

One of the rationales for the inclusion of this diagnosis is to reduce what is believed to be a high rate of false diagnosis of childhood bipolar disorder (Margulies, Weintraub, Basile, Grover, & Carlson, 2012). It is too soon to know whether the new category will achieve this goal, and, of course, whether it will create other diagnostic issues.

With regard to occupational therapy interventions, it seems likely that the strategies that are effective in working with children with other kinds of behavior disorders (e.g., ADHD, conduct disorders) are likely to be helpful for these children as well. Particular areas of emphasis would be appropriate emotional expression (perhaps through creative arts), management of anger through alternate mechanisms (e.g., physical activity), and positive engagement in age-appropriate and expected occupations (Bazyk, 2011). Educational interventions to assist parents and teachers in managing the child's anger may also be helpful.

Major Depressive Disorder, Single and Recurrent Episodes

Major depressive episodes characterize both the bipolar and depressive disorders. The diagnostic criteria for specific episodes are identical, regardless of the condition in which they appear. Distinctions among bipolar and depressive disorders are made on the basis of the frequency and duration of the episodes and whether or not they are accompanied by manic or hypomanic episodes. The diagnostic criteria were described in the previous chapter, but they are repeated here because of their centrality to major depressive disorder (APA, 2013). It is helpful to keep in mind that because depressive disorders can be diagnosed on the basis of a single major depressive episode, the diagnostic criteria are the same for both depressive disorders and bipolar disorders in which depressive episodes occur.

For a diagnosis of major depressive episode (and/or depressive disorder), the individual must show five symptoms that include depressed mood or anhedonia and four other manifestations of depression (APA, 2013). Those other manifestations may include weight loss without attempting to do so, insomnia or hypersomnia almost every day, fatigue or lack of energy, feelings of guilt or worthlessness, difficulty concentrating, and/or repeated suicidal ideation. The symptoms must cause distress and functional impairment, they must be distinguished from grief reaction following a loss, and they must occur almost every day for at least 2 weeks.

The duration and depth of feeling are important in distinguishing major depression from the kind of normal sadness everyone experiences at times over the course of daily life. Breaking up with a boyfriend or girlfriend, being laid off from a job, and other unhappy life events may cause sadness, sleep difficulties, poor appetite, and tearfulness. However, most people gradually rebound from those feelings without major interruptions in their lives. If the symptoms become more severe and persistent, the individual may well meet the criteria for major depressive disorder. Other signs of major depression may include hopelessness, somatic complaints, anxiety, irritability or anger, psychomotor agitation, fatigue, and impaired cognition.

Other diagnoses, such as bipolar I or II or schizoaffective disorder, must be ruled out, and the major depressive diagnosis is not appropriate if there has ever been a manic or hypomanic episode. Frequent comorbid conditions include the anxiety disorders, substance use disorders, and personality disorders.

The major depressive diagnosis can be specified as mild, moderate, or severe; with psychotic features; in partial or full remission; with anxious distress; mixed, melancholic, atypical, mood-congruent or mood-incongruent psychotic features; with catatonia; with peripartum onset; and/or with seasonal pattern.

A significant change from the revised fourth edition of the DSM (DSM-IV-TR; APA, 2000) is the removal of the bereavement exclusion. This notation in the previous edition of the DSM indicated that individuals who experienced a recent significant loss should not be diagnosed with major depressive disorder, unless the symptoms persisted for more than 2 months. Now, however, an individual presenting with the symptoms of major depressive disorder may be diagnosed even if there is an immediate loss that might explain the condition. The rationale was that anyone with symptoms of major depressive disorder might need support and intervention, even immediately after a loss, and that bereavement and major depression can coexist (Pies, 2013). However, others feel that this diagnosis pathologizes what is a normal human process (Stetka & Correll, 2013).

Etiology

A vast amount of research has investigated the origins of major depressive disorder. It is clear that there is a genetic component (Jabbi, Korf, Ormel, Kema, & den Boer, 2009), although the precise characteristics of the genetic factors are not yet established (Wray et al., 2012). Depressive disorders seem somewhat less genetically associated than bipolar disorders (Belmaker & Agam, 2008), with a twin heritability rate at approximately 37%. This suggests that other mechanisms are also factors.

Among the other factors with significant support is the hypothesis that depressive disorder is the result of monoamine deficiency (Belmaker & Agam, 2008). Emotion and cognition are mediated by monoamines, leading to speculation that these substances are insufficient in individuals with depression. These individuals respond to medications that increase monoamines, which is a finding that supports this hypothesis.

Some researchers have focused on the possibility that major depressive disorder is associated with viral infection, although the hypothesis is unsupported at present (Hornig et al., 2012). Similarly, there has been some investigation of the possibility that this disorder is the result of an inflammatory process (Krishnadas & Cavanagh, 2012), and, in fact, approximately one third of individuals with major depression have elevated markers for inflammation. Whether inflammation is a cause, a consequence, or simply a co-occurring phenomenon is yet not known.

The genetic hypothesis is also supported by findings of strong family histories of major depressive disorder (Dunner, 2008). However, this finding also suggests a social and environmental component. Stress, in particular, seems to be a major factor (Belmaker & Agam, 2008). For example, a substantially elevated risk of major depressive disorder exists in individuals with a history of physical, emotional, or sexual abuse.

Also a strong association exists between depression and a number of physical disorders, including Parkinson's disease (Starkstein et al., 2008), cancer (Pirl, Greer, Temel, Yeap, & Gilman, 2009), and asthma (Van Lieshout, Bienenstock, & MacQueen, 2009). In addition, cardiovascular disease is strongly associated with depression (Mast, 2010). Mast (2010) suggested that such vascular depression is a unique syndrome that reflects heightened risk for cerebrovascular incidents and cognitive impairment. In such cases, there are undoubtedly situational factors contributing to the depression, although it is possible there are neurological or biological factors as well. Depressive disorders are frequently comorbid with anxiety disorders (Dunner, 2008).

Depressive disorders are far more frequently diagnosed in women than in men (Harkness et al., 2010). It appears this may be due in part to greater experience of stressful life events in young adulthood. On the other hand, it is also possible that women are more willing to seek help.

Prognosis

Outcomes for major depressive disorder vary, with some individuals ultimately doing well, experiencing few recurrences and better postepisode function, and others having a chronic and severe course (Rhebergen et al., 2012). In general, younger females with fewer childhood traumas and fewer somatic symptoms do better than older individuals with early age of onset. Accompanying physical symptoms are associated with poor outcome (Huijbregts et al., 2010). Another prognostic factor is the extent of positive emotion expressed by the individual during depressive episodes (Morris, Bylsma, & Rottenberg, 2009). More positive emotion is associated with better outcome.

At 1 year postdiagnosis, approximately 40% of individuals have persistent symptoms (Wang, Patten, Currie, Sareen, & Schmitz, 2012). These individuals were likely to report long working hours, with accompanying work-family conflict; negative thinking; and coexisting social phobia. The severity of the episode and severe symptoms of depressed mood, intense sadness, and anorexia, for example, were also prognostic factors for recurrence.

Implications for Function and Treatment

Symptoms that occurred in more than 50% of depressed clients included reduced energy, impaired concentration, anorexia, initial insomnia, loss of interest, difficulty starting activities, worrying, subjective agitation, slowed thinking, difficulty making decisions, terminal insomnia, suicidal ideation or plans, weight loss, tearfulness, slowed movements, irritability, and feeling one will never get well.

During a major depressive episode, function in all occupations is likely to be affected (Bender, 2011). Individuals struggle with self-care, instrumental activities of daily living, work, leisure, play, sleep, and social occupations (Godard, Grondin, Baruch, & Lafleur, 2011). The degree of occupational deficit is, to some extent, associated with the demands of the individual's circumstances. For example, an individual with a cognitively challenging job (a university professor, perhaps, or a business executive) would have substantially greater work deficits than an individual with a less cognitively demanding, more routine kind of work (Figure 6-1). However, in either case, deficits would almost certainly extend to all areas of daily life.

The major skill deficits during a major depressive episode are cognitive, particularly executive function (Wagner, Doering, Helreich, Lieb, & Tadić, 2012) and memory (Maeshima et al., 2012). Memory deficits tend to persist, even when individual episodes of depression remit. In fact, the degree of neurocognitive deficits may be prognostic (Gallagher, Robinson, Gray, Porter, & Young, 2007), with worse symptoms during each episode that are associated with worse outcomes.

Emotional regulation is significantly impacted (Leppänen, 2006). In particular, individuals with major depressive disorder focus greater attention on negative than positive emotion and remember negative emotion more consistently. There is also some degree of motor slowing, which is somewhat similar to that found in Parkinson's disease (Lohr, May, & Caligiuri, 2013).

One significant issue that may require special attention in working with individuals with major depression is concern about sexual function (IsHak et al., 2013). Sexual interest is typically decreased during a depressive episode, and many of the medications used to treat

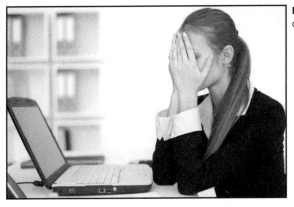

Figure 6-1. Depression has negative consequences for work. (©2014 Shutterstock.com.)

depression have significant sexual side effects. Therefore, there is a strong likelihood that this occupation will be impacted by both the disorder and the treatment. In fact, some individuals choose not to take antidepressant medication because of the sexual side effects.

A number of potential directions exist for the treatment of individuals with major depressive disorder. Major depression is one of the disorders for which psychopharmacology is well-established, with a wide array of medications from which to choose (Parikh et al., 2009). As will be discussed in Chapter 21, these drugs fall into a number of different classifications with somewhat different actions. On the whole, these drugs address issues with neurotransmission.

Psychotherapeutic approaches also have strong supporting evidence (Georgiades et al., 2012). In particular, psychodynamic and **cognitive behavioral therapies (CBT)** are useful in resolving individual episodes and reducing the risk of recurrence. CBT has been studied extensively and shows significant benefits (Feliciano, Segal, & Vair, 2011).

CBT focuses on identifying thought patterns that are dysfunctional and on identifying strategies for reframing them. For example, one young woman in the midst of a major depressive episode indicated it was clear to her that there was no hope for improvement. The therapist helped her to determine that there was no realistic way to know whether or not there was hope, and that assuming the worst almost ensured that outcome. The therapist and the client worked toward strategies that allowed the client to focus on smaller units of events and to make more balanced assessments of the probability of satisfying outcomes for these smaller units. The client was able to focus on taking a test in class the next day, rather than focusing on her academic pursuits as a whole, and to mentally review the steps she had taken to prepare to do well. Over time, these new thought strategies became somewhat more habitual and her pessimism decreased.

Other forms of psychotherapy that have shown some value include mindfulness-based cognitive therapy, which is a CBT-related strategy (Fresco, Flynn, Mennin, & Haigh, 2011). Evidence suggests that the most effective interventions incorporate both medication and psychotherapy (Georgiades et al., 2012; Parikh, et al., 2009). The impact of the two combined appears at approximately the sixth week of treatment; however, over time, psychotherapy appears to be more effective in maintaining improvement (Georgiades et al., 2012). It is noteworthy that CBT may be effective when delivered online, as well as in person (Parikh et al., 2009).

Complementary and alternative strategies have been examined for efficacy. Hypnotherapy shows some value (Alladin, 2012). Other complementary and alternative approaches that have shown sufficient evidence to suggest they may be helpful include omega-3 fatty acids, St John's wort (*Hypericum*), folate, S-adenosyl-L-methionine, acupuncture, and mindfulness psychotherapies (Freeman et al., 2010).

Exercise has been examined in a number of reasonably well designed studies. Findings suggest that moderate exercise is effective in improving quality of life, social functioning, and physical functioning (Mota-Pereira et al., 2011). Light therapy is also effective, particularly when administered in the morning (Martiny et al., 2012). It is noteworthy for individuals who do not respond well to medications or who find their side effects unacceptable that a number of other helpful interventions are available.

Another treatment, typically used as a last resort in individuals with intractable depression is **electroconvulsive therapy** (ECT; Huuhka et al., 2012). ECT was one of the earliest bio-medical interventions for a variety of severe mental disorders (Shorter & Healy, 2007). In its early form, a large dose of electrical current was administered without anesthesia for lengthy courses—sometimes as many as 30 or 40 treatments for a given individual. Although it was beneficial for some individuals, ECT administration seemed barbaric, and for several decades it was abandoned almost entirely. However, more recently, it has had resurgence in treating individuals who do not respond to other forms of intervention (Huuhka et al., 2012). The treatment is now administered under anesthesia, and a typical course is approximately six to eight treatments. ECT is effective for some individuals with severe, intractable depression, although there is also a high rate of relapse of approximately 40%.

Due to the life-altering consequences of major depression, an important strategy is preven-tion (Muñoz, Beardslee, & Leykin, 2012). Such prevention is possible through a variety of strategies, including those focused on mitigating risk factors, such as family history, poverty, exposure to violence, and child or spousal abuse. Among the suggested interventions are cog-nitive behavioral strategies, parent training, and screening for postpartum depression.

Implications for Occupational Therapy

Occupational therapy has a major role in ameliorating depression and addressing func-tional deficits. Depression makes function difficult for the individual (Creek, 2006), and occupations are all affected during major depressive episodes. Individuals with major depres-sion struggle with self-care, work, leisure, sleep, and sexual occupations; depression has been defined as a combination of skill and habit deficits (Rogers & Holm, 2000). At the level of specific skills, cognition is almost always impaired. Concentration and problem-solving abil-ity are diminished. Sensory perceptual skill is usually not affected—except in the presence of hallucinations—although perceptions can be skewed by the client's tendency to look for signs that he or she is unworthy. Psychomotor activity is often either slowed or speeded. Social and communication skills are often poor, leading to significant interpersonal difficulty. Those around the individual may become more hostile, anxious, and rejecting in response to the behavior of the depressed individual. Thus, the behavior of the depressed person sets a cycle of disturbed interaction.

Habit deficits include problems with instrumental activities of daily living and with per-sonal care (Rogers & Holm, 2000). It may be that depressed individuals lack motivation and interest in these activities or that they are too fatigued to complete them. Regardless of the reason, individuals who are depressed often fail to accomplish self-care activities at a socially acceptable level.

Social and emotional support are essential in depression (Reblin & Uchino, 2008). Unfortunately, the lethargy that characterizes the disorder makes it likely that the individual will not participate fully in social interaction, which can lead to social isolation. A particular challenge is addressing marital issues when one partner is depressed (Rehman, Gollan, & Mortimer, 2008). Although spouses and others may be supportive initially, they may become more irritated with the individual's behavior over time if the symptoms of depression persist.

As noted previously, physical activity seems to have value in ameliorating depressive symptoms (Mata et al., 2011). Because exercise has numerous other health benefits, there is no reason not to try it when it is not medically contraindicated. One issue in implementing exercise programs with individuals who are depressed is the lack of motivation that characterizes the disorder.

Occupational therapists can focus on assisting the client to find gratifying activities that improve self-esteem and increase motivation. Individuals who are depressed are typically lethargic and apathetic, so finding occupations that are meaningful can be vital. In many situations, this requires an understanding of the values, beliefs, and meaningful spiritual practices that might provide motivation.

In addition, activities that provide opportunities for self-expression are valuable, as individuals who are depressed may be reluctant or unable to put their feelings into words. Art or other creative activities can provide a valuable outlet for such emotions. One very timid woman experiencing depression was asked to participate on a woodworking project. After a few half-hearted taps, she began to pound the hammer, shouting with great enthusiasm, "This is for my husband, this is for my boss, this is for the dog...." She was then better able to express her rage about feeling taken advantage of by those around her.

Social skills training may be helpful to individuals who are depressed (Thase, 2012), particularly those who never acquired social skills because of prolonged, early-onset depression. In addition, activities that ensure positive reinforcement from others can be of great value. One woman who was depressed spent a week baking cookies every day for the other clients in a day-treatment center. She thoroughly enjoyed their appreciation. At the end of the week, she was able to say, "Now I think I'll do something for me," and she began to knit a scarf for herself. She chose a bright cheery yellow that was in marked contrast to the drab browns and grays she had been wearing.

Occupational therapy has been used to address depression-related dysfunction in work (Nieuwenhuijsen et al., 2008). Although there is no adequate research to validate the effectiveness of such interventions, there is reason to believe that occupational therapy can help individuals improve their function at work. Specific strategies might include assistance in identifying valued work, structuring tasks, developing coping mechanisms for work-related stress, and finding satisfaction in interaction with coworkers. Another aspect of depression for which occupational therapy can be valuable is in establishing positive sleep patterns. Sleep disturbance—a common occurrence in mood disorders—can affect function and quality of life (Krystal, Thakur, & Roth, 2008); thus, an intervention to support adequate rest can have a significant impact. These interventions include examining bedtime rituals to avoid those that interrupt sleep and maximize those that support sleep, as well as developing strategies to address nighttime anxiety.

Assisting individuals in creating meaningful and satisfying patterns of occupational engagement is central to success in addressing depression. Additional interventions to accomplish this goal are discussed in the sections that follow, as they are consistent with recommended interventions for other mood disorders.

Persistent Depressive Disorder (Dysthymia)

Persistent depressive disorder is a more chronic—but typically less severe—condition than major depressive disorder. In the DSM-5 (APA, 2013), it combines the characteristics of two DSM-IV-TR (APA, 2000) conditions: chronic major depressive disorder and dysthymic disorder. The diagnostic criteria include depressed mood most of the time, with two or more other symptoms of depression that may include appetite changes, poor sleep, fatigue or low energy, low self-esteem, difficulty concentrating, and feelings of hopelessness (APA, 2013). These symptoms must have persisted for at least 2 years, with no more than a 2-month period during which the individual was symptom free.

The diagnosis is not made if the person has had a manic or hypomanic episode, and other conditions must be ruled out. The conditions that may be considered are cyclothymic disorder, schizoaffective disorder, delusional disorder, schizophrenia, and medical and substance abuse problems. In addition—and important for occupational therapy—the symptoms must cause distress or functional impairments.

The diagnostic criteria include specifiers for anxious distress; mixed, melancholic, atypical, or psychotic features; and peripartum onset. The diagnosis can also reflect partial or full remission; early or late onset; and mild, moderate, or severe symptoms. Finally, the diagnosis can describe specific characteristics of the depression in the context of major or intermittent major depressive episodes or as a pure dysthymic syndrome that has never included a major depressive episode.

Etiology

The origins of dysthymic disorder are less clear than those of major depressive disorder (Sansone & Sansone, 2009). It may be that the etiology is the same, and there is some evidence for a genetic factor in the development of the disorder, but there is no clear evidence to indicate the precise nature of a genetic origin. There is also evidence that, like major depressive disorder, stress and dysfunctional social circumstances are also contributing factors.

Prognosis

Although the disorder is less severe than major depressive disorder, it is also relatively intractable (Sansone & Sansone, 2009). One study reported that over a 5-year follow up period, 70% of individuals diagnosed with dysthymic disorder experienced depressive symptoms, compared with 40% of individuals with major depressive disorder (McQueen, 2009). When dysthymic disorder onset is early in life, it is likely to be a persistent condition (Sansone & Sansone, 2009). One reason for this may be that the symptoms are insidious, making it somewhat difficult to distinguish a period of exacerbation from normal daily emotion and behavior. In contrast, major depressive disorder symptoms are significant and easily recognizable.

Many factors make the prognosis worse, including history of sexual abuse, poor relationships with parents, comorbid mental disorders (e.g., anxiety and substance use disorders), less education, a family history of depression, and low self-efficacy (Sansone & Sansone, 2009).

Implications for Function and Treatment

Function is generally impaired to a mild or moderate degree in individuals with dysthymia. Although they typically hold jobs and have social relationships and interests, these activities are not maintained at optimal levels because of lethargy and lack of interest. Their constant depression wears on those around them, and they may lose friends as a result of their inability to enjoy activities or take pleasure in people. The chronicity of the disorder is a problem, as individuals tend to feel bad for long periods of time without relief.

Treatment for dysthymia is somewhat more problematic than for major depressive episodes (Young, Klap, Shoai, & Wells, 2008). Medication has been used with some success, although the widely touted selective serotonin reuptake inhibitors have side effects, including sexual dysfunction, which make them less ideal for some individuals. In addition, recent evidence suggests serotonin reuptake inhibitors may be less effective than initially thought. In any case, some experimentation is required to find the right drug and dose—a process that can take time and be frustrating to the individual. Cognitive behavioral therapy and psychotherapy have both been reported as somewhat helpful. A mixture of these therapies may be most effective (Sansone & Sansone, 2009).

Implications for Occupational Therapy

In general, interventions that are indicated for individuals with major depressive disorder are also indicated for individuals with dysthymic disorder. Identifying meaningful occupations, encouraging active participation, identifying strategies for understanding, expressing, and reframing emotional responses are all strategies that may ameliorate depressive symptoms. CBT focused on specific occupations can be helpful, as can psychoeducational interventions focused on learning to manage a chronic disorder.

Premenstrual Dysphoric Disorder

In the DSM-IV (APA, 1994), premenstrual dysphoric disorder (PDD) was included in the list of diagnoses found in the appendix as requiring added research. Premenstrual dysphoric disorder has been moved to the depressive disorder cluster in the DSM-5 (APA, 2013) based on a significant (although still inconclusive) body of research over the past decade. Diagnostic criteria include five or more symptoms before and during menses, including **emotional lability**—rapid and severe mood swings, irritability, depressed mood, anxiety, decreased interest in activities, poor concentration, lethargy, changes in appetite and sleep, feelings of being overwhelmed or out of control, and physical symptoms such as breast tenderness, joint pain, bloating, or weight gain (APA, 2013). The symptoms occur during most menstrual cycles for at least 1 year and improve immediately following menstruation. The condition must also interfere with the individual's daily function.

It is important to rule out major depression, cyclothymia, dysthymia, substance use, or any other medical condition.

Etiology

The precise etiology of PDD is not well understood. The presence of major depressive disorder is one risk factor (Accortt, Kogan, & Allen, 2013), as are poor physical health and psychological distress (Tschudin, Bertea, & Zemp, 2010).

Among the many hypothesized causes of PDD are genetics, hormonal and/or steroid influences, neurotransmitter alterations, nutrition and micronutrients, immunologic factors, and psychosocial factors, such as stress (Pérez-López, Chedraui, Pérez-Roncero, López-Baena, & Cuadros-López, 2009).

Prognosis

Over the long term, PDD resolves with the onset of menopause (Pérez-López et al., 2009). In the interim, a variety of mechanisms exist for minimizing symptoms, although no single treatment completely eliminates them.

Implications for Function and Treatment

Women with PDD show cognitive and functional impairments (Epperson, 2013). In particular, emotional regulation is impaired, with accompanying increased bilateral reactivity in the amygdala (Gignell, Morell, Bannbers, Wikström, & Sundström Poromaa, 2012).

Irritability may be the result of sleep disturbance (Shechter, Lespérance, Kin, Ng, & Boivin, 2012). Working memory has also been demonstrated to be impaired (Yen et al., 2012).

Women with severe PDD have higher absenteeism from work and lower productivity than other workers (Heinemann, Minh, Heinemann, Lindermann, & Filonenko, 2012); this finding is consistent globally.

Neither psychotropic medications nor CBT was found to be helpful in treating individuals with PDD (Kleinstäuber, Witthöft, & Hiller, 2012). Generally, treatment focuses on symptom management and reduction of distress during the menstrual cycle (Pérez-López et al., 2009). Diet, especially avoidance of high glycemic foods during menses, and exercise seem beneficial. Psychotropic medications may be tried in spite of a lack of evidence of their effectiveness. In addition, some clinicians advocate use of birth control medications to help regulate hormone balance.

Implications for Occupational Therapy

Because much of the treatment of PDD focuses on symptom management, occupational therapy may help to educate the client and assist her in developing habits and patterns that will minimize exacerbations. For example, the occupational therapist may work with the client to identify an exercise regimen that is appealing to the individual and is sufficiently intense to contribute to symptom reduction. In addition, strategies for managing work tasks through energy efficient activity may be helpful in avoiding the work-related functional consequences of the disorder. Table 6-2 shows the diagnostic criteria and functional implications of the various depressive disorders.

Cultural Considerations

A significant body of literature (cf., Bäärnhielm, 2013; Csordas, Storck, & Strauss, 2008; Lackey, 2008) focuses on cultural factors in depression and other psychiatric disorders. Individuals from Hispanic backgrounds are likely to emphasize the social aspects of both etiology and treatment for depression, whereas Native Americans focus on balance with the environment (Csordas et al., 2008). For example, Kuwaiti students showed greater religiosity and depression than American students, who had higher mean scores on happiness and love of life (Abdel-Khalek & Lester, 2013), and individuals from Turkey were more likely to present with somatic symptoms than individuals from Sweden (Bäärnhielm, 2013).

In the United States, significant disparities exist among racial groups in rates of depression, with African Americans being more likely to experience depression (Skarupski et al., 2005). This effect is found even when poverty, education, and other social determinants of health are controlled. Rates of suicidal behavior also differ among groups (Goldston et al., 2008) and may be the result of differing stressors and cultural distrust of help-seeking.

Not only do symptoms differ, but **explanatory models** differ as well (Grover et al., 2012). Explanatory models are the conceptualizations that individuals have regarding the causes of their symptoms. In India, depression may be attributed to karma, rather than to genetics. The differences in the explanatory model, in addition to other factors, suggest that it may be helpful to craft interventions that are sensitive to cultural difference, and there is evidence that such strategies are, in fact, more effective (Kaslow et al., 2010).

Cultural factors are also prevalent in the diagnosis, understanding, and treatment of PDD (Tschudin et al., 2010). For example, the rates of individuals diagnosed with PDD are considerably lower in East Asia than in the United States (Schatz, Hsiao, & Liu, 2012).

TABLE 6-2		
DIAGNOSTIC CRITERIA AND FUNCTIONAL CONSEQUENCES: DEPRESSIVE DISORDERS		
DISORDER	*DIAGNOSTIC CRITERIA (APA, 2013)*	*IMPLICATIONS FOR FUNCTION*
Disruptive mood dysregulation disorder	Frequent excessive temper outbursts, inappropriate for developmental stage Angry or irritable mood most of the time Lasts at least 12 months in at least two settings Onset before age 10, with diagnosis between age 6 and 18	School and social occupations disrupted. May interfere with play Deficits in emotional skills
Major depressive disorder	Five symptoms of which one is either depressed mood or anhedonia. Other symptoms may include: • Weight loss or anorexia • Insomnia or hypersomnia • Fatigue or lethargy • Feelings of guilt • Difficulty concentrating • Suicidal ideation or attempt Distress and dysfunction Not a grief reaction	Difficulty with social, work, leisure occupations May have reduced ability to manage activities of daily living (ADL) and instrumental activities of daily living (IADL) Habits, roles, routines deteriorate during major depressive episodes Motor, process, and communication slowing All improve between episodes
Persistent depressive disorder (dysthymia)	Depressed mood much of the time over at least 2 years At least two persistent symptoms: • Appetite changes (poor eating or overeating) • Sleep disruption • Fatigue or low energy • Low self-esteem • Poor concentration • Feelings of hopelessness No manic or hypomanic episode or cyclothymic disorder	Same as major depressive disorder but less severe More persistent and chronic
		(continued)

TABLE 6-2 (CONTINUED)		
DIAGNOSTIC CRITERIA AND FUNCTIONAL CONSEQUENCES: DEPRESSIVE DISORDERS		
DISORDER	*DIAGNOSTIC CRITERIA (APA, 2013)*	*IMPLICATIONS FOR FUNCTION*
Premenstrual dysphoric disorder	At least five symptoms during most menstrual cycles, improving after menstruation At least one of: • Emotional lability • Irritability, anger • Depressed mood • Anxiety, tension And other possible symptoms: • Decreased interest in activities • Difficulty concentrating • Lethargy or fatigue • Change in appetite • Sleep changes • Feelings of being overwhelmed • Breast tenderness, joint or muscle pain, a sensation of bloating Distress and dysfunction	Deficits in work occupations in particular, possibly social and leisure Possibly cognitive and emotional regulation skills Remit during weeks between menstrual periods

These differences impact occupational therapy intervention because of the effect of culture on occupational preferences and enactment. For example, in some countries, autonomy and independence have less salience than in the United States (Marbell & Grolnick, 2013). In Ghana, for example, parent–child interactions emphasize communal, group-focused behaviors. When children enter school, where more individualistic values are promoted, parent–child relationships can suffer, leading to depression in the children.

Lifespan Considerations

Special note should be made about depression in children and youth. These diagnoses are becoming more common in children and adolescents (Moreno et al., 2007), and childhood depression can have serious, lifelong consequences (Miller, 2007).

Children who are depressed may present with symptoms that reflect their developmental stage, including anxiety, school phobias, or difficulty sleeping. School refusal or negative behaviors are also common signs of depression (Frühe et al., 2012). School and social function are likely to be impaired. At the same time, it may be difficult for children to articulate the problem (or even state that it exists). As with adults, low self-esteem is common. Teens often become sullen and withdrawn—a behavior that should not be written off as "just a phase," as adolescents are at considerable risk for depression (Cronin, 2001).

Play therapy may help the child to express feelings nonverbally. It appears that for children, symptoms differ depending on the severity of the depression; higher levels of depression are associated with psychomotor and appetite disturbance, as well as suicidal ideation (Cole et al., 2011). Adolescents benefit from opportunities of self-expression (perhaps through creative arts), social activities, and sports that may offer opportunities to build self-confidence. Intervention must be sensitive to the age and stage of the individual child. Involving parents in the treatment process is important, especially with younger children (Luby, Lenze, & Tillman, 2012).

At the other end of the age spectrum, mood disorders are also very common (Wu, Schimmele, & Chappell, 2012). One notable difference is that the gender disparity in the rates of diagnosis is reduced in older populations (Harkness et al., 2010). A variety of life circumstances appear to have either contributory or mediating effects on depression in later life. For example, older adults who are employed have lower rates of depression. Although this may be an artifact (that is, those who are not depressed are less likely to choose to retire because they have more energy), it suggests the importance of continuing to have valued occupations in late life (Christ et al., 2007).

The presentation of depression in later life can be quite different than in younger individuals. In particular, care providers need to recognize that symptoms of dementia may reflect depression. Dementia that is characterized by poverty of response and lethargy typifies late-life depression for some individuals. One specific presentation of depression in later life is vascular depression, an event that occurs in approximately one third of stroke clients (O'Donoghue & Ryan, 2011). This condition is a reminder of the extent to which physical and mental disorders are linked. Although there is evidence that depression in late life has a biological component, there is also evidence that negative life events contribute to the development of the disorder (Kraaij, Arensman, & Spinhoven, 2002).

Older adults who are depressed demonstrate a number of functional deficits (Lenze et al., 2005) and report poor quality of life. They also report poor health and decreased independence. Three effective treatments for depression in late life are psychotherapy, pharmacotherapy, and ECT (O'Donoghue & Ryan, 2011). Occupational therapy can make a significant difference for elders in both terms of enhancing patterns of meaningful occupations and providing strategies such as assistive devices that support function (Mann et al., 2008). In fact, evidence exists that suicide risk among older adults is associated with their feelings of being burdens to their families (John & Cukrowicz, 2011). Interventions to assist elders in maintaining independence and a sense of meaning may ameliorate these feelings. Expressive therapies, including life review writing, can foster such sense of meaning (Chippendale & Bear-Lehman, 2012).

Identifying and Managing Suicide Risk

Suicide is a particular concern related to mood disorders (Hawton, Casañas, Comabella, Haw, & Saunders, 2013). In 2007, the National Institute of Mental Health (NIMH) reported that suicide was the 10th leading cause of death in the United States, with 11.3 deaths for every 100,000 people. The rate of suicide attempts was 11 times the number of completed suicides (NIMH, n.d.). Suicide rates are particularly high among older adults and adolescents.

Approximately 60% of all suicides are associated with depression. Many individuals with depression or bipolar disorder contemplate suicide, and those who appear to have active suicidal intent may require hospitalization to prevent them from harming themselves. There is also some evidence that suicide risk is higher during exacerbations of premenstrual dysphoric disorder (Pilver, Libby, & Hoff, 2013). The problem of suicidal intent is a concern because the antidepressant medications that may be used to treat the disorder can be lethal if taken in too large a dose, thus requiring careful monitoring—especially before the drugs have taken effect in elevating mood, which is a process that can take several weeks.

Professionals who work with depressed individuals must be aware of the potential for suicide, and they should note the presence of suicidal risk in these individuals and take the necessary precautions to prevent it (Rihmer, & Gonda, 2012). Professionals should ask the individual directly whether he or she is suicidal and determine whether he or she has a plan of action. If a plan exists, assessing the extent to which it can be lethal is important. An individual with a loaded gun in the car is at higher risk than one who is thinking about finding someone who can get him or her some pills. Because many suicidal individuals are actually looking for an "avenue of escape" (Tummey, 2001, p. 41), they may well answer honestly and accept assistance in finding other, less damaging, methods to resolve their difficulties.

Although the responsibility for assessing a client's suicidal ideation falls primarily to the main therapist (i.e., team leader or psychiatrist), other professionals must also be alert to suicide risk in clients (NIMH, n.d.). Particular suicide risk factors include the following:

- Having a clear and feasible plan
- Showing sudden significant improvement in mood (this may signify that they have made a decision to act)
- Showing early signs that medication is effective (the individual has increased energy to act)

Suicide precautions include careful monitoring, often in inpatient settings, and removal of means to cause death until the individual is clearly no longer actively suicidal (Tummey, 2001). Contracting with the client (i.e., having the client agree he or she will not make any suicide gesture) is also helpful (Drew, 2001). Although most suicide attempts are made with drugs and guns, access to other lethal substances and sharp implements should be monitored as well.

Occupational therapists should be sensitive to the use of sharp tools and toxic solvents by suicidal clients in their care. A belief exists that some single-car accidents are, in fact, suicide attempts; therefore, it may be necessary to monitor driving—especially when accompanied by drinking—in suicidal individuals. Occupational therapists should report any expressions of suicidal ideation to the primary therapist without delay and should never assume that these are idle threats. It is also useful to be aware that occupational therapy interventions might focus on engagement in occupation for adolescents (Ramey et al., 2010) and social support (Kleiman & Liu, 2013), both of which have been shown to reduce suicide risk.

Children and adolescents, as well as adults, who are depressed are at risk of suicide (Kerr, Reinki, & Eddy, 2013). A wish to reunite with a deceased loved one or to punish an adult is a common motivation for suicide attempts in this age group. Teens who become sullen and withdrawn should be watched carefully. It should not be assumed that the adolescent is just "going through a phase." One particular dilemma in working with children and adolescents who are depressed is there is strong evidence that psychotropic medications can inaugurate suicidal impulses in these individuals. Particular vigilance is needed when younger clients are given these drugs (Olfson & Marcus, 2008).

Suicide risk is also high among individuals with HIV or at high risk of acquiring HIV (e.g., homosexuals and intravenous drug users; Shelton et al., 2006). Individuals with physical illnesses that cause significant pain are at high risk for suicide as well. Another high-risk group is older adults, among whom the suicide rate is almost twice that of younger adults (Crumpacker, 2008). It is hypothesized that stressors, such as loss of spouse, retirement, and reduced economic circumstances, contribute to this risk.

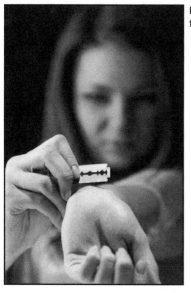

Figure 6-2. Suicides cause significant emotional pain for friends, family, and staff involved in care. (©2014 Shutterstock.com.)

The staff in inpatient settings will need to deal with the feelings of other clients, as well as their own, when a suicide attempt or completed suicide occurs in the unit. Although precautions can reduce the incidence, individuals who are determined to complete a suicide are quite difficult to stop (Figure 6-2). However, the majority of suicide attempts are a cry for help. Careful attention to warning signs can reduce the incidence of both attempts and completed suicides. In either case, it is important to recognize that although suicide attempts and completed suicides express the individual's pain, they are also an expression of anger, which can be challenging for family, friends, and staff to address—in the individual and in themselves.

Internet Resources

American Academy of Child and Adolescent Psychiatry Depression Resource Center
http://www.aacap.org/AACAP/Families_and_Youth/Resource_Centers/Depression_Resource_Center/Home.aspx
Good resource for professionals and families, with a focus on depression in young people.

Depression and Bipolar Support Alliance
http://www.dbsalliance.org/site/PageServer?pagename=education_resources
A self-help organization with a specific focus on mood disorders. Includes many helpful links.

Medscape
http://www.medscape.com/resource/depression
Medscape is a terrific source of information about all things medical. It does require a sign in, but it is free. The site frequently updates current knowledge about a wide range of medical topics, lectures, continuing medical education offerings, and other resources.

National Library of Medicine, PubMed Health
http://www.ncbi.nlm.nih.gov/pubmedhealth/PMH0002844/
Links to other helpful sources of information. Also links to research/evidence reviews and other PubMed resources.

CASE STUDY

Mary Phillips is a 53-year-old African American widow. She has four children, ranging in age from 16 to 25. Two of her daughters live with her, along with four grandchildren, who are between 1 and 5 years old. One of Mrs. Phillips' daughters had to leave her abusive husband and has been unemployed and living with Mrs. Phillips. The daughter is unmotivated and lethargic, and she has been unable to get herself organized to find a job and move out. Mrs. Phillips has encouraged her to seek care, but the daughter has resisted, and Mrs. Phillips has taken primary responsibility for looking after the grandchildren, given her daughter's difficulty in doing so. The other daughter in the home tries to help with the children and the housework, but she holds two minimum wage jobs so is often unavailable.

The other two children live nearby, but Mrs. Phillips sees them infrequently. When she calls to ask how they are doing, they report that they're "very busy" and that they will visit soon. However, they rarely follow up on this promise.

Because her children and grandchildren need her help, she has little time for friends. This lack of social connection is troubling to her, but she does not have time to build a social network. Although she attends church every Sunday, she has stopped her involvement in the sisterhood. She is a member of an African American sorority, but she has not participated actively in the past several years.

Mrs. Phillips used to be an elementary school teacher, but she quit when her third child was born. Her husband was an accountant. He died 4 years ago and left Mrs. Phillips with a fairly comfortable pension. She has been reluctant to go back to work, given her home responsibilities, although she often feels bored and at loose ends. She has been lethargic and unmotivated since her husband's death. She finds herself frequently tearful, and she has lost weight. Her pastor suggested several times that she might have a thyroid condition, and he has urged her to get a checkup. She finally seeks help from a physician in a primary care walk-in clinic because she has had great difficulty sleeping and is exhausted.

The physician gives Mrs. Phillips a careful examination and can find no physical reason for her lack of energy and difficulty sleeping. He refers her to a psychiatrist. Although somewhat reluctant to go, Mrs. Phillips finally makes an appointment. The psychiatrist diagnoses depression and provides her with antidepressant medication and a referral to occupational therapy.

An occupational profile interview with the occupational therapist reveals that Mrs. Phillips used to have a lot of valued occupations, but she currently feels obligated to her family and feels guilty when she does not give them enough of her time and attention. She also feels guilty about her resentment of her children and grandchildren, and she feels sad that she does not have warmer feelings toward them.

THOUGHT QUESTIONS

1. What functional deficits are evident in Mrs. Phillips' current situation?
2. Of these deficits, which might be most critical to first address?
3. What are some factors in Mrs. Phillips' history that could help structure a meaningful occupational profile?
4. Do you feel that Mrs. Phillips might be at risk for suicide? What factors lead you to this conclusion?

References

Abdel-Khalek, A., & Lester, D. (2013). Mental health, subjective well-being, and religiosity: Significant associations in Kuwait and USA. *Journal of Muslim Mental Health, 7*(2), 64-76.

Accortt, E.E., Kogan, A.V., & Allen, J.J. (2013). Personal history of major depression may put women at risk for premenstrual dysphoric symptomatology. *Journal of Affective Disorders, 150*(3), 1234-1237.

Alladin, A. (2012). Cognitive hypnotherapy for major depressive disorder. *American Journal of Clinical Hypnosis, 54*(4), 275-293.

American Psychiatric Association. (1994). *Diagnostic and statistical manual of mental disorders* (4th ed.). Washington, DC: Author.

American Psychiatric Association. (2000). *Diagnostic and statistical manual of mental disorders* (4th ed., text revision). Washington, DC: Author.

American Psychiatric Association. (2013). *Diagnostic and statistical manual of mental disorders* (5th ed.). Washington, DC: Author.

Bäärnhielm, S. (2013). Depression and 'somatization' among two divergent cultural groups. In S. Barnow & N. Balkir (Eds.), *Cultural variations in psychopathology: From research to practice* (pp. 154-172). Cambridge, MA: Hogrefe.

Bazyk, S. (2011). *Mental health promotion, prevention and intervention with children and youth: A guiding framework for occupational therapy*. Washington, DC: American Occupational Therapy Association.

Belmaker, R.H., & Agam, G. (2008). Mechanisms of disease: Major depressive disorder. *The New England Journal of Medicine, 358*(1), 55-68.

Bender, A. (2011). Restoring function in MDD: Balancing efficacy and tolerability to optimally manage major depressive disorder. *Canadian Journal of Diagnosis, 28*, 13-20.

Chippendale, T., & Bear-Lehman, J. (2012). Effect of life review writing on depressive symptoms in older adults: A randomized controlled trial. *American Journal of Occupational Therapy, 66*, 438-446.

Christ, S.L., Lee, D.J., Fleming, L.E., LeBlanc, W.G., Arheart, K.L., Chung-Bridges, K., . . . McCollister, K.E. (2007). Employment and occupation effects on depressive symptoms in older Americans: Does working past age 65 protect against depression? *Journal of Gerontology: Social Sciences, 62B*(6), S399-S403.

Cole, D.A., Cai, L., Martin, N., Findling, R., Youngstrom, E., Garber, J., . . . Forehand, R. (2011). Structure and measurement of depression in youths: Applying item response theory to clinical data. *Psychological Assessment, 23*, 819-833.

Copeland, W.E., Angold, A., Costello, E.J., & Egger, H. (2013). Prevalence, comorbidity, and correlates of DSM-5 proposed disruptive mood dysregulation disorder. *American Journal of Psychiatry, 170*(2), 173-179.

Creek, J. (2006). Living with depression: Function, activity and participation. *Mental Health Occupational Therapy, 11*(2), 47-49.

Cronin, A.F. (2001). Psychosocial and emotional domains. In J. Case-Smith (Ed.), *Occupational therapy for children* (4th ed., pp. 413-452). St. Louis, MO: Mosby.

Crumpacker, D.W. (2008). Suicidality and antidepressants in the elderly. *Baylor University Medical Center Proceedings, 21*, 373-377.

Csordas, T.J., Storck, M.J., & Strauss, M. (2008). Diagnosis and distress in Navajo healing. *Journal of Nervous and Mental Disease, 196*, 585-596.

Deibler, M.W. (2013, May 17). The DSM-5 is not crazy. *Slate*. Retrieved from http://www.slate.com/articles/health_and_science/medical_examiner/2013/05/defense_of_the_dsm_5_new_diagnoses_for_picking_bingeing_and_tantrums.html.

Drew, B.L. (2001). Self-harm behavior and no-suicide contracting in psychiatric in-patient settings. *Archives of Psychiatric Nursing, 15*(3), 99-106.

Dunner, D.L. (2008). Major depressive disorder. In S.H. Fatemi & P.J. Clayton (Eds.), *The medical basis of psychiatry* (3rd ed., pp. 73-83). Totowa, NJ: Humana.

Epperson, C.N. (2013). Premenstrual dysphoric disorder and the brain. *American Journal of Psychiatry, 170*(3), 248-252.

Feliciano, L., Segal. D.L., & Vair, C.L. (2011). Major depressive disorder. In K.H. Sorocco & S. Lauderdale (Eds.), *Cognitive behavior therapy with older adults: Innovations across care settings* (p. 31-64). New York, NY: Springer.

Freeman, M.P., Fava, M., Lake, J., Trivedi, M.H., Wisner, K.L., & Mischoulon, D. (2010). Complementary and alternative medicine in major depressive disorder: The American Psychiatric Association Task Force report. *Journal of Clinical Psychiatry, 71*(6), 669-681.

Fresco, D.M., Flynn, J.J., Mennin, D.S., & Haigh, E.A.P. (2011). Mindfulness-based cognitive therapy. In J.D. Herbert & E.M. Forman (Eds.), *Acceptance and mindfulness in cognitive behavior therapy: Understanding and applying the new therapies* (pp. 57-82). Hoboken, NJ: John Wiley & Sons.

Frühe, B., Allgaier, A., Pietsch, K., Baethmann, M., Peters, J., Kellnar, S., . . . Schulte-Körne, G. (2012). Children's depression screener (ChilD-S): Development and validation of a depression screening instrument for children in pediatric care. *Child Psychiatry and Human Development, 43*(1), 137-151.

Gallagher, P., Robinson, L.J., Gray, J.M., Porter, R.J., & Young, A.H. (2007). Neurocognitive function following remission in major depressive disorder: Potential objective marker of response? *Australian & New Zealand Journal of Psychiatry, 41*(1), 54-61.

Georgiades, M., Kyloudis, P.L., Rekleiti, M., Bagiatis, V., Wozniak, G., & Roupa, Z. (2012). Cumulative effect of psychotherapy in remission of symptomatology of major depressive disorder. *Health Science Journal, 26*(1), 45-59.

Gignell, M., Morell, A., Bannbers, E., Wikström, J, & Sundström Poromaa, I. (2012). Menstrual cycle effects on amygdala reactivity to emotional stimulation in premenstrual dysphoric disorder. *Hormones and Behavior, 62*(4), 400-406.

Godard, J., Grondin, S., Baruch, P., & Lafleur, M.F. (2011). Psychosocial and neurocognitive profiles in depressed patients with major depressive disorder and bipolar disorder. *Psychiatry Research, 190*(2-3), 244-252.

Goldston, D.B., Molock., S.D., Whitbeck, L.B., Murakami, J.L., Zayas, L.H., & Hall, G.C.N. (2008). Cultural considerations in adolescent suicide prevention and psychosocial treatment. *American Psychologist, 63*(2), 14-31.

Grover, S., Kumar, V., Chakrabarti, S., Hollikati, P., Singh, P., Tyagi, S., . . . Avasthi, A. (2012). Explanatory models in patients with first-episode depression: A study from North India. *Asian Journal of Psychiatry, 5*(3), 251-257.

Harkness, K.L., Alavi, N., Monroe, S.M., Slavich, G.M., Gotlib, I.H., & Bagby, R.M. (2010). Gender differences in life events prior to onset of major depressive disorder: The moderating effect of age. *Journal of Abnormal Psychology, 119*(4), 791-803.

Hawton, K., Casañas, I., Comabella, C., Haw, C., & Saunders, K. (2013). Risk factors for suicide in individuals with depression: A systematic review. *Journal of Affective Disorders, 147*(1-3), 17-28.

Heinemann, L.A.J., Minh, T.D., Heinemann, K., Lindermann, M., & Filonenko, A. (2012). Intercountry assessment of the impact of severe premenstrual disorders on work and daily activities. *Health Care for Women International, 33*(2), 109-124.

Hornig, M., Briese, T., Licinio, J., Khabbaz, R.F., Altschuler, L.L., Potkin, S.G., . . . Lipkin, W.I. (2012). Absence of evidence for bornavirus infection in schizophrenia, bipolar disorder and major depressive disorder. *Molecular Psychiatry, 17*(5), 486-493.

Huijbregts, K.M.L., van der Feltz-Cornelis, C.M., van Marwijk, H.W.J., de Jong, F.J., van der Windt, D.A.W.M., & Beekman, A.T.F. (2010). Negative association of concomitant physical symptoms with the course of major depressive disorder: A systematic review. *Journal of Psychosomatic Research, 68*(6), 511-519.

Huuhka, K., Viikki, M., Tammentie, T., Tuohimaa, K., Björkqvist , M., Alanen, H., . . . Kampman, O. (2012). One-year follow-up after discontinuing maintenance electroconvulsive therapy. *Journal of ECT, 28*(4), 225-228.

IsHak, W., William, C., Christensen, S., Sayer, G., Ha, K., Li, N., . . . Cohen, R.M. (2013). Sexual satisfaction and quality of life in major depressive disorder before and after treatment with citalopram in the STARD Study. *Journal of Clinical Psychiatry, 74*(3), 256-261.

Jabbi, M., Korf, J., Ormel, J., Kema, I.P., & den Boer, J.A. (2009). Investigating the molecular basis of major depressive disorder etiology: A functional convergent genetic approach. In R. Kvetňanský, G., Aguilera, D. Goldstein, D. Goldstein, D. Jezova, O. Krizanova, . . . K. Pacak (Eds.), *Stress, neurotransmitters, and hormones: Neuroendocrine and genetic mechanisms* (pp. 42-56). New York, NY: New York Academy of Sciences.

John, D.R., & Cukrowicz, K.C. (2011). The mediating effect of perceived burdensomeness on the relation between depressive symptoms and suicide ideation in a community sample of older adults. *Aging & Mental Health, 15*, 214-220.

Kaslow, N.J., Leiner, A.S., Reviere, S., Jackson, E., Bethea, K., Bhaju, J., . . . Thompson, M.P. (2010). Suicidal, abused African American women's response to a culturally informed intervention. *Journal of Counseling and Clinical Psychology, 78*, 449-458.

Kerr, D.C.R., Reinki, W.M., & Eddy, J.M. (2013). Trajectories of depressive symptoms and externalizing behaviors across adolescence: Associations with histories of suicide attempt and ideation in early adulthood. *Suicide and Life-Threatening Behavior, 43*(1), 50-66.

Kleiman, E.M., & Liu, R.T. (2013). Social support as a protective factor in suicide: Findings from two nationally representative samples. *Journal of Affective Disorders, 150*(2), 540-545.

Kleinstäuber, M., Witthöft, M., & Hiller, W. (2012). Cognitive-behavioral and pharmacological interventions for premenstrual syndrome or premenstrual dysphoric disorder: A meta-analysis. *Journal of Clinical Psychology in Medical Settings, 19*(3), 308-319.

Kraaij, V., Arensman, E., & Spinhoven, P. (2002). Negative life events and depression in elderly persons: A meta-analysis. *Journal of Gerontology: Psychological Sciences, 57B*, P87-P94.

Krishnadas, R., & Cavanagh, J. (2012). Depression: An inflammatory illness? *Journal of Neurology, Neurosurgery & Psychiatry, 83*(5), 495-502.

Krystal, A.D., Thakur, M., & Roth, T. (2008). Sleep disturbance in psychiatric disorders: Effects on function and quality of life in mood disorders, alcoholism, and schizophrenia. *Annals of Clinical Psychiatry, 20*(1), 39-46.

Lackey, G.F. (2008). "Feeling blue" in Spanish: A qualitative inquiry of depression among Mexican immigrants. *Social Science and Medicine, 67*, 228-237.

Lenze, E.J., Schulz, R., Martire, L., Zdaniuk, B., Glass, T., Kop, W., . . . Reynolds, C.F. (2005). The course of functional decline in older people with persistently elevated depressive symptoms: Longitudinal findings from the cardiovascular health study. *Journal of the American Geriatric Society, 53*, 569-575.

Leppänen, J.M. (2006). Emotional information processing in mood disorders: A review of behavioral and neuroimaging findings. *Current Opinion in Psychiatry, 19*(1), 34-39.

Lohr, J.B., May, T., & Caligiuri, M.P. (2013). Quantitative assessment of motor abnormalities in untreated patients with major depressive disorder. *Journal of Affective Disorders, 146*(1), 84-90.

Luby, J., Lenze, S., & Tillman, R. (2012). A novel early intervention for preschool depression: Findings from a pilot randomized controlled trial. *Journal of Child Psychology and Psychiatry, 53*, 313-322.

Maeshima, H., Baba, H., Nakano, Y., Satomura, E., Namekawa, Y., Takebayashi, N., . . . Arai, H. (2012). Residual memory dysfunction in recurrent major depressive disorder—A longitudinal study from Juntendo University Mood Disorder Project. *Journal of Affective Disorders, 143*(1-3), 84-8.

Mann, W.C., Johnson, J.L., Lynch, L.G., Justiss, M.D., Tomita, M., & Wu, S.S. (2008). Changes in impairment level, functional status, and use of assistive devices by older people with depressive symptoms. *American Journal of Occupational Therapy, 62*, 9-17.

Marbell, K.N., & Grolnick, W.S. (2013). Correlates of parental control and autonomy support in an interdependent culture: A look at Ghana. *Motivation and Emotion, 37*(1), 79-92.

Margulies, D.M., Weintraub, S., Basile, J., Grover, P.J., & Carlson, G.A. (2012). Will disruptive mood dysregulation disorder reduce false diagnosis of bipolar disorder in children? *Bipolar Disorders, 14*(5), 488-496.

Martiny, K., Refsgaard, E., Lund, V., Lunde, M., Sørensen, L., Thougaard, B., . . . Bech, P. (2012). A 9-week randomized trial comparing chronotherapeutic intervention (wake and light therapy) to exercise in major depressive disorder patients treated with duloxetine. *Journal of Clinical Psychiatry, 73*(9), 1234-1242.

Mast, B.T. (2010). Vascular depression: Cardiovascular implications for mental health. In K.E. Whitfield (Ed.), *Annual review of gerontology & geriatrics* (pp. 135-154). New York, NY: Springer.

Mata, J., Thompson, R.J., Jaeggi, S.M., Buschkuehl, M., Jonides, J., & Gotlib, I.H. (2011). Walk on the bright side: Physical activity and affect in major depressive disorder. *Journal of Abnormal Psychology, 121*(2), 297-308 .

McQueen, D. (2009). Depression in adults: Some basic facts. *Psychoanalytic Psychotherapy, 23*(3), 225-235.

Miller, A. (2007). Social neuroscience of child and adolescent depression. *Brain and Cognition, 65*(1), 47-68.

Moreno, C., Laje, G., Blanco, C., Jiang, H., Schmidt, A.B., & Olfson, M. (2007). National trends in the outpatient diagnosis and treatment of bipolar disorder in youth. *Archives of General Psychiatry, 64*, 1032-1039.

Morris, B.H., Bylsma, L.M., & Rottenberg, J. (2009). Does emotion predict the course of major depressive disorder? A review of prospective studies. *British Journal of Clinical Psychology, 48*(3), 255-273.

Mota-Pereira, J., Carvalho, S., Silverio, J., Fonte, D., Pizarro, A., Teixeira, J., . . . Ramos, J. (2011). Moderate physical exercise and quality of life in patients with treatment-resistant major depressive disorder. *Journal of Psychiatric Research, 45*(12), 1657-1659.

Muñoz, R.F., Beardslee, W.R., & Leykin, Y. (2012). Major depression can be prevented. *American Psychologist, 67*(4), 285-295.

National Institute of Mental Health. (n.d.). *Statistics.* Retrieved from http://www.nimh.nih.gov/health/publications/suicide-in-the-us-statistics-and-prevention/index.shtml.

Nieuwenhuijsen, K., Bültmann, U., Neumeyer-Gromen, A., Verhoeven, A.C., Verbeek, J.H.A., & van der Feltz-Cornelis, C.M. (2008). Interventions to improve occupational health in depressed persons. *Cochrane Database of Systematic Reviews*, Issue 2, CD006237.

O'Donoghue, M., & Ryan, P. (2011). Depression and ageing: Assessment and intervention. In P. Ryan & B.J. Coughlan (Eds.), *Ageing and older adult mental health: Issues and implications for practice* (pp. 127-142). New York, NY: Routledge/Taylor & Francis.

Olfson, M., & Marcus, S.C. (2008). A case-control study of antidepressants and attempted suicide during early phase treatment of major depressive episodes. *Journal of Clinical Psychiatry, 69*, 425-432.

Parikh, S.V., Segal, Z.V., Grigoriadis, S., Ravidindran, A.V., Kennedy, S.H. Lam, R.W., . . . Patten, S.B. (2009) Canadian Network for Mood and Anxiety Treatments (CANMAT) clinical guidelines for the management of major depressive disorder in adults. II. Psychotherapy alone or in combination with antidepressant medication. *Journal of Affective Disorders, 117*(Suppl. 1), S15-S25.

Pérez-López, F.R., Chedraui, P., Pérez-Roncero, G., López-Baena, M.T., & Cuadros-López, J.L. (2009). Premenstrual syndrome and premenstrual dysphoric disorder: Symptoms and cluster influences. *Open Psychiatry Journal, 3*, 39-49.

Pies, R.W. (2013, January 24). Bereavement does not immunize against major depression. *Medscape.* Retrieved from http://www.medscape.com/viewarticle/777960.

Pilver, C.E., Libby, D.J., & Hoff, R.A. (2013). Premenstrual dysphoric disorder as a correlate of suicidal ideation, plans, and attempts among a nationally representative sample. *Social Psychiatry and Psychiatric Epidemiology, 48*(3), 437-446.

Pirl, W.F., Greer, J., Temel. J.S., Yeap, B.Y., & Gilman, S.E. (2009). Major depressive disorder in long-term cancer survivors: Analysis of the national comorbidity survey replication. *Journal of Clinical Oncology, 27*(25), 4130-4134.

Ramey, H.L., Busseri, M.A., Khanna, N., Hamilton, Y.N., Résau Ado Ottawa, Y.N., & Rose-Krasnor, L. (2010). Youth engagement and suicide risk: Testing a mediated model in a Canadian community sample. *Journal of Youth and Adolescence, 39*(3), 243-258.

Reblin, M., & Uchino, B.N. (2008). Social and emotional support and its implications for health. *Current Opinion in Psychiatry, 21*, 201-205.

Rehman, U.S., Gollan, J., & Mortimer, A.R. (2008). The marital context of depression: Research, limitations, and new directions. *Clinical Psychology Review, 28*, 179-198.

Rhebergen, D., Lamers, F., Spijker, J., de Graaf, R., Beekman, A.T.F., & Penninx, B.W.H.H. (2012). Course trajectories of unipolar depressive disorders identified by latent class growth analysis. *Psychological Medicine, 42*(7), 1383-1396.

Rihmer, Z., & Gonda, X. (2012). Prevention of depression-related suicides in primary care. *Psychiatria Hungarica, 27*(2), 72-81.

Rogers, J.C., & Holm, M.B. (2000). Daily-living skills and habits of older women with depression. *Occupational Therapy Journal of Research, 20*(Suppl. 1), 68S-85S.

Sansone, R.A., & Sansone, L.A. (2009). Dysthymic disorder: Forlorn and overlooked? *Psychiatry (Edgmont), 6*(5), 46-50.

Schatz, D.B., Hsiao, M., & Liu, C. (2012). Premenstrual dysphoric disorder in East Asia: A review of the literature. *International Journal of Psychiatry in Medicine, 43*(4), 365-380.

Shechter, A., Lespérance, P., Kin, N. M. K., Ng, Y., & Boivin, D.B. (2012). Nocturnal polysomnographic sleep across the menstrual cycle in premenstrual dysphoric disorder. *Sleep Medicine, 13*(8), 1071-1078.

Shelton, A.J., Atkinson, J., Risser, J.M.H., McCurdy, S.A., Useche, B., & Padgett, P.M. (2006). The prevalence of suicidal behaviours in a group of HIV-positive men. *AIDS Care, 18*, 574-576.

Shorter, E., & Healy, D. (2007). *Shock therapy: A history of electroconvulsive treatment in mental illness.* New Brunswick, NJ: Rutgers University Press.

Skarupski, K.A., Mendes de Leon, C.F., Bienias, J.L., Barnes, L.L., Everson-Rose, S.A., Wilson, R.S., & Evans, D.A. (2005). Black-white differences in depressive symptoms among older adults over time. *Journal of Gerontology: Psychological Sciences, 60B*(3), P136-P142.

Starkstein, S.E., Merello, M., Jorge, R., Brockman, S., Bruce, D., Petracca, G., & Robinson, R.G. (2008). A validation study of depressive syndromes in Parkinson's disease. *Movement Disorders, 23*(4), 538-546.

Stetka, B.S., & Correll, C.U. (2013). A guide to DSM-5. Retrieved from http://www.medscape.com/viewarticle/803884_10.

Thase, M.E. (2012). Social skills training for depression and comparative efficacy research: A 30-year retrospective. *Behavior Modification, 36*(4), 545-557.

Tschudin, S., Bertea, P.C., & Zemp, E. (2010). Prevalence and predictors of premenstrual syndrome and premenstrual dysphoric disorder in a population-based sample. *Archives of Women's Mental Health, 13*(6), 485-494.

Tummey, R. (2001). A collaborative approach to urgent mental health referrals. *Suicide Prevention, 15*(52), 39-42.

Van Lieshout, R.J., Bienenstock, J., & MacQueen, G.M. (2009). A review of candidate pathways underlying the association between asthma and major depressive disorder. *Psychosomatic Medicine, 71*(2), 187-195.

Wagner, S., Doering, B., Helreich, I., Lieb, K., & Tadić, A. (2012). A meta-analysis of executive dysfunctions in unipolar major depressive disorder without psychotic symptoms and their changes during antidepressant treatment. *Acta Psychiatrica Scandinavica, 125*(4), 281-292.

Wang, J.L., Patten, S.B., Currie, S., Sareen, J., & Schmitz, N. (2012). Predictors of 1-year outcomes of major depressive disorder among individuals with a lifetime diagnosis: A population-based study. *Psychological Medicine, 42*(2), 327-334.

Wray, N.R., Pergadia, M.L., Blackwood, D.H.R., Penninx, B.W.J.H., Gordon, S.D., Nyholt, D.R., . . . Sullivan, P.F. (2012). Genome-wide association study of major depressive disorder: New results, meta-analysis, and lessons learned. *Molecular Psychiatry, 17*(1), 36-48.

Wu, Z., Schimmele, C.M., & Chappell, N.L. (2012). Aging and late-life depression. *Journal of Aging and Health, 24*(1), 3-28.

Yen, J., Chang, S., Long, C., Tang, T., Chen, C., & Yen, C. (2012). Working memory deficit in premenstrual dysphoric disorder and its associations with difficulty in concentrating and irritability. *Comprehensive Psychiatry, 53*(5), 540-545.

Young, A.S., Klap, R., Shoai, R., & Wells, K.B. (2008). Persistent depression and anxiety in the United States: Prevalence and quality of care. *Psychiatric Services, 59,* 1391-1398.

Zepf, F.D., & Holtmann, M. (2012). Disruptive mood dysregulation disorder: Mood disorders. In J.M.Rey (Ed.), *IACAPAP e-textbook of child and adolescent mental health.* Geneva, Switzerland: IACAPAP. Retrieved from http://iacapap.org/wp-content/uploads/E.3-MOOD-DYSREGULATION-072012.pdf.

Anxiety
Disorders

Learning Outcomes

By the end of this chapter, readers will be able to:

- Describe the symptoms of anxiety disorders
- Differentiate among the anxiety disorders on the basis of symptoms and onset
- Identify the causes of anxiety disorders
- Discuss the ways in which anxiety disorders affect daily function
- Describe treatment strategies for anxiety disorders
- Discuss occupational therapy interventions for anxiety disorders

Bonder B.
Psychopathology and Function, Fifth Edition (pp 159-180).
© 2015 SLACK Incorporated.

KEY WORDS

- Psychodynamic
- Successive approximation
- Systematic desensitization
- Panic attack

- Paresthesias
- Derealization
- Depersonalization
- Dissociative

CASE VIGNETTE

Sam Levin is a 7-year-old second-grader who lives with his parents and two older sisters in a suburb of a large southern city. Sam has always been a somewhat shy and reticent child. When he was younger, he got very upset each time his parents went out for the evening, leaving the children with a sitter. He also had great difficulty getting started in preschool. For the first 3 months he was in preschool, he cried for hours after his mother left him. He finally made the adjustment and seemed to like the school thereafter, although after every school holiday he was somewhat reluctant to start back again.

At the start of the current school year, Sam again was reluctant to return to school. He dawdled in the mornings while getting ready and frequently missed the school bus. He complained almost daily of a stomach ache, and began, once again, to cry when he had to leave home. When questioned, he said he was afraid his mother was going to die while he was at school. Indeed, he began to follow her around the house, expressing great worry that she would die.

His parents assumed that as he adjusted to the new school year, his worry would diminish, but the behavior became more pronounced. On two occasions, his mother had to pick him up from school after he became inconsolably upset during routine fire drills. He began to refuse to go outside to play after school and turned down play dates and sleepovers with friends. The behavior has now persisted for several months and shows no signs of abating.

THOUGHT QUESTIONS

1. Do you think that Sam has a mental disorder?
2. What characteristics of the description contribute to your conclusion?
3. How do you think his behaviors might affect his daily function? In what occupations?

ANXIETY DISORDERS

- Separation anxiety disorder
- Selective mutism
- Specific phobia
- Social anxiety disorder (social phobia)

- Panic disorder
- Agoraphobia
- Generalized anxiety disorder

Anxiety disorders, as a group, are characterized by excessive fear and worry. Individuals with these disorders also have associated behaviors that either reflects functional deficits related to the anxiety or behaviors designed to ameliorate the anxiety (American Psychiatric

TABLE 7-1

PREVALENCE OF ANXIETY DISORDERS

DIAGNOSIS	PREVALENCE	GENDER RATIO (M:F)	SOURCE
Separation anxiety	0.9% to 1.9% (adults), 5% (children)	1:1 (clinical settings) More common in women (in the community)	APA, 2013 Ehrenreich, Santucci, & Weinrer, 2008
Selective mutism	0.03% to 1%	1:1	APA, 2013
Specific phobias	8.7%	1:2	Kessler, Chiu, Demler, & Walters, 2005
Social anxiety disorder (social phobia)	7%	1:1.5 to 1:2.2	APA, 2013 Lampe, 2009
Panic disorder	2.7%	1:2	Kessler et al., 2005
Agoraphobia	0.8%	1:2	Kessler et al., 2005
Generalized anxiety disorder	3.1%	1:2	Kessler et al., 2005

Association [APA], 2013). The fifth edition of the *Diagnostic and Statistical Manual of Mental Disorders* (DSM-5) has moved some disorders into this cluster (e.g., separation anxiety disorder, selective mutism) from their prior classification of disorders of infancy, childhood, and adolescence. This cluster reflects the recognition that although there are some conditions—particularly the neurodevelopmental disorders that, by definition, emerge early in life—most, including psychotic, bipolar, depressive, and anxiety disorders, may be seen in children as well as in adults. It also reflects the recognition that adults may experience separation anxiety and other disorders that were previously categorized as disorders of childhood. Some of the conditions previously included in this cluster have been moved out of the anxiety disorders cluster. Specifically, obsessive-compulsive disorders and stress-related disorders now have separate chapters, even though anxiety is a key symptom in all of them. Those disorders were deemed sufficiently different in presentation and etiology to be described separately, and they will be discussed in Chapters 8 and 9. Table 7-1 shows the prevalence of the anxiety disorders.

Separation Anxiety Disorder

Separation anxiety disorder reflects extreme anxiety of an individual that is related to separation from others to whom the person is attached. The anxiety must be inappropriate for the individual's developmental stage (APA, 2013). For this diagnosis to be made, at least three signs of excessive anxiety must be demonstrated at times when the individual faces separation from an important figure. These include excessive distress when thinking about or experiencing a separation from major people in one's life; worry about losing these people or about unlikely events (like being kidnapped) that would cause separation; refusal to participate in activities away from home; excessive fear of being alone; and/or frequent nightmares or physical complaints when separation occurs. The symptoms must be persistent over at least 4 weeks for children or 6 months for adults, and the symptoms must cause distress or functional impairment.

The condition must be differentiated from depression and substance use disorders, and it may coexist with each of these.

Etiology

Separation anxiety disorder is hypothesized to have two major etiological factors—genetics and environment (Drake & Ginsberg, 2012; Roberson-Nay, Eaves, Hettema, Kendler, & Silberg, 2012). A clear familial pattern exists, and genetic studies have shown a pattern similar to that found in other anxiety disorders (Roberson-Nay et al., 2012). It is estimated that genetic factors contribute approximately 30% to the total risk, family dynamics of 20%, and personal and other environmental factors account for the remainder (Drake & Ginsberg, 2012).

Early indicators of the disorder in a child's behavior exist; these children typically exhibit excessive anxiety around strangers at an early age, well beyond the normal stranger anxiety that children experience at 1 to 2 years of age (Lavallee et al., 2011). Considerable evidence exists that the quality of the parent-child relationship is a factor, particularly in issues of inadequate or ineffective attachment (Brumariu & Kerns 2008). It appears that insecure attachment is the result of unpredictable adult behavior, which leads to hypervigilance in the child. Becker and Ginsburg (2011) found that anxious mothers, compared with those who are not anxious, were more likely to expect their child to experience distress during a social-evaluative task and that this maternal anxiety correlated with increased anxiety in the child. The disorder can also emerge as a result of a life stressor. Parents in the middle of a divorce, for example, may find that their child develops separation anxiety. One sixth-grader had to be dragged to the school bus in the mornings for nearly 1 year while her father was being treated for cancer. As his health improved, the girl's condition abated.

Prognosis

Although the symptoms of separation anxiety disorder may diminish over time, the accompanying anxiety is typically chronic and is predictive of risk for adult anxiety disorder, substance abuse, and suicide (Bittner et al., 2007). One study found that separation anxiety disorder symptoms did not cause significant impairment, but it tended to continue over time, especially in older children (Foley et al., 2008).

Implications for Function and Treatment

A variety of functional impairments accompany separation anxiety disorder, most notably in school and social occupations (Drake & Ginsberg, 2012). Children may become emotionally distraught when required to separate from home and/or parents (Figure 7-1). Home life is also disrupted, as the child's clingy, sometimes irritable behavior can be challenging for parents (Muroff & Ross, 2011). As the child's school and social occupations suffer, self-concept can be damaged as well. Children with separation anxiety disorder typically have skill deficits in emotional regulation. They are more likely than nonanxious children to interpret situations that are ambiguous as threatening (Cannon & Weems, 2010).

Several psychotherapeutic interventions have demonstrated value (Drake & Ginsberg, 2012). In particular, cognitive behavioral therapy (CBT) that includes psychoeducation can improve the family environment and reduce anxiety. Additional components of CBT that enhance positive outcomes are contingency management, problem solving skills, gradual in vivo exposure, cognitive restructuring, relaxation skills, and relapse prevention. CBT can be

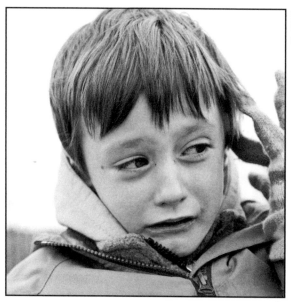

Figure 7-1. Children with separation anxiety have great difficulty coping with their emotions. (©2014 Shutterstock.com.)

provided to the child or to the family as a whole. It is not clear which therapy has a superior outcome, but both are helpful.

Although CBT is supported by research as the most efficacious intervention for separation anxiety disorder, trials of medication may be warranted when CBT is not effective. In particular, selective serotonin reuptake inhibitors (SSRIs) and other classes of antidepressants have been helpful in some situations (Jurbergs & Ledley, 2005).

Implications for Occupational Therapy

As noted, children with separation anxiety disorder experience significant difficulty in school and social occupations. These difficulties can be exacerbated by how the child's behavior is be interpreted by others. For example, Crawford and Manassis (2011) found that the social difficulties these children display can lead to peer victimization (e.g., bullying), which may further increase anxiety.

For these reasons, occupational therapy interventions should focus on supporting school and social occupations. Practice managing anticipated events and the development of coping strategies (e.g., meditation, guided imagery, and role playing) may help to reduce anxiety and increase self-confidence. Support and education for families can be of great help in reducing symptoms of anxiety (Beesdo, Pine, Lieb, & Wittchen, 2010), particularly in families where overprotection is an issue. Parents benefit from learning how their own anxiety may contribute to the child's anxiety.

Selective Mutism

Selective mutism reflects an unwillingness to speak in certain settings. It assumes that there is no clear reason—such as hearing impairment—that results in an inability to produce speech. Rather, it is to some extent a choice by the individual. Diagnostic criteria includes the following: repeated failure to speak in a setting where speech is expected, the individual speaks in other settings; failure to speak interferes with function; failure to speak is not the result of language difference; and the disturbance lasts at least 1 month (APA, 2013).

Most often, the unwillingness to speak that characterizes selective mutism emerges in situations that cause high anxiety for the individual. When there is unwillingness to speak at school, it may be difficult to assess the individual—almost always a child—in terms of academic performance, which sometimes leads to inaccurate identification of requirements for special services. Social interaction with peers can also be a contributing factor if the individual feels worried about his or her ability to manage the situation. In some instances, other forms of communication—gestures, grunts, pointing, writing—may be substituted. The disorder is often accompanied by excessive shyness, social isolation, withdrawal, and other signs of excessive anxiety in interaction with others.

Etiology

Most of the conceptualizations of selective mutism focus on **psychodynamic** explanations, which are focused on the understanding of the underlying psychic phenomena that contribute to the disorder (Bussey & Downey, 2011), especially family dynamics and experience of trauma. There may be conflicts in family relationships or a learned pattern in which the child uses silence as a way to manage anxiety. It is frequently comorbid with social anxiety disorder, suggesting a common etiology.

Temperamental factors, such as shyness and family issues, may be involved. One study found that 37% of the parents of children with selective mutism had social phobias, compared with 14.1% of a control group (Chavira, Shipon-Blum, Hitchcock, Cohan, & Stein, 2007).

It is important to recognize that selective mutism has a different etiology and presentation than the communication disorders described in Chapter 3. Unlike those disorders, which have evidence of a biological component, selective mutism is, by definition, selective or voluntary. Although the child perceives a need for silence, usually to manage his or her anxiety, there are no biological or structural impediments to speech; indeed, the child will have established spoken language and may speak freely in some settings.

Prognosis

With appropriate treatment, selective mutism can be successfully remediated (Bussey & Downey, 2011). Although it is associated with other anxiety disorders that may be more chronic, good evidence exists that most children with selective mutism resume normal speech, particularly if intervention is provided early in the course of the disorder.

Implications for Function and Treatment

Selective mutism usually occurs in some specific settings and not in others. This means that performance will be affected primarily in settings where the child refuses to speak. Frequently, this is school, which means that education is most likely to be impaired (Bussey & Downey, 2011). If the child refuses to speak at home or in other social settings, those occupations would also be affected. Certainly, the child's refusal to speak at school can lead to tension at home.

Early diagnosis and treatment can be helpful as a way to avoid having the choice to remain silent, thus becoming habitual and ingrained (Viana, Beidel, & Rabian, 2009). In addition, early treatment can reduce the negative impact on the child's social and academic occupations (Crundwell, 2006). If left untreated, the disorder can become an accepted part of the child's identity (Omdal, 2008).

Three approaches to treatment exist: intervention with the child, intervention with parents, and intervention with teachers. Intervention with the child should focus on behavioral strategies (Bussey & Downey, 2011), including CBT, as well as operant conditioning that sets up a reinforcement structure for speech, including reward for **successive approximation** (gradual improvement) of expected speech. Group therapy in which the child can practice speech in a safe, supportive environment may be helpful.

Intervention with parents and teachers should focus on their education about the onset and causes of selective mutism, as well as strategies for encouraging speech. For example, expecting children to respond verbally and requiring a verbal response, rather than using gestures, while sympathizing with the child's anxiety, may increase his or her comfort with speaking. Accompanying this treatment with appropriate reinforcement may be helpful.

Implications for Occupational Therapy

Selective mutism is a condition in which the occupational therapist's role in educating others can be of great value. The therapist may be able to help guide parents and teachers in understanding how to best minimize the child's anxiety and encourage appropriate speech.

The occupational therapist also has the opportunity to encourage speech in a safe and welcoming setting. Activities that engage the child's interest, while also requiring speech, can provide opportunities for practice in a low-stress environment. For example, a child might play Go Fish or be encouraged to draw a picture and describe its contents, each of which is a potentially enjoyable activity that requires speech. The ability to provide activities in which speech is not the central focus of attention can diminish anxiety.

Specific Phobia

Specific phobias are anxiety reactions related to one or more particular stimuli. This is a common mental disorder, and most of us know someone who has a profound fear of flying, snakes, or public speaking. An encounter with the feared stimulus can lead to crippling anxiety that makes functioning in that setting almost impossible. Diagnostic criteria, for a period of at least 6 months, include the following: noticeable fear of a particular object or situation with resulting anxiety; avoidance of the stimulus; reactions out of proportion to the actual danger or risk associated with the stimulus; and anxiety and avoidance that cause distress and dysfunction (APA, 2013).

Specifiers allow for greater detail about the nature of the phobia so that each can be described as being related to animals, the natural environment, blood-injection-injury, or situational stimuli. When more than one specifier is present, each would be diagnosed. It is not uncommon to have multiple phobias and approximately 75% of individuals with phobias have at least two (APA, 2013).

As shown in the prevalence table (see Table 7-1), specific phobias are extremely common. They are often associated with depression, other anxiety disorders, and personality disorders. In the latter, the risk of suicide is particularly high (APA, 2013).

Etiology

Specific phobias are believed to be learned through fear conditioning (Coelho & Purkis, 2009). The theory is that exposure to the feared stimulus is associated with an anxiety response (for example, a spider crawls on one's arm, evoking a startle reflex, or a plane flight is unusually turbulent, causing fear) and that anxiety is associated with the stimulus thereafter.

Some speculation exists that these anxiety responses may have provided an evolutionary benefit as a way to avoid danger.

Phobic reactions mimic actual threat reactions (McTeague & Lang, 2012), mobilizing the autonomic nervous system. This reaction is common across the anxiety disorders, but it appears to be least severe in specific phobia, with the primary expressed concern being one of fear of physical harm when exposed to the specific threat.

Prognosis

Because phobias are believed to be learned, they can also be unlearned (Hood & Anthony, 2012). However, in many instances, individuals present for treatment with some other problem, typically another anxiety disorder or depression. In these cases, treatment can be more complex. In addition, the prognosis may depend on the precise nature of the specific phobia, its duration, and the intensity of the reaction.

Implications for Function and Treatment

The functional impairments that are related to specific phobias are dependent on the feared stimulus, its pervasiveness in the individual's life circumstances, and the intensity of the response. For example, a traveling salesperson's work may suffer significantly if she or he has a fear of flying, whereas a retired teacher traveling for pleasure may be perfectly satisfied traveling by train, bus, and car, without any impact on work or other aspects of function. This second example highlights one of the characteristics of specific phobias—the fact that they may not conform to realistic threat. It is well known that air travel is substantially safer than car travel, yet fear of flying is one of the more common phobias.

Some people with phobias find creative ways to deal with them. One young boy wore a ski hat every time he went outdoors, even in the heat of summer. His mother's questioning revealed that he had been startled by a bee that flew close to his ear, and he resolved to keep his ears covered thereafter. The behavior diminished so that by the time he was a teen, he was comfortable being outside wearing a baseball cap, rather than a ski hat.

Treatment for specific phobias tends to be largely psychological (Magee, Erwin, & Heimberg, 2009). Behavioral strategies are most common, including **systematic desensitization** and challenging negative thoughts. Systematic desensitization involves identifying a hierarchy of feared items, and using guided mental imagery to move from the least to the most feared item, while pairing each thought with anxiety reduction techniques, such as deep breathing. Some evidence exists that a single systematic desensitization session may be adequate to remediate the phobia (Hood & Antony, 2012).

Implications for Occupational Therapy

Occupational therapy can assist in direct behavioral interventions that are focused on the phobia. Occupational therapy can also address any functional deficits that may have emerged as a result of the phobia. In situations where the phobia has been prolonged and has had significant functional impact, chances for engagement in meaningful occupations with opportunities for success can ameliorate the negative consequences of the phobia on the individual's self-esteem. For example, an individual whose fear of public speaking has interfered with work can benefit from behavioral strategies to minimize this anxiety, but the individual can also benefit from a focus on strategies to rebuild his or her work reputation through enhanced function in other work-related tasks.

Social Anxiety Disorder (Social Phobia)

Social anxiety disorder is closely associated with separation anxiety and selective mutism. All three disorders are characterized by significant anxiety in specific situations, in this case, social encounters. Although separation anxiety and selective mutism are disorders that often begin in childhood, social anxiety disorder may also emerge in adulthood. The diagnostic criteria include a period of at least 6 months with excessive and consistent fear and anxiety in some or all social situations, fear of being negatively evaluated, avoidance of social encounters, and anxiety out of proportion to the threat (APA, 2013). The only added specifier for social anxiety disorder is that it occurs only in performance situations.

An individual who only occasionally becomes anxious in social situations would not be diagnosed with social anxiety disorder. However, in an individual who is diagnosed with the disorder, the intensity of the fear and anxiety may vary. For instance, the individual might always feel anxious at parties and avoid them whenever possible, but will find them less difficult if among people he or she knows well.

Etiology

Social anxiety disorder is thought to be caused by a combination of biological and psychosocial factors (Bandelow et al., 2004). Specifically, social anxiety disorder is associated with early traumatic life events (for example, bullying or victimization at school), parental rearing styles (overcontrolling or ineffectively attached), family history of mental disorders, and birth risk. Genetic factors are thought to account for between 30% and 60% of the risk for social anxiety disorder (Lampe, 2009). It appears that these factors affect neurotransmission, especially of norepinephrine, dopamine, and serotonin (Fink et al., 2009). Introversion neuroticism and trait anxiety have also been associated with social anxiety disorder.

Additional risk factors include discontentedness with the absence of a partner, loneliness, self-rated low intelligence, not feeling part of a whole, unhappiness, low quality of life, and low meaningfulness (Flensborg-Madsen, Tolstrup, Sørensen, & Mortensen, 2012). The last factor (low meaningfulness) is particularly relevant to occupational therapy. It is important to distinguish social anxiety from ordinary shyness, which some speculate is an evolutionary tactic with performance benefits (Cain, 2013).

Prognosis

One of the first hurdles in improving outcomes of social anxiety disorder is encouraging the individual to seek treatment. Only about 20% of individuals with diagnosable social anxiety seek treatment (Lampe, 2009). A number of reasons may be responsible for this, including fear of stigma, a preference for trying to address the problem independently, and a sense that there are no useful treatments. However, there is good evidence that treatment can be highly effective (Clark et al., 2006).

Some individuals with social anxiety disorder also have associated substance abuse problems and often use alcohol or other substances to self-medicate for anxiety. This comorbidity is associated with worse outcomes, as the substance abuse is, in itself, problematic (Windle & Windle, 2012).

Implications for Function and Treatment

By definition, functional impairments are in social occupations. The individual avoids social encounters, is uncomfortable in interpersonal interactions, and may struggle in work or school settings that require social skills. The long-term functional consequences can be significant because of the social demands of many occupations (Fink et al., 2009). For example, one mid-career woman had been laid off from her job as an accountant because, as she moved up the ladder, her role increasingly involved interaction with clients. She struggled with such social interactions—as long as she had been able to focus on working with numbers, she performed quite well, but otherwise her performance deteriorated. Now she was confronted with a need to find a new job and was paralyzed by the idea of having to interview. Thus, her anxiety in social situations was no small matter in her life.

Effective treatment appears to incorporate both medication and psychological interventions (Fink et al., 2009; Lampe, 2009). SSRIs have been used with good effect, as have other antidepressant medications. In addition, cognitive behavioral therapy seems effective. However, it seems that the most effective interventions incorporate both treatments modalities.

Implications for Occupational Therapy

One of the contributing factors in social anxiety disorder is lack of meaning. Enabling a client to consider activities that he or she identifies as meaningful can make a significant contribution to improvement. These activities may also provide an opportunity for low stress, low stakes social encounters. For example, participating in an activity or a volunteer activity with a group of other people allows for a focus on the activity, with the social elements being less central. Anxiety may be less prominent if the social interaction is less prominent.

Therapists can also focus on specific skill building to enhance social skills and confidence. Having clients construct a list of conversation topics, role-play interactions, and receive supportive feedback can reduce anxiety. It may also be that interaction with individuals from a different generation (e.g., volunteering at a preschool or senior center) may be less anxiety provoking and provide opportunities for practice and positive feedback.

Panic Disorder

Note that the anxiety disorders considered so far are characterized by extreme anxiety, fear, or avoidance. None requires (or even mentions) the occurrence of **panic attacks**. However, panic disorder is a diagnosis made only in the presence of recurrent panic attacks—surges of significant fear and discomfort that may last several minutes or longer. Specific diagnostic criteria consist of repeated panic attacks that involve at least four symptoms of panic, including palpitations, sweating, shaking, a feeling of shortness of breath or choking, chest pain, nausea, dizziness, chills, **paresthesias** (numbness or tingling), **derealization** (feelings of unreality) or **depersonalization** (feeling of being detached from oneself), or a fear of dying (APA, 2013). In addition, the individual worries about having additional panic attacks and engages in maladaptive behavior to avoid them.

There are two major reasons that recurrent panic attacks are so disturbing. One is the actual experience, which is frightening and extremely unpleasant. The second is the persistent worry that another such attack may occur. These attacks are not typically related to a particular stimulus, so avoiding snakes or flying, which might help to reduce anxiety in the case of a specific phobia, would not be effective in the case of panic disorder. However, the individual may try to identify a trigger and avoid any situation suspected of contributing to the occurrence of an attack.

Etiology

Panic disorder has been hypothesized as a neurological disorder (Zwanzger, Domschke, & Bradwejn, 2012) that is characterized by either flawed neuronal circuitry or flawed neurotransmitters. Imaging studies have focused on the role of the amygdala and the prefrontal cortex, and the most consistent neurochemical finding is elevated corticotropin-releasing factor (Mathew, Price, & Charney, 2008). A strong genetic component also seems to be a likely factor (Cosci, 2012). It may be that this and other anxiety disorders are the evolutionary consequence of a "fight or flight" response gone awry (Grillon, 2008). Environmental factors, including relationships between the individual and his or her parents, seem to be factors in at least some cases (Bögels & Phares, 2008).

Anxious individuals seem to remember threatening events more frequently and with more intensity than those who are not anxious (Mitte, 2008; Richter et al., 2012), and they make decisions to avoid risk (Maner et al., 2007).

Prognosis

Prognosis is variable, but on the whole, panic disorder is relatively intractable (Batelaan et al., 2010). Some individuals have an almost subclinical presentation, and these individuals do better. According to Batelaan et al. (2010), 43% of those with panic disorder had more than 24 panic attacks during a 3-month period. Both men and women who reported low self-esteem had a worse course.

Another study found that at 9-year follow-up, only 50% of individuals with panic disorder reported either partial or complete remission (Svanborg, Bäärnhielm, Åberg Wistedt, & Lützen, 2008). Those who had improved were helped by understanding themselves and the mechanisms of the illness, thus enhancing their ability to think flexibly and changing their focus from avoidance coping to approach coping. Such individuals reported that a helpful relationship with the health care provider had been of assistance in achieving these behavioral changes.

Implications for Function and Treatment

Function is dependent on the severity of the disorder. In some individuals, functional impairment is minimal. Although one experiences extreme discomfort during panic attacks, he or she may be relatively symptom-free between attacks and have long periods without problems. In other instances, function is severely impaired, particularly work and social participation, including marital relationships (Davidoff, Christensen, Khalili, Nguyen, & IsHak, 2012).

Generally speaking, activities of daily living remain intact, although instrumental activities of daily living may be impaired by an unwillingness to leave the house. For example, some individuals experience panic attacks while driving and, as a result, refuse to drive. Repetitive thoughts intrude on daily life (Watkins, 2008). Because of these functional impairments and the unpleasantness of each panic attack, quality of life is negatively affected (Davidoff et al., 2012).

The most effective treatment of panic disorder is a combination of psychotropic medications and cognitive behavioral treatment (Kircher et al., 2013). Medications include some of the tricyclic antidepressants, SSRIs, and anti-anxiety agents. Behavioral interventions include systematic desensitization, which is useful but sometimes quite stressful to the individual. This involves pairing increasingly anxiety-provoking stimuli with relaxation methods to reduce the incidence of panic and to provide the individual with a sense of control of the symptoms. A growing body of evidence exists that cognitive behavioral therapy is effective (Rufer et al., 2010). Relaxation therapy is also an effective behavioral intervention. In addition, psychodynamic therapy has some demonstrated value (Gibbons, Crits-Christoph, & Hearon, 2008). Overall, treatment is relatively effective, even when accompanied with coexisting depression. However, as noted, exacerbations are common.

Implications for Occupational Therapy

Occupational therapy can support cognitive behavioral interventions (Lambert, Caan, & McVicar, 2008). In addition, occupational therapy can be helpful in reconsidering performance patterns and working toward substituting effective habits and routines for individuals who are dysfunctional. Inaccurate sensory processing may contribute to anxiety, so thoughtfully structured sensory perceptual interventions may be of value.

Panic Attack (Specifier)

Although, as indicated previously, a panic attack is not an assumed component of other anxiety disorders, many disorders may be accompanied by panic attacks. Posttraumatic stress disorder, depressive disorders, and substance use disorders are among the mental disorders that may be associated with panic attacks. In addition, some medical conditions, including heart disease and some respiratory and gastrointestinal disorders, may also be associated with panic attacks (APA, 2013). The symptoms are the same as those listed in the panic disorder section, although the requirements about frequency, duration, and post–panic attack behavior are not necessarily included.

Agoraphobia

For some individuals with panic disorder, agoraphobia is the next step in a life that is increasingly circumscribed by anxiety or worry about anxiety. Although preexisting panic attacks are not a necessary feature of agoraphobia, at least 30% of individuals with the condition have previously had these attacks. The diagnostic criteria for agoraphobia include severe anxiety or fear about at least two situations that require going outside (using public transportation or driving, being in open spaces, being in enclosed spaces, being in a crowd, or being outside the home alone); avoidance of these situations because of fear of inability to escape if the person has a panic attack; the situations almost always cause anxiety; the anxiety is out of proportion to the real danger of the feared situation; and the fear causes distress or dysfunction (APA, 2013). The disorder can be diagnosed whether panic disorder is also present, and if the individual meets the criteria for both, both should be diagnosed.

Etiology

Agoraphobia is a severe condition, but its origin is not well understood. Risk factors include early experiences of loss, childhood separation or school anxiety, and recent experience of loss (Kessler, Chiu, Demler, & Walters, 2005). A family history of anxiety disorders is also predictive. In addition, childhood respiratory disease and temperamental emotional reactivity at age 3 are predictive (Craske, Poulton, Tsao, & Plotkin, 2001).

Prognosis

Agoraphobia is usually chronic, with periods of exacerbation and remission (McTeague & Lang, 2012; Smitts, O'Cleirgh, & Otto, 2005). Some individuals may also find that as one situation becomes less anxiety provoking, another replaces it. The disorder can be intractable; in particular, comorbidity with other mental disorders is prognostic of poor outcome (Smitts et al., 2005).

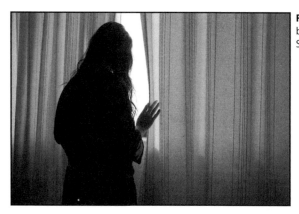

Figure 7-2. Individuals with agoraphobia may fear leaving the house. (©2014 Shutterstock.com.)

Implications for Function and Treatment

Agoraphobia can be extremely disabling (Smitts et al., 2005). Approximately 60% of individuals with agoraphobia report significant difficulty with daily activities and 50% are dissatisfied with one or more life domains (Cramer, Torgersen, & Kringlen, 2005). Although underlying skills (cognitive, sensory, and motor) appear to be intact, the interaction of the disorder with skills is not well understood. It is possible that some sort of sensory change may occur, but this is not well researched, and flaws in processing anxiety may exist that lead to misinterpretation or misunderstanding of the environment (Hayward & Wilson, 2007).

Performance is severely impaired in those occupations requiring movement to public places, such as grocery stores, offices, and shopping malls. Individuals with agoraphobia have difficulty with most occupations. Individuals often cannot work because they fear leaving the house (Figure 7-2). Their social lives may become quite circumscribed, and they are fearful of any activity that requires them to be in new situations, although they may be able to maintain activities of daily living and those instrumental activities of daily living functions that do not require leaving the home. Their families may be involved in the condition as well. In one extreme case, the individual's husband reported that no one in the family was allowed to use the upstairs portion of the house, as this would precipitate a panic attack for the individual. Because the bedrooms were all upstairs, the family had to move beds into the living room.

In some instances, the individual may be able to go out with one trusted companion (e.g., a friend or spouse). Performance patterns are excessively entrenched, as these patterns are experienced by the individual as reducing anxiety, and such patterns are typically avoidant (i.e., the individual has a routine that reduces new or unfamiliar experiences).

Treatments for agoraphobia include behavioral fear reduction and avoidance reduction procedures (Van Apeldoorn et al., 2010). Cognitive behavioral treatments help (Butler, Chapman, Forman, & Beck, 2006; White et al., 2012), as do psychotropic medications, including SSRIs, which reduce anxiety (Dinan, 2006). However, these interventions are most effective in concert (Van Apeldoorn et al., 2010).

Increasingly, technology-supported interventions are being tried (Bee et al., 2008), including computer-based therapy and group therapy via the Internet. These interventions may be helpful for individuals who refuse to leave their homes. In addition, some complementary and alternative strategies, including hypnotherapy, are also implemented on occasion, with some evidence of positive outcome (Kraft, 2011).

Implications for Occupational Therapy

Occupational therapy can be helpful for individuals with agoraphobia (Dunk, 2004) as it is important for these individuals to refocus attention toward positive engagement in occupations. Providing supportive environments in which to gradually develop or reestablish previously valued occupational patterns may ameliorate the symptoms of the disorder. Because some individuals with agoraphobia are able to leave the home more comfortably with a trusted companion, a graduated program of activities outside the home accompanied by a friend, family member, or the therapist, can help the individual to gain increased confidence in new environments.

Generalized Anxiety Disorder

Generalized anxiety disorder is a rough parallel in anxiety disorders to dysthymic disorder in the depressive disorders. It is a chronic, fairly constant, but lower-level anxiety disorder, compared with panic disorder or other disorders that have episodes of extreme anxiety and avoidance. The diagnostic criteria include excessive worry and anxiety most days for at least 6 months; the anxiety is hard to control and causes distress or dysfunction; and the individual has three noticeable symptoms that may include restlessness, being easily fatigued, difficulty concentrating, irritability, tension, or sleep disturbance (APA, 2013). In general, the level of dysfunction and distress is less than in other anxiety disorders, but it is still sufficient to cause distress on a regular basis. Unlike panic attacks, which remit in a few minutes, the generalized anxiety that characterizes this disorder is persistent as a low-level unease that continues for hours or days at a time.

Generalized anxiety disorder is characterized by a generalized state of anxiety or worry in the absence of specific reason. The individual may worry excessively about the state of his or her health or about finances when there is no realistic basis for the concern. However, the diagnosis is not made if substance abuse or depression might be the cause of the anxiety, although mild depressive symptoms may be present. Generalized anxiety disorder is usually a chronic disorder, although any functional impairment is mild (Hoffman, Dukes, & Wittchen, 2008). Quality of life is negatively affected for generalized anxiety disorder because of the relatively constant underlying anxiety the individual experiences.

Etiology

The etiology of generalized anxiety disorder is not well understood, although it appears likely to have at least some genetic component (Schienle, Hettema, Cáceda, & Nemeroff, 2011). The observed biological mechanism involves dysfunction in the amygdala and various prefrontal cortical regions of the brain. Activity in the amygdala is heightened during anticipation of unpleasant stimuli but occurs also in those that are ambiguous, suggesting a generally heightened state of awareness.

In addition, almost certainly environmental, family, and personality factors exist that contribute to the disorder (Lightfoot, Seay, & Goddard, 2010), and there may well be learned response elements. Parenting style that is overcontrolling or lacking in warmth may be factors (Drake & Ginsberg, 2012).

Prognosis

Generalized anxiety disorder tends to be relatively chronic (Drake & Ginsberg, 2012), particularly if left untreated. Individuals with the disorder typically experience exacerbations and remissions, depending on the level of stress in their lives at any given point in time (Hoffman et al., 2008).

Implications for Function and Treatment

Unlike some of the more severe anxiety disorders, generalized anxiety disorder is not associated with severe dysfunction. Nevertheless, individuals with generalized anxiety disorder experience noticeable disability (Bobes, Caballero, Vilardaga, & Rejas, 2011). They report less participation in meaningful activities and lower quality of life, compared with individuals without a mental disorder (Michelson, Lee, Orsillo, & Roemer, 2011). Evidence of impairment exists in most life roles (Barrera & Norton, 2009), in particular work, social and family, and leisure participation.

Treatment recommendations will, by now, sound familiar. The two best validated approaches are psychotropic medication, especially SSRIs, and cognitive behavioral therapy (Van Apeldoorn et al., 2010). As is true for other anxiety disorders, a combination of these two interventions seems to be the most effective.

Implications for Occupational Therapy

Occupational therapists may see individuals with this disorder in the context of treatment for other conditions, and they should be aware that even low levels of anxiety can interfere with motivation and ability to comprehend and follow instructions. Generalized anxiety disorder is a chronic disorder for which management strategies that enable individuals to cope with ongoing symptoms support performance. Reframing life challenges, participating in exercise and other activities that refocus energy and attention, energy conservation strategies, and other management mechanisms can help individuals to redirect their attention away from their worries and toward occupations that meet their needs for meaning. Mindfulness interventions can support emotional regulation and reduce anxiety (Mankus, Aldao, Kerns, Mayville, & Mennin, 2013). Table 7-2 shows the main symptoms and functional deficits that occur with anxiety disorders.

Cultural Considerations

A number of conditions exist in other cultures that closely mirror one or more of the DSM-5 (APA, 2013) anxiety disorders. In Japan and Korea, a condition known as *taijin kyofusho* is similar to social phobia, but it has several specific cultural variations (Kim, Rapee, & Gaston, 2008). In this disorder, the focus is on fear of harming others, rather than on the consequences for the individual. Several of the Hispanic cultures describe a condition known as *nervios*, which translates literally to "nerves" (Lewis-Fernandez, Guarnaccia, Patel, Lizardi, & Diaz, 2005). Symptoms include shaking, crying, shouting, and sometimes, **dissociative** experiences, in which the individual detaches from his or her immediate surroundings.

Other culturally-related diagnostic challenges in treating anxiety disorders also exist. It is possible to misdiagnose these disorders due to failure to understand the expected behaviors in other cultures. For example, children from immigrant backgrounds have been found to be more likely than nonimmigrant children to be diagnosed with selective mutism (Toppelberg, Tabors, Coggins, Lum, & Burger, 2005). These findings are almost certainly due to misdiagnoses. It is also important to be aware that some cultural groups would not feel it is acceptable to seek care for social phobia (Hsu & Alden, 2008).

TABLE 7-2

DIAGNOSTIC CRITERIA AND FUNCTIONAL DEFICITS: ANXIETY DISORDERS

DISORDER	DIAGNOSTIC CRITERIA (APA, 2013)	IMPLICATIONS FOR FUNCTION
Separation anxiety disorder	Anxiety as demonstrated by some of the following: • Excessive distress related to a separation from important people or one's home • Excessive worry about losing important people • Excessive worry about unlikely events (like kidnapping or getting lost) that would cause a separation from important people • Reluctance to leave home • Fear of being alone • Physical complaints when separation occurs Persists for at least 4 weeks in children and adolescents, 6 or more months in adults	Deficits in school, play, social occupations Development of emotional skills negatively affected Habits, roles, patterns all negatively affected
Selective mutism	For at least 1 month, failure to speak in settings where speech is expected, in someone who has the ability to speak Associated dysfunction Not the result of lack of knowledge of or comfort with the language	Deficits in any occupation requiring verbal communication in which the individual chooses not to speak
Specific phobia	For at least 6 months, significant fear, out of proportion to danger, of a particular object or situation resulting from previous encounters with the feared stimulus The stimulus is avoided Distress or dysfunction	Dependent on stimulus, may or may not limit any sphere
Social anxiety disorder (social phobia)	At least 6 months of fear or anxiety, out of proportion to threat, about one or more social situations which could involve scrutiny by others Social situations almost always cause anxiety and are avoided	Deficits in any occupation requiring social interaction Habits, roles, and patterns are all negatively affected
		(continued)

	Table 7-2 (continued)	
	DIAGNOSTIC CRITERIA AND FUNCTIONAL DEFICITS: ANXIETY DISORDERS	
DISORDER	*DIAGNOSTIC CRITERIA (APA, 2013)*	*IMPLICATIONS FOR FUNCTION*
Panic disorder	Repeated panic attacks that may include the following: • Palpitations or accelerated heart rate • Sweating, trembling or shaking • Sensation of shortness of breath • Chest pain • Nausea • Dizziness, light-headedness • Chills or sensation of heat, paresthesias • Derealization or depersonalization • Fear of losing control or of dying At least one has been followed by at least 1 month: • Worry about additional panic attacks • Maladaptive behavior changes to avoid another attack	Work, leisure, and activities of daily life (ADL) all negatively affected during attacks Fear of attack may impact any function Negatively affects routines and habits as individual attempt to avoid panic attacks
Agoraphobia	At least 6 months of anxiety or fear about at least two of the following: • Using public transportation (including automobiles) • Being in open spaces • Being in enclosed places • Standing in line or being in a crowd • Being outside the home alone Avoidance of these situations because of fears The specific situation almost always causes fear or anxiety out of proportion to the actual danger Distress or dysfunction	May be mild to severe If mild, limited impairment that occurs primarily in occupations outside familiar/comfortable settings If severe, global impairment
Generalized anxiety disorder	At least 6 months of excessive and frequent anxiety and worry that is difficult to control Anxiety is associated with the following: • Restlessness • Being easily fatigued • Difficulty concentrating • Irritability, tension • Sleep disturbance Distress or dysfunction	Work, leisure, other occupations essentially intact, but persistent anxiety and worry while engaged in occupation Cognition and emotional skills distorted by anxiety Patterns, habits, roles may be circumscribed in an attempt to avoid or manage anxiety

Lifespan Considerations

Anxiety disorders are common among children and adolescents and later in life. Particular attention has been paid to anxiety in children, perhaps because it predicts lifelong outcomes (Hirshfeld-Becker, Micco, Simoes, & Henin, 2008). Childhood and separation anxiety are clear antecedents of adult anxiety and separation anxiety, behavioral inhibition, anxiety sensitivity, and negative affectivity. Children are also subject to posttraumatic stress disorder (Najjar, Weller, Weisbrot, & Weller, 2008).

Evidence about treatment of childhood anxiety emphasizes individual, group, and family-based cognitive behavioral therapy, as well as social skills training for children with social or school phobia (Silverman, Pina, & Viswesvaran, 2008). There is reason to believe that early intervention might reduce the potential for later anxiety disorders.

Among older adults, the prevalence of anxiety disorders has been estimated to be between 1.2% and 15% (Bryant, Jackson, & Ames, 2008). Anxiety symptoms that do not rise to the level of an anxiety disorder are even more common and are found in approximately 15% to 56% of individuals. One particularly challenging aspect of intervention with older adults is the potential for coexisting cognitive deficits that complicate treatment of both conditions (Beaudreau & O'Hara, 2008). Older adults with anxiety disorders have high rates of comorbid conditions, such as personality disorders and depression, and these comorbid conditions also predict coexisting medical conditions (Mackenzie, Reynolds, Chou, Pagura, & Sareen, 2011). Mackenzie et al. (2011) reported that older adults with anxiety disorders have particularly poor quality of life, but they also tend not to seek help, making treatment particularly challenging.

Internet Resources

Anxiety and Depression Association of America
http://www.adaa.org/
Family- and consumer-focused information and materials.

Anxiety Disorders, National Institute of Mental Health
http://www.nimh.nih.gov/health/publications/anxiety-disorders/index.shtml
Includes both consumer and professional information. Good resource for evidence-based information.

Anxiety Disorders Resource Center, American Academy of Child & Adolescent Psychiatry
http://www.aacap.org/AACAP/Families_and_Youth/Resource_Centers/Anxiety_Disorder_Resource_Center/Home.aspx
Resources that are particularly focused on children and adolescents with anxiety disorders and their families. A rich listing of links and references that are targeted to consumers.

CASE STUDY

Diane Hamilton is a 56-year-old wife and mother who lives in a small ranch house in the suburbs of a large Midwestern city. Mrs. Hamilton describes herself as having been a shy and anxious child and a withdrawn and unpopular teenager who preferred to stay at home and read or watch television. She attended community college while living at home, and met her husband when she worked as a veterinary technician at a local pet hospital. She quit her job and stayed at home to raise her three children.

During the years when her children were young, Mrs. Hamilton was very focused on their well-being. She was a devoted mother who sewed her children's clothing, liked to make them special lunches to take to school, and enjoyed conversing with them about their schoolwork and their lives. She was less enthusiastic about going to school or attending their sporting events because she felt uneasy in unfamiliar surroundings. It was easier for her when her husband attended these events with her.

When her youngest child went to college, following the older children, Mrs. Hamilton found that she felt anxious and worried almost all the time. She thought initially that her worry was about her children who were away at school, but she began to feel worried about other parts of her life as well. Her anxiety spiked in the late afternoon when her husband was due home from work. She worried almost daily that he had been in a car accident.

One day her husband was delayed at his office and Mrs. Hamilton became over-wrought. She felt clammy, couldn't breathe, and her heart was pounding. She thought she was having a heart attack and called emergency medical services. A thorough examination in the emergency department found no evidence of a cardiovascular event, and the physician diagnosed a panic attack.

From that point on, Mrs. Hamilton began to have difficulty leaving the house for any purpose. She insisted that her husband do the grocery shopping and run errands because she became clammy and short of breath any time she had to leave home. She has difficulty even going to the back yard to tend her garden—an activity she previously enjoyed. Her husband is supportive, but he is concerned about the ways in which her behavior restricts their activities as a couple. He would like to go to the movies, go out to eat, and even to travel, but she is, at present, unable to do so. He has urged her to seek help.

THOUGHT QUESTIONS

1. Do you think that Mrs. Hamilton has a mental disorder? What are the behaviors and emotions that contribute to your assessment?
2. What functional strengths does Mrs. Hamilton have?
3. In what areas does Mrs. Hamilton have functional deficits?
4. What additional information would be helpful to understand Mrs. Hamilton's emotional state and function?

References

American Psychiatric Association. (2013). *Diagnostic and statistical manual of mental disorders* (5th ed.). Washington, DC: Author.

Bandelow, B., Torrente, A.C., Wedekind, D., Broocks, A., Hajak, G., & Rüther, E. (2004). Early traumatic life events, parental rearing styles, family history of mental disorders, and birth risk factors in patients with social anxiety disorder. *European Archives of Psychiatry and Clinical Neuroscience, 254*(6), 397-405.

Barrera, T.L., & Norton, P.J. (2009). Quality of life impairment in generalized anxiety disorder, social phobia, and panic disorder. *Journal of Anxiety Disorders, 23*(8), 1086-1090.

Batelaan, N.M., de Graaf, R., Spijker, J., Smit, J.H., van Balkom, A.J.L.M., Vollbergh, W.A.M., & Beekman, A.T.F. (2010). The course of panic attacks in individuals with panic disorder and subthreshold panic disorder: A population-based study. *Journal of Affective Disorders, 121*(1-2), 30-38.

Beaudreau, S.A., & O'Hara, R. (2008). Late-life anxiety and cognitive impairment: A review. *American Journal of Geriatric Psychiatry, 16,* 790-803.

Becker, K.D., & Ginsburg, G.S. (2011). Maternal anxiety, behaviors, and expectations during a behavioral task: Relation to children's self-evaluations. *Child Psychiatry and Human Development, 42,* 320-333.

Bee, P.E., Bower, P., Lovell, K., Gilbody, S., Richards, D., Gask, L., & Roach, P. (2008). Psychotherapy mediated by remote communication technologies: A meta-analytic review. *BMS Psychiatry, 8,* 60-68.

Beesdo, K., Pine, D.S., Lieb, R., & Wittchen, H. (2010). Incidence and risk patterns of anxiety and depressive disorders and categorization of generalized anxiety disorder. *Archives of General Psychiatry, 67,* 47-57.

Bittner, A., Egger, H.L., Erkanli, A., Costello, E.J., Foley, D.L., & Angold, A. (2007). What do childhood anxiety disorders predict? *Journal of Child Psychology and Psychiatry, 48,* 1174-1183.

Bobes, J., Caballero, L., Vilardaga, I., & Rejas, J. (2011). Disability and health-related quality of life in outpatients with generalised anxiety disorder treated in psychiatric clinics: Is there still room for improvement? *Annals of General Psychiatry, 10,* 7-24.

Bögels, S., & Phares, V. (2008). Fathers' role in the etiology, prevention, and treatment of child anxiety: A review and new model. *Clinical Psychology Review, 28,* 539-558.

Brumariu, L.E., & Kerns, K.A. (2008). Mother–child attachment and social anxiety symptoms in middle childhood. *Journal of Applied Developmental Psychology, 29,* 393-402.

Bryant, C., Jackson, H., & Ames, D. (2008). The prevalence of anxiety in older adults: Methodological issues and a review of the literature. *Journal of Affective Disorders, 109,* 233-250.

Bussey, R.T., & Downey, J. (2011). Selective mutism: A three-tiered approach to prevention and intervention. *Contemporary School Psychology, 15,* 53-63.

Butler, A.C., Chapman, J.E., Forman, E.M., & Beck, A.T. (2006). The empirical status of cognitive-behavioral therapy: A review of meta-analyses. *Clinical Psychology Review, 26,* 17-31.

Cain, S. (2013). *Quiet: The power of introverts in a world that can't stop talking.* New York, NY: Broadway Books.

Cannon, M.F., & Weems, C.F. (2010). Cognitive biases in childhood anxiety disorders: Do interpretive and judgment biases distinguish anxious youth from their non-anxious peers? *Journal of Anxiety Disorders, 24,* 751-758.

Chavira, D.A., Shipon-Blum, E., Hitchcock, C., Cohan, S., & Stein, M.B. (2007). Selective mutism and social anxiety disorder: All in the family? *Journal of American Academy of Child and Adolescent Psychiatry, 46,* 1464-1472.

Clark, D.M., Ehlers, A., Hackmann, A., McManus, F., Fennell, M., Grey, N., . . . Wild, J. (2006). Cognitive therapy versus exposure and applied relaxation in social phobia: A randomized controlled trial. *Journal of Consulting and Clinical Psychology, 74,* 568-578.

Coelho, C., & Purkis, H. (2009). The origins of specific phobias: Influential theories and current perspectives. *Review of General Psychology, 13*(4), 335-348.

Cosci, F. (2012). The psychological development of panic disorder: Implications for neurobiology and treatment. *Revista Brasileira de Psiquiatria, 34*(Suppl. 1), S09-S19.

Cramer, V., Torgersen, S., & Kringlen, E. (2005). Quality of life and anxiety disorders: A population study. *Journal of Nervous and Mental Disease, 193*(3), 196-202.

Craske, M.G., Poulton, R., Tsao, J.C.I., & Plotkin, D. (2001). Paths to panic disorder/agoraphobia: An exploratory analysis from age 3 to 21 in an unselected birth cohort. *Journal of the American Academy of Child & Adolescent Psychiatry, 40*(5), 556-563.

Crawford, A., & Manassis, K. (2011). Anxiety, social skills, friendship quality, and peer victimization: An integrated model. *Journal of Anxiety Disorders, 25,* 924-931.

Crundwell, R.M.A. (2006). Identifying and teaching children with selective mutism. *Teaching Exceptional Children, 38,* 48-54.

Davidoff, J., Christensen, S., Khalili, D.N., Nguyen, J., & IsHak, W.W. (2012). Quality of life in panic disorder: Looking beyond symptom remission. *Quality of Life Research: An International Journal of Quality of Life Aspects of Treatment, Care & Rehabilitation, 21*(6), 945-959.

Dinan, T. (2006). Therapeutic options: Addressing the current dilemma. *European Neuropsychopharmacology, 16*(Suppl. 2), S119-S127.

Drake, K.L., & Ginsburg, G.S. (2012). Family factors in the development, treatment, and prevention of childhood anxiety disorders. *Clinical Child and Family Psychology Review, 15*(2), 144-162.

Dunk, T. (2004). Focus on research occupational therapy and agoraphobia in community mental health teams. *British Journal of Occupational Therapy, 67*, 446-458.

Ehrenreich, J.T., Santucci, L.C., & Weinrer, C.L. (2008). Separation anxiety disorder in youth: Phenomenology, assessment, and treatment. *Psicologia Conductual, 16*(3), 389-412.

Fink, M., Akimova, E., Spindelegger, C., Hahn, A., Lanzenberger, R., & Kasper, S. (2009). Social anxiety disorder: Epidemiology, biology and treatment. *Psychiatria Danubina, 21*(4), 533-542.

Flensborg-Madsen, T., Tolstrup, J., Sørensen, H.J., & Mortensen, E.L., (2012). Social and psychological predictors of onset of anxiety disorders: Results from a large prospective cohort study. *Social Psychiatry and Psychiatric Epidemiology, 47*(5), 711-721.

Foley, D.L., Rowe, R., Maes, H., Silberg, J., Eaves, L., & Pickels, A. (2008). The relationship between separation anxiety and impairment. *Journal of Anxiety Disorders, 22*(4), 635-641.

Gibbons, M.B., Crits-Christoph, P., & Hearon, B. (2008). The empirical status of psychodynamic therapies. *Annual Review of Clinical Psychology, 4*, 93-108.

Grillon, C. (2008). Models and mechanisms of anxiety: Evidence from startle studies. *Psychopharmacology, 199*, 421-437.

Hayward, C., & Wilson, K.A. (2007). Anxiety sensitivity: A missing piece to the agoraphobia-without-panic puzzle. *Behavior Modification, 31*, 162-173.

Hirshfeld-Becker, D.R., Micco, J.A., Simoes, N.A., & Henin, A. (2008). High risk studies and developmental antecedents of anxiety disorders. *American Journal of Medical Genetics, Part C, Seminars in Medical Genetics, 148*, 99-117.

Hoffman, D.L., Dukes, E.M., & Wittchen, H. (2008). Human and economic burden of generalized anxiety disorder. *Depression and Anxiety, 25*(1), 72-90.

Hood, H.K., & Antony, M.M. (2012). Evidence-based assessment and treatment of specific phobias in adults. In T.E. Davis, T.H. Ollendick, & L. Öst (Eds.), *Intensive one-session treatment of specific phobias* (pp. 19-42). New York, NY: Springer Science + Business Media.

Hsu, L., & Alden, L.E. (2008). Cultural influences on willingness to seek treatment for social anxiety in Chinese- and European-heritage students. *Cultural Diversity and Ethnic Minority Psychology, 14*, 215-223.

Jurbergs, N., & Ledley, D.R. (2005). Separation anxiety. *Psychiatric Annals, 35*(9), 728-735.

Kessler, R.C., Chiu, W.T., Demler, O., & Walters, E.E. (2005). Prevalence, severity, and comorbidity of twelve-month DSM-IV disorders in the National Comorbidity Survey Replication (NCS-R). *Archives of General Psychiatry, 62*(6), 617-627.

Kim, J., Rapee, R.M., & Gaston, J.E. (2008). Symptoms of offensive type Taijin-Kyofusho among Australian social phobics. *Depression and Anxiety, 25*(7), 601-608.

Kircher, T., Arolt, V., Jansen, A., Pyka, M., Reinhardt, I., Kellerman, T., . . . Straube, B. (2013). Effect of cognitive-behavioral therapy on neural correlates of fear conditioning in panic disorder. *Biological Psychiatry, 73*(1), 93-101.

Kraft, D. (2011). The place of hypnosis in psychiatry, part 4: Its application to the treatment of agoraphobia and social phobia. *Australian Journal of Clinical & Experimental Hypnosis, 38*(2), 91-110.

Lambert, R.A., Caan, W., & McVicar, A. (2008). Influences of lifestyle and general practice (GP) care on the symptom profile of people with panic disorder. *Journal of Public Mental Health, 7*, 18-24.

Lampe, L.A. (2009). Social anxiety disorder: Recent developments in psychological approaches to conceptualization and treatment. *Australian and New Zealand Journal of Psychiatry, 43*(10), 887-898.

Lavallee, K., Herren, C., Blatter-Meunier, J., Afdonetto, C. In-Albon, T., & Schneiter, S. (2011). Early predictors of separation anxiety disorder: Early stranger anxiety, parental pathology and prenatal factors. *Psychopathology, 44*(6), 354-361.

Lewis-Fernandez, R., Guarnaccia, P. J., Patel, S., Lizardi, D., & Diaz, N. (2005) Ataque de nervios: Anthropological, epidemiological, and clinical dimensions of a cultural syndrome. In A. M. Georgiopoulos & J.F. Rosenbaum (Eds.), *Perspectives in cross-cultural psychiatry* (pp. 63-85). Philadelphia, PA: Lippincott, Williams & Wilkins.

Lightfoot, J.D., Seay, S., & Goddard, A.W. (2010). Pathogenesis of generalized anxiety disorder. In D.J. Stein, E. Hollander, & B.O. Rothbaum (Eds.), *Textbook of anxiety disorders* (2nd ed., pp. 173-192). Arlington, VA: American Psychiatric Publishing.

Mackenzie, C.S., Reynolds, K., Chou, K., Pagura, J., & Sareen, J. (2011). Prevalence and correlates of generalized anxiety disorder in a national sample of older adults. *American Journal of Geriatric Psychiatry, 19*(4), 305-315.

Magee, L., Erwin, B.A., & Heimberg, R.G. (2009). Psychological treatment of social anxiety disorder and specific phobia. In M.M. Antony & M.B. Stein (Eds.), *Oxford handbook of anxiety and related disorders* (pp. 334-349). New York, NY: Oxford University Press.

Maner, J.K., Richey, J.A., Cromer, K., Mallott, M., Lejuez, C., Joiner, T.E., & Schmidt, N.B. (2007). Dispositional anxiety and risk-avoidant decision making. *Personality and Individual Differences, 42,* 665-675.

Mankus, A.M., Aldao, A., Kerns, C., Mayville, E.W., & Mennin, D.S. (2013). Mindfulness and heart rate vulnerability in individuals with high and low generalized anxiety symptoms. *Behavior Research and Therapy, 51,* 386-391.

Mathew, S.J., Price, R.B., & Charney, D.S. (2008). Recent advances in the neurobiology of anxiety disorders: Implications for novel therapeutics. *American Journal of Medical Genetics, Part C, Seminars in Medical Genetics, 148,* 89-98.

McTeague, L.M., & Lang, P.J. (2012). The anxiety spectrum and the reflex physiology of defense: From circumscribed fear to broad distress. *Depression and Anxiety, 29*(4), 264-281.

Michelson, S.E., Lee, J.K., Orsillo, S.M., & Roemer, L. (2011). The role of values-consistent behavior in generalized anxiety disorder. *Depression and Anxiety, 28*(5), 358-366.

Mitte, K. (2008). Memory bias for threatening information in anxiety and anxiety disorders: A meta-analytic review. *Psychological Bulletin, 134,* 886-911.

Muroff, J., & Ross, A. (2011). Social disability and impairment in childhood anxiety. In D. McKay & E.A. Storch (Eds.), *Handbook of child and adolescent anxiety disorders* (pp. 457-478). New York, NY: Springer Science Business Media.

Najjar, F., Weller, R.A., Weisbrot, J., & Weller, E.B. (2008). Post-traumatic stress disorder and its treatment in children and adolescents. *Current Psychiatry Report, 10*(2), 104-108.

Omdal, H. (2008). Including children with selective mutism in mainstream schools and kindergartens: Problems and possibilities. *International Journal of Inclusive Education, 12,* 301-315.

Richter, J., Hamm, A.O., Pané-Farré, C.A., Gerlach, A.L., Gloster, A.T., Wittchen, H, ... Arolt, V. (2012). Dynamics of defensive reactivity in patients with panic disorder and agoraphobia: Implications for the etiology of panic disorder. *Biological Psychiatry, 72*(6), 512-520.

Roberson-Nay, R., Eaves, L.J., Hettema, J.M., Kendler, K.S., & Silberg, J.L. (2012). Childhood separation anxiety disorder and adult onset panic attacks share a common genetic diathesis. *Depression and Anxiety, 29*(4), 320-327.

Rufer, M., Albrecht, R., Schmidt, O., Zaum, J., Schnyder, U., Hand, I., & Mueller-Pfeiffer, C. (2010). Changes in quality of life following cognitive-behavioral group therapy for panic disorder. *European Psychiatry, 25*(1), 8-14.

Schienle, A., Hettema, J.M., Cáceda, R., & Nemeroff, C.B. (2011). Neurobiology and genetics of generalized anxiety disorder. *Psychiatric Annals, 41*(2), 113-123.

Silverman, W.K., Pina, A.A., & Viswesvaran, C. (2008). Evidence-based psychosocial treatments for phobic and anxiety disorders in children and adolescents. *Journal of Clinical Child and Adolescent Psychology, 37,* 105-130.

Smitts, J.A.J., O'Cleirgh, C.M., & Otto, M.W. (2005). Panic and agoraphobia. In F. Andrasic (Ed.), *Comprehensive handbook of personality and psychopathology: Volume 2: Adult psychopathology* (pp. 121-137). New York, NY: Wiley.

Svanborg, C., Bäärnhielm, S., Åberg Wistedt, A., & Lützen, K. (2008) Helpful and hindering factors for remission in dysthymia and panic disorder at 9-year follow-up: A mixed methods study. *BMC Psychiatry, 8,* 52-61.

Toppelberg, C.O., Tabors, P., Coggins, A., Lum, K., & Burger, C. (2005). Differential diagnosis of selective mutism in bilingual children. *Journal of the American Academy of Child and Adolescent Psychiatry, 44*(6), 592-595.

Van Apeldoorn, F.J., Timmerman, M.E., Mersch, P.P.A., van Hout, W.J.P.J., Visser, S., van Dyck, R., & den Boer, J.A. (2010). A randomized trial of cognitive-behavioral therapy or selective serotonin reuptake inhibitor or both combined for panic disorder with or without agoraphobia: Treatment results through 1-year follow-up. *Journal of Clinical Psychiatry, 71*(5), 574-586.

Viana, A.G., Beidel, D.C., & Rabian, B. (2009). Selective mutism: A review and integration of the last 15 years. *Clinical Psychology Review, 29*(1), 57-67.

Watkins, E.R. (2008). Constructive and unconstructive repetitive thought. *Psychological Bulletin, 134,* 163-206.

White, K.S., Payne, L.A., Gorman, J.M., Shear, M.K., Woods, S.W., Saksa, J.R., & Barlow, D.H. (2012). Does maintenance CBT contribute to long-term treatment response of panic disorder with our without agoraphobia? A randomized controlled clinical trial. *Journal of Consulting and Clinical Psychology, 81*(1), 47-57.

Windle, M., & Windle, R.C. (2012). Testing the specificity between social anxiety disorder and drinking motives. *Addictive Behaviors, 37*(9), 1003-1008.

Zwanzger, P., Domschke, K., & Bradwejn, J. (2012). Neuronal network of panic disorder: The role of the neuropeptide cholecystokinin. *Depression and Anxiety, 29*(9), 762-774.

Obsessive-Compulsive and Related Disorders

Learning Outcomes

By the end of this chapter, readers will be able to:

- Describe the various obsessive-compulsive disorders
- Differentiate among obsessive-compulsive disorders on the basis of symptoms and onset
- Identify the causes of obsessive-compulsive disorders
- Describe functional consequences of obsessive-compulsive disorders
- Describe treatment strategies for obsessive-compulsive disorders
- Discuss occupational therapy interventions for obsessive-compulsive disorders

Bonder B.
Psychopathology and Function, Fifth Edition (pp 181-196).
© 2015 SLACK Incorporated.

CASE VIGNETTE

Alexander Abrams is a 34-year-old plumber who has been hospitalized on an acute care psychiatric ward following a suicide attempt. Mr. Abrams was found by emergency medical personnel in the garage of his bungalow with the door closed and the car running.

He spends his time in a corner of the day room, wearing a hoodie, dark glasses, and a wool scarf around his neck. When brought to see the psychiatrist, he reports that he has no friends, his girlfriend broke up with him, and he has lost his job. He indicates that this has happened because his ears are extremely large and ugly.

The psychiatrist asks Mr. Abrams to remove his hoodie, which he does with great reluctance. The psychiatrist notes two very ordinary ears of normal size and positioned close to his head in the usual spot for ears. When she indicates this to Mr. Abrams, he replies that whenever he asks an acquaintance about his ears, he or she says the same thing, but he cannot accept that they are something other than huge and hugely malformed. He tried to have them surgically altered, but the plastic surgeon refused, noting that there was nothing wrong with them.

Mr. Abrams indicates that he is obsessed with the appearance of his ears, to the point that he often cannot focus on anything else. He indicates that his girlfriend was quite patient with him but finally found it impossible to spend time with him and broke up with him the prior week.

THOUGHT QUESTIONS

1. Do you believe that Mr. Abrams has a mental disorder?
2. If so, what behaviors, thoughts, or other symptoms do you identify as being problematic?
3. Of those symptoms, which might cause Mr. Abrams problems in his daily activities?
4. Are there cultural factors that might affect this situation? If so, what might they be? How might you gather more information about this issue?

OBSESSIVE-COMPULSIVE AND RELATED DISORDERS

- Obsessive-compulsive disorder
- Body dysmorphic disorder
- Hoarding disorder
- Trichotillomania (hair-pulling disorder)
- Excoriation disorder (skin-picking disorder)

The chapter on obsessive-compulsive and related disorders is new to the fifth edition of the American Psychiatric Association's (APA) *Diagnostic and Statistical Manual of Mental Disorders* (DSM-5; APA, 2013). This edition of the DSM separates obsessive-compulsive

TABLE 8-1			
PREVALENCE OF OBSESSIVE-COMPULSIVE DISORDERS			
DIAGNOSIS	PREVALENCE	GENDER RATIO (M:F)	SOURCE
Obsessive-compulsive disorder	1.2% (United States and international)	Slightly higher in women	Kessler, Petukhova, Sampson, Zaslavsky, & Wittchen, 2012
Body dysmorphic disorder	1.7% to 2.4%	Slightly higher in women	Phillips, Menard, Quinn, Didie, & Stout, 2013
Hoarding disorder	Unknown	Unknown	
Trichotillomania	0.6% to ~3%	1:10	Walther, Ricketts, Conelea, & Woods, 2010
Excoriation disorder	1.4%	1:3	APA, 2013

disorder (OCD) from the anxiety disorder cluster, adds two new diagnoses (hoarding disorder and excoriation disorder), and moves trichotillomania from the impulse control disorders. As noted in Chapter 7, the changes in the categorization of the various disorders with a significant anxiety component were made on the basis of specific etiological and behavioral manifestations (Bystritsky, Khalsa, & Shiffman, 2013). In the case of the OCD, the common thread is the existence of obsessive thoughts and compulsive behaviors. Table 8-1 shows the prevalence of the obsessive-compulsive and related disorders.

Obsessive-Compulsive Disorder

Obsessions are thoughts or ideas that are intrusive and anxiety provoking (Pallanti & Hollander, 2008). Most common are obsessions with violence or contamination. The individual may recognize that these ideas are internally derived (i.e., not based on any external event) but is unable to control them and finds that the thoughts intrude while he or she is attempting to do something else. The individual often knows that the obsessive thoughts are unreasonable.

Compulsions are repetitive, purposeful behaviors performed in response to an obsession, with the goal of preventing the discomfort caused by the obsession (Pallanti & Hollander, 2008). However, the activity is either excessive or not realistically helpful in resolving the obsession. An individual with an obsession about contamination may engage in ritual hand washing or laundering of clothing, even though this cannot eliminate all possible contaminants in the environment.

Many individuals with OCD recognize the nature of the obsession and the futility of the compulsion but experience great anxiety or tension when attempting to resist it. If the individual attempts to suppress the compulsion, over time, the individual may become increasingly unwilling to experience the anxiety and thus stop resisting the compulsion.

Depression, anxiety, and avoidance of anxiety-provoking situations commonly accompany the condition. Thus, in addition to engaging in cleanliness rituals, an individual may avoid unfamiliar situations that he or she views as providing further risk of contamination.

OCD includes a number of elements in common with anxiety disorders. In particular, the thoughts and behaviors associated with the condition are linked with significant anxiety, especially when the individual is prevented from acting on the compulsions. Diagnostic criteria include presence of obsessions (i.e., recurrent, intrusive, unwanted thoughts that cause distress), in spite of efforts to control them, and compulsions (i.e., repetitive behaviors or mental acts the individual is driven to perform) intended to reduce anxiety (APA, 2013). The obsessions and compulsions are time consuming and cause distress or dysfunction. A good example of OCD was demonstrated in the movie *As Good as it Gets* (Brooks, Johnson, & Zea, 1997), in which the main character is shown pursuing a variety of hygiene rituals, engaging in compulsive behaviors centered around food, performing rituals like touching door frames repeatedly on leaving or entering his home, and demonstrating many other compulsive behaviors that are clearly intended to reduce his anxiety about interacting with the social and physical environment.

Specifiers clarify whether good, fair, poor, or absent insight exists. The absence of insight may be considered delusional in the sense that the individual is convinced of a fact that does not correlate with reality as observed by others. An additional specifier notes whether there is an associated tic.

OCD must be differentiated from depressive disorders, other anxiety disorders, eating disorders, psychotic disorders, and obsessive-compulsive personality disorder. It may also be comorbid with any of these disorders, as well as substance abuse.

Etiology

OCD has a clear biological component (Pallanti & Hollander, 2008). Serotonin dysregulation is well documented, as are brain changes, including increased blood flow to the orbital–frontal lobes and the basal ganglia (Pallanti & Hollander, 2008). Heredity may also play a role, although this is less pronounced in the etiology of OCD than in many other disorders (Iervolino, Rijsdijk, Cherkas, Fullana, & Mataix-Cols, 2011). It seems that genetic predisposition is associated with specific environmental factors, such as family dynamics, that encourage **neuroticism**, a tendency to experience negative emotions when confronted with threat, frustration, or loss (Taylor, Asmundson, & Jang, 2011).

Prognosis

OCD has a chronic course, with a small proportion of individuals having either partial or complete remission. One study found that at the end of 5 years, only 16.9% of OCD clients experienced full remission, and 22.1% had partial remission (Eisen et al., 2013). Partial remission is associated with high rates of relapse, as was the presence of a coexisting obsessive-compulsive personality disorder.

It has been suggested that OCD has as many as 11 subtypes (Rosario-Campos et al., 2001). One subtype is early onset and is characterized by a higher rate of comorbid tic disorders, more frequently occurring in men, and greater familial association than other subtypes.

Implications for Function and Treatment

Depending on the compulsion, functional impairment may be modest or extreme (Moritz, 2008). Many of us have some ritualistic, almost superstitious, behavior that is minimally disruptive (e.g., wearing a particular item of clothing when taking a test or checking the door

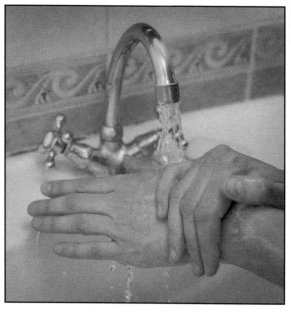

Figure 8-1. An individual with OCD may wash his or her hands until the skin is raw. (©2014 Shutterstock.com.)

lock exactly four times before leaving home). However, in some cases, the compulsion may become the central focus of life (e.g., as in the case of an individual who must wash clothing 13 times before wearing it). Individuals with these kinds of compulsions may be unable to maintain jobs or social relationships or engage in any activity other than the compulsion (Figure 8-1). This is true in spite of the individual's recognition of the disabling nature of the behavior.

Obsessive compulsiveness is often associated with social isolation (Moritz, 2008). However, many of the fears individuals have about the potential for harmful events do not materialize. They are, for example, not likely to commit suicide, engage in criminal behavior, or become addicted to drugs, even though these are common obsessional worries. Although the incidence of suicide and drug abuse is higher in individuals with OCD than in the general population, neither is frequent.

In the area of skills, cognition is the most obviously affected (Nakao et al., 2009). Verbal memory, global attention and psychomotor speed, and visuospatial and executive functions are all impaired. Individuals with OCD have difficulty with learning strategies, perhaps as a result of limited mental flexibility and limited ability to plan their activities (Tükel et al., 2012).

Performance patterns are seriously affected in individuals with OCD. Unlike those psychiatric disorders in which patterns are disrupted, in OCD, patterns are rigid, well-established, and highly dysfunctional (Moritz, 2008). As a result, quality of life is poor for these individuals.

The most effective treatment involves the use of psychotropic medication in combination with cognitive behavioral therapy (CBT; Alsadat, Madani, Kanaifar, Hamid Atashpour, & Bin Habil, 2013; McGuire, Lewin, Horng, Murphy, & Storch, 2012). Medication is prescribed to reduce anxiety and depressive symptoms, whereas CBT focuses on training the individual to reframe distorted thought processes that lead to ineffectual behaviors. As an adjunct to CBT, mindfulness therapy can serve as an additional strategy for addressing ineffective thought processes. Mindfulness requires focusing on immediate thoughts in a structured way, with an emphasis on being in the present. Evidence also exists that adding family intervention to CBT and medication can improve outcomes, especially for children with OCD (Piancentini et al., 2011).

Complementary and alternative treatments, including herbal supplementation and yoga, have some limited evidence of efficacy (Sarris, Camfield, & Berk, 2012). Acupuncture also has been used, again with limited research but some positive findings (Samuels, Gropp, Singer, & Oberbaum, 2008).

Implications for Occupational Therapy

Occupational therapy can focus on both symptom management and the replacement of negative patterns and habits with more helpful ones. Anxiety management, either by diverting attention or through relaxation training, is one strategy. The therapist might, for example, help the individual to identify a pleasurable activity that requires attention (e.g., writing a poem, playing chess). This approach requires the therapist to be sensitive to the possibility that such activity could increase anxiety for some people as they begin to exchange habits and patterns for their compulsive behaviors. Activities that require gross motor action to the point of fatigue may also promote relaxation. When the client is relaxed, it may be possible to focus the individual's attention so that he or she knows what relaxation feels like.

Replacement of habits and patterns can be an essential component of CBT. Individuals with OCD may have limited experience of pleasurable and productive engagement in occupation, in part because so much of their time has been consumed with their compulsions. It is helpful to move gradually—using principles of systematic desensitization—so that the individual can experience the successes that help reduce anxiety and build self-esteem.

Body Dysmorphic Disorder

Individuals with this disorder are preoccupied with perceived flaws in their physical appearance. Most typically, the perceived flaw is one that others either do not see at all or see as a very minor feature.

Specific diagnostic criteria include preoccupation with perceived flaws in appearance that others do not see and repetitive behaviors or acts (i.e., excessive grooming, seeking reassurance, comparing one's appearance with others) because of concern about appearance (APA, 2013). These behaviors are accompanied by significant distress or dysfunction. It is important to rule out eating disorders in particular but also other anxiety, depressive, and psychotic disorders.

Specifiers allow for greater detail about whether the main preoccupation is **muscle dysmorphia** (i.e., preoccupation with the adequacy of muscle mass). Muscle dysmorphia is an added dimension of body dysmorphic disorder (BDD) in the DSM-5 (Murray & Baghurst, 2013). Some concern exists that it may be difficult to discriminate between bodybuilding as a leisure and health-focused activity, and a focus that is more obsessional in nature.

BDD specifiers can also note whether the condition is accompanied by good, fair, poor, or absent insight. As with OCD, the absence of insight is delusional, given that the individual is convinced of a fact that does not correlate with reality as observed by others.

Etiology

The etiology of BDD is almost certainly multifactorial (Feusner, Neziroglu, Wilhelm, Mancusi, & Bohan, 2010); abuse (physical, emotional, sexual) in childhood, learned response (e.g., to teasing about a body part), and cultural factors (differing aesthetic standards between groups) have all been implicated. These factors are consistent with a learned cognition model of behavior.

It is probable that at least some genetic component exists for the development of BDD, although, compared with some of the disorders presented in earlier chapters, this factor makes a smaller contribution to its development (Feusner et al., 2010). Similarly, there are observed changes in neurotransmission, but, again, not to the extent found in the psychotic or mood disorders.

BDD is often comorbid with eating disorders (Kollei, Schieber, de Zwaan, Svitak, & Martin, 2013). Both disorders focus on obsession with perceived physical imperfections.

Similarly, muscle dysmorphia seems to be associated with eating disorders (Grieve, Truba, & Bowersox, 2009). However, it has diagnostic criteria very similar to those for body dysmorphic disorder, which is a more global misperception of the body. Muscle dysmorphia occurs primarily in men and is reflected in a belief that one's muscles are smaller than they actually are. Prognosis, function, and treatment are similar to those for body dysmorphic disorder.

Prognosis

Body dysmorphic disorder tends to be chronic, often with a pattern of exacerbation and remission (Phillips, Menard, Quinn, Didie, & Stout, 2013). In a longitudinal study over 4 years, 85% of individuals with BDD experienced either partial or full remission; however, of those individuals, 29% relapsed. Psychotic features and poor insight are associated with a more chronic course.

Implications for Function and Treatment

Body dysmorphic disorder is associated with an array of functional deficits (Phillips et al., 2013). Quality of life is reported to be poor, and there is a relatively high risk of suicide (IsHak et al., 2012). The disorder does not contribute directly to occupational dysfunction, in that the individual may be capable of managing work, self-care, and other occupations. However, anxiety about personal appearance interferes with social relationships and, by extension, with any aspect of function that might require social interaction (Kelly, Walters, & Phillips, 2010). Because of this anxiety, work may be affected by having difficulty interacting with coworkers, and social participation may be significantly limited.

Patterns, roles, and habits can be impaired by the constant focus on appearance to the exclusion of other, more positive, activities (Figure 8-2). There is reason to believe that cognition is impaired, as the person's perceptions are considerably distorted (Buhlmann, Winter, & Kathmann, 2013; Kollei, Brunhoeber, Rauh, de Zwaan, & Martin, 2012). In particular, it appears that individuals with BDD focus more strongly on individual details in visual stimuli, and they have difficulty responding to global aspects of those stimuli (Feusner et al., 2010).

Individuals with BDD are quite likely to seek plastic surgery, often repeatedly (Sarwer & Spitzer, 2012). A striking example is that of the pop star, Michael Jackson. Early photos of the singer are significantly different when compared with those taken near his death.

Body dysmorphic disorder treatment recommendations focus on CBT, with psychopharmacological intervention to reduce anxiety as CBT is implemented (Neziroglu & Santos, 2013). Medications typically include selective serotonin reuptake inhibitors, as well as antianxiety medications (Phillips et al., 2013). In addition to CBT, family therapy and several forms of psychotherapy have been reported as typical intervention strategies. However, as noted previously, all these interventions have limited success.

Because BDD is at least in part learned, researchers believe it can be remediated with behavioral strategies (Feusner et al., 2010). Operant conditioning strategies may be helpful.

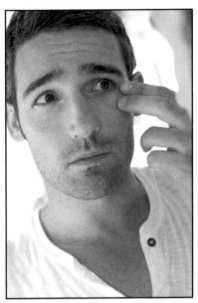

Figure 8-2. People with body dysmorphic disorder are excessively focused on, and critical of, their appearance. (©2014 Shutterstock.com.)

Implications for Occupational Therapy

As is true for many disorders in which habits, roles, and patterns are dysfunctional and distorted, occupational therapy can be valuable in redirecting energy and attention to more helpful performance patterns in individuals with body dysmorphic disorder. As a person reduces his or her focus on physical attributes, new interests, opportunities for meaningful engagement with others, and renewed focus on work, leisure, and social interactions may increase. In particular, individuals with BDD may struggle with social skills. Opportunities for direct practice (through role playing) and less direct practice (through group activities) can provide positive experiences that build self-confidence.

Hoarding Disorder

Reality television has made the general population aware of a disorder that was, until recently, relatively hidden. Some individuals have an obsessive need to collect and an inability to part with possessions. Taken to extremes, these individuals may live in situations so cluttered that their health and safety—and that of others—is at risk. Specific diagnostic criteria include persistent difficulty parting with possessions, even those of no value, accompanied by perceived need to save those objects and experiencing anxiety and distress when attempting to discard them (APA, 2013). These behaviors lead to substantial clutter in living areas. Individuals retain this mass of objects unless others (family, authorities) have cleaned the space—and they then acquire more possessions. The disorder must be distinguished from other anxiety disorders, OCD, personality disorders, and psychosis.

Specifiers clarify whether there is accompanying excessive acquisition (e.g., buying multiple versions of objects and being unable to discard them) and whether there is good, fair, poor, or absent insight.

Etiology

Because hoarding has only recently been accepted as a diagnosis separate from OCD, its etiology is not well understood (Timpano et al., 2013). Among the theories about its emergence are the possibility that it is a learned behavior, reinforced by reduction in anxiety when objects are saved, or that it is a cognitive disorder, reflected in the inability to recognize that one has kept too much (Grisham & Barlow, 2005).

Hoarding disorder mechanisms include some compulsive features, but there is relatively low comorbidity. The disorder may more closely mirror the impulse control disorders discussed in Chapter 16. Another strong comorbid relationship exists with depression, but there is good evidence that hoarding is indeed a separate disorder (Hall, Tolin, Frost, & Steketee, 2013).

Hoarding has been linked to life stressors and trauma (Landau et al., 2011). Severity of hoarding is associated with the frequency of traumatic events. In addition, speculation exists that hoarding is an evolutionary strength run amok (Grisham & Barlow, 2005). Keeping objects that might be needed in a potential situation of scarcity would confer survival benefits in the event the scarcity actually occurred. However, for individuals with hoarding disorder, the acquisition and keeping of objects (and sometimes animals) becomes excessive and overwhelming. Typically, awareness that the behavior is a problem emerges much later than the behavior itself.

Prognosis

Hoarding disorder seems to be relatively chronic and has a progressive course (Grisham & Barlow, 2005). Symptoms typically appear in late adolescence and young adulthood and worsen over the course of life. It is not unusual for the individual's behavior to be called to the attention of authorities, at which point the living space may be cleared. However, as soon as the authorities are no longer involved, accumulation of possessions tends to resume.

Implications for Function and Treatment

A challenge for the diagnosing of hoarding disorder is distinguishing between collecting, a common and often enjoyable leisure (and sometimes work) occupation, and hoarding (Nordsletten & Mataix-Cols, 2012). The magnitude of the hoarding behavior is such that most clinicians in the DSM trials had little difficulty distinguishing between the normative behavior and the disorder.

In the case of animal hoarding, such as the housing of dozens of cats, the dominant issue may be difficulty with social interaction (Patronek & Nathanson, 2009). The individual may transfer his or her interactive needs onto the animals as a way to avoid anticipated disappointment with other humans.

Over time, hoarding can lead to significant dysfunction. Individuals may find it extremely difficult to manage self-care activities, as their living spaces are overwhelmed with objects. They may experience anxiety that causes them to have work-related difficulties and to withdraw from social interaction.

Many of these individuals do not identify themselves as having a problem, and among those who do, it is often articulated in terms of problems organizing their belongings, not of having them in the first place (Grisham & Barlow, 2005). Most often these individuals seek treatment only when family members, neighbors, or friends insist.

The greatest treatment success for hoarding disorder has been reported with cognitive behavioral therapy (Tolin, Frost, & Steketee, 2007). The affected individual needs to learn to reframe his or her beliefs about objects and to practice removing them from the home. As suggested by behavioral strategies about successive approximations, early efforts may need to be modest. For this reason, intervention that occurs before the hoarding behavior has led to unsafe conditions in the home is most helpful. However, there are situations in which the individual must be removed and, in some extreme cases, the home destroyed.

Implications for Occupational Therapy

Little occupational therapy literature exists that addresses specific interventions for individuals with hoarding disorder. Undertaking an occupational profile, helping the client to understand what valued activities might be prevented by the hoarding behavior and encouraging resumption of those valued activities may be of help. Focusing on safety issues and the needs of loved ones might also encourage behavior change. In situations where the individual expresses a willingness to change, teaching and practicing strategies for removing objects and organizing those that remain may be helpful.

Trichotillomania (Hair-Pulling Disorder); Excoriation (Skin-Picking) Disorder

These two disorders are often considered together in the literature. Trichotillomania joined the diagnostic system in the fourth edition of the DSM (DSM-IV; APA, 1994), whereas excoriation disorder is new to the DSM-5 (APA, 2013). These disorders are both characterized by intentional damage to the self, the former through the pulling of hair and the latter by picking at the skin until lesions appear. Some researchers cluster them as "grooming disorders" because they mimic grooming behaviors found in other species (Lovato et al., 2012).

Specific diagnostic criteria for trichotillomania include the recurrent pulling out of hair with accompanying hair loss, in spite of repeated efforts to stop the behavior (APA, 2013). Symptoms cause distress or dysfunction. The disorder must be distinguished from other disorders, such as BDD.

Specific diagnostic criteria for excoriation (skin-picking) disorder include repeated picking at the skin, with resulting sores, in spite of repeated attempts to stop the behavior (APA, 2013). The behavior causes significant distress or dysfunction. The behavior must be distinguished from other physical or mental disorders, such as a psychotic disorder or body dysmorphic disorder.

Etiology

Although the etiology of trichotillomania and excoriation disorders is not well understood, they are hypothesized to emerge on the basis of a number of factors. The disorders' similarity to the grooming behaviors of some other animal species has led to speculation about a lingering evolutionary component (Zuchner et al., 2009). This would lend itself to a genetic explanation for the behavior. Specifically, the genetic component seems to affect neuroregulation. Alternate, or perhaps coexisting, explanations focus on learned emotional regulation.

The behaviors may also reflect a drive for particular sensory experiences (Walther, Ricketts, Conelea, & Woods, 2010). In addition, anxiety may lead to a set of cognitive beliefs that contribute to reduce unpleasant emotion.

Prognosis

Both trichotillomania and excoriation disorders seem to be relatively chronic in nature, with exacerbations and remissions over time (APA, 2013).

Implications for Function and Treatment

Function is affected in most spheres of life in individuals with trichotillomania and excoriation disorders. They may experience school or work problems, as well as difficulty in any occupation that requires social interaction (Walther et al., 2010). The individual is likely to be embarrassed by the physical consequences of his or her behavior (bald spots, lesions), although with excoriation disorder it may be possible to hide lesions. The individual may feel unattractive and may experience guilt, shame, pain, isolation, and fear.

The most effective interventions appear to be various behavioral strategies (Neziroglu, Hsia, & Yaryura-Tobias, 2000). Habit reversal therapy (Walther et al., 2010) that focuses on awareness, establishment of competing responses (e.g., using one's hands for something else so they are not free to engage in the pulling or picking behavior), and social support are all strategies that have some benefit. Medication seems to be of limited value.

Implications for Occupational Therapy

Trichotillomania and excoriation disorders have little concrete information in the occupational therapy literature. It is reasonable to assume that therapists can be helpful in implementing behavioral strategies, particularly insofar as these help the individual to redirect behavior to more functional, purposeful occupations. It is undoubtedly valuable to have the individual engaged in occupations that keep his or her hands and attention occupied and focused elsewhere. Table 8-2 shows the diagnostic criteria and functional implications of the obsessive-compulsive and related disorders.

Cultural Considerations

OCD appears to have a fairly consistent presentation across cultures, although the research confirming this is limited (Matsunaga, & Seedat, 2011). Some differences have been noted in the content of the obsessions (Fontenelle, Mendlowicz, Marques, & Versiani, 2004).

The prevalence of BDD seems to vary somewhat based on ethnicity, with Whites and Latinos being somewhat more likely to have the disorder than Black, Native American, or Asian individuals (Boroughs, Krawczyk, & Thompson, 2010). To some extent, this may be the result of differing cultural values. Kanayama and Pope (2011) suggested, for example, that Japanese and Chinese cultures place less importance on physical strength, which may explain the much lower rates of muscle dysmorphia found in these two cultures.

Lifespan Considerations

School-age children (or their parents) who have OCD may attempt to hide the behaviors out of embarrassment or fear of peer victimization. Early treatment is important because the disorder can compromise school function, social development, and play, contributing to long-term functional consequences (Helbing & Ficca, 2009). OCD may also manifest somewhat differently in children, with rage sometimes being seen as the primary symptom (Storch et al., 2012). Such acting out can also compromise school, social, and home life.

In later life, consequences of these relatively chronic disorders are apparent in the long-term impact on work life, social networks, and other areas of function. Because individuals with OCD often experience the disorder over a lifetime, they have worse symptoms and poorer quality of life than individuals with less chronic mental disorders (Pulular, Levy, & Stewart, 2013).

TABLE 8-2

DIAGNOSTIC CRITERIA AND FUNCTIONAL IMPLICATIONS: OBSESSIVE-COMPULSIVE AND RELATED DISORDERS

DISORDER	DIAGNOSTIC CRITERIA (APA, 2013)	IMPLICATIONS FOR FUNCTION
Obsessive-compulsive disorder	Presence of obsessions and/or compulsions The obsessions and/or compulsions are time consuming or cause distress or dysfunction	Disorder may be moderate to severe Work, leisure, social, activities of daily life/instrumental activities of daily life (ADL/IADL) all negatively affected Dysfunctional roles, habits, and routines Impaired process skills Motor and communication skills typically not affected
Body dysmorphic disorder	Preoccupation with one or more perceived flaws or defects in appearance that are not visible to others Repetitive behaviors or thoughts related to concerns about appearance Distress or dysfunction Not an eating disorder	Deficits in social occupations, and any activity or occupation requiring social skills Roles, habits, routines all negatively affected, particularly in terms of grooming
Hoarding disorder	Significant difficulty parting with possessions associated with distress or anxiety if required to discard them Results in an accumulation of possessions that significantly clutter living areas, interfering with their use	Deficits in all occupations related to ADL/IADL, leisure, social, and potentially work Habits, routines, roles all negatively affected
Trichotillomania	Recurrent pulling out of hair, with hair loss accompanied by repeated attempts to stop the behavior Distress or dysfunction	Deficits in any occupation that requires social interaction
Excoriation disorder	Repeated skin picking with resulting sores or lesions accompanied by repeated attempts to stop the behavior Distress or dysfunction	Deficits in any occupation that requires social interaction

CASE STUDY

Jaime Olivares is a 28-year-old single man from Puerto Rico who lives in a small apartment in a run-down neighborhood in New York. His parents live in a suburb of New York City and call him regularly to see how he is doing. They also bring him groceries and provide other services because Mr. Olivares is very reluctant to leave his apartment building. His mother brings him food almost every day because he is very particular about what he will eat. There are only two or three traditional Puerto Rican dishes he will consume, and only if his mother fixes them. If she does not bring a meal, he will subsist on one particular brand of premade tortillas and bottled water.

Mr. Olivares spends most of each day in the building laundry room, where he washes every article of clothing a minimum of seven times after it has been worn. Unlike the rest of the apartment building, the laundry room is spotless because as Mr. Olivares waits for each wash cycle to finish, he cleans the room repeatedly.

Mr. Olivares works part time from his apartment as a computer support technician. He is highly skilled, but can work only a few hours a day because so much of his time is consumed by his need to wash his clothes repeatedly. He has few friends, although he does email a few of his former high school classmates from time to time. He takes anti-anxiety medication and is very responsible about the medication schedule. However, he does not find the medication particularly helpful.

His parents have become increasingly concerned about him because they are getting older and finding it more difficult to provide support for him. They are worried about what will happen when they are not around to help. When they consulted with Mr. Olivares' doctor, the physician recommended that he see both a psychiatrist and an occupational therapist. Cultural values made them all reluctant to involve a psychiatrist, but they were comfortable with the idea of seeing an occupational therapist.

The occupational therapist undertakes an occupational profile with Mr. Olivares but has difficulty identifying any occupations that are meaningful to him. Consistent with characteristics of anxiety disorders, his most habitual activity—clothes washing—is not satisfying, except as a way to reduce anxiety. Working with the therapist, Mr. Olivares begins the process of exploring various activities. He and the therapist focus initially on his computer activities, as these offer him opportunities to expand his horizons without increasing his anxiety by requiring him to leave his apartment. They also begin to explore more helpful mechanisms to manage his anxiety, including meditation and physical exercise. The therapist encourages him to consider purchasing a Nintendo Wii to provide a bridge from computer activities to physical activity.

As Mr. Olivares finds himself able to focus on activities other than washing his clothes, the therapist initiates a discussion of his eating habits. Together they explore mechanisms for increasing his comfort with a wider range of foods and ways he can begin to prepare his own food, rather than depending on his mother. As one strategy for helping him progress, he and the therapist explore nutritional factors related to good health. To support this effort, his mother makes him a cookbook of the several recipes he can consume comfortably, noting the brands of each ingredient she uses so that he can mimic her food preparation. This enables her to reduce the frequency with which she must prepare food for him, and he very gradually expands his food horizons to include a more balanced diet.

(continued)

CASE STUDY (CONTINUED)

THOUGHT QUESTIONS

1. What behavioral and emotional issues suggest that Mr. Olivares has a mental disorder?
2. What strengths do you see in Mr. Olivares' occupational profile?
3. What areas seem particularly problematic?
4. What cultural factors support Mr. Olivares' improvement, and what factors might interfere?

Internet Resources

American Association for Marriage and Family Therapy
http://www.aamft.org/imis15/content/Consumer_Updates/Obsessive-Compulsive_Disorder.aspx
Focuses on family issues associated with OCD and other anxiety disorders.

American Psychiatric Association
http://www.psychiatry.org/obsessive-compulsive-disorder
This site provides numerous resources for consumers and professionals.

International OCD Foundation
http://www.ocfoundation.org/
A self-help organization with a wide array of resources for individuals with OCD, their families, and for health care professionals.

Mayo Clinic
http://www.mayoclinic.com/health/body-dysmorphic-disorder/DS00559
Although it is difficult to find resources focused on body dysmorphic disorder, this Mayo Clinic site has a good overview, as well as a number of links and some publication listings.

National Institute of Mental Health
http://www.nimh.nih.gov/health/topics/obsessive-compulsive-disorder-ocd/index.shtml
Another in the National Institute of Mental Health series on mental disorders, this site has information for consumers and professionals.

References

Alsadat, M., Madani, N., Kanaifar, N., Hamid Atashpour, S., & Bin Habil, M. (2013). The effects of mindfulness group training on the rate of obsessive-compulsive disorder symptoms on the women in Isfahan City (Iran). *International Medical Journal, 20*(1), 13-37.

American Psychiatric Association. (1994). *Diagnostic and statistical manual of mental disorders* (4th ed.). Washington, DC: Author.

American Psychiatric Association. (2013). *Diagnostic and statistical manual of mental disorders* (5th ed.). Washington, DC: Author.

Boroughs, M.S., Krawczyk, R., & Thompson, K. (2010). Body dysmorphic disorder among diverse racial/ethnic and sexual orientation groups: Prevalence estimates and associated factors. *Sex Roles, 63*(9-10), 725-737.

Brooks, J.L., Johnson, B., & Zea, K. (Producers), & Brooks, J.L. (Director). (1997). *As good as it gets* [Motion picture]. United States: Gracie Films.

Buhlmann, U., Winter, A., & Kathmann, N. (2013). Emotion recognition in body dysmorphic disorder: Application of the reading the mind in the eyes task. *Body Image, 10*(2), 247-250.

Bystritsky, A., Khalsa, S.S., & Shiffman, J. (2013). Current diagnosis and treatment of anxiety disorders. *Pharmacy and Therapeutics, 38*(1), 41-44, 57

Eisen, J.L., Sibrava, N.J., Boisseau, C.L., Mancebo, M.C., Stout, R.L., Pinto. A., & Rasmussen, S.A. (2013). Five-year course of obsessive-compulsive disorder: Predictors of remission and relapse. *Journal of Clinical Psychiatry, 74*(3), 233-239.

Feusner, J.D., Neziroglu, F., Wilhelm, S., Mancusi, L., & Bohan, C. (2010). What causes BDD? Research findings and a proposed model. *Psychiatric Annals, 40*(7), 349-355.

Fontenelle, L.F., Mendlowicz, M.V., Marques, C., & Versiani, M. (2004). Trans-cultural aspects of obsessive-compulsive disorder: A description of a Brazilian sample and a systematic review of international clinical studies. *Journal of Psychiatric Research, 8*(4), 403-411.

Grieve, F.C., Truba, N., & Bowersox, S. (2009). Etiology, assessment, and treatment of muscle dysmorphia. *Journal of Cognitive Psychotherapy, 23*(4), 306-314.

Grisham, J.R., & Barlow, D.H. (2005). Compulsive hoarding: Current research and theory. *Journal of Psychopathology and Behavioral Assessment, 27*(1), 45-52.

Hall, B.J., Tolin, D.F., Frost, R.O., & Steketee, G. (2013). An exploration of comorbid symptoms and clinical correlates of clinically significant hoarding symptoms. *Depression and Anxiety, 30*(1), 67-76.

Helbing, M.C., & Ficca, M. (2009). Obsessive-compulsive disorder in school-age children. *Journal of School Nursing, 25*(1), 15-26.

Iervolino, A.C., Rijsdijk, F.V., Cherkas, L., Fullana, M.A., & Mataix-Cols, D. (2011). A multivariate twin study of obsessive-compulsive symptom dimensions. *Archives of General Psychiatry, 68*(6), 637-644.

IsHak, W.W., Bolton, M.A., Bensoussan, J.C., Dous, G.V., Nguyen, T.T., Powel-Hicks, A.L., . . . Ponton, K.M. (2012). Quality of life in body dysmorphic disorder. *CNS Spectrums: The International Journal of Neuropsychiatric Medicine, 17*(4), 167-175.

Kanayama, G., & Pope, H.G. (2011). Gods, men, and muscle dysmorphia. *Harvard Review of Psychiatry, 19*(2), 95-98.

Kelly, M.M., Walters, C., & Phillips, K.A. (2010). Social anxiety and its relationship to functional impairment in body dysmorphic disorder. *Behavior Therapy, 41*, 143-153.

Kessler, R.C., Petukhova, M., Sampson, N.A., Zaslavsky, A.M., & Wittchen, H. (2012). Twelve-month and lifetime prevalence and lifetime morbid risk of anxiety and mood disorders in the United States. *International Journal of Methods in Psychiatric Research, 21*(3), 169-184.

Kollei, I., Brunhoeber, S., Rauh, E., de Zwaan, M., & Martin, A. (2012). Body image, emotions and thought control strategies in body dysmorphic disorder compared to eating disorders and healthy controls. *Journal of Psychosomatic Research, 72*(4), 321-327.

Kollei, I., Schieber, K., de Zwaan, M., Svitak, M., & Martin, A. (2013). Body dysmorphic disorder and nonweight-related body image concerns in individuals with eating disorders. *International Journal of Eating Disorders, 46*(1), 52-59.

Landau, D., Iervolino, A.C., Pertusa, A., Santo, S., Singh, S., & Mataix-Cols, D. (2011). Stressful life events and material deprivation in hoarding disorder. *Journal of Anxiety Disorders, 25*, 192-202.

Lovato, L., Ferrão, Y.A., Stein, D.J., Shavitt, R.G., Fontenelle, L.F., Vivian, A., . . . Cordioli, A.V. (2012). Skin picking and trichotillomania in adults with obsessive-compulsive disorder. *Comprehensive Psychiatry, 53*(5), 562-568.

Matsunaga, H., & Seedat, S. (2011). Obsessive-compulsive spectrum disorders: Cross-national and ethnic issues. In E. Hollander, J. Zohar, P.J. Sirovatka, & D.A. Regier (Eds.), *Obsessive-compulsive spectrum disorders: Refining the research agenda for DSM-V* (pp. 205-221). Arlington, VA: American Psychiatric Association.

McGuire, J.F., Lewin, A.B., Horng, B., Murphy, T.K., & Storch, E.A. (2012). The nature, assessment, and treatment of obsessive-compulsive disorder. *Postgraduate Medicine, 124*(1), 152-165.

Moritz, S. (2008). A review on quality of life and depression in obsessive-compulsive disorder. *CNS Spectrums: The International Journal of Neuropsychiatric Medicine, 13*(9, Suppl. 14), 16-22.

Murray, S.B., & Baghurst, T. (2013). Revisiting the diagnostic criteria for muscle dysmorphia. *Strength & Conditioning Journal, 35*(1), 69-74.

Nakao, T., Nakagawa, A., Yoshiura, T., Nakatani, E., Nabeyama, M., Sanematsu, M., . . . Kanba, S. (2009). Duration effect of obsessive-compulsive disorder on cognitive function: A functional MRI study. *Depression & Anxiety, 26*(9), 814-823.

Neziroglu, F., Hsia, C., & Yaryura-Tobias, J.A. (2000). Behavioral, cognitive, and family therapy for obsessive-compulsive and related disorders. *Psychiatric Clinics of North America, 23*(3), 657-670.

Neziroglu, E., & Santos, N.M. (2013). Advances in the treatment of body dysmorphic disorder. *International Journal of Cognitive Therapy, 6*(2), 138-149.

Nordsletten, A.E., & Mataix-Cols, D. (2012). Hoarding versus collecting: Where does pathology diverge from play? *Clinical Psychology Review, 32*(3), 165-176.

Pallanti, S., & Hollander, E. (2008). Obsessive-compulsive disorder spectrum as a scientific "metaphor." *CNS Spectrum, 13*(Suppl. 14), 6-15.

Patronek, G.J., & Nathanson, J.N. (2009). A theoretical perspective to inform assessment and treatment strategies for animal hoarders. *Clinical Psychology Review, 29*(3), 274-281.

Piancentini, J., Bergman, L., Chang, S., Langley, A., Peris, T., Wood, J.J., & McCraken, J. (2011). Controlled comparison of family cognitive behavioral therapy and psychoeducation/relaxation training for child obsessive-compulsive disorder. *Journal of the American Academy of Child & Adolescent Psychiatry, 50*, 1149-1161.

Phillips, K.A, Menard, W., Quinn, E., Didie, E.R., & Stout, R.L. (2013). A 4-year prospective observational follow-up study of course and predictors of course in body dysmorphic disorder. *Psychological Medicine, 43*(5), 1109-1117.

Pulular, A., Levy, R., & Stewart, R. (2013). Obsessive and compulsive symptoms in a national sample of older people: Prevalence, comorbidity, and associations with cognitive function. *American Journal of Geriatric Psychiatry, 21*(3), 263-271.

Rosario-Campos, M.C., Leckman, J.F., Mercadante, M.T., Shavitt, R.G., Prado, H.S., Sada, P., . . . Miguel, E.C.(2001). Adults with early-onset obsessive-compulsive disorder. *American Journal of Psychiatry, 158*, 1899-1903.

Samuels, N., Gropp, C., Singer, S.R., & Oberbaum, M. (2008). Acupuncture for psychiatric illness: A literature review. *Behavioral Medicine, 34*, 55-62.

Sarris, J., Camfield, D., & Berk, M. (2012). Complementary medicine, self-help, and lifestyle interventions for obsessive compulsive disorder (OCD) and the OCD spectrum: A systematic review. *Journal of Affective Disorders, 138*(3), 213-221.

Sarwer, D.B., & Spitzer. J.C. (2012). Body image dysmorphic disorder in persons who undergo aesthetic medical treatments. *Aesthetic Surgery Journal, 32*(8), 999-1009.

Storch, E.A., Jones, A.M., Lack, C.W., Ale, C.M., Sulkowski, M.L., Lewin, A.B., . . . Murphy, T.K. (2012).Rage attacks in pediatric obsessive-compulsive disorder: Phenomenology and clinical correlates. *Journal of the American Academy of Child & Adolescent Psychiatry, 51*(6), 582-592.

Taylor, S., Asmundson, G.J.G., & Jang, K.L. (2011). Etiology of obsessive-compulsive symptoms and obsessive-compulsive personality traits: Common genes, mostly different environments. *Depression and Anxiety, 28*(10), 863-869.

Timpano, K.R., Rasmussen, J., Exner, C., Rief, W., Schmidt, N.B., & Wilhelm, S. (2013). Hoarding and the multi-faceted construct of impulsivity: A cross-cultural investigation. *Journal of Psychiatric Research, 47*(3), 363-370.

Tolin, D.F., Frost, R.O., & Steketee, G. (2007). *Buried in treasures: Help for compulsive acquiring, saving, and hoarding.* New York, NY: Oxford University Press

Tükel, R., Gürvit, H., Ertekin, B., Aslantaş, O. Serap, E. Erhan, B., . . . Atalay, F. (2012). Neuropsychological function in obsessive-compulsive disorder. *Comprehensive Psychiatry, 53*(2), 167-175.

Walther, M.R., Ricketts, E.J. Conelea, C.A., & Woods, D.W. (2010). Recent advances in the understanding and treatment of trichotillomania. *Journal of Cognitive Psychotherapy, 24*(1), 46-64.

Zuchner, S., Wedland, J.R., Ashley-Koch, A.E., Collins, A.L., Tran-Viet, K.N., Quinn, K., . . . Murphy, D.L. (2009). Multiple rare SAPAP3 missense variants in trichotillomania and OCD. *Molecular Psychiatry, 14*, 6-9.

Trauma-Related and Stressor-Related Disorders

Learning Outcomes

By the end of this chapter, readers will be able to:
- Describe the various trauma- and stressor-related disorders
- Differentiate among trauma- and stressor-related disorders on the basis of symptoms and onset
- Identify the causes of trauma- and stressor-related disorders
- Discuss the prevalence of trauma- and stressor-related disorders
- Describe treatment strategies for stressor-related disorders
- Discuss occupational therapy interventions for trauma- and stressor-related disorders

Bonder B.
Psychopathology and Function, Fifth Edition (pp 197-214).
© 2015 SLACK Incorporated.

KEY WORDS

- Dissociative
- Depersonalization

- Derealization
- Prolonged exposure therapy

CASE VIGNETTE

Hnub Khaab is a 38-year-old Hmong refugee who was recently given permission to immigrate to the United States. She was born in a refugee camp in Thailand, where she has lived with her parents and three siblings. Because the family remained in Thailand at the end of the Vietnam War, they lost their refugee status and were unable to come to the United States. A new policy established in 2003 changed this and the family decided to immigrate. However, they had heard stories from Hmong refugees returning from the United States about gangs and violence. Ms. Khaab is frightened by these stories, and she is anxious about the move. Like the rest of her family, she does not read and has very limited education. Her parents, who are now in their 70s, both recall the war with terror. They have nightmares and wake screaming in the night. Ms. Khaab is now terrified about staying in Thailand and about moving to the United States.

THOUGHT QUESTIONS

1. Do you think that Ms. Khaab has a mental disorder?
2. If so, what behaviors or feelings led you to that conclusion?
3. What areas of performance seem particularly impaired?
4. Are there cultural factors in this situation? If so, what do they contribute to the situation?

TRAUMA- AND STRESSOR-RELATED DISORDERS

- Reactive attachment disorder
- Disinhibited social engagement disorder

- Posttraumatic stress disorder
- Acute stress disorder
- Adjustment disorders

The common thread among these disorders is that the symptoms result from a severe traumatic or stressful event. Although studies exist that examine the possibility that some people have a biological predisposition to difficulty coping with trauma, the overarching etiology is based on an external factor or factors. The disorders in this cluster have been moved from other categories to create a new grouping. For example, posttraumatic stress disorder (PTSD) was previously included in the anxiety disorders category. Table 9-1 shows the prevalence of the trauma- and stressor-related disorders.

TABLE 9-1

PREVALENCE OF TRAUMA- AND STRESSOR-RELATED DISORDERS

DIAGNOSIS	PREVALENCE	GENDER RATIO (M:F)	SOURCE
Reactive attachment disorder	1.4% in a deprived population		Minnis, Marwick, Arthur, & McLaughlin, 2013
Disinhibited social engagement disorder	Not yet established		
Posttraumatic stress disorder	23% of individuals experiencing significant trauma	More frequent in women	Haagsma et al., 2012 APA, 2013
Acute stress disorder	7% to 33% of individuals experiencing trauma	More frequent in women	Bryant et al., 2011 APA, 2013
Adjustment disorders	2.9% in primary care client population		Fernández et al., 2012

Reactive Attachment Disorder and Disinhibited Social Engagement Disorder

Reactive attachment disorder and disinhibited social engagement disorder emerge from a similar set of circumstances (Gleason et al., 2011). Although the behavioral manifestations of the two conditions are essentially polar opposites, the resultant functional deficits are quite similar. For this reason, the diagnostic criteria for each disorder will be presented here, followed by a combined section addressing function and intervention.

Reactive attachment disorder (RAD) is a condition found most often in children who have experienced traumatic life circumstances in early life, typically institutionalization, severe abuse, or other experiences of "pathological care" (Follan et al., 2011; Figure 9-1). Follan et al. (2011) found that these children have distorted and problematic interactions with adults, particularly in the areas of "cuddliness with strangers; comfort-seeking from strangers, unpredictable reunion responses and frozen watchfulness" (p. 523). Not only do they tend to show excessive friendliness to strangers, they are also distant and distrustful with individuals they may know well.

Diagnostic criteria for RAD include a pattern of either disinhibited or withdrawn behavior toward caregivers, such as failure to seek comfort when distressed; social and emotional disturbance that is demonstrated by minimal social or emotional response to others; limited positive affect; and episodes of irritability, sadness, or fearfulness (American Psychiatric Association [APA], 2013). A history may exist of extremely inadequate care, including social neglect or deprivation, changes in caregivers that limit stable attachment, and residence in settings (e.g., institutions) that limit interaction with adults. Specifiers indicate whether the disorder is persistent, as well as the severity of the disorder.

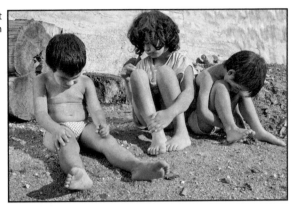

Figure 9-1. Children in institutions may not have adequate opportunity to bond with adult caregivers. (©2014 Shutterstock.com.)

Disinhibited social engagement disorder is new to the fifth edition of the *Diagnostic and Statistical Manual of Mental Health Disorders* (DSM-5; APA, 2013) and reflects a similar etiology with very different behavioral consequences, compared with RAD. In this case, the diagnostic criteria include a behavior pattern in which the child interacts with unfamiliar adults while displaying reduced reticence, overly familiar behavior, diminished checking in with adult caregiver, inappropriate willingness to go with strangers, and social disinhibition (APA, 2013). The child has had extremes of inadequate care, including social neglect or deprivation and residence in a setting that limits interaction with adults. Therefore, children with RAD respond to deprivation by withdrawing, whereas children with disinhibited social engagement disorder respond by inappropriate and excessive social interaction.

Children with RAD or disinhibited social engagement disorder have usually resided in situations where caregiving is distant and inadequate during important developmental periods, such as in the case of some children adopted from Russian and Romanian orphanages. Alternatively, the child may have been shunted from foster home to foster home, without having the experience of building a close, trusting relationship with a caring adult.

Etiology

For these two disorders, the etiology is in the diagnostic criteria. The child must have had the kind of deprived or traumatic caregiving that produces the behavioral and emotional symptoms. That said, there are differences of opinion about both the origin and the nature of the resultant behaviors. For example, some speculate that the behavior may carry an evolutionary advantage, and thus is a coping strategy, rather than a mental disorder (Balbernie, 2010). Although some consensus exists that the precipitant is inadequate care during critical periods in development of social interactions, there is also speculation that the disorders have neurological consequences that affect core brain and social functions (Minnis, Marwick, Arthur, & McLaughlin, 2006).

Prognosis

The prognosis for RAD is not good (Kay & Green, 2012). Because disinhibited social engagement disorder is a new label, little information about its prognosis exists, although there is reason to believe that the long-term outcome is similar. Although children placed in stable, loving environments may show improvement in behavior and emotional expression, there is speculation that particular aspects of these social relationships develop at particular periods during child development and may remain permanently impaired. Certainly, parents of children adopted from difficult backgrounds may find that these children never establish the kinds of warm, close relationships the parents attempt to foster (Harris, Thompson, & Mauldin, 2007; Stinehart, Scott, & Barfield, 2012).

Implications for Function and Treatment

RAD and disinhibited social engagement disorder affect multiple areas of occupation. In particular, children with these disorders have significant difficulty in social and educational settings. Their social skills are inadequate to the demands of the learning environment, often contributing to bullying—with the child either being bullied or becoming a bully (Raaska, Lapinleimu, et al., 2012). Also, a high incidence of learning disorders exists among these children, compounding their difficulties with everyday functioning (Raaska, Elovainio, et al., 2012).

Most typically, children with these disorders come to the attention of therapists, school counselors, and other health care professionals when they have been placed in a more stable environment, such as when they have been adopted. It is typical for these children to struggle with adjustment to family life, even in the presence of supportive and concerned adoptive parents (Raaska, Elovainio, et al., 2012; Wimmer, Vonk, & Reeves, 2010). The children, as they get older, may also struggle in work settings and have impulse and conduct issues that lead to legal troubles.

For example, a family adopted two Russian brothers, aged 7 and 9, who had lived most of their lives in an institution after being abandoned by their alcoholic mother. The adoptive family was aware that the boys might experience challenges adjusting to their new environment, and they were involved and supportive in helping the boys to make the change. Nevertheless, the boys had significant, ongoing school difficulties, frequent altercations with their adoptive parents, and, in the case of the younger brother, such frequent encounters with the juvenile justice system that the magistrate recognized him on sight.

A variety of interventions have been attempted in these children, all with mixed success at best. Family therapy is an obvious first choice because of the centrality of the issues around attachment to caregivers (Wimmer et al., 2010). In particular, a form of family therapy called *attachment therapy* has been suggested. It focuses explicitly on strategies to encourage effective and helpful attachment between parents and children.

Behavior management therapy has also been recommended (Buckner, Lopez, Dunkel, & Joiner, 2008). The specific focus is on developing systematic strategies for addressing problem behaviors, with reinforcement of appropriate social interactions. Typically, this therapy must be enacted by the parents, with guidance from professionals as needed.

Implications for Occupational Therapy

An initial occupational therapy intervention may be preparing foster and adoptive parents for the behaviors they might expect to minimize initial shock and family chaos. Direct instruction about parenting, particularly about behavior management strategies and behavior modification, can minimize initial adjustment difficulties. However, it is also important to help parents establish realistic expectations to minimize their disappointment if they cannot establish the hoped-for relationships. The family that adopted two Russian brothers described previously had been prepared for the initial difficulties they experienced, but they had limited success in establishing relationships with the boys.

Modeling, role-playing, and problem solving can help the parents to cope more effectively. Play therapy with the children can have multiple benefits (O'Connor, 2011), such as providing opportunities for expression of emotion through nonverbal mechanisms, particularly where the foster or adopted child is not a native English speaker. Opportunities for stress relief through physical activity can also be helpful. Play situations may reduce the threat of social encounters, shifting the focus from the child to the activity. Gross motor play may have beneficial effects in terms of coping in the classroom, and may help the child to develop positive interests.

Posttraumatic Stress Disorder

By definition, the emergence of this disorder always follows an event that was a major life stress—one that must be more severe and unusual than those found in everyday life. Distress following a divorce would not be considered PTSD, whereas distress following a life-threatening fire might. The trauma may involve a threat to one's life or the lives of one's family, destruction of one's home, victimization during a crime, or seeing someone else severely injured or killed. The trauma may be something that occurs only to the individual (e.g., cases of sexual or physical abuse) or to groups of individuals (e.g., Holocaust survivors).

PTSD was identified following the Vietnam War as a result of the large numbers of combat veterans who had extreme difficulty readapting to civilian life. However, it should be noted that the syndrome certainly existed prior to this time (e.g., "shell shock" during World War I; Tierney, 2000). World War II veterans who were prisoners of war showed signs of psychological distress long after the event (Yoder, Tuerk, & Acierno, 2010). Among the events that have been associated with PTSD in individuals is involvement with homicide, war, torture, automobile accident, or natural disaster (Seides, 2010). In addition, hospitalization in an intensive care unit (Griffiths, Fortune, Barber, & Young, 2007), surviving childhood cancer (Lee & Santacroce, 2007), and sexual abuse (Fogler, Shipherd, Clarke, Jensen, & Rowe, 2008) have been described as precipitating PTSD. PTSD is also seen in individuals whose occupational role is to assist victims of trauma, such emergency medical personnel.

The trauma is usually accompanied by extreme feelings of terror and helplessness, and a primary characteristic of PTSD is reexperiencing both the event and such feelings in ways that are recurrent and intrusive. The individual may have bad dreams or experience these feelings of terror and helplessness at unpredictable times and in unpredictable places. As this occurs, the individual begins to avoid the situations that seem to stimulate the feeling or to develop a diminished ability to respond to the world as a mechanism for avoiding the unpleasant emotions.

Individuals who have this disorder have disturbed sleep, exaggerated startle reflexes, poor concentration, and extreme irritability, which is often accompanied by aggression. The disorder frequently occurs in conjunction with depression or anxiety. Substance abuse is also a commonly coexisting condition, perhaps as the individual attempts to self-medicate to reduce symptoms (Durai et al., 2011).

The diagnostic criteria for PTSD in individuals aged 6 years and older include exposure to actual or threatened death, serious injury, or sexual violence, either by direct experience, witnessing the event in person, learning of a traumatic event that happened to a close friend or family member, or experiencing repeated or extreme exposure to details of a traumatic event (as in the case of first responders or police; APA, 2013). Intrusive symptoms associated with the trauma are in evidence, including recurrent, intrusive memories of the trauma; nightmares; and dissociative reactions in which one feels the events are recurring, accompanied by intense distress and physiological reactions. In addition, the individual persistently avoids stimuli associated with the traumatic event and experiences negative alterations in cognition and mood after the event, including difficulty remembering important aspects of the trauma and distorted beliefs about oneself, others, or the world. Notably, there is decreased interest or participation in important activities, along with feelings of detachment. The individual often experiences altered arousal, such as irritability, angry outbursts, reckless behavior,

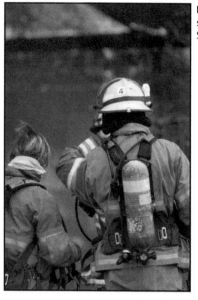

Figure 9-2. Emergency personnel experience repeated exposure to traumatic events that can contribute to PTSD. (©2014 Shutterstock.com.)

hypervigilance, sleep difficulties, or exaggerated startle reflex. The symptoms persist for at least 1 month and cause distress or dysfunction.

Specifiers can clarify whether **dissociative** symptoms, altered sense of reality, or inability to remember aspects of the event exist. These symptom can include **depersonalization** or **derealization**. Depersonalization is a sense of being outside oneself, watching oneself act. Derealization is a sense that the world is somehow unreal. In children aged 6 years or younger, the trauma may be acted out in play situations, and dreams and flashbacks may be symbolic, lacking the specific content of the trauma.

Etiology

A traumatically stressful event is a necessary precondition to the emergence of this disorder. The event may include anything ranging from natural disasters, involvement in combat, physical or sexual abuse, or other highly traumatic and stressful events. Emergency personnel have repeated exposure to traumatic events and may develop PTSD over time (Figure 9-2). Depending on the severity of the event, a single event—as was the case with 9/11—can contribute to long-term PTSD.

It is not clear why some individuals are susceptible to PTSD, whereas others who have similar experiences are not. A variety of premorbid personality traits seem associated with the probability of developing PTSD (Breslau, Troost, Bohnert, & Luo, 2013). For example, psychological resilience seems to be a moderating factor (Nemeroff et al., 2006). Styles of learning, which are associated with coping mechanisms, also appear to be personality factors that increase the probability of developing PTSD in the event of exposure to a traumatic event (Lommen, Engelhard, Sijbrandij, van den Hout, & Hermans, 2013).

PTSD may have genetic predisposition (Wilker & Kolassa, 2012), and neurological changes occur in multiple memory circuits with the development of PTSD (Peres, McFarlane, Nasello, & Moores, 2008). In particular, function of the hippocampus is impaired (Nemeroff et al., 2006).

An important factor for occupational therapists is the increasing recognition that PTSD may occur in individuals who have experienced a traumatic injury or other medical condition

(Griffiths et al., 2007; Lee & Santacroce, 2007; Spitzer et al., 2009). Burn victims (Ehde, Patterson, Wiechman, & Wilson, 2000), cancer clients, and individuals with spinal cord injuries (Otis, Marchand, & Courtois, 2012) often show evidence of PTSD, which can complicate recovery from the physical injury. For example, individuals remembering the experience of being burned may have agitated movement that can compromise skin grafts.

Prognosis

Many individuals with PTSD improve over time and, depending on the individual's personality and the type of trauma, access to helpful therapeutic support can reduce symptoms. However, for a substantial group of individuals, the disorder is chronic. One study of clients who experienced major physical trauma found that 2 years after the event, the prevalence of PTSD was 20% (Haagsma et al., 2012).

By definition, PTSD must last at least 1 month, but it may persist for long periods of time. For example, World War II prisoners of war showed high levels of depression 40 years after the war (Rintamaki, Weaver, Elbaum, Klama, & Miskevics, 2009).

Good prognosis is predicted by healthy premorbid function, less severe and briefer trauma, and good social support (Miller, 2000). Women are more likely to have a good outcome than men (Haagsma et al., 2012). Some individuals with PTSD develop a comorbid substance abuse disorder, which probably is the result of efforts to self-medicate to reduce anxiety (Johnson, 2008). The acute form of PTSD may be somewhat more responsive to treatment than more chronic forms (Bisson, 2007; Miller, 2000). Children with PTSD as a result of abuse, invasive medical procedures (e.g., cancer treatment), or refugee experiences often show later signs of personality disorder (Tierney, 2000).

Implications for Function and Treatment

Depending on the severity of PTSD, function may be moderately or severely impaired. Some individuals continue to hold jobs and maintain social and leisure activities. Because a defining characteristic of PTSD is the avoidance of any stimulus that might cause the individual to remember the event, some individuals find that their function is circumscribed. If the trauma occurred in a place that is difficult to avoid, the resultant PTSD may be quite disabling. Many individuals with PTSD find it difficult or impossible to work (Wald & Taylor, 2009). Similarly, some individuals find that reexperiencing the event is frequent and that the accompanying fears are severe, leading to significant disability. Social function can be greatly affected as a result of both the individual's anxiety and the irritability and anger they direct toward others.

Children who have experienced trauma may have difficulty functioning well in school (Uguak, 2010). Skill areas, such as cognition, are impaired as intrusive thoughts affect concentration. Social and academic occupations are also affected.

Where the trauma has been severe and prolonged, rage, depression, and humiliation may persist for years (Moser, Cahill, & Foa, 2010). For example, abused children may show signs of trauma throughout adulthood. More than one-third of abused women in a homeless shelter had symptoms of PTSD (Humphreys, Lee, Neylan, & Marmar, 2001), suggesting that these women were unable to manage work and activities of daily life.

Strong evidence exists that **prolonged exposure**, a type of cognitive behavioral therapy (CBT), is highly effective (Foa, Gillihan, & Bryant, 2013). Many studies conducted in independent research laboratories have demonstrated that prolonged exposure is effective for most types of trauma, for most individuals, and across cultures. Prolonged exposure is similar to behavioral strategies of systematic desensitization in which the individual constructs a hierarchy from not at all traumatic to very traumatic and envisions these in association with meditation or other relaxation techniques. Trauma-focused CBT is effective for children and adolescents as well (Smith et al., 2013).

Group and other psychodynamic therapies may also be helpful (Schottenbauer, Glass, Arnkoff, & Gray, 2008), particularly those in which the individual can talk with others who have had similar experiences. Antianxiety or antidepressant medication may be used, although it is concerning that a substance abuse disorder may emerge as the individual seeks to relieve tension. Another concern is that the use of medications has not been adequately studied in individuals with PTSD (Sheerin, Seim, & Spates, 2012). Behavioral and cognitive interventions are preferred for this reason because they appear to be somewhat more effective (Foa et al., 2013; Gerearts & McNally, 2008). Hypnosis, other mindfulness techniques (Lynn, Malakataris, Condon, Maxwell, & Cleere, 2012), and qigong, and tai chi (Grodin, Piwowarczyk, Fulker, Bazazi, & Saper, 2008) may also be helpful and may be particularly appealing to individuals from non-U.S. cultural groups, particularly Asian cultures.

In cases of sexual or physical abuse, remediation of the situation that led to the disorder is an important component of treatment. The abuser must be treated or the child must be removed from his or her presence and sometimes removed from the family. In cases of natural disasters, children who receive supportive intervention immediately tend to have better outcomes than if treatment is delayed (Deering, 2000). Similarly, women who are in abusive relationships do best when they can escape the situation and learn adaptive mechanisms for coping with their anxiety and their life situations (Woods & Isenberg, 2001).

One clear finding is that the sooner intervention for PTSD is started, the more likely it is to be helpful (Bisson, 2007). The reasons for this are not well understood, although it may be that prompt treatment reduces the likelihood that reactions and behavior will become habitual. Dropout rates from treatment, regardless of type, are high (Schottenbauer, Glass, Arnkoff, Tendick, & Gray, 2008). Efforts to understand these findings have been hampered by methodological inconsistency in the research literature.

Implications for Occupational Therapy

Occupational therapists use a variety of approaches when working with individuals with trauma- and stressor-related disorders. Several goals are prominent. First, anxiety management is essential. Relaxation, either by diverting attention or through relaxation training, is one strategy. The therapist might, for example, help the individual to identify a pleasurable activity that requires attention (e.g., writing a poem, playing chess). Yoga can be effective in managing stress as well (Stoller, Greuel, Cimini, Fowler, & Koomar, 2012). Activities that require gross motor action to the point of fatigue may also promote relaxation. However, the therapist must be sensitive to the possibility that any activity could increase anxiety for some people.

For individuals with PTSD, opportunities to express emotion are important. These individuals often benefit from talking with others who have had the experience and from nonverbal expressive activities. One such client, a rape victim, progressed over time from drawing horrible monsters in stormy skies to drawing pleasant pastoral scenes. She found the activity both relaxing and cathartic.

Goals may focus on specific performance skills (e.g., setting goals, managing time) or on symptom management (e.g., stress management strategies; Precin, 2011). In children, the skills that promote resilience are important to assess and develop (Precin & Lopez, 2011). For example, practice identifying emotions and managing them, perhaps through a creative activity, as well as opportunities to learn to use social support, can reduce anxiety.

As anxiety is resolved, attention must be paid to substituting new activities that are satisfying. Individuals may need with help reestablishing social ties, work activities, or leisure pursuits. Individuals with PTSD report restrictions in participation in most occupations and that resuming participation in work and leisure increases enjoyment and perceived competence (Tuchner, Meiner, Parush, & Hartman-Maeir, 2010).

Acute Stress Disorder

Acute stress disorder has symptoms almost identical to those of PTSD, but the duration is shorter. Symptoms must last at least 3 days (although they usually emerge immediately after the trauma), but if they last for 1 month or longer, the diagnosis would be changed to PTSD. Diagnostic criteria for acute stress disorder include exposure to actual or threatened death, serious injury, or sexual violation; witnessing a trauma; learning about a trauma that has affected a close friend or family member; or experiencing repeated or extreme exposure to trauma, as in the case of first responders or police (APA, 2013). The individual must have at least nine symptoms reflecting intrusion (e.g., recurrent intrusive thoughts or distressing dreams), such as negative mood, **dissociative** symptoms (i.e., altered sense of reality or inability to remember aspects of the event), avoidance symptoms, or arousal symptoms (e.g., sleep disturbance, irritability or angry outbursts, hypervigilance, difficulty concentrating), leading to significant distress or dysfunction.

Etiology, implications for function, treatment, and occupational therapy intervention are quite similar to those for PTSD. Although some speculation exists that acute stress disorder may be a precursor to PTSD, existing research has not supported that contention (Bryant, Friedman, Spiegel, Ursano, & Strain, 2011). A significant factor is that acute stress disorder has a better prognosis than PTSD, particularly if treatment is implemented quickly. Both supportive counseling and cognitive behavioral therapies can be effective in helping an individual process trauma in its immediate aftermath (Nixon, 2012). Including anxiety management techniques in particular can be helpful (Koucky, Galovski, & Nixon, 2012). It is important to note that the dropout rate from CBT is considerably higher than from supportive counseling.

One caution about early intervention is the recognition that some degree of reaction to trauma is normal and expected (Koucky et al., 2012). For this reason, some suggest that treatment might be delayed until 2 weeks after the event, given that many people cope with the early distress without the need for intervention. The obvious challenge in making a decision about delaying treatment is that early treatment is associated with better outcomes, at least for PTSD.

Adjustment Disorders

In the fourth edition of the DSM (DSM-IV; APA, 1994), adjustment disorder was not included in the stress-related disorders, and was, in fact, used primarily as a diagnosis for individuals who had immediate life issues that were causing distress, making it something of a "wild card" diagnosis (Baumeister & Kufner, 2009). In the new conceptualization, adjustment disorder is considered a response to stress, so that it fits most closely with PTSD and the other trauma- and stress-related disorders (Strain & Friedman, 2011). One hope with regard to this move is that the reclassification will promote more research on an important but often overlooked diagnosis.

Diagnostic criteria for adjustment disorders include emotional or behavioral symptoms associated with specific stressors (APA, 2013). The symptoms must be clinically significant and include distress out of proportion to the severity of the stressor and impairment in important areas of function. Normal bereavement is excluded, and the symptoms of adjustment disorder generally abate within 6 months after the stressor has ended. For example, if an adjustment disorder follows a job loss, the expectation is that within 6 months the individual would resume normal function and mood, assuming that there has been resolution of the unemployment. Depression and anxiety are common co-occurring mental disorders.

Specifiers indicate whether the disorder is accompanied by depression, anxiety, mixed anxiety and depression, disturbance of conduct, or mixed disturbance of emotions and conduct.

Etiology

As is true with the other trauma- and stress-related disorders, a stressor of some type must be present. However, for adjustment disorder, the stressor is less severe and more typical of daily life. For example, an individual coping with a divorce would almost certainly not be diagnosed with PTSD (unless, of course, physical or sexual abuse has occurred), but he or she might be diagnosed with adjustment disorder if he or she was excessively distressed in comparison to the usual reaction and had associated functional deficits. The specific characteristics of the stressor and the individual that are required to trigger an adjustment disorder are not clear (Baumeister, Maercker, & Casey 2009).

In addition to the presence of a stressor, undoubtedly some personal or environmental factors exist that contribute to the reaction (Faudino, Fergusson, & Horwood, 2013). The presence of a dysfunctional parent–adolescent relationship predicts future adjustment disorder risk for the adolescent.

Overall, there is a low rate of recognition of the condition, in part because adjustment disorder is often used as a residual category. In addition, there is poor delineation from other disorders or, on the other end of the spectrum, from normal stress responses (Casey & Doherty, 2012).

Prognosis

In general, adjustment disorder has a good prognosis, although individuals who have had difficulty adjusting to one stressor may have difficulty if they encounter subsequent stressors. For example, someone who struggled with a divorce may later have similar difficulty if she or he is laid off from work.

Implications for Function and Treatment

Adjustment disorder includes some degree of dysfunction in one or more occupations. These occupations are often social and/or work related, as the individual may have difficulty concentrating, interacting calmly with others, and organizing tasks. Because the stressors are often related to work or social life, it is not surprising that the individual would struggle with function in the occupation that generates stress. These individuals report higher levels of stress than those with anxiety disorders (Fernández et al., 2012), which is another factor that can interfere with function.

Short-term psychotherapy is effective in reducing the distress associated with adjustment disorder (Ben-Itzhak et al., 2012). The impact of psychotherapy seems to be that it increases coping skills and minimizes defense mechanisms (Kramer, Despland, Michel, Drapeau, & de Roten, 2010). Psychotherapy also reduces depression in adolescents with adjustment disorder (Kottai, 2012).

Cognitive behavioral therapy has demonstrated value in individuals with adjustment disorder (van der Heiden & Melichior, 2012). Perhaps the most effective approach is a combination of behavioral therapy, including cognitive restructuring, relaxation training, behavioral activation, and self-monitoring, together with one or more psychotherapeutic interventions, such as supportive psychotherapy, family therapy, psychoeducation, existential psychotherapy, and interpersonal psychotherapy (Kottai, 2012).

Implications for Occupational Therapy

Two main areas of focus exist for occupational therapy. The first focus is on symptom management, particularly activities that might reduce stress, redirect attention from symptoms, or allow for expression of emotions. Expressive arts, such as writing and story-telling, are examples of this intervention strategy (Duffy, 2010). The second area of focus is enhancing coping skills, including stress management and, as needed, enhancing specific skills that may be deficient and thus contributing to the stressor. If an individual has lost his or her job, a focus on constructing a resume, learning how to network, and developing other job seeking skills may help the individual to feel more in control of the future and may help resolve the stressor. Table 9-2 summarizes the diagnostic criteria and functional implications of the trauma- and stressor-related disorders.

Cultural Considerations

PTSD is clearly a diagnosis that applies across cultures (Hinton & Lewis-Fernandez, 2011). Practitioners working with immigrant groups should be alert to the possibility of PTSD, as well as to the potential for its expression in somewhat varied forms in some cultural groups (Alaszewski & Coxon, 2008). For example, for some groups, overt expression of anxiety may be unacceptable, leaving individuals to demonstrate their worries through withdrawal or excessive lethargy instead. Individuals from some cultural groups are more likely to express their distress through depersonalization, whereas in others, intrusive thoughts may be more prominent. The unique experiences of some cultural groups—in terms of living with war, deprivation, or other forms of constant threat—are also important factors for care providers to recognize. For refugees, the experiences that led them to leave their home countries, such as war or famine, are compounded by the stress of being in an unfamiliar environment, sometimes with no expectation of ever returning home.

Lifespan Considerations

Reactive attachment disorder and disinhibited social engagement disorder are largely disorders of childhood and adolescence, although their impact can be long term. A substantial subset of these individuals later develops conduct disorders, personality disorders, or other mental disorders associated with difficulty with social interaction. PTSD can occur at any age, although as indicated previously, young children may well have somewhat different symptoms than adults. In particular, reliving of the experience and the intrusive dreams may have less specific content.

In later life, PTSD and adjustment disorders are also common, although there is evidence that PTSD symptoms tend to lessen in later life (Clapp & Beck, 2012). It is unclear whether this is the result of older adults' tendency to minimize psychological symptoms or some buffering effects of later life. For older adults, PTSD presents with somewhat different symptoms, notably greater cognitive symptoms. Although some concern exists about the effectiveness of CBT and other treatments in working with older adults with PTSD, Clapp and Beck (2012) found CBT to be equally helpful for adults and older adults.

	TABLE 9-2	
DIAGNOSTIC CRITERIA AND FUNCTIONAL IMPLICATIONS: STRESS AND TRAUMA-RELATED DISORDERS		
DISORDER	*DIAGNOSTIC CRITERIA (APA, 2013)*	*IMPLICATIONS FOR FUNCTION*
Reactive attachment disorder	Inhibited or withdrawn behavior toward caregivers such that the child rarely seeks or responds to comfort Social and emotional disturbance that might include the following: • Minimal social responsiveness • Limited positive affect • Irritability, sadness, or fearfulness Child has experienced extreme insufficient care that is responsible for the behavior	Social occupations significantly and negatively affected, with accompanying damage to school occupations Self-care may be intact (and age appropriate) assuming some level of teaching/training has been provided Social skills, emotional regulation significantly impaired
Disinhibited social engagement disorder	The child interacts inappropriately with unfamiliar adults, perhaps including the following: • Reduced reticence • Excessively familiar behavior • Social disinhibition Associated with extreme insufficient care that is responsible for the disturbed behavior	Social occupations significantly and negatively affected, with accompanying damage to educational occupations Self-care may be intact (and age appropriate) assuming some level of teaching/training has been provided Social skills, emotional regulation significantly impaired
Posttraumatic stress disorder	Exposure to actual or threatened death, serious injury, or sexual violence Intrusive symptoms, lasting at least one month, associated with the traumatic event such as the following: • Intrusive memories of the trauma • Dreams related to the trauma • Feeling the events are recurring (in children, may occur during play)	May be mild to marked Most typical deficits are in social, work, and leisure occupations Habits, routines, and roles are negatively affected by periodic exacerbations and anxiety
		(continued)

TABLE 9-2 (CONTINUED)		
DIAGNOSTIC CRITERIA AND FUNCTIONAL IMPLICATIONS: STRESS AND TRAUMA-RELATED DISORDERS		
DISORDER	*DIAGNOSTIC CRITERIA (APA, 2013)*	*IMPLICATIONS FOR FUNCTION*
Posttraumatic stress disorder (continued)	Avoidance of stimuli associated with the trauma Negative change in cognition and mood associated with the trauma Alterations in arousal	Process skills are negatively affected by intrusive thoughts Motor and communication skills are intact
Acute stress disorder	Same as posttraumatic stress disorder, but duration of the disturbance is 3 days to 1 month after the trauma	May be mild to marked although more likely to be marked because of immediacy of stressor Most typical deficits are in social, work, and leisure occupations Habits, routines, and roles are negatively affected by periodic exacerbations and anxiety Process skills are negatively affected by intrusive thoughts Motor and communication skills are intact
Adjustment disorders	Development of emotional or behavioral symptoms in response to specific stressors within 3 months of the onset of those stressors Dysfunction and distress Does not include normal bereavement Symptoms resolve within 6 months of the end of the stressor	Deficits occur most often in social, work and leisure occupations Habits, roles and routines may be negatively affected Less likely to affect skills

CASE STUDY

Nadia was adopted from a Romanian orphanage when she was 3 years old. Her adoptive parents, Mr. and Mrs. Miller, knew there was a possibility of various kinds of health problems, so they had a physician perform an examination. The physician found no evidence of fetal alcohol syndrome and felt that Nadia was quite healthy overall. Her physical development has been normal; however, from the time the Millers brought her to the United States, she has had social difficulties, impulsivity, and violent outbursts with no evidence of remorse. She has also shown manipulative and controlling behaviors and frequently tells lies. When she started school, her teachers also saw these behaviors and referred her to the school psychologist and occupational therapist for evaluation. They found that she had normal intelligence and normal cognitive and language skills, and they felt her behavior was associated with reactive attachment disorder.

The school team recommended attachment therapy and school accommodations. The school psychologist saw Nadia in individual counseling for approximately 1 year, but Nadia showed little improvement in dysfunctional behaviors. At that point, the Millers sought help from a private counselor. The counselor worked with Nadia and the Millers on behavioral strategies, which the family reports have been moderately helpful. The Millers are deeply distressed that Nadia has shown so little improvement. Although they find her friendly and charming, she has never progressed to any deeper relationship with her parents—or, to the best of their knowledge, anyone else. They are hurt that she does not seem appreciative of their efforts over the 5 years since her adoption.

THOUGHT QUESTIONS

1. How do you think the occupational therapist might approach assessment? What particular information might the therapist need to be able to frame an intervention plan?
2. On the basis of the information above, what would you anticipate about Nadia's interactions with her peers at school?
3. What, if anything, might the occupational therapist do to help the Millers cope with their concerns?

Internet Resources

Dart Foundation Gateway to Post Traumatic Stress Disorder Resources
http://ptsdinfo.org/
Associated with Gift from Within. Provides a vast array of resources.

Gift From Within
http://giftfromwithin.org/
An international organization focused on support and resources for individuals with PTSD. This site addresses many forms of PTSD, beyond military issues.

National Alliance on Mental Illness
http://www.nami.org/Template.cfm?Section=posttraumatic_stress_disorder&Template=/ContentManagement/ContentDisplay.cfm&ContentID=123108.
National Alliance on Mental Illness has been listed in other chapters as well. Its focus is on providing support for individuals with a wide range of mental disorders, with particular emphasis on self-help.

National Center for PTSD

http://www.ptsd.va.gov/

A site sponsored by the U.S. Department of Veteran's Affairs. Much of the information is most relevant to military personnel, but some of the links and resources would be helpful more generally.

References

Alaszewski, A., & Coxon, K. (2008). The everyday experience of living with risk and uncertainty. *Health Risk & Society, 10*(5), 413-420.

American Psychiatric Association. (1994). *Diagnostic and statistical manual of mental disorders* (4th ed.). Washington, DC: Author.

American Psychiatric Association. (2013). *Diagnostic and statistical manual of mental disorders* (5th ed.). Washington, DC: Author.

Balbernie, R. (2010). Reactive attachment disorder as an evolutionary adaptation. *Attachment & Human Development, 12*(3), 265-281.

Baumeister, H., Maercker, A., & Casey, P. (2009). Adjustment disorder with depressed mood: A critique of its DSM-IV and ICD-10 conceptualisations and recommendations for the future. *Psychopathology, 42*, 139-147.

Baumeister, H.K., & Kufner, K. (2009). It is time to adjust the adjustment disorder category. *Current Opinion in Psychiatry, 22*(4), 409-412.

Ben-Itzhak, S., Bluvstein, I., Schreiber, S., Ahronov-Zaig, I., Maor, M., Lipnik, R., & Bloch, M. (2012). The effectiveness of brief versus intermediate duration psychodynamic psychotherapy in the treatment of adjustment disorder. *Journal of Contemporary Psychotherapy, 42*(4), 249-256.

Bisson, J.I. (2007). Post-traumatic stress disorder. *Occupational Medicine, 57*, 399-403.

Breslau, N., Troost, J.P., Bohnert, K., & Luo, Z. (2013). Influence of predispositions on post-traumatic stress disorder: Does it vary by trauma severity? *Psychological Medicine, 43*(2), 381-390.

Bryant, R.A., Friedman, M.J., Spiegel, D., Ursano, R., & Strain, J. (2011). A review of acute stress disorder in DSM-5. *Depression and Anxiety, 28*, 802-817.

Buckner, J.D., Lopez, C., Dunkel, S., & Joiner, T. (2008). Behavior management training for the treatment of reactive attachment disorder. *Child Maltreatment, 13*(3), 289-297.

Casey, P., & Doherty, A. (2012). Adjustment disorder: Implications for ICD-11 and DSM-5. *British Journal of Psychiatry, 201*(2), 90-92.

Clapp, J.D., & Beck. J.G. (2012). Treatment of PTSD in older adults: Do cognitive-behavioral interventions remain viable? *Cognitive and Behavioral Practice, 19*(1), 126-135.

Deering, C.G. (2000). A cognitive developmental approach to understanding how children cope with disasters. *Journal of Child and Adolescent Psychiatric Nursing, 13*(1), 7-16.

Duffy, J.T. (2010). A heroic journey: Re-conceptualizing adjustment disorder through the lens of the hero's quest. *Journal of Systemic Therapies, 29*(4), 1-16.

Durai, U., Nalla, B., Chopra, M.P., Coakley, E., Llorente, M.D., Kirchner, J.E., . . . Levkoff, S.E. (2011). Exposure to trauma and posttraumatic stress disorder symptoms in older veterans attending primary care: Comorbid conditions and self-rated health status. *Journal of the American Geriatrics Society, 59*(6), 1087-1092.

Ehde, D.M., Patterson, D.R., Wiechman, S.A., & Wilson, L.G. (2000). Post-traumatic stress symptoms and distress 1 year after burn injury. *Journal of Burn Care and Rehabilitation, 21*, 105-111.

Faudino, A., Fergusson, D.M., & Horwood, L.J. (2013). The quality of parent/child relationships in adolescence is associated with poor adult psychosocial adjustment. *Journal of Adolescence, 36*(2), 331-340.

Fernández, A., Mendive, J.M., Salvador-Carulla, L., Rubio-Valera, M.V., Luciano, J., Pinto-Meza, A.M., . . . DASMAP Investigators. (2012). Adjustment disorders in primary care: Prevalence, recognition and use of services. *The British Journal of Psychiatry, 201*(2), 137-142.

Foa, E.B., Gillihan, S.J., & Bryant, R.A. (2013). Challenges and successes in dissemination of evidence-based treatments for posttraumatic stress: Lessons learned from prolonged exposure therapy for PTSD. *Psychological Science in the Public Interest, 14*(2), 65-111.

Fogler, J.M., Shipherd, J.C., Clarke, S., Jensen, J., & Rowe, E. (2008). The impact of clergy-perpetrated sexual abuse: The role of gender, development, and posttraumatic stress. *Journal of Child Sexual Abuse, 17*, 329-358.

Follan, M., Anderson, S., Huline-Dickens, S., Lidstone, E., Young, D., Brown, G., & Minnis, H. (2011). Discrimination between attention deficit hyperactivity disorder and reactive attachment disorder in school aged children. *Research in Developmental Disabilities, 32*(2), 520-526.

Gerearts, E., & McNally, R.J. (2008). Forgetting unwanted memories: Directed forgetting and thought suppression methods. *Acta Psychologica, 127*, 614-622.

Gleason, M.M., Fox, N. A., Drury, S., Smyke, A., Egger, H.L., Nelson, C.A., . . . Zeanah, C.H. (2011). Validity of evidence-derived criteria for reactive attachment disorder: Indiscriminately social/disinhibited and emotionally withdrawn/inhibited types. *Journal of the American Academy of Child & Adolescent Psychiatry, 50*(3), 216-231.

Griffiths, J., Fortune, G., Barber, V., & Young, J.D. (2007). The prevalence of post-traumatic stress disorder in survivors if ICU treatment: A systematic review. *Intensive Care Medicine, 33*, 1506-1518.

Grodin, M.A., Piwowarczyk, L., Fulker, D., Bazazi, A.R., & Saper, R.B. (2008). Treating survivors of torture and refugee trauma: A preliminary case series using qigong and t'ai chi. *Journal of Alternative and Complementary Medicine, 14*, 801-806.

Haagsma, J.A., Ringburg, A.N., van Lieshout, E.M.M., van Beek, E.F., Patka, P., Schipper, I.B., & Polinder, S. (2012). Prevalence rate, predictors and long-term course of probable posttraumatic stress disorder after major trauma: A prospective cohort study. *BMC Psychiatry, 12*, 236-252.

Harris, C.A., Thompson, C.L., & Mauldin, G.R. (2007) 'Why does she behave this way?': Reactive attachment disorder. In S.M. Dugger & L. Carlson (Eds.), *Critical incidents in counseling children* (pp. 23-32). Alexandria, VA: American Counseling Association.

Hinton, D.E., & Lewis-Fernandez, R. (2011). The cross-cultural validity of posttraumatic stress disorder: Implications for DSM-5. *Depression and Anxiety, 28*, 783-801.

Humphreys, J., Lee, K., Neylan, T., & Marmar, C. (2001). Psychological and physical distress of sheltered battered women. *Health Care for Women International, 22*, 401-414.

Johnson, S.D. (2008). Substance use, post-traumatic stress disorder and violence. *Current Opinion in Psychiatry, 21*, 242-246.

Kay, C., & Green, J. (2012). Reactive attachment disorder following early maltreatment: Systematic evidence beyond the institution. *Journal of Abnormal Child Psychology, 41*(4), 571-581.

Kottai, S.R. (2012). Effects of multiple psychotherapeutic interventions in the treatment of adjustment disorder with prolonged depressive reaction in teenaged girls. *Indian Journal of Community Psychology, 8*(1), 100-112.

Koucky, E.M., Galovski, T.E., & Nixon, R.D.V. (2012). Acute stress disorder: Conceptual issues and treatment outcomes. *Cognitive and Behavioral Practice, 19*(3), 437-450.

Kramer, U., Despland, J., Michel, L., Drapeau, M., & de Roten, Y. (2010). Change in defense mechanisms and coping over the course of short-term dynamic psychotherapy for adjustment disorder. *Journal of Clinical Psychology, 66*(12), 1232-1241.

Lee, Y.L., & Santacroce, S.J. (2007). Posttraumatic stress in long-term young adult survivors of childhood cancer: A questionnaire survey. *International Journal of Nursing Studies, 44*, 1406-1417.

Lommen, M.J.J., Engelhard, I.M., Sijbrandij, M., van den Hout, M.A., & Hermans, D. (2013). Pre-trauma individual differences in extinction learning predict posttraumatic stress. *Behaviour Research and Therapy, 51*(2), 63-67.

Lynn, S.J., Malakataris, A., Condon, L., Maxwell, R., & Cleere, C. (2012). Post-traumatic stress disorder: Cognitive hypnotherapy, mindfulness, and acceptance-based treatment approaches. *American Journal of Clinical Hypnosis, 54*(4), 311-330.

Miller, J.L. (2000). Post-traumatic stress disorder in primary care practice. *Journal of the American Academy of Nurse Practitioners, 12*, 475-485.

Minnis, H., Macmillan, S., Pritchett, R., Young, D., Wallace, B., Butcher, J., . . . Gillberg, C. (2013). Prevalence of reactive attachment disorder in a deprived population. *The British Journal of Psychiatry, 202*(5), 342-346.

Minnis, H., Marwick, H., Arthur, J., & McLaughlin, A. (2006). Reactive attachment disorder—A theoretical model beyond attachment. *European Child & Adolescent Psychiatry, 15*(6), 336-342.

Moser, J.S., Cahill, S.P., & Foa, E.B. (2010). Evidence for poorer outcome in patients with severe negative trauma-related cognitions receiving prolonged exposure plus cognitive restructuring: Implications for treatment matching in posttraumatic stress disorder. *Journal of Nervous and Mental Disease, 198*(1), 72-75.

Nemeroff, C.B., Bremner, J.D., Foa, E.B., Mayberg, H.S., North, C.S., & Stein, M.B. (2006). Posttraumatic stress disorder: A state-of-the-art review. *Journal of Psychiatric Research, 40*, 1-21.

Nixon, R.D.V. (2012). Cognitive processing therapy versus supportive counseling for acute stress disorder following assault: A randomized pilot trial. *Behavior Therapy, 43*(4), 825-836.

O'Connor, K. (2011). Integrating ecosystemic play therapy and theraplay in the treatment of attachment disorders. In A.A. Drewes, S.C. Bratton, & C.E. Schaefer (Eds.), *Integrative play therapy* (pp. 297-324). Hoboken, NJ: John Wiley & Sons.

Otis, C., Marchand, A., & Courtois, F. (2012). Risk factors for posttraumatic stress disorder in persons with spinal cord injury. *Topics in Spinal Cord Injury Rehabilitation, 18*(3), 253-263.

Peres, J.F., McFarlane, A., Nasello, A.G., & Moores, K.A. (2008). Traumatic memories: Bridging the gap between functional neuroimaging and psychotherapy. *Australian and New Zealand Journal of Psychiatry, 42,* 478-488.

Precin, P.J. (2011). Occupation as therapy for trauma recovery: A case study. *Work, 38*(1), 77-81.

Precin, P.J., & Lopez, A. (2011). Posttraumatic stress disorder and occupational performance: Building resilience and fostering occupational adaptation. *Work, 38*(1), 33-38.

Raaska, H., Elovainio, M., Sinkkonen, J., Matomäki, J., Mäkipää, S., & Lapinleimu, H. (2012). Internationally adopted children in Finland: Parental evaluations of symptoms of reactive attachment disorder and learning difficulties—FINADO study. *Child: Care, Health and Development, 38*(5), 697-705.

Raaska, H., Lapinleimu, H., Sinkkonen, J., Salmivallim C., Matomäki, J., Mäkipää, J., & Elovainio, M. (2012). Experiences of school bullying among internationally adopted children: Results from the Finnish Adoption (FINADO) study. *Child Psychiatry and Human Development, 43*(4), 592-611.

Rintamaki, L.S., Weaver, F.M., Elbaum, P.L., Klama, E.N., & Miskevics, S.A. (2009). Persistence of traumatic memories in World War II prisoners of war. *Journal of the American Geriatrics Society, 57*(12), 2257-2262.

Schottenbauer, M.A., Glass, C.R., Arnkoff, D.B., & Gray, S.H. (2008). Contributions of psychodynamic approaches to treatment of PTSD and trauma: A review of the empirical treatment and psychopathology literature. *Psychiatry, 71,* 13-34.

Schottenbauer, M.A., Glass, C.R., Arnkoff, D.B., Tendick, V., & Gray, S.H. (2008). Nonresponse and dropout rates in outcome studies on PTSD: Review and methodological considerations. *Psychiatry, 71,* 134-168.

Seides, R. (2010). Should the current DSM-IV-TR definition for PTSD be expanded to include serial and multiple microtraumas as aetiologies? *Journal of Psychiatric and Mental Health Nursing, 17*(8), 725-731.

Sheerin, C.M., Seim, R.W., & Spates, C.R. (2012). A new appraisal of combined treatments for PTSD in the era of psychotherapy adjunctive medications. *Journal of Contemporary Psychotherapy, 42*(2), 69-76.

Smith, P., Perrin, S., Dalgleish, T., Meiser-Stedman, R., Clark, D.M., & Yule, W. (2013). Treatment of posttraumatic stress disorder in children and adolescents. *Current Opinion in Psychiatry, 26*(1), 66-72.

Spitzer, C., Barnow, S., Völzke, H., John, U., Freyberger, H.J., & Grabe, H.J. (2009). Trauma, posttraumatic stress disorder, and physical illness: Findings from the general population. *Psychosomatic Medicine, 71*(9), 1012-1017.

Stinehart, M.A., Scott, D.A., & Barfield, H.G. (2012). Reactive attachment disorder in adopted and foster care children: Implications for mental health professionals. *Family Journal, 20*(4), 355-360.

Stoller, C.C., Greuel, J.H., Cimini, L.S., Fowler, M.S., & Koomar, J.A. (2012). Effects of a sensory-enhanced yoga on symptoms of combat stress in deployed military personnel. *American Journal of Occupational Therapy, 66,* 59-68.

Strain, J.J., & Friedman, M.J. (2011). Considering adjustment disorders as stress response syndromes for DSM-5. *Depression and Anxiety, 28,* 818-823.

Tierney, J.A. (2000). Post-traumatic stress disorder in children: Controversies and unresolved issues. *Journal of Child and Adolescent Psychiatric Nursing, 13*(4), 147-158.

Tuchner, M., Meiner, Z., Parush, S., & Hartman-Maeir, A. (2010). Relationships between sequelae of injury, participation, and quality of life in survivors of terrorist attacks. *OTJR: Occupation, Participation & Health, 30*(1), 29-38.

Uguak, U.A. (2010). The importance of psychosocial needs for the posttraumatic stress disorder (PTSD) and displaced children in schools. *Journal of Instructional Psychology, 37*(4), 340-351.

van der Heiden, C., & Melichior, K. (2012). Cognitive-behavioral therapy for adjustment disorder: A preliminary study. *Behavior Therapist, 35*(3), 57-60.

Wald, J., & Taylor, S. (2009). Work impairment and disability in posttraumatic stress disorder: A review and recommendations for psychological injury research and practice. *Psychological Injury and Law, 2*(3-4), 254-262.

Wilker, S., & Kolassa, I. (2012). Genetic influences on posttraumatic stress disorder (PTSD): Inspirations from a memory-centered approach. *Psychiatria Danubina, 24*(3), 278-279.

Wimmer, J.S.E., Vonk, M., & Reeves, P.M. (2010). Adoptive mothers' perceptions of reactive attachment disorder therapy and its impact on family functioning. *Clinical Social Work Journal, 38*(1), 120-131.

Woods, S.J., & Isenberg, M.A. (2001). Adaptation as a mediator of intimate abuse and traumatic stress in battered women. *Nursing Science Quarterly, 14,* 215-221.

Yoder, M.S., Tuerk, P.W., & Acierno, R. (2010). Prolonged exposure with a World War II veteran: 60 years of guilt and feelings of inadequacy. *Clinical Case Studies, 9*(6), 457-467.

Dissociative Disorders

Learning Outcomes

By the end of this chapter, readers will be able to:
- Describe the various dissociative disorders
- Differentiate among dissociative disorders on the basis of symptoms and onset
- Identify the causes of dissociative disorders
- Describe treatment strategies for dissociative disorders
- Discuss occupational therapy interventions for dissociative disorders

Bonder B.
Psychopathology and Function, Fifth Edition (pp 215-224).
© 2015 SLACK Incorporated.

KEY WORDS

- Positive dissociative symptoms
- Negative dissociative symptoms
- Malingering
- Integration
- Fusion
- Dissociative fugue

CASE VIGNETTE

Mary Bligh is a 28-year-old woman who has been in and out of therapy for the past 5 years. She had a troubled childhood, during which she was removed from her parents after they were discovered to be abusing her physically. She was then placed in foster care and remained in such care until she aged out at 18 years old. While in foster care, she finished high school but also had a number of episodes of depression during adolescence, and she began cutting her arms and legs. Her foster parents arranged therapy for her, and she gradually improved.

Shortly after she turned 18 years old, she married and got a job as a checker at a local grocery store. For the next 5 years, she did reasonably well but then became depressed and started cutting herself again. Her husband was concerned, but he was unable to convince her to seek treatment. Then, in the past 6 months, she developed periods of complete amnesia and was reported by her boss to have missed work. She cannot account for the time during which she was not at work, and she has had other "memory lapses," during which she is unaware of how much time has passed or where she is. She notes that her closet contains clothing that she does not recall buying and feels the clothing is not her style. She has become increasingly upset and made a serious suicide attempt. Her husband insisted that she seek care.

THOUGHT QUESTIONS

1. Do you think Mrs. Bligh has a mental disorder?
2. Which of her behaviors or feelings led you to that conclusion?
3. What do you think might be the functional consequences of her behavior?

DISSOCIATIVE DISORDERS

- Dissociative identity disorder
- Dissociative amnesia
- Depersonalization/derealization disorder

Dissociation is a defense or emergency mechanism that is an individual's attempt to prevent being overwhelmed by awareness of trauma (Gentile, Dillon, & Gillig, 2013). It emerges in individuals who are subjected to repeated trauma that they cannot control, so they "remove" themselves psychically. The diagnosis of dissociation disorder is somewhat controversial (Gillig, 2009), with some clinicians asserting that it is a willful form of malingering, rather than a true dissociative phenomenon. Previously known as multiple personality disorder,

TABLE 10-1			
PREVALENCE OF DISSOCIATIVE DISORDERS			
DISORDER	*PREVALENCE*	*GENDER RATIO (M:F)*	*SOURCE*
Dissociative identity disorder	1% to 5% of clients in psychiatric programs 0.08% to 2.8% of the general population		Spiegel et al., 2011
Dissociative amnesia	1.8% to 7.3%		Spiegel et al., 2011
Depersonalization/ derealization disorder	2%	1:1	APA, 2013

dissociative disorder is one of the mental disorders that has had numerous representations in the media, for example, in *The Three Faces of Eve* (Johnson, 1957) and *Fight Club* (Linson, Chaffin, & Bell, 1999).

Dissociation can be thought of as a disruption in the normal integration of psychological functioning in memory, identity, consciousness, and motor control. According to Spiegel et al. (2011), dissociation disorder is, "in essence, aspects of psychobiological functioning that should be associated, coordinated, and/or linked are not" (p. 826). Dissociation may be characterized by **positive dissociative symptoms** (i.e., unpleasant intrusions into awareness or behavior with associated loss of continuity in experience) or **negative dissociative symptoms** (i.e., inability to access information or control functions).

The fifth edition of the *Diagnostic and Statistical Manual of Mental Disorders* (DSM-5; American Psychiatric Association [APA], 2013) identifies the following three main forms of dissociation: dissociative identity disorder (DID) in which there is a splitting of personal identity into two or more states; dissociative amnesia, in which the individual loses memory for periods of time; and derealization/depersonalization, in which the person feels as if he or she is outside his or her own experience or outside of reality. Table 10-1 shows the prevalence of these disorders.

Dissociative Identity Disorder

DID is diagnosed on the basis of disruption of identity manifested by two or more personality states (APA, 2013). The different states lead to a discontinuous sense of self, as well as changes in affect and function. Gaps in recall of events and personal information exist beyond what would be considered ordinary forgetting, and the symptoms cause distress. It is also important to confirm that the dissociation is not part of a cultural or religious practice or, in children, fantasy play.

The disorder must be distinguished from major depressive disorder, bipolar disorder, post-traumatic stress disorder (PTSD), or psychotic disorders, and it must be confirmed that it is not the result of a medical condition, such as a seizure disorder. Because this disorder is often portrayed in the popular media, there is also the potential for **malingering**; that is, the individual pretending to be ill to derive some secondary gain.

In addition, it is important to be aware that the mental disorders listed earlier may be comorbid with DID. Depression is common, and there is a high risk for suicidal behavior.

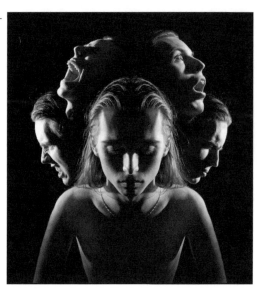

Etiology

DID is almost always preceded by childhood trauma or abuse (Gentile et al., 2013; Spiegel et al., 2011). The resulting development of two or more personality states has been hypothesized to be a consequence of either psychodynamic or neurological causes (Biswas, Chu, Perez, & Gutheil, 2013). Reasonably good evidence exists from functional magnetic resonance imaging studies that changes in cognition accompany personality shifts (Savoy, Frederick, Keuroghlian, & Wolk, 2012; Simone Reinders, Willemsen, Vos, den Boer, & Nijenhuis, 2012). It is noteworthy that studies of childhood abuse have also demonstrated psychobiological alterations in abused children (Spiegel et al., 2011).

Prognosis

With appropriate treatment, younger individuals with DID may improve substantially (Myrick et al., 2012). Older individuals tend to have less positive outcomes, perhaps as a result of a longer duration of the disorder.

Implications for Function and Treatment

Individuals with DID may experience periods of extreme dysfunction (Brand, Lanius, Vermetten, Loewenstein, & Spiegel, 2012). Dysfunction tends to be global (Mueller-Pfeiffer et al., 2012), as the separate personalities typically do not communicate and are often quite disparate in terms of personal presentation (Figure 10-1). To some extent, function is dependent on the frequency and duration of the appearance of the different personalities. If a dominant personality is present most of the time, function may be somewhat better than if there are regular brief appearances of the various personalities.

Dissociation is considered to be an adaptive reaction to a dysfunctional situation. A child in an abusive situation might cope by removing himself or herself emotionally from that situation. This can then become the child's main coping mechanism as he or she matures.

For children with one of the dissociative disorders, functional limitations may be a result of consequences of the dissociation, not the dissociation itself (Spiegel et al., 2011). Spiegel et al. (2011) presented the example of a child whose teacher becomes angry when the child's dissociation results in an inability to recall important information taught in school, even though he or she is capable of learning that information under normal circumstances.

At the level of skills, dissociation—like other forms of posttraumatic symptoms—may affect executive function; changes in function of the prefrontal cortex, hippocampus, amygdala, and related structures are evident during dissociative episodes (Spiegel et al., 2011).

The overall goal of treatment is **integration** of the personalities because they are each aware of the others and find ways to communicate internally to allow the individual to function (International Society for the Study of Trauma and Dissociation, 2011). Integration is reflected by acceptance of the thoughts and feelings of all the personalities as being part of the individual (Gentile et al., 2013). This may be a complete **fusion**, in which the alter egos are completely incorporated into the dominant personality. The process can be characterized as including the following three phases:

1. Establishing safety, stabilization, and symptom reduction

2. Confronting, working through, and integrating traumatic memories

3. Identity integration and rehabilitation (Brand et al., cited in Gentile et al., 2013, p. 26)

Psychodynamic treatments may focus on reframing the dissociation in a positive light as a useful coping strategy that has protected the individual. This can be helpful in establishing a positive therapeutic relationship and helping the individual feel sufficiently comfortable to share his or her experiences. This, in turn, allows for consideration of integration of the two or more personalities. Sometimes the process is helped through hypnotherapy as well (Kluft, 2012).

Although psychopharmacology has not been established as being effective for DID, atypical (or second-generation) antipsychotic drugs that block both dopamine and serotonin receptors may help to treat comorbid anxiety, depression, and psychotic symptoms (Brand et al., 2012).

Dissociative Amnesia

In dissociative amnesia, the person loses memory about important parts of his or her own experience—where he or she went, what he or she thought and experienced, and so on (Spiegel et al., 2011). Unlike the signs of DID, no splitting of the personality exists.

Diagnostic criteria for dissociative amnesia include the inability to recall important personal information, especially information of a traumatic nature (APA, 2013). This difficulty causes distress or dysfunction. Specifiers note whether the disorder is accompanied by **dissociative fugue,** which is apparently purposeful travel or wandering, accompanied by amnesia for personal information.

The disorder must be distinguished from PTSD, DID, neurocognitive disorder, substance-related disorders, brain injury or seizure, and malingering. Dissociative amnesia can be comorbid with depression, anxiety, PTSD, and several of the personality disorders.

Etiology

As with DID, dissociative amnesia appears to have an adaptive function in helping the individual cope with traumatic events. The frontal cortex, hippocampus, and occipital cortex seem to be associated with retrieval of autobiographical memory and are altered in individuals with dissociative amnesia (Spiegel et al., 2011). The occipital changes may be associated with visual memory deficits that are hypothesized to be involved in autobiographical memory (Henning-Fast et al., 2008).

Prognosis

Some individuals are successfully treated for dissociative amnesia. In these individuals, the altered brain activation disappears as memories are recovered (Kikuchi et al., 2010).

Implications for Function and Treatment

Typically, dissociative amnesia is associated with loss of biographical memory and identity, but other knowledge about facts and events is unchanged (Henning-Fast et al., 2008). There is lower global functioning in these individuals (Mueller-Pfeiffer et al., 2012).

Again, treatment is predominantly psychotherapeutic, and focuses on building strategies for dealing with trauma in less damaging ways.

Depersonalization/Derealization Disorder

Diagnostic criteria for depersonalization/derealization disorder include recurrent experiences of depersonalization or derealization (APA, 2013); reality testing is intact, but the symptoms cause distress or dysfunction.

Etiology

As is true for the other dissociative disorders, the etiology of depersonalization/derealization disorder seems to be childhood trauma (Cox & Swinson, 2002).

Prognosis

Depersonalization and derealization are closely tied to panic disorder (Cox & Swinson, 2002). Individuals with both disorders have a worse course than those with one or the other.

Implications for Function and Treatment

In general, there do not appear to be substantial functional impairments for these individuals (Mueller-Pfeiffer et al., 2012). If the symptoms are tied to a panic disorder, treatment of that disorder may to help ameliorate the depersonalization and derealization.

Implications for Occupational Therapy for the Dissociative Disorders

In the early stages of treatment for dissociative disorders, it can be helpful to provide opportunities for nonverbal expression of emotion. Providing art activities—drawing, painting, sculpting—can offer a safe way to express difficult emotions or those emotions that the client may not be aware of him- or herself. Occupational therapy has a significant role in the later stages of intervention when the focus may be on emotional, social, and vocational concerns (International Society for the Study of Trauma and Dissociation, 2011). Clients may need coaching and practice associated with managing a work environment, coping with daily problems without dissociating, and generally managing the stresses and challenges of daily life. It is worth emphasizing here that it is particularly important for all the members of the treatment team to work closely, as any perceived inconsistency or splitting among clinicians can be threatening to the client with a dissociative disorder. Table 10-2 summarizes the diagnostic criteria and functional implications of the dissociative disorders.

TABLE 10-2		
DIAGNOSTIC CRITERIA AND FUNCTIONAL IMPLICATIONS: DISSOCIATIVE DISORDERS		
DISORDER	DIAGNOSTIC CRITERIA (APA, 2013)	IMPLICATIONS FOR FUNCTION
Dissociative identity disorder	Disruption of identity, with presence of two or more personality states, resulting in a disjointed sense of self Changes in affect and functioning Gaps in recall of events and personal information, Distress and/or dysfunction	Poor work, social functioning Emotional regulation and social skills negatively affected May be some personality states that show cognitive and emotional regulation deficits
Dissociative amnesia	Inability to recall important personal information usually of a traumatic nature, not reflective of normal forgetting Significant distress and/or dysfunction	Potential for all spheres of occupation to be negatively affected as a result of loss of memory Social, cognitive, and emotional regulation skills may be impaired
Depersonalization/ derealization disorder	Repeated experiences of depersonalization, derealization, or both Significant distress and/or dysfunction	Most often work and social occupations negatively affected Cognitive, social, and emotional regulation skills impaired

Cultural Considerations

In some cultures, DID is experienced as a possession (APA, 2013). Somewhat different symptoms or presentations occur in some cultures, including more frequent trance states (Seligman & Kirmayer, 2008). However, considerable debate exists about whether dissociative disorders have a cultural component. Sierra-Siegert and David (2007) suggested that the disorders are found more frequently in individualistic (mostly Western) societies. Other findings suggest that dissociation is biologically based (McFarlane, 2013) and may not actually have a cultural component (Ross, Schroeder, & Ness, 2013).

Lifespan Considerations

DID is believed to be rare in children (Boysen, 2011). This seems reasonable given the belief that the disorder is an outcome of severe, repeated, long-term trauma. However, it has also been argued that the disorder is often overlooked in children and may, in fact, be more common than has been reported in the literature (Sar, Middleton, & Dorahy, 2012).

Relatively little has been written about dissociative disorders in later life (cf., Rosik, 1997). Holocaust survivors are among those particularly at risk for dissociative disorders (Yehuda et al., 1996), but here, too, the literature is sparse and relatively old.

CASE STUDY

Mrs. Fujimori is a 60-year-old Japanese woman who has been treated periodically over the past 10 years for depression and anxiety. She has periods of intense anxiety, insomnia, tearfulness, and poor concentration. Over the past year, she has had increasing trouble with her memory, which is demonstrated by her leaving the stove on, getting into the shower fully clothed, and putting the newspaper in the freezer. Her son was concerned that she was developing dementia and moved back home to look after her.

The son discovered that, for the most part, her function was not severely impaired. She was able to shop, cook, pay bills, and manage her medical care, and her strange behaviors were episodic and inconsistent. The son did note that sometimes his mother seemed to be "not present," almost as if she was sleepwalking during the day. Mrs. Fujimori also reported that she would sometimes find that she had walked for a significant distance without recalling having done so. These behaviors have made her increasingly anxious and depressed.

Mrs. Fujimori saw a neurologist, at her son's request. The neurologist obtained psychological testing, which did not show performance typical of dementia. Mrs. Fujimori was clearly worried about her dependence on her son and the peculiar and, to her, inexplicable periods she could not remember. The neurologist found nothing on a computed tomography scan, magnetic resonance imaging scan, or electroencephalogram that would explain her symptoms. The neurologist thought her cognitive difficulties might be consistent with her long-standing depression, which can, in older adults, present itself with symptoms similar to dementia.

The neurologist referred Mrs. Fujimori to a psychiatrist, who learned that she had a very difficult childhood. By her report, her father believed in severe corporal punishment, and her mother felt her role was to support her husband. Mrs. Fujimori developed severe anxiety that had numerous obsessive-compulsive features. As a way to escape her family situation, Mrs. Fujimori married young, only to discover that her husband was also abusive to both her and to her children.

THOUGHT QUESTIONS

1. Are there features in Mrs. Fujimori's behavior and emotions that are consistent with the symptoms described for the disorders in this chapter?
2. What more would you want to know to be able to clarify a diagnosis?
3. What do you perceive as the most pressing functional problems?

Internet Resources

American Association for Marriage and Family Therapy
http://www.aamft.org/imis15/content/Consumer_Updates/Dissociative_Identity_Disorder.aspx

This resource has pages for numerous mental disorders, with information for both consumers and professionals.

Zur Institute Dissociative Identity Disorder Resources
http://www.zurinstitute.com/dissociative_identity_disorder_resources.html
The Zur Institute is a commercial purveyor of continuing education for psychologists and other mental health professionals. However, this resource page is free and helpful and includes numerous listings for professionals and some for families.

References

American Psychiatric Association. (2013). *Diagnostic and statistical manual of mental disorders* (5th ed.). Washington, DC: Author.

Biswas, J., Chu, J.A., Perez, D.L., & Gutheil, T.J. (2013). From the neuropsychiatric to the analytic: Three perspectives on dissociative identity disorder. *Harvard Review of Psychiatry, 21*(1), 41-51.

Boysen, G.A. (2011). The scientific status of childhood dissociative identity disorder: A review of published research. *Psychotherapy and Psychosomatics, 80*(6), 329-334.

Brand, B.L., Lanius, R., Vermetten, E., Loewenstein, R.J., & Spiegel, D. (2012). Where are we going? An update an assessment, treatment, and neurobiological research in dissociative disorders as we move toward the DSM-5. *Journal of Trauma and Dissociation, 13*(1), 9-31.

Cox, B.J., & Swinson, R.P. (2002). Instrument to assess depersonalization-derealization in panic disorder. *Depression and Anxiety, 15*(4), 172-175.

Gentile, J.P., Dillon, K.S., & Gillig, P.M. (2013). Psychotherapy and pharmacotherapy for patients with dissociative identity disorder. *Innovations in Clinical Neuroscience, 10*(2), 22-29.

Gillig, P.M. (2009). Dissociative identity disorder: A controversial diagnosis. *Psychiatry, 6*(3), 24-29.

Henning-Fast, K., Meister, F., Frodl, T., Beraldi, A., Padberg, F., Engel, R.R., . . . Meindl, T. (2008). A case of persistent retrograde amnesia following a dissociative fugue: Neuropsychological and neurofunctional underpinnings of loss of autobiographical memory and self-awareness. *Neuropschologia, 46*, 2993-3005.

International Society for the Study of Trauma and Dissociation. (2011). Guidelines for treating dissociative identity disorder in adults, third revision: Summary version. *Journal of Trauma & Dissociation, 12*(2), 188-212.

Johnson, N. (Producer), & Johnson, N. (Director). (1957). *The three faces of Eve* [Motion picture]. United States: 20th Century Fox.

Kikuchi, H., Jujii, T., Abe, N., Suzuki, M., Takagi, M., Mugikura, S., . . . Mori, E. (2010). Memory repression: Brain mechanisms underlying dissociative amnesia. *Journal of Cognitive Neuroscience, 22*(3), 602-613.

Kluft, R.P. (2012). Hypnosis in the treatment of dissociative identity disorder and allied state: An overview and case study. *South African Journal of Psychology, 42*(2), 146-155.

Linson, A., Chaffin, C., & Bell, R.G. (Producers), & Fincher, D. (Director). (1999). *Fight club* [Motion picture]. United States: 20th Century Fox.

McFarlane, A.C. (2013). Biology not culture explains dissociation in posttraumatic stress disorder. *Biological Psychiatry, 73*(4), 296-297.

Mueller-Pfeiffer, C., Ruifbach, K., Perron, N., Wyss, D., Kuuenzler, C., Prezowowsky, C., . . . Rufer, M. (2012). Global functioning and disability in dissociative disorders. *Psychiatry Research, 200*(2-3), 475-481.

Myrick, A.C., Brand, B.L., McNary, S.W., Classen, C.C., Lanius, R., Loewenstein, R.J., . . . Putnam, F.W. (2012). An exploration of young adults' progress in treatment for dissociative disorder. *Journal of Trauma & Dissociation, 13*(5), 582-595.

Rosik, C.H. (1997). Geriatric dissociative identity disorder. *Clinical Gerontologist: The Journal of Aging and Mental Health, 17*(3), 63-66.

Ross, C.A., Schroeder, E., & Ness, L. (2013). Dissociation and symptoms of culture-bound syndromes in North America: A preliminary study. *Journal of Trauma & Dissociation, 14*, 224-235.

Sar, V., Middleton, W., & Dorahy, M.J. (2012). The scientific status of childhood dissociative identity disorder: A review of published research. *Psychotherapy and Psychosomatics, 81*(3), 183-184.

Savoy, R.L., Frederick, B.B., Keuroghlian, A.S., & Wolk, P.C. (2012). Voluntary switching between identities in dissociative identity disorder: A functional MRI case study. *Cognitive Neuroscience, 3*(2), 112-119.

Seligman, R., & Kirmayer, L.J. (2008). Dissociative experience and cultural neuroscience: Narrative, metaphor and mechanism. *Culture, Medicine and Psychiatry, 32*(1), 31-64.

Sierra-Siegert, M., & David, A.S. (2007). Depersonalization and individualism: The effect of culture on symptom profiles in panic disorder. *Journal of Nervous and Mental Disease, 195*(12), 989-995.

Simone Reinders, A.A.T., Willemsen, A.T.M., Vos, H.P.J., den Boer, J.A., & Nijenhuis, E.R. (2012). Fact or facti-
tious? A psychobiological study of authentic and simulated dissociative identity states. *PLoS ONE, 7*(6),
e39279.
Spiegel, D., Loewenstein, R.J., Lewis-Fernández, R., Sar, V., Simeon, D., Vermetten, E., . . . Dell, P.F. (2011).
Dissociative disorders in DSM-5. *Depression and Anxiety, 28*, 824-852.
Yehuda, R., Elkin, A., Binder-Byrnes, K., Kahana, B., Southwick, S.M., Schmeidler, J., & Giller, E.L. (1996).
Dissociation in aging Holocaust survivors. *American Journal of Psychiatry, 153*(7), 935-940.

Somatic Symptom and Related Disorders

Learning Outcomes

By the end of this chapter, readers will be able to:

- Describe the signs of somatic symptom and related disorders
- Differentiate among the somatic symptom and related disorders on the basis of signs and onset
- Identify the causes of the somatic symptom and related disorders
- Discuss the ways in which somatic symptom and related disorders affect daily function
- Describe treatment strategies for somatic symptom and related disorders
- Discuss occupational therapy interventions for somatic symptom and related disorders

Bonder B.
Psychopathology and Function, Fifth Edition (pp 225-237).
© 2015 SLACK Incorporated.

KEY WORDS

- Somatic
- Hypochondriasis
- Munchausen syndrome

CASE VIGNETTE

Mark Reynolds is a 35-year-old married bank executive. For the past several years, he has had repeated episodes in which he has physical symptoms that he believes are related to a serious physical illness. Three years ago, he had a 9-month period during which he complained of severe headaches, and he was sure he had a brain tumor. One year ago, he had stomach pain and nausea and believed he had stomach cancer. For the past 6 months, he has had symptoms that have convinced him he has lung cancer. He complains of shortness of breath, dizziness, and chest pain, and frequently feels pan-icky while experiencing these symptoms. He has undergone an array of tests, including repeat chest x-rays and two magnetic resonance imaging scans. Mr. Reynolds's physician has assured him repeatedly that he does not have cancer, and the tests have continued to show no sign of disease, but he has now become convinced that he has tuberculosis. His fears have been triggered by recurrent symptoms of shortness of breath and dizzi-ness, as well as a sense of exhaustion. He has extensively researched both lung cancer and tuberculosis and spends much of his day on the Internet looking for new informa-tion. The time spent on this activity has caused his productivity at work to suffer, and he has been cautioned by his boss that his work is unacceptable. Despite repeated reassurance from his physician, Mr. Reynolds is convinced that the tests have missed something, so he visits his general practitioner on a weekly basis, with each consultation taking an average of 20 minutes before he is suitably reassured.

THOUGHT QUESTIONS

1. Do you think that Mr. Reynolds has a mental disorder? What other information would help you determine this?
2. What characteristics of the description contribute to your conclusion?
3. How do you think his behaviors might affect his daily function beyond what is described? In what performance areas?

SOMATIC SYMPTOM AND RELATED DISORDERS

- Somatic symptom disorder
- Illness anxiety disorder
- Conversion disorder (functional neurological symptom disorder)
- Psychological factors affecting other medical conditions
- Factitious disorder

The disorders in this cluster are all characterized by the presence of or worry about **somatic** (bodily) symptoms that cannot be explained by a clear physical etiology. A large number of individuals frequently seek medical attention for symptoms that have no discernible biological

TABLE 11-1			
PREVALENCE OF SOMATIC SYMPTOM AND RELATED DISORDERS			
DIAGNOSIS	*PREVALENCE*	*GENDER RATIO (M:F)*	*SOURCE*
Somatic symptom disorder	3% to 5% of clients in medical practices		Savino & Fordtran, 2006
Illness anxiety disorder	1.3% to 10%		APA, 2013
Conversion disorder	Unknown		APA, 2013
Psychological factors affecting other medical conditions	Uncertain		APA, 2013
Factitious disorder	8% of hospitalized clients	1:8	Catalina, Macias, & Gómez de Cos, 2008

basis or for reassurance necessitated by intrusive worry about physical illness. Table 11-1 shows the prevalence of these disorders.

It is important to be careful in making these diagnoses of somatic symptom or related disorders, as there are certainly times when a biological basis does exist but is not readily identifiable. For example, until recently it was thought that celiac disease was a childhood disorder, and adults presenting with vague, intermittent gastrointestinal symptoms for which no cause could be identified were at risk of being diagnosed with a somatoform disorder (the term used in previous editions of the *Diagnostic and Statistical Manual of Mental Disorders* [DSM]). However, in the past decade, a blood test has been developed that now makes diagnosis easier. This has led to the finding that just under 1% of the adult population worldwide has celiac disease (Gujral, Freeman, & Thomson, 2012), meaning that, for people with celiac disease, those apparently psychosomatic symptoms were the result of a clear physical disorder. Similarly, multiple sclerosis may present initially with mild and intermittent symptoms that can present a diagnostic challenge, which might tempt some physicians to assume the individual has a mental disorder.

In addition, the absence of an underlying physical cause does not mean that the individual is not suffering. The physical and psychological signs of the somatic symptom disorders are difficult for the individual to manage, and it is important to find ways to ameliorate the client's discomfort.

Somatic Symptom Disorder

Somatic symptom disorder, formerly somatoform disorder, is characterized by the client seeking medical care for physical symptoms in the absence of a clear biological explanation (Sharma & Manjula, 2013). One significant change from previous versions of the DSM is the emphasis on the psychological aspects of the client's concerns (Voigt et al., 2012), particularly the client's response to physical symptoms—worry, anxiety, excessive concern—rather than on the existence of physical symptoms that are not associated with physical findings. It is the anxiety about the reported physical symptoms, rather than the symptoms themselves that is most important (Creed, 2011).

Diagnostic criteria for somatic symptom disorder include one or more distressing somatic symptoms that cause distress or dysfunction, with excessive thoughts, feelings, or behaviors related to the symptoms (American Psychiatric Association [APA], 2013). These symptoms might include persistent thoughts about the seriousness of the symptoms, persistent worry, and excessive time focused on the somatic symptoms. Although the somatic symptoms that are the focus of concern may change over time, the worry persists for at least 6 months. Specifiers note whether pain is the main symptom, whether the disorder is persistent, and whether it is mild, moderate, or severe. It is important to rule out medical conditions, panic and other anxiety disorders, depressive disorders, illness anxiety disorder, and body dysmorphic disorder, among others.

Etiology

A number of theories exist about the etiology of somatic symptom disorder. In some instances, the etiology appears to be a response to severe trauma (Punamäki, Qouta, & El Sarraj, 2010), similar to the mechanism for posttraumatic stress disorder. Brain changes are associated with the somatic disorders (Garcia-Campayoa, Fayed, Serrano-Blanco, & Roca, 2009; Stein & Muller, 2008), particularly in the dorsolateral prefrontal, insular, rostral anterior cingulate, premotor, and parietal cortices, which are associated with perception of pain.

Prognosis

The somatic symptom disorder may be chronic (Sharma & Manjula, 2013), although it has been reported that as many as 75% of clients show some recovery (Olde Hartman et al., 2009). Somatic symptom disorder is associated with high rates of absenteeism from work, high medical costs, and poor long-term outcomes (Hoedeman, Blankenstein, Krol, Koopmans, & Groothoff, 2010). Somatic symptoms, especially stomach aches, in adolescence are predictive of later development of depression (Bohmen et al., 2012).

Implications for Function and Treatment

Somatic symptom disorder has substantial functional implications (Sharma & Manjula, 2013). Because of its chronicity, the individual may struggle to hold a job, in part because of high levels of absenteeism. Social relationships can be challenging because of the individual's self-involvement that is focused on his or her own physical health. Another implication for social interaction is that others may find the individual's persistent complaints unpleasant so that they avoid the person. One family described an aunt who complained from her teenage years about pain, shortness of breath, and a conviction that her death was imminent—right up until the moment she died at age 97. Self-care may be altered or hampered by constant worry about various somatic symptoms.

Cognitive behavioral treatment, particularly with associated emphasis on adaptive coping skills, such as self-management, can be helpful (Prior & Bond, 2013). Psychotropic medications are often prescribed, particularly tricyclic antidepressants, serotonin reuptake inhibitors (SSRIs), and serotonin and noradrenaline reuptake inhibitors (Somashekar, Jainer, & Wuntkal, 2013). Atypical antipsychotic medications and some herbal remedies have also been used with some success.

Implications for Occupational Therapy

Little has been written in the occupational therapy literature specifically about the somatic disorders as a focus of treatment. As discussed in Chapter 23, many of the generally helpful approaches to intervention may have value in working with these individuals. Understanding their functional limitations in the context of what they need and want to do, assisting them to develop meaningful occupations that redirect attention from their physical symptoms, and supporting them in acquiring effective coping mechanisms can all be valuable strategies.

Illness Anxiety Disorder

Clients with illness anxiety disorder are likely to believe that any bodily symptom they may have is an indication of a catastrophic illness (Weck, Neng, Richtberg, & Stangier, 2012). They are more likely than individuals with no mental disorder or with an anxiety disorder to make this leap in logic from symptom to severe illness. This misinterpretation of symptoms is a characteristic specific to this disorder, which, in previous editions of the DSM, was known as **hypochondriasis**. A stigma is associated with illness anxiety disorder because many primary care providers—the first-line providers of care for these individuals—may find them difficult (Reese, 2013). However, for the majority of individuals who worry about their health and experience vague symptoms, reassurance resolves their concerns. It is the small number of clients whose anxiety persists who need more intensive intervention.

The symptoms of illness anxiety disorder include preoccupation and anxiety about having or getting a serious illness in the absence of somatic symptoms and is accompanied by excessive health-related behaviors such as repeated checks for signs of illness or by maladaptive avoidance of doctors and hospitals (APA, 2013). These preoccupations and behaviors persist for at least 6 months, although the illness that is the focus of attention may change. Specifiers clarify whether the individual is care-seeking or care-avoidant. Medical conditions must be ruled out as must anxiety, depressive, and psychotic disorders. The illness anxiety disorder is often comorbid with personality disorders.

Etiology

Two major theories exist about the etiology of this disorder. The first is cognitive behavioral and suggests that the individual has biased attention and memory processes. These processes focus on physical symptoms that serve as stimuli for beliefs about health threats and result in significant anxiety (Gropalis, Bleichardt, Hiller, & Witthöft, 2012).

The second cluster of theories focuses on neurological changes associated with pain perception (Fishbain, Lewis, Gao, Cole, & Rosomoff, 2009). Dysfunction in the limbic and frontal-striatal regions of the brain may be present (van den Heuvel et al., 2011).

Prognosis

To some extent, prognosis depends on the severity of the condition (Olde Hartman et al., 2009). Recovery rates between 30% and 50% have been reported, and long-term use of SSRIs is associated with greater recovery (Schweitzer, Zafar, Pavlicova, & Fallon, 2011).

Implications for Function and Treatment

Illness anxiety disorder is associated with social dysfunction and deficits in work occupations (Sharma & Manjula, 2013). As is true for somatic symptom disorder, individuals with this diagnosis tend to use substantial medical resources as they seek treatment for the perceived physical threats and for the anxiety they feel about their physical condition. Clients may also spend a great deal of time searching for information about their presumed illness, often to the detriment of their other occupations (Figure 11-1).

Figure 11-1. The Internet has made it easier to search for symptoms of illness. (©2014 Shutterstock.com.)

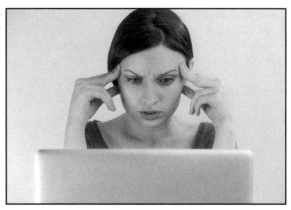

Several psychosocial treatments have some supporting evidence. Within limits, psychoeducational strategies may help individuals to understand the illness more accurately (Weck et al., 2012). Attention training (Weck, Neng, & Stangier, 2013) and mindfulness-based cognitive behavioral therapy also seem helpful (McManus, Surawy, Muse, Vazquez-Montes, & Williams, 2012).

As noted previously, long-term treatment with SSRIs seems helpful (Schweitzer et al., 2011). A combination of medication and cognitive behavioral therapy may be the most effective (Sørensen, Birket-Smith, Wattar, Buemann, & Salkovskis, 2011).

Implications for Occupational Therapy

Again, there is little specific information about occupational therapy approaches for individuals with illness anxiety disorder. However, the interventions described here and in Chapter 23 can apply.

Conversion Disorder (Functional Neurological Symptom Disorder)

Unlike the two previously described somatic disorders, individuals with conversion disorder have neurological symptoms (e.g., paralysis, blindness, seizures) for which there is no evidence of actual neurological impairment. Typically, the neurological symptoms do not fit the characteristic presentation of a neurological disorder (cf., Daum & Aybek, 2013). The individual is not consciously faking (as in the case of factitious disorder, described later). For example, one young woman complained of a severe hearing impairment that occurred very suddenly. No neurological explanation could be found, but her behavior was consistent with an inability to hear. At the same time, the symptoms were idiosyncratic and did not fit precisely with the typical circumstances associated with hearing impairment.

The diagnostic criteria for conversion disorder include one or more symptoms of altered motor or sensory function (e.g., visual impairment, paralysis), with clinical findings that do not show physiological causes for the symptoms (APA, 2013). Specifiers note the symptom type (e.g., weakness or paralysis, abnormal movement, swallowing symptoms, anesthesia or sensory loss, mixed symptoms), whether the episode is acute (less than 6 months) or persistent (more than 6 months), and whether there is a psychological stressor. The disorder must be distinguished from neurological disorders, malingering, somatic symptom disorder, dissociative disorder, depression, and panic disorder, among others.

Etiology

One theory is that conversion disorder represents a displacement of an emotion the individual cannot experience consciously or put into words (Kaplan et al., 2013). It is possible that conversion disorder is associated with childhood trauma (Kozlowska, 2007). Anxiety associated with unexpressed emotions may affect cortical ties between the controlling neural circuitry and the networks that regulate anxiety (Bryant & Das, 2012). It is believed that the neurobiology of conversion disorder relates to dysfunction of the anterior cingulate and posterior parietal cortices (Perez, Barsky, Daffner, & Silbersweig, 2012).

Prognosis

Prognosis for conversion disorder is generally good in children and adolescents (Pehlivantürk & Unal, 2002). This is particularly true when the disorder is diagnosed early, and no accompanying anxiety or depressive disorder is noted. For adults, the prognosis is good when intervention allows the individual to learn coping strategies to reduce distress and to develop alternate strategies for seeking attention (Ovsiew, 2003).

Implications for Function and Treatment

Function is impacted to the extent that the individual's physical symptoms affect their ability to work, accomplish self-care tasks, or engage in social interaction. Social relationships can be negatively affected by the individual's need for attention, expressed through physical symptoms.

Treatment strategies for conversion disorder focus on learning new methods for managing emotional expression and needs (Ovsiew, 2003). Medication is indicated when there is accompanying depression or anxiety.

Implications for Occupational Therapy

When occupational therapists see individuals with conversion disorder, it is typically in the context of a physical dysfunction referral. A challenge in framing occupational therapy intervention is that the individual does not conform to the usual pattern for the diagnosed difficulty and, because the origin is psychogenic, it does not respond to the usual interventions for physical limitations. Although there is little information specific to intervention for this disorder, emphasizing emotional management and the establishment of more productive, meaningful occupational patterns may be helpful.

Psychological Factors Affecting Other Medical Conditions

The diagnostic criteria for psychological factors affecting other medical conditions disorder include the presence of a medical condition with psychological factors that affect the medical condition (APA, 2013). The factors may affect the medical condition's course, they may interfere with treatment, and they may increase health risk. Specifiers note whether the disorder is mild, moderate, severe, or extreme. Adjustment disorder and somatic symptom disorder must be ruled out, and, by definition, a physical disorder is comorbid.

Psychological factors affecting other medical conditions disorder is a somewhat different condition than the others described in this chapter and elsewhere in this text. It exists only in the context of a medical condition and is characterized by psychosocial symptoms of some variety that affect the course of treatment and recovery from the accompanying medical condition (Sirri, Fabbri, Fava, & Sonino, 2007). For example, an individual with a cardiovascular problem might have an accompanying depression. The depressive symptoms make it more difficult to participate in rehabilitation for the cardiovascular problem as a result of the lethargy and hopelessness that characterize depression. Likewise, an individual with an anxiety disorder might have substantially more difficulty than others managing diabetes, as the anxiety might contribute to excessive concern about diet or contribute to an inability to focus on the important elements of disease management.

As discussed in Chapter 2, it is quite common for occupational therapists to encounter individuals in any health care setting who have psychological symptoms that affect the course of treatment. Such symptoms must be among the considerations in framing an intervention that enables the individual to gain or resume those occupations that are important to him or her.

Factitious Disorder

Unlike the previously discussed somatic disorders, in factitious disorder, the individual is aware that he or she is not actually ill. As distinct from malingering, in which the individual is quite aware of his or her motivation for the behavior, the individual with factitious disorder is not conscious of the underlying motivation for wanting to assume the sick role (McCullumsmith & Ford, 2011). The factitious disorder can present with the individual as the sick person, or as imposed on another, almost always a child (Kozlowska, Foley, & Savage, 2012).

Two types of factitious disorder exist: one imposed on the self and one imposed on another. Diagnostic criteria for factitious disorder imposed on self include falsifying symptoms, causing an injury or disease to oneself, or presenting oneself as injured or ill as an intentional deception that has no obvious external reward (APA, 2013). Specifiers note whether this is a single episode or repeated episodes.

Diagnostic criteria for factitious disorder imposed on another include the same symptoms as imposed on the self, except they are imposed on someone else, typically a child in one's care or another individual (e.g., an aging parent) for whom one has caregiving responsibility (APA, 2013). The most typical situations involve children. Again, specifiers note whether this is a single or recurrent episode. It is important to keep in mind that it is the perpetrator, not the victim who is diagnosed. This disorder frequently appears in the literature as **Munchausen syndrome**.

Etiology

Most theories center on the individual's need for attention, care, or to satisfy another emotional need that is not evident to others (Kozlowska et al., 2012).

Prognosis

The prognosis for these disorders is poor (Huffman & Stern, 2003). Although some individuals have a few episodes and then improve, on the whole, the disorder is a long-term condition that is difficult to treat. Among other issues, these individuals are likely to switch providers when one refuses to accommodate the client's demand for care (e.g., hospitalization or drugs). This starts the cycle again in a new setting where the condition has not been identified.

Implications for Function and Treatment

Factitious disorder is found relatively frequently in inpatient hospital settings, with one study finding that 8% of hospitalized clients fit the criteria for the disorder (Catalina, Macias,

& Gómez de Cos, 2008). In that study, the most typical presentation was exaggeration of psychological symptoms. The individuals studied also had problematic relationships with the other clients and with care providers.

Treatment ideally uses diverse strategies, including family therapy, cognitive behavioral therapy, and expressive therapies, such as writing and art (Kozlowska et al., 2012).

Among the concerns with regard to intervention is determining—when the condition is factitious disorder by proxy—whether the situation rises to the level of child abuse and must be reported to child protective services (Frye & Feldman, 2012). This is an issue for every professional involved in the situation.

Implications for Occupational Therapy

One challenging situation that may involve occupational therapists is the increase in cases of factitious disorder by proxy in school settings (Frye & Feldman, 2012). Parents may come with requests for evaluation and accommodation for their children in the absence of any real need. Although there has not been a great deal of research reported in the occupational therapy literature with regard to specific interventions for individuals with somatic disorders, it is possible that providing opportunities for emotional expression through more positive mechanisms, as well as strategies to help the individual redirect attention to a more meaningful constellation of occupations, may be beneficial. Table 11-2 summarizes the diagnostic criteria and functional implications of the somatic symptom disorders.

Cultural Considerations

There is little cultural perspective with regard to the somatic disorders (Fritzsche, Xudong, & Schaefert, 2011). A number of cultural syndromes have symptoms similar to those listed for somatic disorders, which include *ataque de nervios* (attack of nerves) in Latinos; *falling-out*, *blacking-out*, and *indisposition* found among Caribbeans of African descent and Southern African Americans; and *kyol goeu* among Cambodians (Brown and Lewis-Fernández, 2011). However, unlike the syndromes described in the DSM-5, these disorders may be considered acceptable expressions of severe distress among those of the cultural group, rather than mental disorders.

Lifespan Considerations

In children, unexplained somatic symptoms often accompany anxiety disorders (Hofflich, Hughes, & Kendall, 2006). Recall that separation anxiety is often characterized by complaints of stomach aches and other relatively invisible physical symptoms that the child may describe as a strategy for being permitted to remain at home. It is essential to understand the social environment and to focus on reducing exposure to violence or abuse, environmental toxins, and other environmental issues that might contribute to somatic expressions of distress. In addition, children with somatic symptoms are likely to have dysfunctional educational experiences—in part because of frequent absences—and to be disproportionately involved in the juvenile justice and welfare systems.

In later life, substantial comorbidity exists among various mental disorders and, in particular, of depression, anxiety, and many other long-term mental disorders along with the somatic disorders. In addition, symptoms of depression and anxiety are frequently somaticized (Crayer et al., 2005).

TABLE 11-2

DIAGNOSTIC CRITERIA AND FUNCTIONAL IMPLICATIONS: SOMATIC DISORDERS

DISORDER	DIAGNOSTIC CRITERIA (APA, 2013)	IMPLICATIONS FOR FUNCTION
Somatic symptom disorder	Excessive worries or behaviors related to somatic symptoms lasting more than 6 months	Mild to moderate in most instances Work deficits associated with absenteeism, distraction as a result of worry May be cognitive and emotional regulation deficits
Illness anxiety disorder	At least 6 months of preoccupation with serious illness and anxiety about health not associated with somatic symptoms Repeated checks for signs of illness or avoidance of doctors, hospitals, etc.	Mild to moderate in most instances Work deficits associated with absenteeism, distraction as a result of worry May be cognitive and emotional regulation deficits
Conversion disorder	One or more symptoms of altered motor or sensory function Clinical findings that are not consistent with the symptom	Limitations dependent on specific symptoms, but typically work, self-care, and social Skill deficits in cognition, emotional regulation, social and motor skills
Psychological factors affecting other medical conditions	Psychological or behavioral factors accompanying a medical condition that affect the medical condition by: • Affecting the course of the medical condition • Interfering with treatment • Influencing the pathophysiology, cause, exacerbation of the disorder or the need for medical treatment	Dependent on specific medical condition, its severity, and the interaction between the medical and mental disorders May well affect function over time if the disorder delays or interferes with effective treatment
Factitious disorder (self or another)	Falsifying physical or psychological symptoms, or causing an injury or disease to oneself, associated with deception Presenting oneself as injured, impaired, or ill when there is no actual cause No obvious external reward	Moderate to severe Work, social, self-care, leisure all impaired because of constant need for medical attention Cognitive, emotional regulation, and social skills impaired Motor skills may be impaired depending on nature of false disorder

CASE STUDY

Ruth Arthur is a 30-year-old, married, White teacher, with a 6-year-old daughter. Mrs. Arthur is a frequent figure in the local hospital's emergency department (ED), to which she brings her daughter at least once a month for medical care. Most of the time, the daughter has a fever of unknown origin; occasionally she is brought in for dehydration from vomiting and diarrhea. The daughter has been hospitalized repeatedly to seek the source of these symptoms, but the medical staff have been unable to identify a cause, in spite of extensive and repeated tests.

Mrs. Arthur is, by all accounts, a devoted and concerned parent. She is frequently tearful when she arrives at the ED, convinced that her daughter is mortally ill. Indeed, the daughter is thin, wan, and unresponsive on most occasions, and she does, repeatedly, have a high fever. Mrs. Arthur stays with her daughter, placing cold compresses on her forehead, urging her to drink, and smiling hopefully at each medical staff member who enters their cubicle.

The physicians in charge are perplexed by the case because of their inability to discern a cause for the frequent illnesses. Over time they have learned that Mrs. Arthur had a difficult childhood with an apparently abusive father. She has indicated she wants to spare her daughter such trauma, and she seems grateful for the attention and concern of the medical staff. She has told them on more than one occasion that she used to take her daughter to another ED where the staff were less supportive.

THOUGHT QUESTIONS

1. Do you think Mrs. Arthur has a mental disorder?
2. What behaviors or emotions does she demonstrate that lead you to that conclusion?
3. How do you think the behavior described here might affect Mrs. Arthur's function in daily life? What about her daughter's function?
4. What role, if any, do you think occupational therapy might have in this situation?

Internet Resources

Australian Government Department of Veteran's Affairs
http://at-ease.dva.gov.au/professionals/mental-health-advice-book/part-3-assessment-formulation-and-treatment-of-common-mental-health-problems-amongst-veterans/4-somatic-symptom-disorders-chapter/

A site posted by the Australian government that offers a concise description of somatic disorders, along with various online resource links. Provides a listing of many other mental disorders for which there are links to descriptions and resources.

Brauser, D. (2013). Medscape: Somatic Symptom Disorders Debate Rages On
http://www.medscape.com/viewarticle/781189

Medscape is a rich resource for information on an array of topics related to mental disorders (and to all things medical). One must create a user login, but the site is free.

References

American Psychiatric Association (APA, 2013). *Diagnostic and statistical manual of mental disorders* (5th ed.). Washington, DC: Author.

Bohman, H., Jonsson, U., Päären, A., von Knorring, L., Olsson, G., & von Knorring, A. (2012). Prognostic significance of functional somatic symptoms in adolescence: A 15-year community-based follow-up study of adolescents with depression compared with healthy peers. *BMC Psychiatry, 12*, 90-108.

Brown, R.J., & Lewis-Fernández, R. (2011). Culture and conversion disorder: Implications for DSM-5. *Psychiatry: Interpersonal and Biological Processes, 74*(3), 187-206.

Bryant, R.A., & Das, P. (2012). The neural circuitry of conversion disorder and its recovery. *Journal of Abnormal Psychology, 121*(1), 289-296.

Catalina, M.L., Macias, V., & Gómez de Cos, Q. (2008). Prevalence of factitious disorder with psychological symptoms in hospitalized patients. *Actas Españolas de Psiquiatría, 36*(6), 345-349.

Crayer, R.A., Mulsant, B.H., Lenze, E.J., Rollman, B.L., Dew, M. A., Kelleher, K., . . . Reynolds, C.F., III (2005). Somatic symptoms in elderly patients with medical comorbidities. *International Journal of Geriatric Psychiatry, 20*(10), 973-982.

Creed, F. (2011). The relationship between somatic symptoms, health anxiety, and outcome in medical outpatients. *Psychiatric Clinics of North America, 34*(3), 545-564.

Daum, C., & Aybek, S. (2013). Validity of the "drift without pronation" sign in conversion disorder. *BMC Neurology, 13*, 31. doi:10.1186/1471-2377-13-31.

Fishbain, D.A., Lewis, J.E., Gao, J., Cole, B., & Rosomoff, R.S. (2009). Is chronic pain associated with somatization/hypochondriasis? An evidence-based structured review. *Pain Practice, 9*(6), 449-467.

Fritzsche, K., Xudong, Z., & Schaefert, R. (2011). Crazy like us?—The proposed diagnosis of complex somatic symptom disorders in DSM-V from a cross-cultural perspective. *Journal of Psychosomatic Research, 71*(4), 282-283.

Frye, E.M., & Feldman, M.D. (2012). Factitious disorder by proxy in educational settings: A review. *Educational Psychology Review, 24*(1), 47-61.

Garcia-Campayoa, J., Fayed, N., Serrano-Blanco, A., & Roca, M. (2009). Brain dysfunction behind functional symptoms: Neuroimaging and somatoform, conversive, and dissociative disorders. *Current Opinion in Psychiatry, 22*(2), 224-231.

Gropalis, M., Bleichardt, G., Hiller, W., & Witthöft, M. (2012). Specificity and modifiability of cognitive biases in hypochondriasis. *Journal of Consulting and Clinical Psychology, 81*(3), 558-565.

Gujral, N., Freeman, H.J., & Thomson, A.B.R. (2012). Celiac disease: Prevalence, diagnosis, pathogenesis and treatment. *World Journal of Gastroenterology, 18*(42), 6036-6059.

Hoedeman, R., Blankenstein, A.H., Krol, B., Koopmans, P.C., & Groothoff, J.W. (2010). The contribution of high levels of somatic symptom severity to sickness absence duration, disability and discharge. *Journal of Occupational Rehabilitation, 20*(2), 264-273.

Hofflich, S.A., Hughes, A.A., & Kendall, P.C. (2006). Somatic complaints and childhood anxiety disorders. *International Journal of Clinical and Health Psychology, 6*(2), 229-242.

Huffman, J.C., & Stern, T.A. (2003). The diagnosis and treatment of Munchausen's syndrome. *General Hospital Psychiatry, 25*(5), 358-363.

Kaplan, M.J., Dwivedi, A.K., Privitera, M.D., Isaacs, K., Hughes, C., & Bowman, M. (2013). Comparisons of childhood trauma, alexithymia, and defensive styles in patients with psychogenic non-epileptic seizures vs. epilepsy: Implications for the etiology of conversion disorder. *Journal of Psychosomatic Research, 75*(2), 142-146.

Kozlowska, K. (2007). The developmental origins of conversion disorders. *Clinical Child Psychology and Psychiatry, 12*, 487-510.

Kozlowska, K., Foley, S., & Savage, B. (2012). Fabricated illness: Working within the family system to find a pathway to health. *Family Process, 51*(4), 570-587.

McCullumsmith, C.B., & Ford, C.V. (2011). Simulated illness: The factitious disorders and malingering. *Psychiatric Clinics of North America, 34*(3), 621-641.

McManus, F., Surawy, C., Muse, K., Vazquez-Montes, M., & Williams, J.M.G. (2012). A randomized clinical trial of mindfulness-based cognitive therapy versus unrestricted services for health anxiety (hypochondriasis). *Journal of Consulting and Clinical Psychology, 80*(5), 817-828.

Olde Hartman, T.C., Borghuis, M.S., Lucassen, P.L.B.J., van der Laar, F.A., Speckens, A.E., & van Weel, C. (2009). Medically unexplained symptoms, somatisation disorder and hypochondriasis: Course and prognosis. A systematic review. *Journal of Psychosomatic Research, 66*(5), 363-377.

Ovsiew, F. (2003). What is wrong in conversion disorder? *Journal of Neurology, Neurosurgery & Psychiatry, 74*(5), 557-557.

Pehlivantürk, B., & Unal, F. (2002). Conversion disorder in children and adolescents: A 4-year follow-up study. *Journal of Psychosomatic Research, 52*(4), 187-191.

Perez, D.L., Barsky, A.J., Daffner, K., & Silbersweig, D.A. (2012). Motor and somatosensory conversion disorder: A functional unawareness syndrome? *Journal of Neuropsychiatry and Clinical Neurosciences, 24*(2), 141-151.

Prior, K.N., & Bond, M.J., (2013). Somatic symptom disorders and illness behaviour: Current perspectives. *International Review of Psychiatry, 25*(1), 5-18.

Punamäki, R., Qouta, S.R., & El Sarraj, E. (2010). Nature of torture, PTSD, and somatic symptoms among political ex-prisoners. *Journal of Traumatic Stress, 23*(4), 532-536.

Reese, S. (2013, April 24). Frustrated by patients with hypochondria? What to do. *Medscape*. Retrieved from http://www.medscape.com/viewarticle/782234.

Savino, A.C., & Fordtran, J.S. (2006). Factitious disease: Clinical lessons from case studies at Baylor University Medical Center. *Proceedings of Baylor University Medical Center, 19*(3), 195-208.

Schweitzer, P.J., Zafar, U., Pavlicova, M., & Fallon, B.A. (2011). Long-term follow-up of hypochondriasis after selective serotonin reuptake inhibitor treatment. *Journal of Clinical Psychopharmacology, 31*(3), 365-368.

Sharma, M.P., & Manjula, M. (2013). Behavioural and psychological management of somatic symptom disorders: An overview. *International Review of Psychiatry, 25*(1), 116-124.

Sirri, L., Fabbri, S., Fava, G.A., & Sonino, N. (2007). New strategies in the assessment of psychological factors affecting medical conditions. *Journal of Personality Assessment: Special Issue: Personality Assessment in Medical Settings, 89*(3), 216-228.

Somashekar, B., Jainer, A., & Wuntkal, B. (2013). Psychopharmacotherapy of somatic symptoms disorders. *International Review of Psychiatry, 25*(1), 107-115.

Sørensen, P., Birket-Smith, Watter, U., Buemann, I., & Salkovskis, P. (2011). A randomized clinical trial of cognitive behavioural therapy versus short-term psychodynamic psychotherapy versus no intervention for patients with hypochondriasis. *Psychological Medicine, 41*(2), 431-441.

Stein, D.J., & Muller J. (2008). Cognitive-affective neuroscience of somatization disorder and functional somatic syndromes: Reconceptualizing the triad of depression-anxiety-somatic symptom. *CNS Spectrum, 13*, 379-384.

van den Heuvel, O.A., Mataix-Cols, D., Zwitser, G., Cath, D.C., van der Werf, Y.D., Groenewegen, H.J., . . . Veltman, D.J. (2011). Common limbic and frontal-striatal disturbances in patients with obsessive compulsive disorder, panic disorder and hypochondriasis. *Psychological Medicine, 41*(11), 2399-2410.

Voigt, K., Wollburg, E., Weinmann, N., Herzog, A., Meyer, B.L., & Gernot Löwe, B. (2012). Predictive validity and clinical utility of DSM-5 somatic symptom disorder—Comparison with DSM-IV somatoform disorders and additional criteria for consideration. *Journal of Psychosomatic Research, 73*(5), 345-350.

Weck, F., Neng, M.M.B., Richtberg, S., & Stangier, U. (2012). Dysfunctional beliefs about symptoms and illness in patients with hypochondriasis. *Psychosomatics: Journal of Consultation Liaison Psychiatry, 53*(2), 148-154.

Weck, F., Neng, J.M., & Stangier, U. (2013). The effects of attention training on the perception of bodily sensations in patients with hypochondriasis: A randomized controlled pilot trial. *Cognitive Therapy and Research, 37*(3), 514-520.

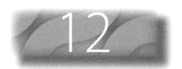

Feeding and Eating Disorders

Learning Outcomes

By the end of this chapter, readers will be able to:
- Describe the symptoms of feeding and eating disorders
- Identify the causes of feeding and eating disorders
- Describe treatment strategies for feeding and eating disorders
- Discuss the occupational perspective on feeding and eating disorders, including specific intervention considerations

Bonder B.
Psychopathology and Function, Fifth Edition (pp 239-256).
© 2015 SLACK Incorporated.

KEY WORDS

- Overcorrection
- Exchange
- Anorexia
- Self-transcendence

- Binge eating
- Dialectical behavioral therapy
- Invalidating environment
- Integrative response therapy

CASE VIGNETTE

Mary Joseph is a 27-year-old home health aide. She lives with her widowed mother. Much of her life revolves around binge eating and vomiting, sometimes as much as 10 times per day. She exercises at least 3 hours each day and becomes anxious when she cannot do so. She spends as much as $200 per day on food and has frequently stolen money from her mother to help cover this cost. She has come into treatment because she is depressed about what she describes as her "chaotic" life. She has lost two previous jobs because she took unauthorized breaks to binge and vomit, and she indicates she has no friends. Her only leisure activity is bingeing and purging.

THOUGHT QUESTIONS

1. Do you believe that Ms. Joseph has a mental disorder?
2. If so, what behaviors, thoughts, or other symptoms do you identify as problematic?
3. Of those symptoms, which might cause Ms. Joseph problems in her work?
4. Can you tell what cultural factors might be important in this situation? How might you gather more information to respond more fully to this question?

FEEDING AND EATING DISORDERS

- Pica
- Rumination disorder
- Avoidant/restrictive food intake disorder

- Anorexia nervosa
- Bulimia nervosa
- Binge-eating disorder

The feeding and eating disorders reflect behaviors that include amount, frequency, and patterns of eating. Their common thread is some form of unusual and unhealthful food-related behavior that is accompanied by feelings of anxiety, guilt, or depression. These disorders are quite common and are increasing in the context of the current obesity epidemic in the United States. Table 12-1 shows the prevalence of these disorders.

Pica

Pica is the label for behavior involved in eating nonfood. Examples include the impulsive and consistent eating of dirt, coins, articles of clothing, and so on. When it occurs, it is often

TABLE 12-1			
PREVALENCE OF FEEDING AND EATING DISORDERS			
DIAGNOSIS	PREVALENCE	GENDER RATIO (M:F)	SOURCE
Pica	Unclear		APA, 2013
Rumination disorder	Unknown		APA, 2013
Avoidant/restrictive food intake disorder	Unclear	1:1	APA, 2013
Anorexia nervosa	0.3%	More women	Hoek, 2006
Bulimia nervosa	1%	More women	Hoek, 2006
Binge-eating disorder	3.5% (women); 2% (men)		Hudson, Hiripi, Pope, & Kessler, 2007

in the context of a developmental disability (Williams & McAdams, 2012). Pregnant women also have relatively high rates of pica related to food cravings (Thihalolipavan, Candalla, & Ehrlich, 2013). The behavior can be quite dangerous, either immediately because of possible intestinal obstruction or laceration, or over the long term because of associated nutritional deficits and chronic damage to the alimentary system.

Diagnostic criteria for pica include persistently eating nonfood items over a period of at least 1 month in an individual for whom the behavior is not developmentally appropriate and when the behavior is not culturally or socially normative (American Psychiatric Association [APA], 2013). The only specifier is whether the condition is in remission. The condition must be distinguished from anorexia or suicidal behavior. It is often comorbid with autism, intellectual disability, and occasionally schizophrenia (Sinha & Mallick, 2010).

Etiology

In individuals with developmental disorders, pica may emerge as an "automatically reinforced behavior" (Carter, 2009, p. 143). This means the individual finds that the behavior meets some unspecified need, and this encourages the individual to continue it. Because pica is considered a normal behavior in infants and toddlers, it seems possible that some find the behavior sufficiently reinforcing that it continues beyond the developmentally expected period (Ali, 2001). The disorder also has some elements in common with other eating disorders and with obsessive-compulsive disorders (Hergüner, Özyıldırım, & Tanidir, 2008).

Prognosis

Pica disorder is self-limiting in pregnant women. When the pregnancy ends, the cravings and associated behaviors also end. In individuals with intellectual disabilities, behavioral interventions can dramatically reduce the incidence of the behavior (Williams, Kirkpatrick-Sanchez, Enzinna, Dunn, & Borden-Karasack, 2009), although it is difficult to eliminate entirely.

Implications for Function and Treatment

In children with intellectual disabilities, function is impaired because of the primary diagnosis. Pica may well reflect difficulty with impulse control (Hergüner & Hergüner, 2010). Depending on the severity of the impulse and the frequency with which it is enacted, most other aspects of function may be impaired or, conversely, may be relatively unaffected.

The most helpful treatment is behavioral (Williams & McAdams, 2012). An initial step may be placing the individual in a safe environment where the substance(s) typically ingested is not available. For some individuals, reinforcement protocols that reward helpful eating patterns may be adequate (Williams, et al., 2009), whereas in others, restrictive procedures that set behavioral limits may be needed. Specifically, strategies include alternate sensory reinforcement, environmental enrichment, visual screening, and **overcorrection**. Overcorrection involves requiring the individual to take a number of relatively distasteful actions each time the pica occurs. In one study, participants were required to spit out a nonedible item, use a toothbrush soaked with mouthwash, and complete positive practice acts (e.g., floor-mopping; Williams & McAdams, 2012). For some individuals, **exchange** procedures, in which the individual is presented with a preferred alternative to the nonfood object (e.g., a cookie), may be helpful (Carter, 2009).

Implications for Occupational Therapy

Among the recommended strategies for the treatment of pica is encouragement of alternative behaviors (Williams & McAdams, 2012). Occupational therapists may be able to help redirect behaviors in more positive directions (i.e., providing alternate sensory reinforcement and environmental enrichment). Providing opportunities for emotional expression can also be helpful.

Rumination Disorder

Rumination disorder is relatively rare and occurs most frequently in infants (Katz & DeMaso, 2011). It occasionally occurs in adults, and it is most typically diagnosed in adults with intellectual disability. The disorder is characterized by regurgitating food into the mouth. In other words, the person does not vomit in the traditional sense, but brings food back from stomach to the mouth repeatedly.

The diagnostic criteria for rumination disorder include repeated regurgitation over at least 1 month (APA, 2013). The only specifier is whether the condition is in remission. It must be distinguished from medical conditions that might explain the symptoms, such as anorexia, bulimia, or another eating disorder. It can occur in conjunction with an anxiety disorder as well as some medical conditions.

Etiology

Not only is this rumination disorder rarely diagnosed, it is also poorly understood. It is speculated as being the result of neonatal stressors such as lack of stimulation for the infant, neglect, and high-stress family situations (Katz & DeMaso, 2011).

Prognosis

Rumination disorder may well disappear on its own. It is responsive to behavioral treatments (Katz & DeMaso, 2011).

Implications for Function and Treatment

Rumination disorder may result in failure to thrive, anemia, and other medical conditions that may affect the infant's developmental progress. Treatment is largely behavioral (Katz & DeMaso, 2011).

Implications for Occupational Therapy

Occupational therapists are often involved in working with infants with various feeding disorders. Behavioral strategies used for other feeding disorders may be helpful. In addition, addressing the root causes (providing adequate stimulation, dealing with family issues) may ameliorate the problem.

Avoidant/Restrictive Food Intake Disorder

Avoidant/restrictive food intake disorder is the new name for a feeding disorder of infancy or early childhood (Bryant-Waugh, 2013). The most significant change is that it no longer is restricted to childhood presentations. The new diagnosis was developed with the "aim of improving clinical utility by adding more detail about the nature of the eating disturbance as well as widening the criteria to be appropriate across the age range" (Bryant-Waugh, 2013, p. 420). Because it is a new disorder, relatively little information exists about it (Kriepe & Palomaki, 2012).

Diagnostic criteria for avoidant/restrictive food intake disorder include an eating distur-bance resulting in failure to meet nutritional needs (i.e., weight loss or, in children, failure to meet expected weight gain; nutritional deficiency; and need for supplemental nutrition) that leads to interference with function (APA, 2013). The eating problem is not associated with lack of available food or some culturally normative behavior, and the child has a normal body image. The only specifier is whether the disorder is in remission. The condition must be dis-tinguished from other eating disorders, autism, phobias, and medical conditions.

Relatively little is known (or at least recorded) about the etiology, prevalence, prognosis, and treatment of avoidant/restrictive food intake disorder. As it enters common use, it will be interesting to see whether a distinction can be made between eaters who are simply picky and those who have a disorder that leads to nutritional deficiency. It is important to be aware that the criteria specify functional deficits. As is true for pica, it seems probable that occupational therapy interventions might be helpful in assisting individuals to adopt healthier and more functional eating patterns and for identifying more positive ways to express emotions.

Anorexia Nervosa

Anorexia nervosa is something of a misnomer, since **anorexia** means, literally, without appetite. Individuals with anorexia actually have appetites, but expend a great deal of energy controlling their eating. They monitor their food intake rigorously to the point that it is insuf-ficient to provide adequate nutrition. For example, a client might spend all day deciding what to eat for dinner, settling on a single lettuce leaf with mustard. As shown in Figure 12-1, over time the individual becomes quite emaciated. At the same time, he or she may well perceive his or her body as being overweight. This inaccurate body image is typical in anorexia.

The modification of diagnostic criteria for anorexia nervosa provides an interesting study of evolution in the understanding of etiology of mental disorders. At the time of the condi-tion's inception in the 1980s, the diagnostic criteria were predicated on an assumption of

Figure 12-1. Typical body appearance for someone with anorexia. (©2014 Shutterstock.com.)

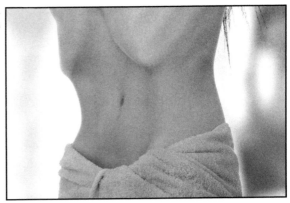

family dysfunction as the source of the disorder (Herpetz-Dahlmann, Seitz, & Konrad, 2011). As described by Herpetz-Dahlmann et al. (2011), wording of the criteria, "refusal to maintain" appropriate body weight, "denial" of the seriousness of the disorder, suggested a willful element that has since been called into question. In the fifth edition of the *Diagnostic and Statistical Manual of Mental Disorders* (DSM-5; APA, 2013), that wording has been altered to reflect a less judgmental stance, one that focuses on the behavior without implying blame directed at the client.

Diagnostic criteria for anorexia nervosa include restriction of caloric intake resulting in significant low body weight, accompanied by an intense fear of gaining weight or being fat, disturbed body image, excessive concern about body weight, and/or lack of recognition of the seriousness of the low body weight (APA, 2013). Specifiers note whether the disorder is the restrictive type, binge eating/purge type, whether it is in partial or full remission, and whether it is mild, moderate, severe, or extreme. Anorexia must be distinguished from bulimia, substance use disorders, schizophrenia, anxiety disorders, and medical conditions. It is often accompanied by depression or anxiety disorders.

Etiology

As noted previously, the understanding of the etiology of anorexia nervosa has changed over time. On the whole, the idea that it is a response to family patterns characterized by enmeshment and overprotectiveness has largely been discarded (Herpetz-Dahlmann et al., 2011). Increasingly, the view is that physiological factors play a major role, although the specifics of those factors have not yet been fully explained. For example, because of the clear family patterns, considerable exploration exists of the possibility of a genetic component, but as of yet the nature of any genetic contribution has not been identified. The best current explanation is a multifactorial one that includes prenatal factors (genetics and hormonal exposure in utero), personality traits (perfectionism, rigidity), and developmental factors (stressful life events, cultural values).

In particular, evidence exist that prematurity accompanied by early trauma leads to alterations in biological responses to stress and poor resilience in the presence of subsequent stressors (Favaro, Tenconi, & Santonasto, 2010). It appears that healthy siblings of individuals with anorexia have less need for approval, greater ability to persist, less anger and interpersonal distrust, and greater self-transcendence (Amianto, Abbate-Daga, Morando, Sobrero, & Fassino, 2010). **Self-transcendence** is the ability to redirect one's focus away from the self to become immersed in relationships with others or in important tasks. This low need for approval and greater self-transcendence may protect the siblings who do not develop the disorder.

Among the specific changes noted in individuals with anorexia nervosa are alterations in dopamine (Kontos & Theochari, 2012). However, findings are contradictory, with studies finding normal, increased, and decreased dopamine. As the disorder progresses, the effects of starvation on neurological function may contribute to further deterioration.

Prognosis

Data suggest a mixed picture with regard to outcome of anorexia nervosa. In one study, 12% of participants had a poor outcome (their anorexia persisted), and 39% met the criteria for at least one mental disorder. One in four had no paid employment (Wentz, Gillberg, Anckarsäter, Gillber, & Råstam, 2009). Poor outcome was associated with premorbid obsessive-compulsive personality disorder, early age of onset, and autistic symptoms.

Comorbid depression and anxiety are also associated with poorer outcomes (Hughes, 2012). Anorexia nervosa is associated with a high lifetime mortality. Assessment and treatment of psychiatric comorbidity, especially alcohol misuse, may be a pathway to better long-term outcomes (Papadopoulos, Ekbom, Brandt, & Ekselius, 2009). Men have better outcomes, possibly because of lower comorbidity (Lindblad, Lindberg, & Hjern, 2006).

Implications for Function and Treatment

Anorexia nervosa is associated with an array of functional deficits in most occupations (Quiles-Cestari, Ribeiro, & Pilot, 2012). Sexual dysfunction is common (Castinellini et al., 2012), as are problematic family relationships (Kyriacou, Treasure, & Schmidt, 2008). In particular, family caregivers report stress as a result of the challenges of caring for the individual. It is noteworthy that some vocational categories predispose people to anorexia, in particular gymnastics, dancing, and wrestling (Cogan, 2009).

At the level of skills, there are issues in a number of areas. These include emotional processing deficits (Hambrook et al., 2011), impaired cognitive flexibility (Sato et al., 2013), and visuo-proprioceptive integration deficits reflected in the erroneous body image of these individuals (Case, Wilson, & Ramachandran, 2012).

It is important to keep in mind that anorexia nervosa is a mental disorder, with potential severe body function/body system deficits. Nutrition-related issues, such as osteoporosis, are common (Mehler, Cleary, & Gaudiani, 2011). In addition, the condition can lead to excess mortality, as some individuals quite literally starve themselves to death. One young man, a six-foot tall wrestler, weighed 67 pounds just before his death. Before he passed, he indicated he thought he was almost at his target weight.

Therapeutic approaches include medical management to address nutritional deficits, in addition to psychodynamic therapy (Blank & Latzer, 2004) that is focused on boundary and control issues. Cognitive behavioral therapy has been used with some success (McCann, McCormick, Bowers, & Hoffman, 2010), as has the use of nontraditional antipsychotic medications to address dopamine dysfunction (Kontos & Theochari, 2012). In all probability, a multidimensional approach is most helpful (Jimerson & Pavelski, 2000) including family therapy, cognitive behavioral therapy, psychodynamic therapy, and psychopharmacological interventions.

Implications for Occupational Therapy

Occupational therapy assessment for individuals with eating disorders is helpful when it emphasizes occupational engagement (Abeydeera, Willis, & Forsyth, 2006). Individuals with anorexia may be involved in occupations that are dysfunctional, particularly patterns that emphasize rigid and obsessive focus on eating.

Building a therapeutic alliance is important (Orchard, 2003), as is true in working with any client. Occupational therapists may support behavioral programs implemented by primary therapists for individuals with anorexia and bulimia. The occupational therapist may, for example, assist the client in developing acceptable leisure pursuits that de-emphasize food. In addition, the therapist may provide social skills training to remediate difficulties these individuals have in developing and maintaining satisfying relationships. Therapists also offer stress management techniques and opportunities for self-expression through the expressive arts.

Supportive and educational interventions with caregivers can help reduce stress (Kyriacou et al., 2008), which, in turn, can reduce stress for the individual.

Bulimia Nervosa

Unlike the situation in anorexia nervosa, where body weight is very low, individuals with bulimia nervosa are most often of normal body weight. Their disorder is characterized by repeated episodes of **binge eating**—eating an excessive amount of food in a set time while feeling a lack of control of eating during that time—that they feel incapable of controlling, along with damaging strategies for compensating for overeating (e.g., taking laxatives, inducing vomiting, obsessive exercise). Also, unlike the situation in anorexia, these individuals do not have distorted body image. They tend to not like their bodies, but they do perceive their bodies as they are (Spangler & Allen, 2012).

Diagnostic criteria for bulimia nervosa include binge eating and repeated use of inappropriate mechanisms to compensate for overeating, such as vomiting and taking laxatives (APA, 2013). These behaviors must occur at least weekly for 3 months or more. Self-image is not excessively affected by the behavior. Specifiers clarify whether the disorder is in partial or full remission, and whether it is mild, moderate, severe, or extreme. Anorexia and binge-eating disorder must be ruled out, as well as neurological or medical conditions that might lead to bingeing. Borderline personality disorder, anxiety disorders, and depression are common comorbid conditions.

Etiology

Bulimia nervosa may share an etiology with alcohol and other substance abuse disorders (Carbaugh & Sias, 2010; Yilmaz, Kaplan, & Zawertailo, 2012). Half of all individuals with eating disorders also have substance abuse problems (Carbaugh & Sias, 2010). Among the causes postulated are psychological, environmental, and biological mechanisms. Those affected might be more impulsive, more easily able to develop an addiction, or might live in family environments conducive to the development of both bulimia and substance use disorders. Shared etiological factors for both substance abuse and bulimia include specific personality type, common family history, similar developmental issues, and specific biological vulnerability (Baker, Mazzeo, & Kendler, 2007). Specific personality type is essential to the shared etiology hypothesis because both diagnoses share addiction traits (Baker et al., 2007). These traits include lack of control, craving, and denial. Family history and societal pressures to be thin are also contributing factors in bulimia.

Physiological factors appear to be involved in the development of bulimia as well, including differences in opioid peptide activity (Grilo, Sinha, & O'Malley, 2002) and alterations in the genotypes affecting the serotonin system (Steiger & Bruce, 2007).

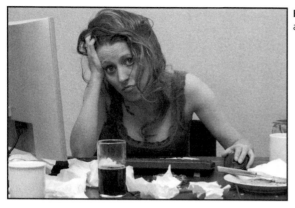

Figure 12-2. Bulimia can interfere with work activities. (©2014 Shutterstock.com.)

Prognosis

Approximately half of clients fully recover from bulimia nervosa, one quarter improves considerably, and the remaining quarter has a chronic and protracted course (Steinhausen & Weber, 2009). Recovery most likely occurs between year 4 and 10 after initial diagnosis and inauguration of treatment. Although these data are encouraging, it is important to be aware that eating disorders and substance abuse have the highest mortality rate of all the mental disorders (Carbaugh & Sias, 2010).

Implications for Function and Treatment

Many occupations are affected because of the centrality of the bingeing and purging behavior. Social interactions can be problematic, and work, school, and leisure are also affected (Figure 12-2).

At the skill level, the individual may have difficulty with emotional regulation (Carbaugh & Sias, 2010). The individual may crave acceptance but be unable to manage social anxiety. Hypersensitivity is common, and the individual may show impulsivity or unpredictability (Carbaugh & Sias, 2010). Starvation and unstable eating patterns affect thoughts and feelings (Woodside & Staab, 2006), and these distortions make positive change difficult.

Cognitive behavioral therapy focused on coping skills and **dialectical behavioral therapy** (DBT) is also useful (Carbaugh & Sais, 2010). DBT "focuses on awareness of problems and choices, mood regulation techniques, and coping skills" (Grilo et al., 2002, p. 157). The focus may be on improving the environment, based on the idea that an invalidating environment may also play a role in dysfunction. An **invalidating environment** is "defined by its tendency to negate, punish, and/or respond erratically and inappropriately to private experiences independent of the validity of the actual behavior" (Barlow, 2008, p. 373). These environments contribute to the individual's behavior by creating a sense of uncertainty, unpredictability, or hostility in the individual's interaction with social or physical surroundings. Another DBT strategy is for the therapist to play devil's advocate by presenting alternate scenarios that differ from the client's expectations. This may help the client reframe specific situations or beliefs.

Implications for Occupational Therapy

Any of the strategies described previously for helping individuals with anorexia nervosa would apply in working with individuals with bulimia. In addition, it may be helpful to implement coping skills training, as these individuals may struggle with mood regulation, managing social situations, and interaction with the environment (Carbaugh & Sais, 2010).

Training to address these deficits can be quite helpful. In addition, helping the individual to learn to avoid trigger situations can be essential. One woman who had struggled with bulimia for years had a job in a grocery store. She would leave every day with a bag full of snack foods that she consumed immediately upon her return home. When she got a new job in an office, she found she was better able to control her bingeing impulse because she was not confronted with food so regularly.

Emotional regulation strategies are an important component of successful intervention of bulimia nervosa (Aldao, Nolen-Hoeksema, & Schweizer, 2010). Psychologists may provide various cognitive and problem-solving interventions. Occupational therapists can focus on problem solving in the context of occupations and emotional regulation through engagement in activities. One example of such an activity is yoga, which requires intense concentration and a focus on perceiving one's body state (Carei, Fyfe-Johnson, Breuner, & Brown, 2010). Technological strategies, such as text messaging, can also be helpful to individuals dealing with bulimia by providing consistent social support through encouraging messages from friends and family (Shapiro et al., 2010).

Binge-Eating Disorder

Binge-eating disorder is new to the DSM-5 (APA, 2013), having been included in the appendix of the fourth edition of the DSM (DSM-IV; APA, 1994) as a possible diagnosis requiring added research. Its main difference from bulimia is the absence of purging behavior. Diagnostic criteria for binge-eating disorder include repeated binge eating associated with eating too rapidly, eating when not hungry, eating until uncomfortably full, eating alone because of embarrassment, and feelings of guilt, depression, or distress about the binge eating (APA, 2013). The behavior must occur at least once per week for at least 3 months. Specifiers clarify whether the disorder is in partial or full remission, and whether it is mild, moderate, severe, or extreme. Anorexia, bulimia, bipolar disorder, and straightforward obesity must be ruled out. The disorder often coexists with bipolar, depressive, and anxiety disorders.

Etiology

Social anxiety and self-consciousness cause the individual to feel greater concern about weight, and this concern can increase binge eating frequency (Sawaoka, Barnes, Blomquist, Masheb, & Grilo, 2012). It has been hypothesized that daily challenges and negative affect play a role in binge eating (Haedt-Matt & Keel, 2011; O'Connor, Conner, Jones, McMillan, & Ferguson, 2009). It also seems probable that neurological factors affect both impulse control and satiety (Friederich, Wu, Simon, & Herzog, 2013).

Prognosis

Binge-eating is a disorder that is quite problematic to address, and the behavior contributes to the obesity epidemic in the United States. Younger individuals may do somewhat better (Grilo, Masheb, & Crosby, 2012). Individuals with lower self-esteem, negative affect, and overvaluation of shape and weight were more likely to respond positively to cognitive behavioral therapy.

Implications for Function and Treatment

Binge-eating disorder is accompanied by both physical and social disability (Robinson, 2013). The eating patterns themselves can contribute to this disability, but accompanying obesity can also cause problems. Social skills and family relationships are typically deficient (Verstuyf, Vansteenkiste, Soenens, Boone, & Mouratidis, 2013). Emotional regulation is a particular deficit (Munsch, Meyer, Quartier, & Wilhelm, 2012).

Overall, treatment is very problematic (Hay, 2013). Several novel approaches have been attempted, such as **integrative response therapy**, which is a group-based guided self-help treatment focused on affect regulation (Robinson, 2013).

Other treatments include cognitive behavioral therapy with accompanying medication (Grilo et al., 2012). Antidepressants and anti-epileptic medications have a modest impact (Mitchell, Roerig, & Steffen, 2013).

Implications for Occupational Therapy

Treating binge-eating disorder can be extremely challenging. Occupational therapists are well positioned to provide support in wellness efforts focused on changing behaviors (Pizzi, 2013). Emphasis on healthy occupations that address eating habits (e.g., cooking as a meaningful occupation, social aspects of eating) has the potential to help individuals reframe their eating habits (Forhan & Gill, 2013).

Emerging evidence exists that prevention programs can be effective in changing problematic food-related behaviors in children (Lau, Stevens, & Jia, 2013). Likewise, a growing number of studies focus on obesity prevention and weight reduction for adults. Many of these programs emphasize physical activity, food-related occupations, such as cooking, education about nutrition, and elements of behavior modification to reframe eating and food behaviors. However, it is important to keep in mind that these studies address obesity, not binge-eating disorder. Although it is reasonable to think that strategies might be helpful with individuals with binge-eating disorder, it remains to be demonstrated that this is actually the case. Table 12-2 summarizes the diagnostic criteria and functional consequences of the various feeding and eating disorders.

Cultural Considerations

The various eating disorders are undoubtedly associated with cultural variations. For example, some cultures have a tradition of culturally accepted pica (Ali, 2001). In some African and African American cultures, pregnant women are expected to crave and eat clay.

It has also been suggested that eating disorders reflect a culturally bound syndrome (Keel & Klump, 2003), a suggestion supported by the absence of such disorders in cultures where food is scarce. However, as Western culture is exported to other countries, the rates of eating disorders increase (Vander Wal, Gibbons, & Del Pilar Grazioso, 2008). For example, as the food supply has become more secure in Guatemala, both the presenting symptoms and the underlying dynamics are increasingly similar to the dynamics of food-related disorders in the United States. In the United States, some groups have higher rates of some eating disorders. For example, African American women have higher rates of binge eating than other groups (Hendrickson, Crowther, & Harrington, 2010).

Programming focused on addressing eating disorders must therefore include cultural considerations (Suarez-Balcazar, Friesema, & Lukanova, 2013; Thompson-Brenner et al., 2013). Cooking behavior, meal-related customs, and food choices vary by culture, thus, intervention strategies will be most successful when the relevant values are incorporated.

TABLE 12-2

DIAGNOSTIC CRITERIA AND FUNCTIONAL IMPLICATIONS: FEEDING AND EATING DISORDERS

DISORDER	DIAGNOSTIC CRITERIA (APA, 2013)	IMPLICATIONS FOR FUNCTION
Pica	Persistently eating nonfood items for a period of at least 1 month Inappropriate for developmental level Not culturally or socially normal	Self-care associated with cooking/eating always negatively affected Other areas of function may or may not be impaired
Rumination disorder	Repeatedly regurgitating food over at least 1 month No medical condition explains the disorder Not another eating disorder	Functional consequences typically minor and associated with self-care
Avoidant/restrictive food intake disorder	Eating behavior that causes failure to meet nutritional needs, causing: • Significant weight loss • Reliance on enteral feeding or nutritional supplements • Interference with functioning Not due to lack of available food or by a culturally-normal practice The eating problem is not another eating disorder	Self-care always negatively affected Other occupations may be negatively affected by malnutrition Social performance may be negatively affected Cognition and emotional regulation skills may be negatively affected
Anorexia nervosa	Purposeful limiting of caloric intake causing significant low body weight Fear of gaining weight Inaccurate body image, excessive concern about body weight, lack of recognition of the seriousness of the current low body weight	Self-care is always negatively affected Other areas of performance are often negatively affected by malnutrition Social occupations may be negatively affected Cognition and emotional regulation skills may be negatively affected

(continued)

TABLE 12-2 (CONTINUED)		
DIAGNOSTIC CRITERIA AND FUNCTIONAL IMPLICATIONS: FEEDING AND EATING DISORDERS		
DISORDER	DIAGNOSTIC CRITERIA (APA, 2013)	IMPLICATIONS FOR FUNCTION
Bulimia nervosa	Repeated episodes of binge eating with a sense of lack of control over eating Inappropriate mechanisms to compensate for the overeating (e.g., self-induced vomiting, laxatives) Occurs at least once a week for 3 months Self-image is not influenced by body weight Not anorexia	Self-care always negatively affected Other areas of occupation may be negatively affected, including work Social and leisure occupations may be negatively affected Cognition and emotional regulation skills may be negatively affected
Binge-eating disorder	Repeated episodes (at least once a week for at least 3 months) of binge eating including a sense of lack of control The episodes may include such symptoms as: • Eating too fast • Eating large amounts when not hungry • Eating alone because of embarrassment • Feeling disgusted with oneself, depressed, or guilty Distress about binge eating Not anorexia or bulimia	Self-care always negatively affected Social and leisure occupations may be negatively affected Cognition and emotional regulation skills may be negatively affected

Lifespan Considerations

Several of the eating disorders, notably pica and rumination disorder, occur primarily in children. This means that parents must be involved in treatment strategies, as they control—to a large extent—the availability of food and the specific choices provided to the child. Anorexia and bulimia most often emerge in adolescence, which is a time when interaction between child and parent can be difficult, even in the best of circumstances. Family interventions are important in minimizing the damage done to relationships by the individual's eating difficulties and resultant parental concern.

For older adults, physiological regulation of appetite differs, compared with younger individuals (Thomas, 2009). Changes in neurotransmitter production often cause a decrease in appetite in older adults, which can then lead to malnutrition. In addition, for older adults,

CASE STUDY

Alexandria McCall is a 22-year-old, White, female college student majoring in physical education. She is 5 feet 6 inches tall, and currently weighs 86 pounds. She is well-groomed, clothed in typical college-student attire—jeans, oversized t-shirt, and flip-flops—and has carefully polished fingernails and toenails. Her parents have insisted that she go to the student health center because of their concern about her emaciated appearance, but Alexandria denies that there is anything wrong. She does acknowledge that she has sometimes experienced irregular heartbeat and that she no longer menstruates, but she claims that her vigorous exercise (she is a gymnast) is probably the cause of these symptoms.

Alexandria's parents note that she has lost a considerable amount of weight, and on her visits home she seems to be constantly monitoring her food intake. Her eating is quite sparse, although she seems very focused on food and talks about it constantly. They confirm that Alexandria is a talented gymnast and that she has competed nationally. However, they point out that in the past year she has stopped competing and now seems to have no extracurricular activities. She has always been an excellent student, but her grades have dropped recently.

Alexandria firmly denies that her weight loss is serious. She describes herself as "obese" and says that her food monitoring is an effort to lose weight, as she knows that obesity is dangerous. She denies any use of laxatives or other purging behavior, and she denies feeling depressed. She indicates that she has few friends, but she does not mind this because she is "very busy" exercising.

THOUGHT QUESTIONS

1. What functional deficits are evident in Alexandria's current situation? Of these deficits, which might be most critical to first address?
2. What are some factors in Alexandria's history that could help structure a meaningful occupational profile?
3. What would be the highest priority in helping Alexandria to regain a level of function that is supportive of her needs?
4. Do you think Alexandria has a mental disorder? If so, what?
5. What cultural factors do you think might be important in this situation?

when appetite has decreased, it is difficult to increase it again. Ten percent of men and 20% of women over age 65 have lower caloric intake than the recommended daily allowance, and 16% to 18% of community-living older adults consume fewer than 1000 calories per day. These findings may be associated with lower expenditure of calories, but it is difficult to consume adequate nutrients at such a low intake. Anorexia of aging adults is qualitatively different from that of younger adults because it is not typically associated with conscious choice but instead with the variety of age-related changes that reduce appetite and pleasure in food. Attention to enhanced appeal of food and to the social aspects of eating can be helpful. One older woman who lived alone was severely underweight. When she moved to an assisted living facility where meals were provided in a family-style environment, she found mealtime pleasant and regained an appetite.

Internet Resources

Eating Disorders Resource Center
http://www.edrcsv.org/
One of several self-help and consumer-focused organizations that provides resources for individuals and families dealing with eating disorders.

Eating Disorders Resources Organization
http://eatingdisordersresources.org/
Another self-help and consumer-focused organization that provides resources for individuals and families dealing with eating disorders.

Medline Plus Eating Disorder Resources
http://www.nlm.nih.gov/medlineplus/ency/article/002171.htm
Medline and the National Library of Medicine that sponsors it are excellent resources for consumers and for professionals.

National Eating Disorders Organization
http://www.nationaleatingdisorders.org/
One of several self-help and consumer-focused organizations that provides resources for individuals and families dealing with eating disorders.

References

Abeydeera, K., Willis, S., & Forsyth, K. (2006). Occupation focused assessment and intervention for clients with anorexia. *International Journal of Therapy and Rehabilitation, 13*, 296.

Aldao, A., Nolen-Hoeksema, S., & Schweizer, S. (2010). Emotion-regulation strategies across psychopathology: A meta-analytic review. *Clinical Psychology Review, 30*, 217-237.

Ali, Z. (2001). Pica in people with intellectual disability: A literature review of aetiology, epidemiology and complications. *Journal of Intellectual and Developmental Disability, 26*(3), 205-215.

American Psychiatric Association. (1994). *Diagnostic and statistical manual of mental disorders* (4th ed.). Washington, DC: Author.

American Psychiatric Association. (2013). *Diagnostic and statistical manual of mental disorders* (5th ed.). Washington, DC: Author.

Amianto, F., Abbate-Daga, G., Morando, S., Sobrero, C., & Fassino, S. (2010). Personality development characteristics of women with anorexia nervosa, their healthy siblings, and controls: What prevents and what relates to psychopathology? *Psychiatry Research, 187*(3), 401-408.

Baker, J.H., Mazzeo, S.E., & Kendler, K.S. (2007). Association between broadly defined bulimia nervosa and drug use disorders: Common genetic and environmental influences. *International Journal of Eating Disorders, 40*, 673-678.

Barlow, D.H. (Ed.). (2008). *Clinical handbook of psychological disorders: A step-by-step treatment manual.* (4th ed.). New York, NY: Guilford Press.

Blank, S., & Latzer, Y. (2004). The boundary-control model of adolescent anorexia nervosa: An integrative approach to etiology and treatment? *American Journal of Family Therapy, 32*(1), 43-54.

Bryant-Waugh, R. (2013). Avoidant restrictive food intake disorder: An illustrative case example. *International Journal of Eating Disorders, 46*(5), 420-423.

Carbaugh, R.J., & Sias, S.M. (2010). Comorbidity of bulimia nervosa and substance abuse: Etiologies, treatment issues, and treatment approaches. *Journal of Mental Health Counseling, 32*(2), 125-138.

Carei, T.R., Fyfe-Johnson, A.L., Breuner, C.C., & Brown, M.A. (2010). Randomized controlled clinical trial of yoga in the treatment of eating disorders. *Journal of Adolescent Health, 46*, 346-351.

Carter, S.L. (2009). Treatment of pica using a pica exchange procedure with increasing response effort. *Education and Training in Developmental Disabilities, 44*(1), 143-147.

Case, L.K., Wilson, R.C., & Ramachandran, V.S. (2012). Diminished size—weight illusion in anorexia nervosa: Evidence for visuo-proprioceptive integration deficit. *Experimental Brain Research, 217*(1), 9-87.

Castinellini, G., Lelli, L., Lo Sauro, C., Fioravanti, G., Vignozzi, L., Maggi, M., . . . Ricca, V. (2012). Anorectic and bulimic patients suffer from relevant sexual dysfunctions. *Journal of Sexual Medicine, 9*(10), 2590-2599.

Cogan, K.D. (2009). Eating disorders. In K.F. Hays (Ed.), *Performance psychology in action: A casebook for working with athletes, performing artists, business leaders, and professionals in high-risk occupations* (pp. 183-202). Washington, DC: American Psychological Association.

Favaro, A., Tenconi, E., & Santonasto, P. (2010). The interaction between perinatal factors and childhood abuse in the risk of developing anorexia nervosa. *Psychological Medicine, 40*(4), 657-665.

Forhan, M., & Gill, S. (2013). Cross-border contributions to obesity research and interventions: A review of Canadian and American occupational therapy contributions. *Occupational Therapy in Health Care, 27*(2), 129-141.

Friederich, H., Wu, M., Simon, J.J., & Herzog, W. (2013). Neurocircuit function in eating disorders. *International Journal of Eating Disorders, 46*(5), 425-432.

Grilo, C.M., Masheb, R.M., & Crosby, R.D. (2012). Predictors and moderators of response to cognitive behavioral therapy and medication for the treatment of binge eating disorder. *Journal of Consulting and Clinical Psychology, 80*(5), 897-906.

Grilo, C.M., Sinha, R., & O'Malley, S.S. (2002). Research update: Eating disorders and alcohol use disorders. *Alcohol Research and Health, 26,* 151-160.

Haedt-Matt, A.A., & Keel, P.K. (2011). Revisiting the affect regulation model of binge eating: A meta-analysis of studies using ecological momentary assessment. *Psychological Bulletin, 137,* 660-681.

Hambrook, D., Oldershaw, A., Rimes, K., Schmidt, U., Tchanturia, K., Treasure, J., . . . Chalder, T. (2011). Emotional expression, self-silencing, and distress tolerance in anorexia nervosa and chronic fatigue syndrome. *British Journal of Clinical Psychology, 50*(3), 310-325.

Hay, P. (2013). A systematic review of evidence for psychological treatments in eating disorders: 2005-2012. *International Journal of Eating Disorders, 46*(5), 462-469.

Hendrickson, H.C., Crowther, J.S., & Harrington, E.F. (2010). Ethnic identity and maladaptive eating: Expectancies about eating and thinness in African American women. *Cultural Diversity and Ethnic Minority Psychology, 16,* 87-93.

Hergüner, S., & Hergüner, A.S. (2010). Pica in a child with attention deficit hyperactivity disorder and successful treatment with methylphenidate. *Progress in Neuro-Psychopharmacology & Biological Psychiatry, 34*(6), 1155-1156.

Hergüner, S., Özyıldırım, I., & Tanidir, C. (2008). Is pica an eating disorder or an obsessive-compulsive spectrum disorder? *Progress in Neuro-Psychopharmacology & Biological Psychiatry, 32*(8), 2010-2011.

Herpetz-Dahlmann, B., Seitz, J., & Konrad, K. (2011). Aetiology of anorexia nervosa: From a "psychosomatic family model" to a neuropsychiatric disorder? *European Archives of Psychiatry and Clinical Neuroscience, 261*(Suppl. 2), S177-S181.

Hoek, H.W. (2006). Incidence, prevalence and mortality of anorexia nervosa and other eating disorders. *Current Opinion in Psychiatry, 19*(4), 389-394.

Hudson, J.I., Hiripi, E., Pope, H.G., & Kessler, R.C. (2007). The prevalence and correlates of eating disorders in the National Comorbidity Survey Replication. *Biological Psychiatry, 61,* 348-358.

Hughes, E.K. (2012). Comorbid depression and anxiety in childhood and adolescent anorexia nervosa: Prevalence and implications for outcome. *Clinical Psychologist, 16*(1), 15-24.

Jimerson, S.R., & Pavelski, R. (2000). The school psychologist's primer on anorexia nervosa: A review of research regarding epidemiology, etiology, assessment, and treatment. *California School Psychologist, 5,* 65-77.

Katz, E.R., & DeMaso, D.R. (2011). Rumination disorder. In R.M. Kliegman, R.E. Behrman, B.F. Stanton, J.W. St. Geme III, N.F. Schor, & R.E. Behrman (Eds.), *Nelson textbook of pediatrics* (19th ed., chapter 21.1, pp. 70-71). Philadelphia, PA: Saunders Elsevier.

Keel, P.K., & Klump, K.L. (2003). Are eating disorders culture-bound syndromes? Implications for conceptualizing their etiology. *Psychological Bulletin, 129*(5), 747-769.

Kontos, D., & Theochari, E. (2012). Dopamine in anorexia nervosa: A systematic review. *Behavioural Pharmacology, Special issue: Pharmacological Approaches to Deeding Behaviour and Eating Disorders. 23*(5-6), 496-515.

Kriepe, R.E., & Palomaki, A. (2012). Beyond picky eating: Avoidant/restrictive food intake disorder. *Current Psychiatry Reports, 14*(4), 421-431.

Kyriacou, O., Treasure, J., & Schmidt, U. (2008). Understanding how parents cope with living with someone with anorexia nervosa: Modeling the factors that are associated with carer distress. *International Journal of Eating Disorders, 41*(3), 233-242.

Lau, C., Stevens, D., & Jia, J. (2013). Effects of an occupation-based obesity prevention program for children at risk. *Occupational Therapy in Health Care, 27*(2), 163-175.

Lindblad, F., Lindberg, L., & Hjern, A. (2006). Anorexia nervosa in young men: A cohort study. *International Journal of Eating Disorders, 39*(8), 662-666.

McCann, E., McCormick, L., Bowers, W., & Hoffman, V. (2010). Cognitive behavioral therapy and non-specific supportive clinical management in individuals with longstanding anorexia nervosa. *Minerva Psichiatrica, 51*(3), 219-229.

Mehler, P.S., Cleary, B.S., & Gaudiani, J.L. (2011). Osteoporosis in anorexia nervosa. *Eating Disorders: The Journal of Treatment & Prevention, 19*(2), 194-202.

Mitchell, J.E., Roerig, J., & Steffen, K. (2013). Biological therapies for eating disorders. *International Journal of Eating Disorders, 46*(5), 470-477.

Munsch, S., Meyer, A.H., Quartier, V., & Wilhelm, F.H. (2012). Binge eating in binge eating disorder: A breakdown of emotion regulatory process? *Psychiatry Research, 195*(3), 118-124.

O'Connor, D.B., Conner, M.T., Jones, F.A., McMillan, B.R.W., & Ferguson, E. (2009). Exploring the benefits of conscientiousness: An investigation of the role of daily stressors and health behaviours. *Annals of Behavioural Medicine, 37,* 184-196.

Orchard, R. (2003). With you, not against you: Applying motivational interviewing to occupational therapy in anorexia nervosa. *British Journal of Occupational Therapy, 66*(7), 325-327.

Papadopoulos, F.C., Ekbom, A., Brandt, L., & Ekselius, L. (2009). Excess mortality, causes of death and prognostic factors in anorexia nervosa. *British Journal of Psychiatry, 194*(1), 10-17.

Pizzi, M.A. (2013). Obesity, health and quality of life: A conversation to further the vision in occupational therapy. *Occupational Therapy in Health Care, 27*(2), 78-83.

Quiles-Cestari, L.M., Ribeiro, R., & Pilot, P. (2012). The occupational roles of women with anorexia nervosa. *Revista Latino-Americana de Enfermagem (RLAE), 20*(2), 235-242.

Robinson, A. (2013). Integrative response therapy for binge eating disorder. *Cognitive and Behavioral Practice, 20*(1), 93-105.

Sato, Y., Saito, N., Utsumi, A., Aizawa, E., Shoji, T., Izumiyama, M., . . . Fukudo, S. (2013). Neural basis of impaired cognitive flexibility in patients with anorexia nervosa. *PLoS ONE, 8*(5), e61108. doi:10.1371/journal.pone.0061108.

Sawaoka, T., Barnes, R.D., Blomquist, K.K., Masheb, R.M., & Grilo, C.M. (2012). Social anxiety and self-consciousness in binge eating disorder: Associations with eating disorder psychopathology. *Comprehensive Psychiatry, 53*(6), 740-745.

Shapiro, J.R., Bauer, S., Andrews, E., Pielsky, E., Bulik-Sullivan, B., Hamer, R.M., & Bulik, C.M. (2010). Mobile therapy: Use of text-messaging in the treatment of bulimia nervosa. *International Journal of Eating Disorders, 43,* 513-519.

Sinha, M., & Mallick, A.K. (2010). Pica in the backdrop of psychiatric disorders: A complex etiology. *International Medical Journal, 17*(1), 21-23.

Spangler, D.L., & Allen, M.D. (2012). An fMRI investigation of emotional processing of body shape in bulimia nervosa. *International Journal of Eating Disorders, 45*(1), 17-25.

Steiger, H., & Bruce, K.R. (2007). Phenotypes, endophenotypes, and genotypes in bulimia spectrum eating disorders. *Canadian Journal of Psychiatr/La Revue canadienne de psychiatrie, 52*(4), 220-227.

Steinhausen, H., & Weber, S. (2009). The outcome of bulimia nervosa: Findings from one-quarter century of research. *American Journal of Psychiatry, 166*(12), 1331-1341.

Suarez-Balcazar, Y., Friesema, J., & Lukanova, V. (2013). Culturally competent interventions to address obesity among African American and Latino children and youth. *Occupational Therapy in Health Care, 27*(2), 113-128.

Thihalolipavan, S., Candalla, B.M., & Ehrlich, J. (2013). Examining pica in NYC pregnant women with elevated blood lead levels. *Maternal and Child Health Journal, 17*(1), 49-55.

Thomas, D.R. (2009). Anorexia: Aetiology, epidemiology and management in older people. *Drugs & Aging, 26*(7), 557-570.

Thompson-Brenner, H., Franko, D.L., Thompson, D.R., Grilo, C.M. Boisseau, C.L., Roehrig, J.P., . . . Wilson, G.T. (2013). Race/ethnicity, education, and treatment parameters as moderators and predictors of outcome in binge eating disorder. *Journal of Consulting and Clinical Psychology, 81*(4), 710-721. doi:10.1037/a0032946.

Vander Wal, J.S., Gibbons, J.L., & Del Pilar Grazioso, M. (2008). The sociocultural model of eating disorder development: Application to a Guatemalan sample. *Eating Behaviors, 9*(3), 277-284.

Verstuyf, J., Vansteenkiste, M., Soenens, B., Boone, L., & Mouratidis, A. (2013). Daily ups and downs in women's binge eating symptoms: The role of basic psychological needs, general self-control, and emotional eating. *Journal of Social and Clinical Psychology, 32*(3), 335-361.

Wentz, E., Gillberg, I.C., Anckarsäter, H., Gillber, C., & Råstam, M. (2009). Adolescent-onset anorexia nervosa: 18-year outcome. *British Journal of Psychiatry, 194*(2), 168-174.

Williams, D.E., Kirkpatrick-Sanchez, S., Enzinna, C., Dunn, J., & Borden-Karasack, D. (2009). The clinical management and prevention of pica: A retrospective follow-up of 41 individuals with intellectual disabilities and pica. *Journal of Applied Research in Intellectual Disabilities, Special Issue: Restrictive Behavioural Practices, 22*(2), 210-215.

Williams, D.E., & McAdam, D., (2012). Assessment, behavioral treatment, and prevention of pica: Clinical guidelines and recommendations for practitioners. *Research in Developmental Disabilities, 33*(6), 2050-2057.

Woodside, B.D., & Staab, R. (2006). Management of psychiatric comorbidity in anorexia nervosa and bulimia nervosa. *CNS Drugs, 20,* 655-663.

Yilmaz, Z., Kaplan, A.S., & Zawertailo, L.A. (2012). Bulimia nervosa and alcohol use disorder: Evidence for shared etiology and neurobiology. *Current Psychiatry Reviews, 8*(1), 69-81.

Elimination Disorders

Learning Outcomes

By the end of this chapter, readers will be able to:
- Describe the symptoms of elimination disorders
- Identify the causes of the elimination disorders
- Describe treatment strategies for elimination disorders
- Discuss the occupational perspective on elimination disorders, including specific intervention considerations

Bonder B.
Psychopathology and Function, Fifth Edition (pp 257-264).
© 2015 SLACK Incorporated.

KEY WORDS

- Enuresis
- Encopresis

CASE VIGNETTE

Tim is a 7-year-old whose parents and teachers describe him as a bright and capable student. He was born full term, without any complications during pregnancy, labor, or delivery, when his mother was 35 years old. However, when he was in preschool, he was found to have low muscle tone and somewhat delayed motor development. He received physical and occupational therapy until he started kindergarten. No history of medical problems or abuse was noted, and he was advanced in most areas of development, other than some motor delay. His parents have become increasingly concerned because they have found stool stains in his clothing approximately twice per week. His parents tried punishment, but this has been ineffective and has caused both Tim and his parents considerable stress. They also tried rewarding him when his underwear was clean, but this had no impact either. They now feel they do not know what to do.

THOUGHT QUESTIONS

1. Do you believe that Tim has a mental disorder?
2. If so, what behaviors, thoughts, or other symptoms do you identify as problematic?
3. Of those symptoms, which might cause Tim difficulty in his daily life?

ELIMINATION DISORDERS

- Enuresis
- Encopresis

Elimination disorder is one of the categories in the *Diagnostic and Statistical Manual of Mental Disorders* (DSM) that includes relatively few diagnoses. Yet, they are important because of their frequency, especially in children, and the potential impact on function and quality of life for both the child and the family (Kushnir, Kushnir, & Sadeh, 2013). Table 13-1 shows the prevalence of these elimination disorders.

Enuresis

Enuresis is an inability or unwillingness to control urination. Its most common form is nocturnal (Kushnir et al., 2013). In approximately 70% of cases, the child never achieved nighttime urinary continence; in the remaining cases, the child did achieve control and maintained it for several months before regressing. Diagnostic criteria for enuresis include repeated involuntary or intentional voiding of urine in bed or on clothing that causes distress or dysfunction (American Psychiatric Association [APA], 2013). The behavior must occur at least twice per week for 3 months in an individual who is at least 5 years old (or an equivalent

TABLE 13-1			
PREVALENCE OF ELIMINATION DISORDERS			
DIAGNOSIS	*PREVALENCE*	*GENDER RATIO (M:F)*	*SOURCE*
Enuresis	At age 6: 3% to 6% At age 10: 7% to 9%	2:1	Kushnir et al., 2013
Encopresis	3% of children under age 12	2:1	Coehlo, 2011

developmental level). Specifiers note whether this is nocturnal only, diurnal only, or both nocturnal and diurnal. It is important to rule out medical conditions or medication side effects. Common co-occurring disorders include developmental disabilities, autistic spectrum disorders, and sleep disorders.

Etiology

A clear genetic factor exists in development of enuresis, with children whose mothers had the condition being 3.6 times more likely than others to have the disorder (Kiddoo, 2012). It is also significantly more common in boys, who, in the normal course of development, acquire bladder control at a later age than girls. Enuresis almost certainly has a neurological component, as children who have enuresis are likely to be deep sleepers but are also prone to sleep disruption. It is important to rule out medical conditions, such as urinary tract infections, back malformation, and other physiological contributors (von Gontard, 2006).

Prognosis

With appropriate treatment, the prognosis of enuresis is quite good (Kiddoo, 2012). Even without treatment, approximately 15% of children with enuresis each year will spontaneously improve (von Gontard, 2006).

Implications for Function and Treatment

Although the disorder may seem relatively minor and self-limiting, enuresis can have substantial impact on overall functioning (Cox, 2009). Children may become socially isolated, avoiding sleepovers or daytime visits to friends' homes. In some cases, the problem may be related to issues about using the toilet, rather than related to bladder control. The child may fear being locked in (or not having privacy), may struggle with clothing, or may not be able to sit on the toilet properly. These concerns can feel humiliating, and the child may experience significant self-esteem issues. In addition, if the condition is stressful to parents, family tensions may be contributing factors as well.

Treatment options are relatively well established and effective. Health education for the child and parent can be of great value (Cox, 2009), particularly if focused on understanding how the urinary system works and how control develops. Other treatment choices include lifestyle and environmental modifications, as well as medication use.

Lifestyle modifications include strategies to manage the condition so that the child can participate in normal childhood activities (Cox, 2009). Developing strategies for managing activities like sleepovers and modifying habits such as fluid intake patterns, may be helpful in minimizing the damage to the child's self-esteem. A bed alarm can wake the child so that he or she can get to the toilet. Medical interventions include desmopressin and tricyclic antidepressants. Desmopressin and behavior modification, either alone or in combination, have been found to be equally effective (Fera, Lelis, Glashan, Pereira, & Bruschini, 2011).

A number of alternative therapies have been used, including hypnotherapy, acupuncture, chiropractic treatment, and psychotherapy. However, limited evidence supports these treatments (Glazener, Evans, & Cheuk, 2011).

It is important to note that the majority of the literature focuses on unintentional enuresis. The situation is significantly different when the failure to control the bladder is intentional. Although less common, the behavior may be associated with conduct disorder, autism, attention-deficit/hyperactivity disorder, or other disorders of childhood (Gontkovsky, 2011). In these cases, intervention to address the comorbid condition is essential.

Implications for Occupational Therapy

A significant role exists for occupational therapy in addressing enuresis, such as providing advice to parents about environmental interventions and strategies for maintaining the child's self-esteem. This may include providing advice about waterproof mattresses and bed protectors, strategies for getting the child to the toilet during the night, and encouragement to establish a bedtime routine that includes a visit to the bathroom before bed. All these strategies can be helpful in both managing the condition and giving the child and parents a sense of control over the situation (Cox, 2009).

Children are often able to predict their own improvement (Ronen, Hamama, & Rosenbaum, 2013). They may recognize their increased personal motivation to learn to manage the condition, and making the prediction and achieving the goal can be very reinforcing.

Encopresis

Encopresis is the term used to describe withholding feces and ignoring the need to defecate (Coehlo, 2011). Encopresis is typically associated with constipation and with leakage that soils clothing. Initially the child ignores the need to defecate, and eventually, he or she loses the ability to recognize the impulse. Diagnostic criteria for encopresis include repeated defecation, either voluntary or involuntary, in inappropriate places in an individual who is at least 4 years old or equivalent developmental level (APA, 2013). The behavior must occur at least once per month for at least 3 months. Specifiers note whether there is accompanying constipation and overflow incontinence. Medical conditions must be ruled out. These children may also have attention-deficit/hyperactivity disorder, conduct disorder, obsessive-compulsive disorder, or cognitive delay.

Etiology

Most research suggests that encopresis results from a combination of risk factors (Coehlo, 2011). These risk factors include an unpleasant experience with toilet training (Figure 13-1), such as pain or parental disapproval. In addition, chronic constipation during infancy, low muscle tone and coordination, slow intestinal motility, and male gender are contributing factors. A poor diet with low dietary fiber and high intake of sugary fluids, stress, low physical activity level, and unpredictable daily routine are also implicated. Many children with encopresis have had at least one bowel event that was uncomfortable or frightening (Cox et al., 2003).

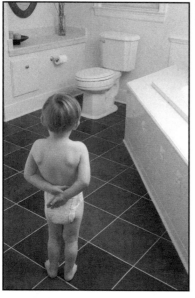

Figure 13-1. Difficult experiences with toilet training can contribute to encopresis. (©2014 Shutterstock.com.)

Prognosis

Unlike enuresis, which has a good prognosis, encopresis can lead to chronic bowel difficulties that persist into adulthood for as many as 30% of those with the childhood condition (Coehlo, 2011). As an individual reaches adolescence, function in most spheres among those who improve is comparable to those who never had encopresis (Hultén, Jonsson, & Jonsson, 2005).

Implications for Function and Treatment

Although there is no immediately obvious reason that function should be affected in other spheres of life, children with encopresis, like children with enuresis, may have difficulty in school, social, and home situations. Children and their families may feel isolated and ostracized (Har & Croffie, 2010).

In general, a combination of intervention strategies is most likely to be helpful. These involve behavior modification (e.g., a specific daily routine, including bathroom time), family education (e.g., to reduce stress and increase comfort with behavioral routines), and bowel management routines (Friman, Hofstadter, & Jones, 2006). Early intervention is essential (McGrath & Murphy, 2004).

Treatment of encopresis can be categorized in six main areas: treatment of bowel impaction as needed, dietary changes, bowel training, behavior management, family support, and medications. Most typically, medications include stool softeners (Coehlo, 2011). Use of strong laxatives used to be recommended, but this has been abandoned as ineffective. Some attempts have been made to use complementary and alternative methods, such as herbal remedies, acupuncture, and hypnotherapy (Culbert & Banez, 2007), although evidence of the effectiveness of these approaches is sparse.

Implications for Occupational Therapy

Occupational therapists often provide treatment for encopresis. They are equipped to identify the readiness signs and developmental skills needed for toilet training (e.g., ability

TABLE 13-2		
DIAGNOSTIC CRITERIA AND FUNCTIONAL IMPLICATIONS: ELIMINATION DISORDERS		
DISORDER	*DIAGNOSTIC CRITERIA (APA, 2013)*	*IMPLICATIONS FOR FUNCTION*
Enuresis	Repeated involuntary or intentional urination in bed or clothing with accompanying distress or dysfunction Chronological or developmental age of at least 5 years	Negatively affects self-care and social occupations May negatively affect school and leisure occupations May be associated with body system/body function deficits
Encopresis	Repeated involuntary or intentional defecation in inappropriate places At least one event each month for at least 3 months Chronological or developmental age of at least 4 years	Negatively affects self-care and social occupations May be associated with body system/body function deficits

to follow simple verbal descriptions, manage clothing) and to provide educational programming for families (Coehlo, 2011). Online instruction is a useful strategy (Ritterband et al., 2006). Multidisciplinary intervention is most helpful (Richards, Macauley, & Tierra, 2009). Table 13-2 summarizes the diagnostic criteria and functional implications of the elimination disorders.

Cultural Considerations

The prevalence of elimination disorders seems fairly consistent across cultures (Kaneko, 2012; Mahmoodzadeh, Amestejani, Karamyar, & Mohammad, 2013). Some differences exist in rate of help seeking. For example, Iranian parents are perhaps less likely to get help (Mahmoodzadeh et al., 2013). Also some differences exist in treatment. For instance, in Japan, treatment is primarily medical (Kaneko, 2012).

Lifespan Considerations

Both enuresis and encopresis are primarily disorders of childhood. When they exist in adults, it is most typically in concert with a developmental or other mental disorder (Matson & Lovullo, 2009).

CASE STUDY

Sammy is a 9-year-old boy who has never achieved nighttime bladder control. He has been dry in the daytime since he was 3 years old, but wets the bed almost nightly. It is not clear how it became known at school, but his classmates are aware of his problem and he is bullied and ostracized. He has one good friend who is supportive and willing to help him stand up to the cruelty of his classmates. His parents are grateful that he has a friend, and do what they can to support this friendship. However, they are otherwise out of ideas for how to help. They have tried limiting his nighttime drinking, and make sure he uses the bathroom before bed, but these efforts have not been successful.

Now Sammy has been invited to spend a week on vacation with his friend, but is embarrassed about his dilemma. He very much wants to go, but fears he will continue to experience nighttime enuresis. He is motivated to deal with the situation and has asked his parents to help him. They decided to start with a consultation with the school nurse.

Sammy reports that he drinks very little during the day. He says that he doesn't want to have to go to the bathroom at school because it is "scary." As a result, he is very thirsty when he gets home, and he drinks quite a bit before supper.

The school nurse recommends that Sammy drink more during the day, and that he begin a regular schedule of bathroom visits. He is encouraged to drink less late in the day. While he is willing to try this, he remains worried about having to use the bathroom at school.

THOUGHT QUESTIONS

1. What functional deficits are evident in Sammy's current situation?
2. What are some factors in Sammy's history that could help frame an intervention?
3. What might an occupational therapist suggest to help resolve the situation?

Internet Resources

MentalHelp.Net: Elimination Disorders: Enuresis
http://www.mentalhelp.net/poc/view_doc.php?type=doc&id=536&cn=5
An article by Barkoukis, Staats Reiss, and Dombeck provides an overview of enuresis, with discussion of issues and treatment.

NYU Child Study Center: Encopresis: Support and Resources
http://www.aboutourkids.org/families/disorders_treatments/az_disorder_guide/elimination_disorders_encopresis/support_resources
This site is focused on helping families learn to manage encopresis.

References

American Psychiatric Association. (2013). *Diagnostic and statistical manual of mental disorders* (5th ed.). Washington, DC: Author.

Coehlo, D.P. (2011). Encopresis: A medical and family approach. *Pediatric Nursing, 37*(3), 107-112.

Cox, D.J., Ritterband, L.M., Quillian, W., Kovatchev, B., Morris, J., Sutphn, J., & Borowitz, S. (2003). Assessment of behavioral mechanisms maintaining encopresis: Virginia Encopresis-Constipation Apperception Test. *Journal of Pediatric Psychology, 28,* 375-382.

Cox, E. (2009). Managing childhood enuresis: An overview. *British Journal of School Nursing, 4(9),* 434-438.

Culbert, T.P., & Banez, G.A. (2007). Integrative approaches to childhood constipation and encopresis. *Pediatric Clinics of North America, 54(6),* 927-948.

Fera, P., Lelis, M.A., Glashan, R., Pereira, S. G., & Bruschini, H. (2011). Desmopressin versus behavioral modifications as initial treatment of primary nocturnal enuresis. *Urologic Nursing, 31(5),* 286-289.

Friman, P.C., Hofstadter, K.L., & Jones, K.M. (2006). A biobehavioral approach to the treatment of functional encopresis in children. *Journal of Early and Intensive Behavior Intervention, 3(1),* 263-272.

Glazener, M.A.C., Evans, H.C.J., & Cheuk, K.L.D. (2011). Complementary and miscellaneous interventions for nocturnal enuresis in children [Review]. *Cochrane Database Systematic Review, 12,* CD005230.

Gontkovsky, S.T. (2011). Prevalence of enuresis in a community sample of children and adolescents referred for outpatient clinical psychological evaluation: Psychiatric comorbidities and association with intellectual functioning. *Journal of Child & Adolescent Mental Health, 23(1),* 53-58.

Har, A.F., & Croffie, J.M. (2010). Encopresis. *Pediatrics in Review, 31(9),* 368-374.

Hultén, I., Jonsson, J., & Jonsson, C. (2005). Mental and somatic health in a non-clinical sample 10 years after a diagnosis of encopresis. *European Child & Adolescent Psychiatry, 14(8),* 438-445.

Kaneko, K., (2012). Treatment for nocturnal enuresis: The current state in Japan. *Pediatrics International, 54(1),* 8-13.

Kiddoo, D.A. (2012). Nocturnal enuresis. *CMAJ: Canadian Medical Association Journal, 184(8),* 908-911.

Kushnir, J., Kushnir, B., & Sadeh, A. (2013). Children treated for nocturnal enuresis: Characteristics and trends over a 15-year period. *Child & Youth Care Forum, 42(2),* 119-129.

Mahmoodzadeh, H., Amestejani, M., Karamyar, M., & Mohammad, N. (2013). Prevalence of nocturnal enuresis in school aged children. The role of personal and parents related socio-economic and educational factors. *Iranian Journal of Pediatrics, 23(1),* 59-64.

Matson, J.L., & Lovullo, S.V. (2009). Encopresis, soiling and constipation in children and adults with developmental disability. *Research in Developmental Disabilities, 30(4),* 799-807.

McGrath, M.I., & Murphy, I. (2004). Empirically supported treatments in pediatric psychology: Constipation and encopresis. *Journal of Pediatric Psychology, 25,* 225-254.

Richards, K., Macauley, R., & Tierra, A. (2009). Encopresis: Multi-disciplinary management. *Journal of Occupational Therapy, Schools & Early Intervention, 2(2),* 96-102.

Ritterband, L.M., Cox, D.J., Gordon, T.L., Borowitz, S.M., Kovatchev, B.P., Walker, L.S., & Sutphen, J.L. (2006). Examining the added value of audio, graphics, and interactivity in an Internet intervention for pediatric encopresis. *Children's Health Care, 35(1),* 47-59.

Ronen, T., Hamama, L., & Rosenbaum, M. (2013). Enuresis—Children's predictions of their treatment's progress and outcomes. *Journal of Clinical Nursing, 22(1-2),* 222-232.

von Gontard, A. (2006). Elimination disorders: Enuresis and encopresis. In C. Gillberg, R. Harrington, & H. Steinhausen (Eds.), *A clinician's handbook of child and adolescent psychiatry* (pp. 625-654). New York, NY: Cambridge University Press.

Sleep–Wake Disorders and Breathing-Related Sleep Disorders

Learning Outcomes

By the end of this chapter, readers will be able to:

- Describe the various sleep disorders
- Differentiate among sleep disorders on the basis of symptoms and onset
- Identify the causes of sleep disorders
- Describe treatment strategies for sleep disorders
- Discuss occupational therapy interventions for sleep disorders

Bonder B.
Psychopathology and Function, Fifth Edition (pp 265-279).
© 2015 SLACK Incorporated.

KEY WORDS

- Hypersomnolence
- Cataplexy
- Hypocretin
- Cheyne-Stokes breathing

- Hypocapnia
- Circadian rhythms
- Sleepwalking
- Sleep terrors

CASE VIGNETTE

Albert Frost is a 46-year-old financial planner. He is married and has two grown sons. Mr. Frost has always been an energetic person, and he is successful in his professional life. He was a college football player who has since engaged in relatively little physical exercise. He recognizes that he has gained more weight than is healthy for him, but he loves to eat and is proud of being a bit of an expert on fine wines. He also enjoys watching sporting events with his sons, and they usually consume quite a bit of beer and pizza while watching.

In the past year, Mr. Frost has found himself frequently very sleepy during the day. He has much less energy than he had in the past and has trouble concentrating at work. His wife, with whom he has a good relationship, started sleeping in the guest bedroom approximately 6 months ago, complaining that he had begun to snore loudly most nights.

At his wife's urging, Mr. Frost has consulted his primary care physician to determine if a cause for his fatigue can be identified. He also wants to know whether he has developed a sinus problem that is causing his snoring. The physician sends him to a local sleep clinic for a sleep study.

THOUGHT QUESTIONS

1. Do you believe Mr. Frost has a mental disorder?
2. What troubling behaviors or emotions is Mr. Frost experiencing that might be consistent with a mental disorder?
3. What functional deficits is Mr. Frost experiencing? What strengths does he demonstrate?

SLEEP–WAKE DISORDERS AND BREATHING-RELATED SLEEP DISORDERS

- Sleep–wake disorders
  - Insomnia disorder
  - Hypersomnolence disorder
  - Narcolepsy
- Breathing-related sleep disorders
  - Obstructive sleep apnea hypopnea
  - Central sleep apnea
  - Sleep-related hypoventilation
  - Circadian rhythm sleep–wake disorders
- Parasomnias
  - Nonrapid eye movement sleep arousal disorders
  - Nightmare disorder
  - Rapid eye movement sleep behavior disorder
  - Restless leg syndrome

TABLE 14-1		
PREVALENCE OF SLEEP DISORDERS		
DIAGNOSIS	*PREVALENCE*	*SOURCE*
Sleep–Wake Disorders		
Insomnia disorder	11% to 12%	National Heart, Blood, & Lung Institute, 2013
Hypersomnolence disorder	1%	APA, 2013
Narcolepsy	0.07%	National Heart, Blood, & Lung Institute, 2013
Breathing-Related Sleep Disorders		
Obstructive sleep apnea hypopnea	4.5%	National Heart, Blood, & Lung Institute, 2013
Central sleep apnea	6% to 7%	National Heart, Blood, & Lung Institute, 2013
Sleep-related hypoventilation	Unknown/uncommon	APA, 2013
Circadian rhythm sleep–wake disorders	1%	APA, 2013
Parasomnias	4% to 67%	Bjorvatn, Grønli, & Pallesen, 2010

The fifth edition of the *Diagnostic and Statistical Manual of Mental Disorders* (DSM-5; American Psychiatric Association [APA], 2013) includes much greater specificity about the various causes and types of sleep disorder, compared with the previous editions of the manual. In part, this is due to improved understanding of the biology and physiology of sleep. Also, we have better understanding that the fatigue associated with sleep disorders has significant negative implications for function. The individual sleep–wake disorders are described below, with implications for function, treatment, and occupational therapy grouped at the end of the chapter, as there are many commonalities across the different disorders.

Diagnosing sleep disorders as mental disorders can be somewhat challenging because they also frequently present as medical conditions (Wing et al., 2012). As a rule, the associated distress and impairment around sleep disorders are the criteria that most clearly warrant a mental disorder diagnosis, and there is frequently, but not always, an accompanying medical diagnosis. In addition, it is important to be aware that sleep–wake disorders are likely to be comorbid with a wide array of other mental disorders, including anxiety, mood, and trauma-related disorders. Table 14-1 shows the prevalence of sleep disorders, which are, as a group, very common.

Insomnia Disorder

Insomnia is very common and often chronic (Neubauer, 2013). Insomnia is problematic in and of itself, but it is also problematic in terms of its impact on quality of life. Individuals with insomnia are often fatigued during the day and struggle to function at work and in their home lives.

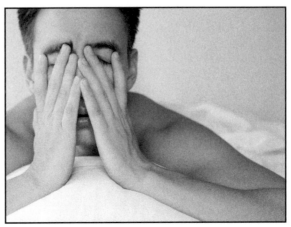

Figure 14-1. Insomnia can cause considerable anxiety. (©2014 Shutterstock.com.)

Diagnostic criteria for insomnia disorder include dissatisfaction with quantity or quality of sleep, particularly reflected in difficulty falling asleep or staying asleep, or experiencing early morning wakening (APA, 2013). For a diagnosis, the sleep disturbance must occur at least three nights per week for at least 3 months, in spite of adequate opportunities for sleep. The sleep disturbance negatively affects function or causes distress (Figure 14-1). Specifiers include whether there is a mental comorbidity, an accompanying medical condition, an additional sleep disorder, and whether the problem is episodic, persistent, or recurrent.

Etiology

Some evidence exists that there is a genetic predisposition for insomnia (Wing et al., 2012). In addition, contributing factors include environmental risk factors, medical and psychiatric comorbidities, and learned behaviors. Several environmental and socioeconomic factors are correlated with the occurrence of insomnia (Wing et al., 2012). For example, shift work can interfere with an individual's ability to establish positive sleep patterns (Mormile, Mazzei, Vittori, Michele, & Squarcia, 2012). Insomnia is often associated with medical conditions (Sarsour, Morin, Foley, Kalsekar, & Walsh, 2010). As discussed in Chapters 6 and 7, individuals with depression or anxiety disorders may have associated insomnia.

Prognosis

For some individuals, insomnia will be self-limiting; and when situational issues associated with the problem are resolved, normal sleep patterns are resumed. For others, treatment is required and can be highly effective (Thase, 2005). Long-term insomnia is associated with an array of functional issues (described in the sections that follow) and individuals should be encouraged to seek help.

Hypersomnolence Disorder

In general, **hypersomnolence** is characterized by daytime sleepiness in an individual who reports adequate sleep at night. Hypersomnolence is common in men with sleep apnea, where the sleepiness probably results from poor quality sleep (Dauvilliers, 2006), but it can also occur in association with a number of medical conditions (e.g., chronic fatigue syndrome) and mental disorders such as depression.

Diagnostic criteria for hypersomnolence disorder include excessive sleepiness, in spite of adequate sleep at night (APA, 2013). The individual experiences periods of falling asleep during the day, a main sleep episode that is not refreshing, and difficulty being awake after abrupt waking. The difficulty must occur at least three times per week for at least 3 months and be associated with distress or dysfunction. Specifiers include whether it occurs with another mental disorder, medical disorder, or sleep disorder, and whether it is acute (1 month), subacute (1 to 3 months), or persistent (more than 3 months).

Etiology

As noted, hypersomnolence is sometimes associated with some version of a sleep disorder, such as sleep apnea. In these situations, although the individual may sleep enough hours to expect to be rested, the quality of sleep may be poor.

Prognosis

Few studies have reported cases of hypersomnolence disorder that are not associated with a comorbid medical or mental disorder diagnosis. When a comorbid condition is present, addressing the primary problem may resolve the issue. However, the prognosis for idiopathic hypersomnolence is not well documented (Masri, Gonzales, & Kushida, 2012).

Narcolepsy

Narcolepsy is, symptomatically, a step beyond hypersomnolence disorder. Although the latter is characterized by excessive daytime sleepiness, narcolepsy is associated with episodes in which the individual unpredictably and unexpectedly falls asleep during the day. These may be brief episodes or more extended ones, and they may occur several times per day every day, or less frequently, perhaps several times per week.

Diagnostic criteria for narcolepsy include recurrent, intense need to sleep, falling asleep, or napping at least three times per week for at least 3 months (APA, 2013). The individual may experience episodes of **cataplexy** at least a few times per month. Cataplexy is characterized by brief, sudden loss of muscle tone when laughing or joking, spontaneous grimaces, and/or global hypotonia. Additional criteria include **hypocretin** deficiency and rapid eye movement sleep for less than 15 minutes. Hypocretin is an excitatory neuropeptide hormone produced in the hypothalamus. Specifiers are quite extensive for this disorder and focused on whether there is cataplexy, hypocretin deficiency, autosomal dominant cerebellar ataxia or deafness, obesity, type 2 diabetes, or other medical conditions, and whether the condition is mild, moderate, or severe.

Etiology

The cause of narcolepsy seems to be a major loss of hypocretin/orexin neurons of the hypo-thalamus, perhaps through some autoimmune mechanism. Hypocretin neurons are associated with the production of neurotransmitters that suppress sleep (Douglass, 2003). This alteration in neurotransmitters may have genetic origins, although it does not appear to be associated with a strong genetic component.

Environmental factors also play a role in narcolepsy. Among those factors identified are flu infections, particularly in the year prior to the onset of symptoms. Psychological stressors also play a role, particularly when these occur prior to puberty (Picchioni, Hope, & Harsh, 2007).

Prognosis

Early diagnosis of narcolepsy plays a significant role in outcome (Ingravallo et al., 2012). Individuals under the age of 30 who were treated tended to have higher educational levels and were more likely to be employed. They also had better overall perceptions of their health and were more often single. All these factors contributed to better outcomes in younger individuals.

Obstructive Sleep Apnea Hypopnea

Obstructive sleep apnea hypopnea (OSAH) is characterized by brief cessation of breathing during sleep, resulting in poor quality sleep and daytime fatigue. It is frequently associated with episodes of snoring and sudden cessation of the snoring due to cessation of breathing, followed by gasping or snorting as breathing resumes. Diagnostic criteria for OSAH include at least five obstructive apneas or hypopneas per hour of sleep, along with nighttime breathing disturbances such as snoring or breathing pauses during sleep (APA, 2013). Daytime sleepiness is present in spite of enough opportunity for sleep. Evidence of 15 or more episodes of apnea or hypopnea per hour of sleep must be present, regardless of other symptoms. Specifiers include indications as to whether the condition is mild, moderate, or severe.

Etiology

OSAH is associated with a particular body type and structure (Okabe et al., 2006). Shape of the jaw and amount of upper airway soft tissue are predictive factors, as is being overweight.

Prognosis

Treatment with continuous positive airway pressure (CPAP) is quite effective, although a significant number of clients find the equipment to be cumbersome and uncomfortable. Many clients discontinue CPAP use, resulting in return to previous, although slightly less severe, symptoms (Young et al., 2013). Quality of life, particularly for those who do not maintain the recommended regimen, tends to be worse than for individuals who do not have the condition (Liu & Li, 2009).

Central Sleep Apnea

The main symptom of central sleep apnea (CSA) is the same as that of OSAH—episodic stoppage of breathing during sleep. The main difference is the absence of a structural reason, such as being overweight (as is seen in OSAH), to explain the disorder. Note, too, that the diagnostic criteria do not specify poor quality of sleep or daytime fatigue, although both are likely to be present.

Diagnostic criteria for CSA include polysomnographic evidence of five or more central apneas per hour of sleep (APA, 2013). Specifiers include noting whether the disorder is idiopathic, includes **Cheyne-Stokes breathing** (periodic crescendo-decrescendo variation in volume), or accompanied by comorbid opioid use.

Etiology

CSA occurs in clinical situations that cause **hypocapnia** (reduced carbon dioxide in the blood) and respiratory instability, such as in heart failure clients, clients suffering from neurological diseases, and idiopathic CSA (Carnevale et al., 2011). CSA can also occur during stays at high altitudes (Lehman et al., 2007).

Prognosis

The prognosis of CSA is somewhat dependent on cause. If it is an underlying heart condition that can be effectively treated, the CSA apnea may abate as well (Lehman et al., 2007). However, in idiopathic cases, treatment may be less effective than in OSAH. CPAP seems less effective in CSA, perhaps because no obvious structural explanation accounts for the sleep apnea.

Sleep-Related Hypoventilation

In the continuum of OSAH, CSA, and sleep-related hypoventilation, sleep-related hypoventilation is the least severe condition. However, due to the fact that sleep-related hypoventilation is most often comorbid with other health conditions, the consequences are as troubling as those of the other breathing-related disorders. Diagnostic criteria for sleep-related hypoventilation include episodes of decreased respiration associated with increased carbon dioxide levels during sleep (APA, 2013). Specifiers include notations about whether the condition is idiopathic, accompanied by congenital central alveolar hypoventilation, and whether the condition is comorbid with a medical disorder.

Etiology

Sleep-related hypoventilation disorder is often associated with other neuromuscular disorders such as muscular dystrophy and multiple sclerosis (Grigg-Damberger, Wagner, & Brown, 2012). In these cases, weakening of the respiratory muscles is responsible for difficulty breathing.

Prognosis

Prognosis is dependent to a large extent on the coexisting medical condition. Disorders such as multiple sclerosis and muscular dystrophy tend to be chronic and progressive, thus improvement in breathing is unlikely. Management typically involves positive pressure ventilation, such as CPAP (Grigg-Damberger et al., 2012).

Circadian Rhythm Sleep–Wake Disorders

Most people have fairly regular **circadian rhythms**; that is, they experience normal daily variation in arousal and fatigue. In some individuals, these rhythms become disrupted, resulting in difficulty falling asleep or staying asleep, or in irregular patterns of sleepiness and alertness. These disrupted sleep patterns lead to fatigue and associated dysfunction.

Diagnostic criteria for circadian rhythm sleep–wake disorders include recurrent sleep disruption due to an alteration of the circadian system; a mismatch between the person's rhythm and the requirements of the social or work environment; excessive sleepiness, insomnia, or both; and distress or dysfunction as a result of these symptoms (APA, 2013). Again, specifiers are numerous and focused particularly on type: delayed sleep phase type (i.e., difficulty falling asleep, familial, or overlapping with non–24-hour sleep–wake type); advanced sleep phase type; irregular sleep–wake type; non–24-hour sleep–wake type; shift-work type; or unspecified type. Notation can also be made about whether the condition is episodic, persistent, or recurrent.

Etiology

Circadian rhythm sleep–wake disorders are caused by degeneration or decreased neuronal activity of suprachiasmatic nucleus neurons, decreased responsiveness of the body's internal clock to signals such as light and activity, and decreased exposure to bright light and structured social and physical activity during the day (Zee & Vitiello, 2009). Many individuals experience the symptoms of circadian rhythm sleep–wake disorders when traveling across time zones (i.e., jet lag), as it can take some time for the internal clock to reset to the new time zone. However, in those situations, the condition is self-limiting and does not cause distress or dysfunction other than 1 or 2 days of fatigue. Shift work is a classic cause of circadian rhythm sleep–wake disorders, and it is particularly problematic in employment situations that require changing shifts from time to time. It is also important to be aware that sleep patterns change naturally over the lifespan, so that older adults are more likely to have sleep–wake difficulty.

Prognosis

For many individuals, the circadian rhythm sleep–wake condition resolves over time, particularly if they can adhere to good sleep hygiene practices. Medication can be used on a short-term basis, but is not helpful over the long term.

Parasomnias

Parasomnias are conditions in which odd or dangerous events happen during sleep, without the individual's awareness (Howell, 2012). Parasomnias seem related to epilepsy in terms of etiology (Tinuper, Bisulli, & Provini, 2012) and most are associated with neuromotor disorders such as Parkinson's disease. Several different manifestations exist, which will be described briefly in this chapter.

Nonrapid Eye Movement Sleep Arousal Disorders

Nonrapid eye movement sleep arousal disorders include **sleepwalking** and **sleep terrors**. Sleepwalking involves repeated episodes of getting up from bed during sleep and moving around. The person is uncommunicative and unresponsive. Sleep terrors are episodes of terror that cause waking from sleep, usually with a panicky scream. In both conditions, the individual typically has no recollection of the episode.

Nightmare Disorder

Nightmare disorder describes a condition in which the individual has frequent, troubling dreams that they remember well upon waking. The individual can be awakened and rapidly becomes oriented, but the sleep disturbance causes distress or dysfunction.

Rapid Eye Movement Sleep Behavior Disorder

An individual with rapid eye movement sleep behavior disorder has repeated periods of arousal during sleep, with vocalization and/or complex motor behaviors, occurring during rapid eye movement sleep. When awakened, the individual is rapidly alert, and their motor

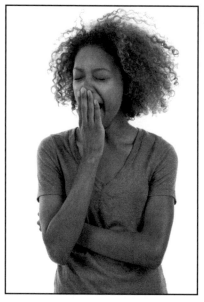

Figure 14-2. Sleep disorders lead to daytime fatigue and difficulty functioning. (©2014 Shutterstock.com.)

activity is abnormal and often violent, possibly causing injury to the person (Brzecka, 2005). Rapid eye movement sleep behavior disorder may be associated with the individual's experience of dreams. It is most common in older men, and it is often associated with neurodegenerative diseases such as Lewy body dementia and Parkinson's disease (Stores, 2008).

Restless Leg Syndrome

Restless leg syndrome is characterized by frequent urge to move the legs, with uncomfortable or unpleasant sensations like a feeling of pins and needles or muscle cramps, with symptoms worsening late in the day or before sleep. The disorder is hypothesized to be the result of abnormalities in medial thalamic metabolism (Rizzo et al., 2012).

Implications for Function and Treatment

Each of the sleep disorders described here interferes with the individual's ability to get enough sleep and restorative sleep. Obvious consequences of sleep disorders are daytime sleepiness and fatigue (Figure 14-2). This, by extension, affects subjective well being (Buysse et al., 2007). Other functional consequences include cognitive impairment and increased health care-related financial burden (Thase, 2005). Excessive sleepiness results in absences from work and higher indirect costs. For example, circadian rhythm problems can lead to a great degree of daytime fatigue so that school and work become impossible to complete (Narita, Echizenya, Takeshima, Inomata, & Shimizu, 2011). Depressive symptoms are common and are associated with lower quality-of-life scores (Ingravallo et al., 2012). Overall, sleep disorders have a profound impact on quality of life, particularly when they are associated with depression and chronic pain (Hajak et al., 2011).

Individuals with sleep disorders have impairment in attention, memory, and executive function (Kielb, Ancoli-Israel, Rebok, & Spira, 2012). Other forms of cognitive impairment are also typical (Edinger, Means, Carney, & Krystal, 2008).

Treatment of sleep disorders using behavioral strategies is effective (Larson, 2012). In particular, cognitive behavioral therapy has demonstrable value (Yang & Hsiao, 2012). A focus on sleep hygiene also can be helpful.

Short-term psychopharmacology with various sleeping medications may work, but use over a protracted period of time is damaging. For some specific sleep disorders, alternative medications can be useful and are less harmful over the long term. For example, for circadian rhythm irregularities, vitamin B_{12}, melatonin, and bright-light therapy, used in combination, work reasonably well (Narita et al., 2011).

Narcolepsy/hypocretin deficiency is treated with stimulants, in addition to antidepressants and behavior modification. These interventions are particularly helpful in children (Mignot, 2012).

Treatment of CSA is challenging because the therapeutic response to CPAP is usually incomplete, with significant residual periodic breathing and sleep fragmentation (Lehman et al., 2007).

Parasomnias can be treated by addressing the underlying primary sleep problems that cause sleep disruption, while also implementing safety precautions to protect clients from harm. Pharmacologic treatment of many parasomnias is also available (Malhotra & Avidan, 2012). Even in the presence of a neurodegenerative disorder, rapid eye movement disorder is usually very treatable. Clonazepam, melatonin, and pramipexole are the medication treatments of choice (Stores, 2008). In general, medications are effective in addressing parasomnias.

Implications for Occupational Therapy

Occupational therapy can provide various concrete interventions to enhance function in individuals who have sleep disorders. Keep in mind that sleep is an important occupation (American Occupational Therapy Association, 2014). In addition, sleep (or the lack thereof) affects other occupations, making it a high priority for intervention. The strategies may be as simple as working to help the client to identify a helpful body position during sleep to minimize sleep apnea (van Kesteren, van Maanen, Hilgevoord, Laman, & de Vries, 2011). Another helpful strategy is providing work simplification and energy conservation mechanisms to help manage fatigue until the underlying cause of the disorder can be addressed.

Sleep hygiene strategies can be helpful in establishing the kinds of habits and patterns that improve the sleep amount and quality (Moss, Lachowski, & Carney, 2013). These strategies include the following:

- Establishing a calm bedtime routine
- Using the bed only for sleep and sex
- Avoiding vigorous exercise too close to bed time
- Making sure the bedroom is dark and at a comfortable temperature for sleep
- Going to sleep and getting up at the same time each day
- Avoiding naps

Establishing these habits can, over time, improve sleep considerably. Table 14-2 summarizes the diagnostic criteria and functional implications of the various sleep disorders.

TABLE 14-2		
DIAGNOSTIC CRITERIA AND FUNCTIONAL IMPLICATIONS: SLEEP–WAKE DISORDERS AND BREATHING-RELATED SLEEP DISORDERS		
DISORDER	*DIAGNOSTIC CRITERIA (APA, 2013)*	*IMPLICATIONS FOR FUNCTION*
Insomnia disorder	Poor sleep quantity or quality associated with difficulty falling asleep, staying asleep, or early morning waking Causes distress or dysfunction Occurs at least three nights per week for at least 3 months	Work, leisure, play, education, social occupations may be negatively affected due to excessive sleepiness Skills negatively affected include cognition, emotional regulation
Hypersomnolence disorder	Excessive sleepiness in spite of at least 7 hours sleep per night, including: • Falling asleep in the day • Unrefreshing sleep • Difficulty being completely awake At least three times a week for at least 3 months Causes distress or dysfunction	Work, leisure, play, education, social occupations are negatively affected due to excessive sleepiness Skills negatively affected include cognition, emotional regulation
Narcolepsy	Repeated intense need to sleep, falling asleep, or napping at least three times a week for at least 3 months, with disruption of REM, or catalepsy	Work, leisure, play, education, social occupations are negatively affected due to excessive sleepiness Skills negatively affected include cognition, emotional regulation
Obstructive sleep apnea hypopnea	One of the following: • Polysomnography of at least five obstructive apneas or hypopneas per hour of sleep • Nighttime breathing disturbances • Daytime sleepiness or fatigue Frequent episodes of apnea or hypopneas each night and every hour of sleep	Work, leisure, play, education, social occupations are negatively affected due to excessive sleepiness Skills negatively affected include cognition, emotional regulation

(continued)

TABLE 14-2 (CONTINUED)		
DIAGNOSTIC CRITERIA AND FUNCTIONAL IMPLICATIONS: SLEEP–WAKE DISORDERS AND BREATHING-RELATED SLEEP DISORDERS		
DISORDER	DIAGNOSTIC CRITERIA (APA, 2013)	IMPLICATIONS FOR FUNCTION
Central sleep apnea	Polysomnographic evidence of five or more central apneas per hour of sleep	Work, leisure, play, education, social occupations are negatively affected due to excessive sleepiness Skills negatively affected include cognition, emotional regulation
Sleep-related hypoventilation	Episodes of decreased respiration associated with increased CO_2 levels during sleep	Work, leisure, play, education, social occupations are negatively affected due to excessive sleepiness Skills negatively affected include cognition, emotional regulation
Circadian rhythm sleep–wake disorders	Sleep disruption from altered circadian system or mismatch between the sleep rhythm and the requirements of the environment Excessive sleepiness or insomnia Causes distress and/or dysfunction	Work, leisure, play, education, social occupations are negatively affected due to excessive sleepiness Skills negatively affected include cognition, emotional regulation
Parasomnias	Abnormal behavioral, experiential, or physiological events during sleep, that may include (among others): • Non-REM sleep arousal disorder • Sleepwalking/night terrors • Nightmare disorder • REM sleep disorder • Restless leg syndrome	Work, leisure, play, education, social occupations are negatively affected due to excessive sleepiness Skills negatively affected include cognition, emotional regulation

Cultural Considerations

Various cultures interpret sleep somewhat differently and engage in a variety of practices around sleep (Worthman, 2011). Where sleep occurs, whether one sleeps alone or with others, cultural meanings assigned to sleep difficulties, and even what constitutes a sleep

---

CASE STUDY

Sharleen Marshall is a 64-year-old woman who has come to the sleep disorders center with complaints of chronic, severe difficulty sleeping that leaves her feeling exhausted during the day. She is a single mother who runs a small bakery, and she now looks after her two young grandchildren while her daughter is at work. Approximately 3 years ago, it appeared that the bakery business would fail, and at that time she began to have sleep difficulties. The bakery is still only marginally profitable, but it provides a modest living. Mrs. Marshall still has the same degree of sleep difficulty. Between looking after her granddaughters and managing her business, Mrs. Marshall has no time for a social life, hobbies, or relaxation. She feels constantly stressed and is struggling to cope.

She has tried a variety of sleep medications, as well as an antidepressant. The sleep medications were initially helpful, but they left her groggy during the day. The antidepressant had numerous side effects that she found unpleasant, so she stopped taking it.

Mrs. Marshall reports that she usually tries to go to bed by approximately 10:30 p.m., but she is often up later baking for the following day. She usually falls asleep right away, but approximately once per week she finds she cannot fall asleep. She wakes up two or three times every night and often cannot go back to sleep. She finds this frustrating and this frustration makes it still more difficult for her to sleep. She gets up around 5:30 a.m. to start her day. A physical examination found no obvious medical problems, other than her self-reported fatigue.

THOUGHT QUESTIONS

1. Are there factors in the description that lead you to believe Mrs. Marshall has a mental disorder? If so, what might it be?
2. What do you believe might be contributing to Mrs. Marshall's difficulty sleeping?
3. What might Mrs. Marshall do in the future to help her sleep better?
4. What are the occupational consequences of her difficulty sleeping?

---

difficulty, are culturally prescribed. For example, in some cultures, early morning waking may be expected and would not be considered a problem. It is important to include an assessment of these cultural factors prior to designing an intervention.

Lifespan Considerations

Some sleep disorders, notably narcolepsy, may first appear in childhood (Nevsimalova, 2009). Early recognition and treatment may reduce the long-term consequences of the disorder. In particular, cooperation between the parents and the school (i.e., teacher) can be important in minimizing functional consequences.

Sleep disorders in children can sometimes be associated with parental problems (Golik et al., 2013). If parents are depressed or anxious, they can subconsciously convey those feelings to their children, who may then mirror their anxiety.

Insomnia is common in older adults, affecting as many as one third of individuals (Hidalgo et al., 2012). Treating older adults with sleep disorders is complicated by their increased sensitivity to medications, concerns about safety (especially falls), and the potential for medications to increase any cognitive deficits the older adult may already have (Uchimura, Kamijo, & Takase, 2012).

Internet Resources

Centers for Disease Control and Prevention
http://www.cdc.gov/sleep/resources.htm; http://www.cdc.gov/Features/Sleep/
Government-sponsored links with background information, links, and resources for professionals and consumers. The second link includes a brief list of sleep hygiene recommendations.

National Library of Medicine
http://www.nlm.nih.gov/medlineplus/sleepdisorders.html
Provides refereed journal articles, links, and information pages.

Seattle Children's Hospital, Research, and Foundation
http://www.seattlechildrens.org/clinics-programs/sleep-disorders/resources/
A focus on information related to children with sleep problems.

References

American Occupational Therapy Association. (2014). Occupational therapy practice framework: Domain & process (3rd ed.). *American Journal of Occupational Therapy, 68*(Suppl. 1), S1-S48.

American Psychiatric Association. (2013). *Diagnostic and statistical manual of mental disorders* (5th ed.). Washington, DC: Author.

Bjorvatn, B., Grønli, J., & Pallesen, S. (2010). Prevalence of different parasomnias in the general population. *Sleep Medicine, 11*(10), 1031-1034.

Brzecka, A. (2005). REM sleep behaviour disorder. *Archives of Psychiatry and Psychotherapy, 7*(4), 27-31.

Buysse, D., Thompson, W., Scott, J., Franzen, P.L., Germain, A., Hall, M.L., . . . Kupfer, D.J. (2007). Daytime symptoms in primary insomnia: A prospective analysis using ecological momentary assessment. *Sleep Medicine, 8*, 198-208.

Carnevale, C., Georges, M., Rabec, C., Tamisier, R., Levy, P., & Pépin, J. (2011). Effectiveness of Adaptive Servo Ventilation in the treatment of hypocapnic central sleep apnea of various etiologies. *Sleep Medicine, 12*(10), 952-958.

Dauvilliers, Y. (2006). Differential diagnosis in hypersomnia. *Current Neurology and Neuroscience Reports, 6*(2), 156-162.

Douglass, A.B. (2003). Narcolepsy: Differential diagnosis or etiology in some cases of bipolar disorder and schizophrenia? *CNS Spectrums, 8*(2), 120-126.

Edinger, J.D., Means, M.K., Carney, C.E., & Krystal, A.D. (2008). Psychomotor performance deficits and their relation to prior nights sleep among individuals with primary insomnia. *Sleep, 31*, 599-607.

Golik, T., Avni, H., Nehama, H., Greenfield, M., Sivan, Y., & Tauman, R. (2013). Maternal cognitions and depression in childhood behavioral insomnia and feeding disturbances. *Sleep Medicine, 14*(3), 261-265.

Grigg-Damberger, M.M., Wagner, L.K., & Brown, L.K. (2012). Sleep hypoventilation in patients with neuromuscular diseases. *Sleep Medicine Clinics, 7*(4), 667-687.

Hajak, G., Petukhova, M., Lakoma, M.D., Coulouvrat, C., Roth, T., Sampson, N.A., . . . Kessler, R.C. (2011). Days-out-of-role associated with insomnia and comorbid conditions in the America Insomnia Survey. *Biological Psychiatry, 70*, 1063-1073.

Hidalgo, J.L., Bravo, B.N., Martínez, I.P., Pretel, F. A., Lapeira, J.T., & Gras, C.B. (2012). Understanding insomnia in older adults. *International Journal of Geriatric Psychiatry, 27*(10), 1086-1093.

Howell, M.J. (2012). Parasomnias: An updated review. *Neurotherapeutics, 9*(4), 753-775.

Ingravallo, F., Gnucci, V., Pizza, F., Vignatelli, L., Govi, A., Dormi, A., . . . Plazzi, G. (2012). The burden of narcolepsy with cataplexy: How disease history and clinical features influence socio-economic outcomes. *Sleep Medicine, 13*(10), 1293-1300.

Kielb, S.A., Ancoli-Israel, S., Rebok, G.W., & Spira, A.P. (2012). Cognition in obstructive sleep apnea-hypopnea syndrome (OSAS): Current clinical knowledge and the impact of treatment. *NeuroMolecular Medicine, 14*(3), 180-193.

Larson, E.B. (2012). Sleep disorders in neurorehabilitation: Insomnia. *Sleep Medicine Clinics, 7*(4), 587-595.

Lehman, S., Antic, N.A., Thompson, C., Catcheside, P.G., Mercer, J., & McEvoy, R.D. (2007). Central sleep apnea on commencement of continuous positive airway pressure in patients with a primary diagnosis of obstructive sleep apnea-hypopnea. *Journal of Clinical Sleep Medicine, 15*(5), 462-466.

Liu, Z., & Li, L. (2009). Quality of life in patients with obstructive sleep apnea/hypopnea syndrome and its related factors. *Chinese Journal of Clinical Psychology, 17*(5), 632-633, 635.

Malhotra, R.K., & Avidan, A.Y. (2012). Parasomnias and their mimics. *Neurologic Clinics, 30*(4), 1067-1094.

Masri, T.J., Gonzales, C.G., & Kushida, C.A. (2012). Idiopathic hypersomnia. *Sleep Medicine Clinics, 7*(2), 283-289.

Mignot, E.J.M. (2012). A practical guide to the therapy of narcolepsy and hypersomnia syndromes. *Neurotherapeutics, 9*(4), 739-752.

Mormile, R., Mazzei, G., Vittori, G.D., Michele, G., & Squarcia, U. (2012). Insomnia and shift-work sleep disorder: A crosstalk between glutamate excitotoxicity and decreased GABAergic neurotransmission? *Sleep and Biological Rhythms, 10*(4), 340-341.

Moss, T.G., Lachowski, A.M., & Carney, C.E. (2013). What all treatment providers should know about sleep hygiene recommendations. *Behavior Therapist, 36*(4), 76-83.

Narita, E., Echizenya, M., Takeshima, M., Inomata, Y., & Shimizu, T. (2011). Core body temperature rhythms in circadian rhythm sleep disorder, irregular sleep–wake type. *Psychiatry and Clinical Neurosciences, 65*(7), 679-680.

National Heart, Blood, and Lung Institute (2013). *Disease statistics.* Retrieved from http://www.nhlbi.nih.gov/about/factbook-10/chapter4.htm.

Neubauer, D.N. (2013). Chronic insomnia. *CONTINUUM: Lifelong Learning in Neurology, 19*(1), 50-66.

Nevsimalova, S. (2009). Narcolepsy in childhood. *Sleep Medicine Reviews, 13*(2), 169-180.

Okabe, S., Ikeda, K., Higano, S., Mitani, H., Hida, W., Kobayashi, T., & Sugawara, J. (2006). Morphologic analyses of mandible and upper airway soft tissue by MRI of patients with obstructive sleep apnea hypopnea syndrome. *Sleep: Journal of Sleep and Sleep Disorders Research, 29*(7), 909-915.

Picchioni, D., Hope, C.R., & Harsh, J.R. (2007). A case-control study of the environmental risk factors for narcolepsy. *Neuroepidemiology, 29*(3-4), 185-192.

Rizzo, G., Tonon, C., Testa, C., Manners, D., Vetrugno, R., Pizza, F., . . . Lodi, R. (2012). Abnormal medial thalamic metabolism in patients with idiopathic restless legs syndrome. *Brain: A Journal of Neurology, 135*(12), 3712-3720.

Sarsour, K., Morin, C.M., Foley, K., Kalsekar, A., & Walsh, J.K. (2010) Association of insomnia severity and comorbid medical and psychiatric disorders in a health plan-based sample: Insomnia severity and comorbidities. *Sleep, 11*, 69-74.

Stores, G. (2008). Rapid eye movement sleep behaviour disorder in children and adolescents. *Developmental Medicine & Child Neurology, 50*(10), 728-732.

Thase, M.E., (2005). Correlates and consequences of chronic insomnia. *General Hospital Psychiatry, 27*(2), 100-112.

Tinuper, P., Bisulli, F., & Provini, F. (2012). The parasomnias: Mechanisms and treatment. *Epilepsia, 53*(Suppl. 7), 12-19.

Uchimura, N., Kamijo, A., & Takase, T. (2012). Effects of eszopiclone on safety, subjective measures of efficacy, and quality of life in elderly and nonelderly Japanese patients with chronic insomnia, both with and without comorbid psychiatric disorders: A 24-week, randomized, double-blind study. *Annals of General Psychiatry, 11*, Article 15.

van Kesteren, E.R., van Maanen, J.P., Hilgevoord, A.A.J., Laman, D.M., & de Vries, N. (2011). Quantitative effects of trunk and head position on the Apnea Hypopnea Index in obstructive sleep apnea. *Sleep: Journal of Sleep and Sleep Disorders Research, 34*(8), 1075-1081.

Wing, Y.K., Zhang, J., Lam, S.P., Li, S.X., Tang, N.L., Lai, K.Y., & Li, A.M. (2012). Familial aggregation and heritability of insomnia in a community-based study. *Sleep Medicine, 13*(8), 985-990.

Worthman, C.M. (2011). Developmental cultural ecology of sleep. In M. El-Sheikh (Ed.), *Sleep and development: Familial and socio-cultural considerations* (pp. 167-194). New York, NY: Oxford University Press.

Yang, C., & Hsiao, F. (2012). Management of sleep disorders—Cognitive behavioral therapy for insomnia. In R.P. Chiang & S.J. Kang (Eds.), *Introduction to modern sleep technology* (pp. 121-136). New York, NY: Springer Science + Business Media.

Young, L.R., Taxin, Z.H., Norman, R.G., Walsleben, J.A., Rapoport, D.M., & Ayappa, I. (2013). Response to CPAP withdrawal in patients with mild versus severe obstructive sleep apnea/hypopnea syndrome. *Sleep: Journal of Sleep and Sleep Disorders Research, 36*(3), 405-412.

Zee, P.C., & Vitiello, M.V. (2009). Circadian rhythm sleep disorder: Irregular sleep wake rhythm. *Sleep Medicine Clinics, 4*(2), 213-218.

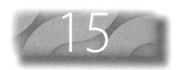

Sexual Dysfunctions, Paraphilic Disorders, and Gender Dysphoria

Learning Outcomes

By the end of this chapter, readers will be able to:

- Describe the symptoms of sexual dysfunctions, paraphilic disorders, and gender dysphoria
- Identify the causes of sexual dysfunctions, paraphilic disorders, and gender dysphoria
- Discuss the functional consequences of these disorders
- Describe treatment strategies for these disorders
- Discuss the occupational perspective on sexual dysfunctions, paraphilic disorders, and gender dysphoria, including specific intervention considerations

Bonder B.
Psychopathology and Function, Fifth Edition (pp 281-299).
© 2015 SLACK Incorporated.

KEY WORDS

- Paraphilias
- Dyspareunia
- Asphyxiaphilia
- Dysphoria

CASE VIGNETTE

Albert Mangiano is a 62-year-old factory manager who has been married for 34 years to his wife Elena, a stay-at-home mother. They have three children, one of whom still lives at home. Until recently, both Mr. Mangiano and his wife would have described their marriage as a happy one, which included a satisfying sex life. However, in the past year, Mr. Mangiano has had increasing difficulty achieving an erection, leaving both him and his wife frustrated. He sought help from his physician who reviewed his medications (for blood pressure and cholesterol) and recommended a trial of Viagra (sildenafil citrate). However, he had limited improvement and was not comfortable taking the medication. Mr. Mangiano believes his problem is not reversible, and he is trying to focus on the many good aspects of the relationship he and his wife have. However, his wife remains frustrated and is insisting that they seek couples counseling. She increasingly wonders whether he has another sex partner, and there has been growing tension in the home as a result.

THOUGHT QUESTIONS

1. Based on the information here, do you think Mr. Mangiano has a medical problem, a psychological problem, both, or neither?
2. Do you think there are solutions in this situation that might satisfy both Mr. Mangiano and his wife?
3. What role might there be for occupational therapy in helping Mr. Mangiano?

SEXUAL DYSFUNCTIONS, PARAPHILIC DISORDERS, AND GENDER DYSPHORIA

- Sexual dysfunctions
  - Delayed ejaculation
  - Erectile disorder
  - Female orgasmic disorder
  - Female sexual interest/arousal disorder
  - Genito-pelvic pain/penetration disorder
  - Male hypoactive sexual desire disorder
  - Premature (early) ejaculation
- Paraphilic disorders
  - Voyeuristic disorder
  - Exhibitionistic disorder
  - Frotteuristic disorder
  - Sexual masochism disorder
  - Sexual sadism disorder
  - Pedophilic disorder
  - Fetishistic disorder
  - Transvestic disorder
- Gender dysphoria

TABLE 15-1		
PREVALENCE OF SEXUAL DYSFUNCTIONS, PARAPHILIC DISORDERS, AND GENDER DYSPHORIA		
DIAGNOSIS	*PREVALENCE*	*SOURCE*
Sexual Dysfunctions		
Delayed ejaculation	8%	Foley, 2009
Erectile disorder	37% of middle aged men	Shaeer & Shaeer, 2012
Female orgasmic disorder	8% to 16%	Robinson et al., 2011
Female sexual interest/ arousal disorder	Estimates vary from 18% to 80%	Basson et al., 2005
Genito-pelvic pain/penetration disorder	Unclear	
Male hypoactive sexual desire disorder	Unclear	
Premature ejaculation	5% to 30%	Giami, 2013
Paraphilic Disorders	Unknown, more common in men	Saleh & Berlin, 2003
Gender Dysphoria	Unclear, estimates between 0.006% and 0.0005%	Conron et al., 2012

This chapter describes three categories from the fifth edition of the *Diagnostic and Statistical Manual of Mental Disorders* (DSM-5; American Psychiatric Association [APA], 2013). Each category addresses difficulties with sexual function or gender identity. The sexual dysfunctions disorders describe problems associated with sexual intercourse, often (but not always) with a biological basis, that cause psychological distress. The paraphilic disorders, on the other hand, are disorders that represent **paraphilias**, which is "intense and persistent sexual interest other than sexual interest in genital stimulation or preparatory fondling with phenotypically normal, physically mature, consenting adult partners" (APA, 2013, p. 685). These are, in other words, situations in which the object of sexual interest or the expression of sexual interest is not typical or socially acceptable. Gender dysphoria is a distinct disorder in which the individual's biological and genetic gender is inconsistent with his or her perceived gender. Such individuals feel trapped in a body of the wrong gender, a feeling that affects sexual interactions, as well as broader issues of gender identity.

It is important to note that these disorders all include a criterion that specifies distress as a diagnostic factor. Certainly in some individuals, for example, low or absent sexual desire is not distressing. Such an individual would be unlikely to seek help, thus would not be diagnosed. It is the individual's (or his or her partner's) sense that a problem exists that leads to a diagnosis and, ideally, treatment. Table 15-1 shows the prevalence of the various sexual dysfunctions, paraphilic disorders, and gender dysphoria.

Delayed Ejaculation

Delayed ejaculation is less well understood than some of the other disorders in this cluster, but it is not uncommon and can be associated with significant psychological distress (Perelman, 2013). Essentially, it is characterized by difficulty ejaculating, or inability to ejaculate, in the presence of adequate sexual stimulation (Abdel-Hamid & Saleh, 2011). Specific diagnostic criteria include either significant delay in or absence of ejaculation on most occasions when intercourse is attempted (APA, 2013). The symptoms must have persisted for at least 6 months and cause distress to the individual. Specifiers clarify whether this is a lifelong or an acquired condition; whether it is generalized or situational; and whether it is mild, moderate, or severe.

Etiology

Delayed ejaculation is strongly associated with both anxiety and depression (Abdel-Hamid & Saleh, 2011), particularly anxiety about sexual performance. If the man's partner also has a sexual issue, such as **dyspareunia**—pelvic or abdominal pain on penetration—he may become anxious about causing pain to his partner, leading to dysfunction for him as well. For many of these individuals, it is possible to reach orgasm through other means (e.g., masturbation); therefore, the problem seems to be associated with inadequate arousal with a partner, rather than an underlying biological difficulty. However, for some, it is associated with taking antidepressant medication (Waldinger, 2010) or other biological factors. Sexual issues are a well-known side effect of the selective serotonin reuptake inhibitors and some other psychotropic medications.

Metz and McCarthy (2007) suggested that there are 10 major causes of delayed ejaculation: five physiological (i.e., physical system factors, illness, injury, drug side effects, lifestyle); four psychological (i.e., psychological system factors, distress, relationship distress, skill deficits); and one mixed source where other sexual issues, such as low desire or partner's dyspareunia, coexist with one or more of the other nine concerns.

Prognosis

Delayed ejaculation can be self-limiting, and it can improve without intervention; however, with treatment, it can be improved considerably.

Implications for Function and Treatment

Sexual performance is, by definition, affected. In addition, social occupations can be impaired by a sense of low self-esteem, as well as the anxiety and depression associated with sexual dysfunction (Foley, 2009). The individual may feel pressure if life circumstances are involved, for example, if the couple is trying to conceive (Foley, 2009).

Treatment of delayed ejaculation includes two main forms: behavioral, particularly helpful with the involvement of the partner (Foley, 2009), and prescribing bupropion, which is helpful in approximately 20% of cases (Abdel-Hamid & Saleh, 2011). Foley (2009) recommended an intersystem approach with the following five components: individual/biological/medical, individual/psychological, dyadic relationship, family of origin, and society/culture/history/religion. As mentioned, the partner almost certainly needs to be involved in addressing the problem (Hartman & Waldinger, 2007).

Erectile Disorder

Erectile disorder is a step beyond delayed ejaculation in that the man is unable to achieve an erection, making typical genital sexual activity impossible. Diagnostic criteria for this disorder include difficulty obtaining or maintaining an erection or decrease in erectile rigidity (APA, 2013). Symptoms must have persisted for at least 6 months and cause distress to the individual. Specifiers clarify whether this is a lifelong or an acquired condition, whether it is generalized or situational, and whether it is mild, moderate, or severe.

Etiology

Erectile dysfunction is quite common and most often affects older men. Causes include diseases (e.g., hypertension and diabetes), lifestyle factors (e.g., obesity), and infectious processes (Shamloul & Ghanem, 2013). Erectile dysfunction is strongly linked to cardiovascular disease as well.

Prognosis

Erectile dysfunction is treatable, particularly if the underlying physiological cause can be identified and reversed. In cases where the cause is a urinary tract infection, limited exercise, or obesity, reversing those circumstances may reverse the erectile dysfunction as well. In cases where the underlying cause cannot be cured—as in the case of diabetes—long-term management of the erectile dysfunction will be required.

Implications for Function and Treatment

There is an obvious functional deficit in sexual performance. This can be associated with lowered self-esteem, anxiety, and deficits in social occupations.

Symptomatic treatment of erectile dysfunction is possible using medication (Buvat et al., 2013). Although medications typically work, they have side effects that some individuals find unacceptable, and they may not be safe for men with cardiovascular problems. Some individuals do not like being dependent on medication and decide to discontinue their use. Although medications are not effective for everyone, they do represent progress in managing the problem.

Female Orgasmic Disorder

An important factor in understanding sexual dysfunctions as mental disorders is that the person must experience sufficient distress to seek help. Only some of the relatively large proportion of women experiencing delayed or absent orgasm report feeling distressed (Robinson, Munns, Weber-Main, Lowe, & Raymond, 2011). Symptoms of female orgasmic disorder include delay, infrequency, reduced intensity, or absence of orgasm on most occasions when intercourse is attempted (APA, 2013). Symptoms must have persisted for at least 6 months and cause distress in the individual. Specifiers clarify whether this is a lifelong or an acquired condition, whether it is generalized or situational, and whether it is mild, moderate, or severe.

Etiology

As is true for the male sexual dysfunctions described, several causes of this difficulty have been hypothesized. The causes range from inadequate tone in the perivaginal muscles to anxiety, illness, neurological conditions, and medications (Robinson et al., 2011).

Prognosis

The prognosis of female orgasmic disorder is generally good if the issue is a psychological one. Behavioral and psychological interventions have been effective for many women. The prognosis is also good if there is an underlying medical problem that can be treated. There is much greater probability of a chronic course if a medical condition is present that cannot be treated.

Implications for Function and Treatment

By definition, a deficit exists in sexual functioning. This is frequently accompanied by social deficits and a potentially negative impact on self-esteem.

Psychological treatments are often effective (Frühauf, Gerger, Schmidt, Maren, & Thomas Barth, 2013). Strategies ranging from psychoanalytic to cognitive behavioral therapies have had positive outcomes. Medical attention to underlying physical problems can also be important (Meston, Hull, Levin, & Sipski, 2004).

Female Sexual Interest/Arousal Disorder

Female sexual interest/arousal disorder is common (Basson, Brotto, Laan, Redmond, & Utian, 2005) but is almost certainly underreported. Its diagnostic criteria include lack of or reduced sexual interest, including absent or reduced erotic fantasies or thoughts, failure to initiate sex and lack of responsiveness to partner's approaches, lack of sexual excitement or pleasure, and reduced sensation during sexual activity (APA, 2013). Symptoms must have persisted for at least 6 months and cause distress to the individual. Specifiers clarify whether this is a lifelong or an acquired condition, whether it is generalized or situational, and whether it is mild, moderate, or severe.

Etiology

As is true for other sexual dysfunctions, the etiology of female sexual interest/arousal disorder is thought to be a complex interaction among physical (e.g., infection, neurological condition) and psychological (e.g., anxiety, lack of information) factors (Basson et al., 2005).

Prognosis

With appropriate treatment, as many as 75% of women report improved sexual functioning (Basson et al., 2005).

Implications for Function and Treatment

Sexual performance is impaired in every instance, with frequent accompanying issues related to social occupations and self-concept.

Female sexual interest/arousal disorder responds well to psychological treatments such as cognitive behavioral therapy, communication skills training, and sex education (Robinson et al., 2011). No obvious drug treatments are available, other than those that address any under-lying physical problem; however, some drugs, including estrogen and testosterone, have been associated with preliminary data suggesting effectiveness.

Genito-Pelvic Pain/Penetration Disorder

The diagnosis of dyspareunia is relatively common, but it is not well understood. Symptoms of genito-pelvic pain/penetration disorder include difficulty with vaginal penetration during sex, pain and fear of pain during intercourse, and tensing of the pelvic floor in anticipation of pain (APA, 2013). Symptoms must persist for at least 6 months and cause distress in the individual. Specifiers clarify whether this is a lifelong or an acquired condition, and whether it is mild, moderate, or severe.

Etiology

In general, genito-pelvic pain/penetration disorder is thought to have three major sources of dyspareunia: physical, psychological, or mixed (Binik, 2010). Anxiety, stress, and tension are among the psychological sources, abdominal abnormalities might be a physical source, and a mixed cause might be consequences of childbirth. The latter situation might occur when inadequate healing following childbirth is accompanied by anxiety about resuming sexual relations (Bertozzi, Londero, Fruscalzo, Driul, & Marchesoni, 2010). Young women may experience discomfort during initial sexual encounters, which contribute to anxiety and subsequent pain (Donaldson & Meana, 2011; Landry & Bergeron, 2009). One complicating factor in understanding the disorder is that the pain symptoms vary greatly.

Prognosis

The fact that the causes of genito-pelvic pain/penetration disorder are mixed and the symptoms are varied, makes clear prognosis somewhat difficult to evaluate. If the cause is self-limiting, and if the woman does not develop significant anticipatory anxiety, the prognosis is likely to be good (Binik, 2010). However, if the cause is obscure, the prognosis might be less positive.

Implications for Function and Treatment

In addition to the expected dysfunction in sexual and social occupations, this and other sexual dysfunctions may affect body image (Pazmany, Bergeron, Oudenhove, Verhaeghe, & Enzlin, 2013).

Treatment of any underlying medical conditions, accompanied by behavioral interventions, can provide considerable relief. Prescribing estrogen is among the medical interventions that have been implemented, and it can be of value, particularly for peri- or postmenopausal women (Krychman, 2011). Much misunderstanding exists about genito-pelvic pain/penetration disorder and the fact that some women decide against seeking treatment is surprising (Donaldson & Meana, 2011).

Male Hypoactive Sexual Desire Disorder

Male hypoactive sexual desire disorder is among the less well-researched sexual disorders. Its diagnostic criteria include persistent lack of sexual thoughts, fantasies, and desire that would normally be consistent with life stage and sociocultural considerations (APA, 2013). The symptoms must persist for at least 6 months and cause distress in the individual. Specifiers clarify whether this is a lifelong or an acquired condition, whether it is generalized or situational, and whether it is mild, moderate, or severe.

Etiology

The cause of limited male sexual desire is almost always psychological in nature (McCarthy & McDonald, 2009). It is hypothesized that one variant is a result of the man's perception that he harbors an unacceptable sexual secret, specifically one of following: an unusual arousal pattern, preference for masturbation as opposed to intercourse, history of sexual trauma, or a conflict about sexual orientation. The more common variant is a result of a loss of confidence in relation to sexual activity that leads to anxiety, embarrassment, and avoidance.

Prognosis

Without treatment, male hypoactive sexual desire disorder is likely to be a persistent problem, but therapy can make a significant difference in outcome (APA, 2013).

Implications for Function and Treatment

Problems with limited sexual desire have significant impact on sexual and social occupations, as well as on psychological well being (McCarthy & McDonald, 2009).

Psychological intervention, particularly couples' therapy, has been demonstrated to be effective (McCarthy & Ginsberg, 2007).

Premature (Early) Ejaculation

Diagnostic criteria for premature (early) ejaculation disorder include a persistent pattern of ejaculation occurring during sex with a partner more rapidly than the individual wants, typically in less than 1 minute (APA, 2013). The symptoms must have persisted for at least 6 months and cause distress in the individual. Specifiers clarify whether this is a lifelong or an acquired condition, whether it is generalized or situational, and whether it is mild, moderate, or severe.

Etiology

Two relatively distinct forms of premature ejaculation exist, one which is a lifelong condition and one which is acquired in later life. A variety of genetic, neurological, psychological, and endocrine factors have been hypothesized as the underlying issue, and probably several coexist when there is a problem. However, evidence about the cause is somewhat contradictory (Bonierbale, 2013). An additional complication is the role of the partner in assessing whether or not a problem exists, as the individual has differing expectations from the sexual experience.

Prognosis

With appropriate treatment, the prognosis is good (APA, 2013).

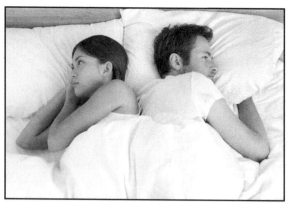

Figure 15-1. Sexual difficulties can contribute to marital strife. (©2014 Shutterstock.com.)

Implications for Function and Treatment

Sexual performance is significantly affected, and social occupations may also suffer as a result. Premature ejaculation disorder can have substantial impact on self-esteem. Any of the sexual disorders described here can have significant negative consequences for close relationships (Figure 15-1).

Psychological interventions—particularly behavioral interventions, in combination with couples therapy—can be highly effective (Althof, 2006). The focus should be not only on addressing the sexual issues but also on efforts to reduce performance anxiety and increase self-confidence. Medications, the selective serotonin reuptake inhibitors in particular, have been effective in some cases (McMahon & Porst, 2011).

Paraphilic Disorders

The sexual dysfunction disorders described previously address difficulties that individuals have during typical sexual intercourse. The paraphilic disorders, on the other hand, describe atypical and dysfunctional attachment or behaviors. The behaviors and urges are considered pathological and may result in legal difficulties for some individuals. Not all the possible paraphilias are listed in the DSM, as it would be impossible to provide a full accounting of every inanimate object or unusual urge that has ever been experienced. A listing and brief description of those paraphilias specifically named in the DSM-5 (APA, 2013) are indicated in the sections that follow, and a summary of the available information about the etiology, prognosis, function, and treatment is presented.

Voyeuristic Disorder

Diagnostic criteria for voyeuristic disorder include repeated intense sexual arousal from observing a person naked or disrobing (with accompanying fantasies or behaviors) and acting on these urges with an individual who is not consenting, or the urges cause distress in functioning (APA, 2013). The diagnosis is made for individuals over the age of 18. Specifiers note whether this occurs in a controlled (institutional) setting and whether it is in full remission.

Exhibitionistic Disorder

Diagnostic criteria for exhibitionistic disorder include repeated intense sexual arousal from exposing one's genitals to an unsuspecting person, either in fantasy or in behavior, and acting on these urges with someone who is not consenting, or the urges cause distress or dysfunction (APA, 2013). Specifiers note whether the behavior occurs in a controlled (institutional) environment and whether it is in full remission.

Frotteuristic Disorder

Diagnostic criteria for frotteuristic disorder include repeated intense sexual arousal from touching or rubbing against a nonconsenting person (APA, 2013). The urges cause distress or dysfunction. Specifiers note whether this occurs in a controlled (institutional) setting and whether it is in full remission.

Sexual Masochism Disorder

Diagnostic criteria for sexual masochism disorder include repeated intense sexual arousal from being humiliated, beaten, or made to suffer, as shown through urges or behaviors that cause distress or dysfunction (APA, 2013). Specifiers clarify whether **asphyxiaphilia**—achieving sexual arousal from restriction of breathing—is present, whether this occurs in a controlled (institutional) environment and whether it is in full remission.

Sexual Sadism Disorder

Diagnostic criteria for sexual sadism disorder include repeated intense sexual arousal from the suffering of another person, manifested through urges or behavior acted upon with a nonconsenting individual or which cause distress or dysfunction (APA, 2013). Specifiers note whether this occurs in a controlled (institutional) setting and whether it is in full remission.

Pedophilic Disorder

Diagnostic criteria for pedophilic disorder include repeated intense sexually arousing fantasies, urges, or behaviors involving sexual activity with a prepubescent child, with distress or interpersonal difficulty resulting from the urges or behaviors (APA, 2013). The individual must be at least 16 years old, and 5 years older than the child or children who are objects of the individual's interest. Specifiers clarify whether the individual is exclusively attracted to children, to which gender he or she is attracted, and whether the behavior is limited to incest.

Fetishistic Disorder

Diagnostic criteria for fetishistic disorder include repeated intense sexual arousal from nonliving objects or specific focus on nongenital body parts through urges or behaviors that cause distress or dysfunction (APA, 2013). Specifiers clarify whether the objects are nonliving or body parts, whether the behavior is occurring in a controlled (institutional) environment, and whether it is in full remission.

Transvestic Disorder

Diagnostic criteria for transvestic disorder include repeated intense sexual arousal from cross-dressing, causing distress or dysfunction (APA, 2013). Specifiers note whether this occurs in a controlled (institutional) setting and whether it is in full remission.

Etiology

A great deal of what is believed about the paraphilic disorders is unproven, with research evidence that is sparse or incomplete. Some evidence exists for dysfunction in hormonal balance, genetic abnormalities, and some neuropsychiatric deficits (Saleh & Berlin, 2003).

Prognosis

In general, the prognosis for paraphilic disorders is not good. They tend to be chronic and stable; that is, not worsening, but not improving (Saleh & Berlin, 2003).

Implications for Function and Treatment

Paraphilic disorders not only reflect dysfunctional sexual and social occupations but they also carry a high risk of legal difficulty (Saleh & Berlin, 2003). In fact, most people who seek treatment do not do so voluntarily but are required by the courts as a condition of probation or parole.

A number of treatments address the paraphilias (Guay, 2009). These include pharmacologic treatments, such as with serotonin and testosterone. Cognitive behavioral therapy has also been used with some success. There is particular concern about individuals incarcerated for their behavior, those who target children, and/or those who are violent. In such cases, both drug treatment and psychotherapy are recommended. However, there is insufficient research about what treatments to use, with whom, when, and for how long (Balon, 2013).

Gender Dysphoria

Gender **dysphoria** reflects a sense of disconnect between a person's biological and genetic gender assignment and his or her perceived gender identity. The term *dysphoria* refers to feeling unwell or uneasy. It is important to recognize that the name for this disorder was carefully selected to avoid the societal bias that such individuals often experience (Fraser, Karasic, Meyer, & Wylie, 2010). Until recently, gender dysphoria was thought to be rare, but as societies have become more open in discussing issues of gender and sexual identity, there is growing recognition that it is not uncommon (Conron, Scott, Stowell, & Landers, 2012).

Most often, the disorder emerges in childhood or adolescence, although it may not be acknowledged until adulthood. Some adolescents later become more comfortable with their assigned gender, whereas others experience persistent dissatisfaction and distress. The period between the ages of 10 and 13 is when a more persistent form of gender dysphoria is likely to develop (Steensma, Biemond, de Boer, & Cohen-Kettenis, 2011).

Diagnostic criteria for children with gender dysphoria include incongruence between one's experienced gender and assigned gender, lasting at least 6 months (APA, 2013). One of the symptoms must be a strong desire to be of the other gender or being insistent that one belongs to the other gender. Other signs in individuals assigned as boys include a preference for cross-dressing; rejection of masculine toys; and avoidance of rough play. In girls, the signs include resistance to wearing female clothing; avoidance of feminine toys; and dislike of feminine activities. And in both males and females, signs include preference for cross-gender roles, toys, and activities in play; preference for playmates of the other gender; strong dislike of one's sexual anatomy; and a desire for sex characteristics that match experienced, opposed to assigned, gender. These symptoms are associated with distress. Specifiers note any disorders of sex development (e.g., congenital adrenogenital disorder).

Diagnostic criteria for gender dysphoria in adolescent and adults include incongruence between experienced gender and assigned gender for at least 6 months (APA, 2013). Symptoms of the perceived incongruence include difference between experienced gender and sex characteristics, a strong desire to be rid of sex characteristics because of this incongruence, a desire to have the sex characteristics of the other gender, a desire to be of the other gender, desire to be treated as the other gender, and a conviction that one has the feelings or reactions of the other gender. These symptoms are associated with distress. Specifiers note whether there is a disorder of sex development and also indicate whether the disorder is posttransition (the individual is living as the other gender, with or without legal gender change) and the individual is preparing for at least one gender reassignment medical procedure.

This gender dysphoria disorder is distinct from transvestism. Although individuals with gender dysphoria may well cross-dress, they do so not to derive sexual pleasure from the behavior, but rather engage in it to create an appearance more consistent with their perceived gender. Likewise, it is not identical to homosexuality, which, it is important to note, is not a mental disorder. The individual may experience sexual attraction to an individual of the same biological gender, but this is in the context of perceiving the self to be the other gender.

Etiology

The gender differentiation process involves complicated genetic and hormonal events. It is increasingly clear that these events can and do unfold in a multitude of ways (Meyer-Bahlburg, 2002). The generally held belief that this is a binary process (i.e., male/female) is not consistent with the apparent biological variability that can occur during the differentiation process. Gender dysphoria is almost certainly a biological phenomenon.

Prognosis

Prognosis for gender dysphoria is variable, dependent on the intervention selected by the individual and the degree of support experienced in his or her social network (Benestad, 2010). A very difficult decision, of course, is to what degree the individual decides to alter his or her gender.

Implications for Function and Treatment

Functional implications for gender dysphoria center largely on social interaction and self-concept. The individual is likely to be perfectly functional in vocational occupations and to have few, if any, skill deficits. However, the individual may struggle to fit in socially and feels uncomfortable and distressed in seeking friendships and sexual relationships. Self-care can be affected if the individual is striving to adjust to a gender change because many self-care activities are associated with gender identity. It is important to note that these individuals often are focused on being the other gender to the greatest extent possible, not on flaunting their different gender identity (Figure 15-2).

The treatment options for individuals with gender dysphoria are relatively straightforward, although the choice is not. Individuals may select to undergo hormone therapy to alter secondary sex characteristics (Wylie, Fung, Boshier, & Rotchell, 2009). Surgical intervention is obviously a more extreme—and irreversible—option, but one that may be the treatment of choice to support the individual's identity. As a general rule, clinicians working with transgender individuals pursuing sex change surgery require the individual to undergo hormone therapy first and to live as the other gender for a period of time before taking a permanent step (De Vries & Cohen-Kettenis, 2012).

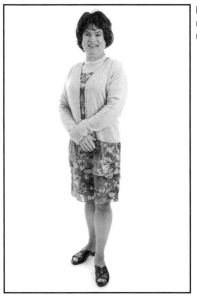

Figure 15-2. Individuals with gender dysphoric disorder are often more interested in living as their perceived gender more than on making a statement. (©2014 Shutterstock.com.)

It is essential for the individual to have opportunities to explore perceptions about gender and identity and to make decisions and choices in a supportive and thoughtful environment (Benestad, 2010). The increasing acceptance of the realities of such situations, along with a number of well-publicized cases (e.g., Chaz Bono), have made the situation somewhat less difficult, but it remains a marginalized and somewhat stigmatized disorder.

It is also important to support the families of individuals with gender dysphoria, as both the initial discussion about the disorder and the subsequent treatment of the individual can be emotionally challenging (Bockting, Miner, Swinburne Romine, Hamilton, & Coleman, 2013). Intervention with employers and friends may also be essential if the individual makes the gender transformation.

Implications for Occupational Therapy Intervention

The *Occupational Therapy Practice Framework* (American Occupational Therapy Association, 2014) identifies sexuality as an important occupation that contributes to meaning in roles, habits, and patterns. Nevertheless, very little has been written about how occupational therapists might provide helpful treatment when the issue is a psychological, as opposed to a physical, dysfunction. Recommendations for working with individuals with physical illnesses and injuries (e.g., multiple sclerosis, cardiovascular disease) emphasize addressing the physical limitations or energy management issues that affect participation (Martinez-Assuncena et al., 2010; Paull, Arndt, Petkovski, Connolly, & Vuong, 2011). Such issues are not likely to be involved in the conditions described in this chapter, but when they are, similar strategies would apply.

It seems probable that for individuals with sexual dysfunction, issues of self-concept and social interaction would be problematic and the individual would benefit from strategies to address these issues, perhaps through the identification of occupations that are his or her particular strengths. Opportunities for emotional expression through nonverbal mechanisms, such as the creative arts, can be helpful for individuals who are not comfortable articulating their feelings or who lack adequate verbal skill or insight to analyze their emotions.

Working with individuals with paraphilic disorders is somewhat more challenging. Identifying occupations that redirect urges into socially acceptable forms is a strategy that may be helpful in conjunction with behavioral strategies. For individuals who are incarcerated, support strategies to prepare them for eventual release can be vital.

For individuals who are dealing with gender dysphoria, occupational therapy focuses on two major areas: self-esteem and self-concept. Occupational therapy also focuses on, where appropriate, learning to live as the other gender. In every society, being male or female is more than simply one's sex characteristics. It is a set of behaviors that are socially prescribed. Although gender roles are more variable than a generation ago, for the individual who wishes to alter gender, identifying ways in which to be comfortable in the new role is a vital strategy.

However, keep in mind that there is limited evidence about the effectiveness of specific occupational therapy interventions with the various sexually related disorders. Focus on occupations can guide intervention; and the documentation of outcomes would help the next generation of therapists. Table 15-2 summarizes the diagnostic criteria and functional deficits associated with sexual dysfunctions, paraphilic disorders, and gender dysphoria.

Cultural Considerations

Significant differences exist among cultures in terms of sexual expression and activity. It is essential that therapists understand the views and values of their clients and avoid imposing their own beliefs. For example, there are differences across cultures with regard to the female orgasm and its acceptability (Laumann et al., 2005). In another example, reports of premature ejaculation were more prevalent among men in Asia-Pacific countries than erectile dysfunction, but self-report is rare for either condition (McMahon, Lee, Park, & Adaikan, 2012).

Likewise, gender identity is strongly mediated by cultural values and beliefs (Benestad, 2010). Although there is evidence of gender dysphoria in many parts of the world, the exact nature of the change in gender roles must be considered in assisting the individual to make helpful choices and adapt to new behaviors.

Lifespan Considerations

Gender dysphoria is most likely to emerge initially in childhood or adolescence, even if it is not acted upon until adulthood (Steensma et al., 2011). Childhood and adolescence are fraught with developmental stressors of many kinds, and those with gender dysphoria face a particularly challenging time. Bullying and social isolation are common (Wallien, Veenstra, Kreukels, & Cohen-Kettenis, 2010), so these young people may struggle with self-esteem more than most.

Aging has a significant impact on sexual functioning, which means sexual dysfunctions are more likely to occur late in life (Foley, 2009). For both genders, development of chronic illnesses, age-related increase in the use of prescription medications, and changes in blood flow and neurological function contribute to sexual performance changes. For men, the result may be periodic delayed ejaculation or erectile dysfunction. For women, decreased estrogen can cause drying and thinning of the genital tissues with associated dyspareunia (Kao et al., 2012).

TABLE 15-2

DIAGNOSTIC CRITERIA AND FUNCTIONAL IMPLICATIONS: SEXUAL DYSFUNCTIONS

DISORDER	DIAGNOSTIC CRITERIA (APA, 2013)	IMPLICATIONS FOR FUNCTION
Delayed ejaculation	At least 6 months of repeated occasions with either significant delay in ejaculation or absence of ejaculation, causing distress	Social interactions impaired Body systems, body functions impaired
Erectile disorder	For at least 6 months, on most occasions when intercourse is attempted: • Difficulty obtaining or maintaining an erection or • Decrease in erectile rigidity Associated distress	Social interactions impaired Body systems, body functions impaired
Female orgasmic disorder	For at least 6 months, one or more of these on most occasions when intercourse is attempted, delay, infrequency, reduced intensity or absence of orgasm Associated distress	Social interactions impaired Body systems, body functions impaired
Female sexual arousal disorder	For at least 6 months, limited sexual interest or arousal Associated distress	Social interactions impaired Body systems, body functions impaired
Genito-pelvic pain/penetration disorder	For at least 6 months, repeated difficulty with vaginal penetration or pain during vaginal intercourse, anxiety about pelvic pain Associated distress	Social interactions impaired Body systems, body functions impaired
Male hypoactive sexual desire disorder	For at least 6 months, limited sexual thoughts, fantasies, or desire for sexual activity Associated distress	Social interactions impaired Body systems, body functions impaired
Premature/early ejaculation	For at least 6 months, pattern of ejaculation occurring within one minute and earlier than the individual wants Associated distress	Social interactions impaired Body systems, body functions impaired

(continued)

TABLE 15-2 (CONTINUED)		
DIAGNOSTIC CRITERIA AND FUNCTIONAL IMPLICATIONS: SEXUAL DYSFUNCTIONS		
DISORDER	*DIAGNOSTIC CRITERIA (APA, 2013)*	*IMPLICATIONS FOR FUNCTION*
Paraphilic disorders	Sexual arousal associated with atypical/unacceptable stimuli or behaviors	Social function impaired May also negatively affect work, self-care Legal difficulties may be associated
Gender dysphoria (adult)	Incongruence between experienced gender and assigned gender with the following: • Desire to be rid of sex characteristics because of this incongruence • Desire to have sex characteristic of or be the other gender • Conviction that one has the feelings or reactions of the other gender Symptoms cause distress	Affects most occupations, particularly social, leisure May affect emotional regulation, cognition

CASE STUDY

Judith Parker is an attractive, divorced 43-year-old woman. She works as a public relations account manager at a large, well-known public relations firm. She and her husband, Ned, divorced 5 years ago after being married for 16 years. They have two sons. The younger son, who is 13 years old, lives with Judith and attends the local middle school. The older son, who is 18 years old, is currently in prison on a drug-related conviction. Ms. Parker's former husband is the first and only man with whom she had sexual intercourse until she started dating Arnold 2 years ago.

Ms. Parker is quite good at her job and has earned several promotions during her time with the company. She recently was again promoted, and she now supervises a major division of the company. She puts in long hours at work, and although she enjoys her job and feels satisfied by it, she also is quite fatigued. Her former husband has gone back to court to ask for additional financial support because of her promotion. Her 13-year-old son is a pleasant and compliant young man, but he has dyslexia and is struggling in school. Judith spends a good bit of time each evening helping him with his homework, and many days she falls into bed exhausted.

Arnold, her new companion, is 44 years old and also divorced. He takes the lead in their sexual relationship, and Judith has had an orgasm only once since they began dating. Arnold is disturbed by this and has convinced Judith to seek help. Ms. Parker is also distressed because she is concerned that her lack of responsiveness may ultimately drive Arnold away, although she is not, herself, particularly interested in sexual activity.

(continued)

CASE STUDY (CONTINUED)

Ms. Parker came to therapy reluctantly, believing there was something seriously wrong with her. She has great difficulty discussing the issue, has a limited sexual vocabulary, and displays considerable reluctance and embarrassment about discussing sex. She reports that her parents were Fundamentalist Christians who never discussed sex or displayed any physical interaction in her presence.

THOUGHT QUESTIONS

1. What disorder do you think Ms. Parker might be experiencing?
2. What specific factors in the description here led you to that conclusion?
3. What functional issues do you think might need to be addressed?

Internet Resources

American Society for Reproductive Medicine

http://www.asrm.org/FACTSHEET_Sexual_Dysfunction_and_Infertility/

Provides both professional and consumer information about sexual dysfunction and infertility.

Emory University School of Medicine

http://medicine.emory.edu/divisions/gen-med-geriatrics/education-geriatrics/edu-resources/sexual-dysfunction.html

Focuses on sexual dysfunctions associated with later life.

MedHelp

http://www.medhelp.org/tags/show/13903/Female-sexual-dysfunction

MedHelp is an online resource for a variety of health-related topics. This page focuses on issues relevant to sexual issues found in women.

References

Abdel-Hamid, I.A., & Saleh, E. (2011). Primary lifelong delayed ejaculation: Characteristics and response to bupropion. *Journal of Sexual Medicine, 8*(6), 1772-1779.

Althof, S. (2006). The psychology of premature ejaculation: Therapies and consequences. *Journal of Sexual Medicine, 3*(Suppl. 4), 324-331.

American Occupational Therapy Association. (2014). Occupational therapy practice framework: Domain & process (3rd ed.). *American Journal of Occupational Therapy, 68*(Suppl. 1), S1-S48.

American Psychiatric Association. (2013). *Diagnostic and statistical manual of mental disorders* (5th ed.). Washington, DC: Author.

Balon, R. (2013). Controversies in the diagnosis and treatment of paraphilias. *Journal of Sex & Marital Therapy, 39*(1), 7-20.

Basson, R., Brotto, L.A., Laan, E., Redmond, G., & Utian, W.H. (2005). Assessment and management of women's sexual dysfunctions: Problematic desire and arousal. *Journal of Sexual Medicine, 2*(3), 291-300.

Benestad, E.E.P. (2010). From gender dysphoria to gender euphoria: An assisted journey. *Sexologies: European Journal of Sexology and Sexual Health/Revue européenne de sexologie et de santé sexuelle, 19*(4), 225-231.

Bertozzi, S., Londero, A.P., Fruscalzo, A., Driul, L., & Marchesoni, D. (2010). Prevalence and risk factors for dyspareunia and unsatisfying sexual relationships in a cohort of primiparous and secondiparous women after 12 months postpartum. *International Journal of Sexual Health, 22*(1), 47-53.

Binik, Y.M. (2010). The DSM diagnostic criteria for dyspareunia. *Archives of Sexual Behavior, 39*(2), 292-303.

Bockting, W., Miner, M., Swinburne Romine, E., Hamilton, A., & Coleman, E. (2013). Stigma, mental health, and resilience among an online sample of the U.S. transgender population. *American Journal of Public Health, 103*(5), 943-951. doi:10.2105/AJPH.2013.301241.

Bonierbale, M. (2013). Evolving concepts in premature ejaculation: Implications for practice. *Sexologies: European Journal of Sexology and Sexual Health/Revue européenne de sexologie et de santé sexuelle, 22*(2), e33-e38.

Buvat, J., Büttner, H., Hatzimouratidis, K., Vendeira, P.A.S., Moncada, I., Boehmer, M., . . . Boess, F.G. (2013). Adherence to initial PDE-5 inhibitor treatment: Randomized open-label study comparing tadalafil once a day, tadalafil on demand, and sildenafil on demand in patients with erectile dysfunction. *Journal of Sexual Medicine, 10*(6), 1592-1602.

Conron, K.J., Scott, G., Stowell, G.S., & Landers, S. (2012). Transgender health in Massachusetts: Results from a household probability sample of adults. *American Journal of Public Health, 102*(1), 118-222.

De Vries, A.L.C., & Cohen-Kettenis, P.T. (2012). Clinical management of gender dysphoria in children and adolescents: The Dutch approach. *Journal of Homosexuality, 59*, 301-320.

Donaldson, R.L., & Meana, M. (2011). Early dyspareunia experience in young women: Confusion, consequences, and help-seeking barriers. *Journal of Sexual Medicine, 8*(3), 814-823.

Foley, S. (2009). The complex etiology of delayed ejaculation: Assessment and treatment implications. In K.M. Hertlein, G.R. Weeks, & N. Gambescia (Eds.), *Systemic sex therapy* (pp. 153-177). New York, NY: Routledge/Taylor & Francis.

Fraser, L., Karasic, D. H., & Meyer, W. J., & Wylie, K. (2010). Recommendations for revision of the DSM diagnoses of gender identity disorders in adults. *International Journal of Transgenderism, 12*, 80-85.

Frühauf, S., Gerger, H., Schmidt, H., Maren, M., & Thomas Barth, J. (2013). Efficacy of psychological interventions for sexual dysfunction: A systematic review and meta-analysis. *Archives of Sexual Behavior, 42*(6), 915-933.

Giami, A. (2013). Social epidemiology of premature ejaculation. *Sexologies: European Journal of Sexology and Sexual Health/Revue européenne de sexologie et de santé sexuelle, 22*(1), e27-e32.

Guay, D.R.P. (2009). Drug treatment of paraphilic and nonparaphilic sexual disorders. *Clinical Therapeutics: The International Peer-Reviewed Journal of Drug Therapy, 31*(1), 1-31.

Hartman, U., & Waldinger, M.D. (2007). Treatment of delayed ejaculation. In S.R. Lieblum (Ed.), *Principles and practices of sex therapy* (4th ed., pp. 241-276). New York, NY: Guilford.

Kao, A., Binik, Y.M., Amsel, R., Funaro, D., Leroux, N., & Khalifé, S. (2012). Biopsychosocial predictors of postmenopausal dyspareunia: The role of steroid hormones, vulvovaginal atrophy, cognitive-emotional factors, and dyadic adjustment. *Journal of Sexual Medicine, 9*(8), 2066-2076.

Krychman, M.L. (2011). Vaginal estrogens for the treatment of dyspareunia. *Journal of Sexual Medicine, 8*(3), 666-674.

Landry, T., & Bergeron, S. (2009). How young does vulvo-vaginal pain begin? Prevalence and characteristics of dyspareunia in adolescents. *Journal of Sexual Medicine, 6*(4), 927-935.

Laumann, E.O., Nicolosi, A., Glasser, D.B., Paik, A., Gingell, C., Moreira, E., & Wang, T. (2005). Sexual problems among women and men aged 40-80 years: Prevalence and correlates identified in the Global Study of Sexual Attitudes and Behaviors. *International Journal of Impotence Research, 17*, 39-57.

Martinez-Assuncena, A., Marnetoft, S., Rovira, T.R., Hernandez-San-Miguel, J., Bernabeu, M., & Martinell-Gispert-Sauch, M. (2010). Rehabilitation for multiple sclerosis in adults (I): Impairment and impact on functioning and quality of life: An overview. *Critical Reviews in Physical & Rehabilitation Medicine, 22*(1-4), 103-177.

McCarthy, B., & Ginsberg, R.L. (2007). Male hypoactive sexual desire disorder: A conceptual model and case study. *Journal of Family Psychotherapy, 18*(4), 29-42.

McCarthy, B., & McDonald, D. (2009). Assessment, treatment, and relapse prevention: Male hypoactive sexual desire disorder. *Journal of Sex & Marital Therapy, 35*(1), 58-67.

McMahon, C.G., Lee, G., Park, J.K., & Adaikan, P.G. (2012). Premature ejaculation and erectile dysfunction prevalence and attitudes in the Asia-Pacific region. *Journal of Sexual Medicine, 9*(2), 454-465.

McMahon, C.G., & Porst, H. (2011). Oral agents for the treatment of premature ejaculation: Review of efficacy and safety in the context of the recent international society for sexual medicine criteria for lifelong premature ejaculation. *Journal of Sex and Medicine, 8*, 2707-2725.

Meston, C.M., Hull, E., Levin, R.J., & Sipski, M. (2004). Disorders of orgasm in women. *Journal of Sexual Medicine, 1*(1), 66-68.

Metz, M.E., & McCarthy, B.W. (2007). The good-enough sex model for couple sexual satisfaction. *Sexual and Relationship Therapy, 22*(3), 351-362.

Meyer-Bahlburg, H.F.L. (2002). Gender assignment and reassignment in intersexuality: Controversies, data, and guidelines for research. *Advances in Experimental Medicine and Biology, 511*, 199-223.

Paull, G., Arndt, P.M., Petkovski, D., Connolly, B., & Vuong, N. (2011). Sexuality and chronic cardiovascular disease—A neglected area of practice: The role of the occupational therapist in a cardiac rehabilitation setting. *Australian Occupational Therapy Journal, 58*(Suppl.), 127.

Pazmany, E., Bergeron, S., Oudenhove, L., Verhaeghe, J., & Enzlin, P. (2013). Body image and genital self-image in pre-menopausal women with dyspareunia. *Archives of Sexual Behavior, 42*(6), 999-1010.

Perelman, M.A. (2013). Delayed ejaculation. *Journal of Sexual Medicine, 10*(4), 1189-1190.

Robinson, B.B.E., Munns, R.A., Weber-Main, A.M., Lowe, M.A., & Raymond, N.C. (2011). Application of the sexual health model in the long-term treatment of hypoactive sexual desire and female orgasmic disorder. *Archives of Sexual Behavior, 40*(2), 469-478.

Saleh, F.M., & Berlin, F.S. (2003). Sexual deviancy: Diagnostic and neurobiological considerations. *Journal of Child Sexual Abuse: Research, Treatment, & Program Innovations for Victims, Survivors, & Offenders, Special issue: Identifying and Treating Sex Offenders: Current Approaches, Research, and Techniques, 12*(3-4), 53-76.

Shaeer, O., & Shaeer, K. (2012). The Global Online Sexuality Survey (GOSS): The United States of America in 2011. Chapter I: Erectile dysfunction among English-speakers. *Journal of Sexual Medicine, 9*(12), 3018-3027.

Shamloul, R., & Ghanem, H. (2013). Erectile dysfunction. *Lancet, 381*(9861), 153-165.

Steensma, T.D., Biemond, R., de Boer, F., & Cohen-Kettenis, P.T. (2011). Desisting and persisting gender dysphoria after childhood: A qualitative follow-up study. *Clinical Child Psychology and Psychiatry, 16*(4), 499-516.

Waldinger, M.D. (2010). Premature ejaculation and delayed ejaculation. In C.B. Risen, S.E. Althof, & S.B. Levine (Eds.), *Handbook of clinical sexuality for mental health professionals* (2nd ed., pp. 267-292). New York, NY: Routledge/Taylor & Francis.

Wallien, M.S.C., Veenstra, R., Kreukels, B.P.C., & Cohen-Kettenis, P.T. (2010). Peer group status of gender dysphoric children: A sociometric study. *Archives of Sexual Behavior, 39*(2), 553-560.

Wylie, K.R., Fung, R., Boshier, C., & Rotchell, M. (2009). Recommendations of endocrine treatment for patients with gender dysphoria. *Sexual and Relationship Therapy, 24*(2), 175-187.

Disruptive, Impulse-Control, and Conduct Disorders

Learning Outcomes

By the end of this chapter, readers will be able to:
- Describe the symptoms of disruptive, impulse-control, and conduct disorders
- Identify the causes of the disruptive, impulse-control, and conduct disorders
- Describe treatment strategies for the disruptive, impulse-control, and conduct disorders
- Discuss the occupational perspective on disruptive, impulse-control, and conduct disorders, including specific intervention considerations

Bonder B.
Psychopathology and Function, Fifth Edition (pp 301-314).
© 2015 SLACK Incorporated.

CASE VIGNETTE

Harry Maloney is a 17-year-old high school junior who is being threatened with expulsion following his most recent outburst at school. Well known to the principal and other teachers and administrators in the school system, Harry has had frequent suspensions throughout his elementary and secondary school years because of his uncontrolled temper outbursts. He has few friends because he often gets into arguments or fights when involved in group activities. The most recent episode began when a science teacher asked Harry to help carry several boxes of laboratory equipment from the office to the classroom. Harry became enraged, threw the boxes, which contained glassware, in the teacher's direction, then began kicking and punching lockers in the hallway.

THOUGHT QUESTIONS

1. What behaviors in this description are cause for concern?
2. Do these behaviors suggest the possibility of a mental disorder?
3. What else might you like to know about Harry and his background?
4. How might Harry's problematic behaviors affect his successful engagement in occupations?

DISRUPTIVE, IMPULSE-CONTROL, AND CONDUCT DISORDERS

- Oppositional defiant disorder
- Intermittent explosive disorder
- Conduct disorder

- Antisocial personality disorder
- Pyromania
- Kleptomania

The common feature of the disruptive, impulse-control, and conduct disorders is the individual's difficulty or inability to manage hostile or disruptive impulses and behaviors as required for socially acceptable interaction. The disorders often emerge in childhood, sometimes in very early childhood, and have significant consequences for the child's function and his or her interactions with others. Among the ways in which the fifth edition of the *Diagnostic and Statistical Manual of Mental Disorders* (DSM-5; American Psychiatric Association [APA], 2013) has changed is that these disorders were previously included with the disorders of infancy, childhood, and adolescence. They were classified, along with attention-deficit/hyperactive disorder (ADHD), as disruptive disorders. As you have seen, ADHD remained with the neurodevelopmental disorders, while a new cluster was framed for the disruptive, impulse-control and conduct disorders. Table 16-1 shows the prevalence of these disorders.

TABLE 16-1			
PREVALENCE OF DISRUPTIVE, IMPULSE-CONTROL, AND CONDUCT DISORDERS			
DIAGNOSIS	*PREVALENCE*	*GENDER RATIO (M:F)*	*SOURCE*
Oppositional defiant disorder	1.3% to 6.9%	Higher in males	Shenk et al., 2012
Intermittent explosive disorder	0.5% to 4.5%	Higher in males	Shenk et al., 2012
Conduct disorder	0.7%	Higher in males	Wichstrøm et al., 2012
Antisocial personality disorder	1%	3:1	APA, 2013
Pyromania	Unknown		
Kleptomania	0.6%	1:3	Talih, 2011

Oppositional Defiant Disorder

Oppositional defiant disorder (ODD) reflects a pattern in children of disobedience, hostility, anger, and defiant behavior particularly focused on authority figures and beyond the bounds of normal childhood behavior (Pardini, Frick, & Moffitt, 2010). These children may be angry and irritable, argumentative and defiant, and/or vindictive. Such children present with difficult classroom behavior, frequent outbursts at home, and difficulties in social situations.

Diagnostic criteria for ODD include a pattern of angry or irritable mood accompanied by argumentative, defiant, or vindictive behavior, lasting at least 6 months, with at least four behavioral manifestations directed at someone other than a sibling (APA, 2013). The behaviors occur more frequently than is normal and cause distress in either the individual or in others. Specifiers note severity.

ODD often coexists with other conditions, including ADHD and developmental disorders (Reimherr, Marchant, Olsen, Wender, & Robison, 2013).

Etiology

ODD is a disorder for which both genetic/biological and environmental circumstances must be present. In particular, children with the identified genetic attributes who experience inconsistent parenting are more likely to display the disorder than children in the same situation without the genetic characteristics (Martel, Nikolas, Jrenigan, Friderici, & Nigg, 2012).

The biological substrate of ODD appears to involve reduced cortisol reactivity to stress, reduced amygdala reactivity to negative stimuli, and altered serotonin and noradrenaline neurotransmission. These contribute to low sensitivity to punishment, which may reduce the child's ability to associate inappropriate behaviors with negative consequences (Matthys, Vanderschuren, & Schutter, 2013). At the same time, the sympathetic nervous system does not react to incentives, and other neurological factors (e.g., low basal heart rate, reduced reactivity of the frontal cortex, and altered dopamine function) reduce responsiveness to reward. Matthys et al. (2013) suggested that this combination of factors predispose the child or adolescent to sensation-seeking behavior, including breaking the rules, delinquency, and drug abuse. Neuroimaging studies confirm functional abnormalities in the amygdala and frontal cortex (Finger et al., 2012).

Early-life environmental risk factors compound these biological risk factors of ODD. In particular, prenatal maternal cigarette smoking, alcohol use, or viral illness; maternal stress and anxiety; low birth weight; early neonatal complications; parental stress; dysfunctional (inconsistent) parenting; and early deprivation or adoption all are implicated in the development of the disorder (Latimer et al., 2012).

Prognosis

ODD is a strong predictor of adult antisocial personality disorder (Finger et al., 2012), as well as conduct disorder and depression (Stepp, Burke, Hipwell, & Loeber, 2012). The frequent emergence of other disorders in later life suggests that early-life irritability is a marker of risk of developing these other conditions (Burke, 2012).

Although ODD is more common in boys, it is also found in girls (Stepp et al., 2012). Here, too, more severe ODD predicted the development of personality disorder in adolescence—more often borderline personality disorder among girls and antisocial personality disorder among boys.

ODD often emerges quite early, before age 2 in some cases. When the disorder appears that early, it is a persistent, life-long condition (Baillargeon, Keenan, & Cao, 2012). ODD is associated with increased risk of adjustment problems during adolescence and adulthood, including academic problems, substance abuse, and antisocial behavior (Séguin & Pilon, 2013). The possibility of poor prognosis and the high social costs of the disorder suggest that careful and early attention should be given to treatment (Cederna-Meko, Koch, & Wall, 2013).

Implications for Function and Treatment

ODD results in dysfunction in many occupations, in particular family/social and academic occupations (Séguin, & Pilon, 2013). These children have chronic social difficulties that result from their hostile and defiant behaviors (Stepp et al., 2012), which affect their relationships with peers as well as authority figures. They frequently engage in bullying behavior, which contributes to their social challenges (Fite, Evans, Cooley, & Rubens, 2014). Self-care activities are less likely to be affected, but play is problematic as a result of difficulty interacting effectively with other children.

At the level of skills, there are clear deficits in executive cognitive function, apparently associated with structural deficits and impairment of the paralimbic system (body system/body function), which relate to cognitive control of emotion (Matthys et al., 2013). In particular, these children seem to have difficulty associating behaviors with negative and positive consequences, making them less responsive to punishment and reward than other children. Therefore, it is difficult for these children to learn appropriate behavior (Matthys, Vanderschuren, Schutter, & Lochman, 2012). Children with ODD also have difficulty with problem solving, attention, and decision making.

Most intervention recommendations for ODD focus on psychotherapeutic efforts. These include cognitive behavioral therapy, parent training, and family therapy (Shenk et al., 2012). Collaborative problem solving has been tried as an intervention with some modest success (Johnson et al., 2012). All of these interventions are focused on social learning (Matthys et al., 2012), and their impact appears to be modest, which may be the result of differences among children, as there are observed individual differences in neurocognitive characteristics among these children. This suggests it is particularly important to design individualized programs based on the individual strengths and weaknesses of each child. Particular emphasis needs to focus on creating an environment in which behaviors have predictable and reasonable consequences.

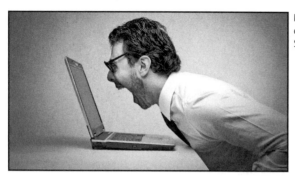

Figure 16-1. Intermittent explosive disorder often persists into adulthood. (©2014 Shutterstock.com.)

Implications for Occupational Therapy

Relatively little has been written about occupational therapy intervention for individuals with ODD. The suggestions provided for treating those with conduct disorder are likely to apply. On the basis of theories of occupation, two major factors would be the emphasis for occupational therapy in relation to ODD. First, there is fairly strong evidence that parenting styles contribute to the development of ODD (Lavigne et al., 2010). Various forms of parent training have been well-documented as effective, and should center on helping parents understand the principles of behavior and social learning, along with specific skills to enhance child cooperation and reduce disruptive behavior. For example, a parent may be inclined to ignore oppositional behavior, conceptualizing it as normal or "what you expect from children." These parents need to understand the dangers of this choice and be provided with strategies (e.g., time out, loss of privileges) that would help the child to understand appropriate behavior. Such information may also be helpful to classroom teachers.

The second major focus, along with parent education efforts, should be on creating highly structured interventions for the children (Larsson et al., 2009). Careful attention to explicit expectations linked repeatedly and consistently with specific outcomes allows children to learn the relationship between their own behavior and desired consequences.

Intermittent Explosive Disorder

Intermittent explosive disorder (IED) most often emerges in childhood or adolescence, but often persists into adulthood (Figure 16-1). IED is characterized by poor impulse control that results in frequent temper outbursts, which can be verbal, physical, or both. Although most people can be pushed to a point at which they lose their tempers, for individuals with IED, the outbursts are more frequent and disproportionate to the perceived stimulus. The majority (82%) of individuals with IED have at least one co-occurring mental condition (Lara, 2007). IED is characterized by recurrent behavioral outbursts that show a failure to manage aggressive impulses through verbal aggression, damage of property, or physical injury to others, occurring at least twice per week over a period of 3 months or more (APA, 2013). These behaviors are out of proportion with any provocation and are not premeditated or goal oriented. The behaviors cause distress and dysfunction and/or legal and financial consequences. The diagnosis is not made in children younger than 6 years old.

Etiology

Several neurocognitive changes have been noted as contributing to IED. These changes include serotonergic abnormalities, particularly in the limbic system and orbitofrontal cortex, with differential activation of the corticolimbic system (Brown University Child & Adolescent Psychopharmacology Update, 2012). In addition, individuals with a first-degree relative with IED are at higher risk of developing the disorder themselves (Harvard Mental Health Letter, 2011). Additional risk factors include male gender and low education and income (Lara, 2007).

Prognosis

IED tends to be chronic. Researchers following individuals with IED longitudinally have found the condition present 20 years after the initial diagnosis (McCloskey, Kleabir, Berman, Chan, & Coccaro, 2010). The anger and hostility appear to contribute to a high risk of physical ailments, most notably cardiovascular disease.

Implications for Function and Treatment

Severe deficits exist in social, academic, and family occupations (McCloskey et al., 2010). The individual's difficulty in controlling his or her temper and frequent violent temper outbursts negatively impacts his or her ability to forge positive relationships. In older individuals, work can also be negatively affected, and these individuals experience frequent legal difficulties.

Treatment typically involves both cognitive behavioral therapy and medication (Brown University Child & Adolescent Psychopharmacology Update, 2012). In particular, antidepressants, mood stabilizers, and antipsychotic drugs can reduce aggressive outbursts (Harvard Mental Health Letter, 2011). Helpful cognitive behavioral therapy emphasizes cognitive restructuring, coping skills, and relaxation training.

Implications for Occupational Therapy

The guidelines described for ODD and conduct disorder are likely to be equally appropriate for working with individuals with IED. If the individual is a child, working with the parents can be helpful. In older individuals, there may be no strong social network as a result of the person's behavior; in such cases, intervention will focus largely on that person. Emphasizing emotional control strategies, appropriate expression of emotions, and focusing on personal strengths can supplement and complement other therapeutic interventions.

Conduct Disorder

Conduct disorder (CD), unlike ODD, is characterized by a pattern of violating the rights of others, as well as violating the norms and expectations for the behavior of one's age. The temper outbursts found in ODD are not as evident in CD. On the other hand, these individuals may be violent toward other people or animals, destructive of property, and defiant of parental and societal rules.

Diagnostic criteria for CD include a persistent pattern of behavior that violates the rights of others or the rules of conduct, including aggression toward people and animals, destruction of property, and deceitfulness or theft (APA, 2103). At least three episodes must occur in a 1-year period, and the behaviors must be associated with dysfunction. Specifiers are fairly extensive, including indication of childhood, adolescent, or unknown onset, and whether there are limited **prosocial** emotions, such as conscience and concern about others. The specifiers indicate whether there is lack of remorse or guilt, lack of empathy, lack of concern about performance, deficient affect, and the severity of the disorder.

Antisocial personality disorder must be ruled out. CD often occurs in concert with substance use disorders, ADHD, intellectual disabilities, and learning disabilities.

Etiology

CD is characterized by subtle neurological deficits, such as poor verbal abilities and lowered inhibitory control (Moffitt, 2006). Gray matter volume reductions in the areas that process socioemotional stimuli have also been reported (Fairchild et al., 2011). These neurological deficits may lead to callous/unemotional traits (Mandy, Skuse, Steer, St Pourcain, & Oliver, 2013; Matthys et al., 2012).

Cognitive deficits are associated with family histories of antisocial behavior and either harsh or inconsistent parenting (Odgers et al., 2008). These forms of parenting lead to difficulties in developing social skills and understanding and acting on rules for appropriate conduct.

Although some individuals develop CD in childhood, there is also an adolescent-onset form. In this case, individuals do not show delinquent behavior until adolescence, and they are less likely to have either family dysfunction or neurological deficits (Moffitt, 2006; Odgers et al., 2008). In this later onset, the etiology may be adolescent rebellion in the context of poor parental monitoring and peer pressure.

Prognosis

On the whole, prognosis for CD is poor, especially if there is associated alcohol or substance abuse (Freestone, Howard, Coid, & Ullrich, 2013). Children with CD have a high probability of developing adult antisocial or borderline personality disorders and encountering financial and legal difficulties. Early onset of the behavior predicts a worse outcome, including a high potential for violence and criminal behavior over time (Webbink, Vujic, Koning, & Martin, 2012).

CD has a somewhat better outlook when onset is during adolescence. These young people may transition to work roles, find more acceptable peers, and in general become more mature (Odgers et al., 2008). However, they do have a higher rate of criminal behavior and functional impairments than peers without conduct disorder.

The prognosis is particularly grim for individuals with CD who show callous/unemotional traits. They appear to become more disruptive over time, with or without treatment (Haas et al., 2011).

Implications for Function and Treatment

Individuals with CD have functional impairments across many occupations. They struggle at school, have difficulty with peer relationships, have problems transitioning to adult roles of work and family life, and are at high risk for criminal behavior (Moffitt, 2006). The social impairments are particularly notable (Greene et al., 2002). For example, girls with conduct disorder are more likely to bully their peers than girls without the disorder (Pardini, Stepp, Hipwell, Stouthamer-Loeber, & Loeber, 2012). These girls typically have tense relationships with parents, as caretakers find managing children and adolescents with CD quite stressful (Manor-Binyamini, 2012).

Preventive interventions have been attempted with children showing early signs of CD, including poor anger management and callous/unemotional behavior. These efforts have had mixed success at best (Dishion et al., 2008).

Many interventions focus on educating parents about the best management strategies. These include a focus on positive parent-child interaction, as well as consistency in discipline (Thomas & Zimmer-Gembeck, 2007). Because these children typically do not respond to punishment, use of positive reinforcement to encourage prosocial behavior may be more helpful.

Implications for Occupational Therapy

Occupational therapists work with children with CD in several ways. First, the child's energy may be channeled to more appropriate activities, along with copious reinforcement for acceptable behavior. Expectations for behavior during such activities must be carefully identified, and reasonable positive or negative reinforcement should be systematically provided. Engagement in recreation (Webster-Stratton, 2000) as a way to provide experiences of success in acceptable activities can be of value.

Opportunities for appropriate expression of emotion appear to be helpful (Mpofu & Crystal, 2001), as children with CD are often unable to express feelings adequately and are inclined to act out their anger. Providing alternative strategies for emotional expression through play, art, music, or movement may be effective. Experiences of success in positive activities can be of great value in building a more positive self-concept. Teaching anger management and self-regulation in school settings may have value in preventing CD (Maas, Mason, & Candler, 2008), as well as for treating it.

Parent training can be effective when parents lack the adequate skills to manage their children (Dishion et al., 2008; Maughan & Rutter, 2001; Woolfenden, Williams, & Peat, 2001). Parents can be taught to provide appropriate reinforcement of positive behaviors and to ensure negative consequences to reduce problem behaviors. Evidence exists that these interventions can be provided through booklets and other media, as well as in face-to-face interaction (Montgomery, Bjornstad, & Dennis, 2006).

Coexisting conditions with CD must be considered. If comorbid, ADHD should be addressed, as described in Chapter 3. Specific learning disabilities should also be remediated if necessary.

Antisocial Personality Disorder

As was noted in a previous chapter, some personality disorders appear twice in the DSM-5 (APA, 2013). They are listed in the chapter with markers most closely associated with their characteristics, and then again in the chapter on personality disorders. Antisocial personality disorder will be covered in detail in Chapter 19, with the other personality disorders.

Pyromania

Both **pyromania**—deliberate fire setting—and **kleptomania**—irresistible impulses to steal—are impulse control disorders that reflect urges that are socially unacceptable, damaging to others, and destructive to the individual as well.

Diagnostic criteria for pyromania include deliberate fire setting on more than one occasion, tension or emotional arousal before setting the fire, fascination with or attraction to fire and its contexts, and pleasure or relief when setting fires or participating in their aftermath (APA, 2013). The pyromania disorder would not be diagnosed if the fires are set for gain or for political expression.

Pyromania is a very rare disorder in its pure form; that is, when there is no coexisting mental disorder (Doley, 2003). One study found that individuals who set fires had a number of additional, possibly primary, diagnoses, including low IQ (20%), psychosis (52%), personality disorder (52%), and substance abuse disorder (61%; Lindberg, Holi, Tani, & Virkkunen, 2005). This has led some clinicians and researchers to question whether pyromania exists as a separate entity. Research on the disorder is difficult because individuals who are believed to have pyromania are almost always discovered through their involvement in the legal system.

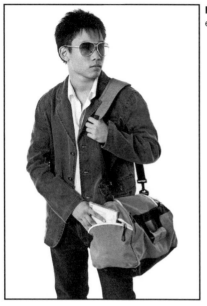

Figure 16-2. Many adolescents and college students report an episode of shoplifting. (©2014 Shutterstock.com.)

The disorder is associated with impulsivity, social dysfunction, and poor cognitive flexibility and executive function (Parks et al., 2005). It appears that some psychopharmacological agents, such as olanzapine and sodium valproate may improve the functional deficits and reduce unacceptable impulses.

Kleptomania

Kleptomania reflects repeated episodes of stealing. Although many adolescents and college students report at least one episode of theft or shoplifting (Figure 16-2), this behavior does not rise to the level of kleptomania because the majority of these occurrences are single episodes, not repeated irresistible urges (Grant, Odlaug, Schreiber, Chamberlain, & Kim, 2013).

Diagnostic criteria for kleptomania include inability to resist an impulse to steal objects that are not needed, a sense of tension before the theft, and pleasure or relief after committing the theft (APA, 2013). The behavior is not focused on expressing anger or vengeance, nor is it the result of a hallucination or delusion.

The etiology of kleptomania is not well understood (Grant et al., 2013). A strong link exists to depression, anxiety, and eating disorders (Talih, 2011), the latter of which are also impulse control disorders. A variety of psychoanalytic theories have focused on childhood trauma, abuse, or neglect, as well as sexual repression. The link with anxiety has caused some researchers to speculate that kleptomania may be associated with neuropsychiatric factors or that it may be related to substance abuse.

Kleptomania has significant impact on function, particularly because it often results in legal difficulties for the individual (Grant, Odlaug, Davis, & Kim, 2009). These individuals experience social and vocational impairments and poor quality of life. They also have a high rate of suicide.

Most reports about intervention focus on psychopharmacological approaches, including use of memantine (Grant et al., 2013), naltrexone, topiramate, lithium, valproate, and trazodone (Talih, 2011). Table 16-2 provides a summary of the diagnostic criteria and functional deficits associated with the disruptive, impulse-control, and conduct disorders.

TABLE 16-2

DIAGNOSTIC CRITERIA AND FUNCTIONAL IMPLICATIONS: DISRUPTIVE, IMPULSE CONTROL, AND CONDUCT DISORDERS

DISORDER	DIAGNOSTIC CRITERIA (APA, 2013)	IMPLICATIONS FOR FUNCTION
Oppositional defiant disorder	At least a 6-month pattern of angry or irritable mood accompanied by defiant behavior, argumentativeness, and/or vindictiveness, greater than normal behavior Distress in the individual or in others	Negatively affects school, social, and work occupations Difficulty in areas of interpersonal skills, emotional regulation Poor enactment of roles, patterns Expression of problematic habits
Intermittent explosive disorder	Repeated behavioral outbursts out of proportion to provocation that show a failure to manage aggressive impulses that may include verbal aggression and/or damage to property or physical injury to others or animals The behavior is not premeditated or intended to accomplish a particular objective Distress, dysfunction, and/or legal or financial consequences The individual is at least 6 years old	Negatively affects school, social, and work occupations Difficulty in areas of interpersonal skills, emotional regulation Poor enactment of roles, patterns Expression of problematic habits
Conduct disorder	Pattern of behavior that violates the rights of others and may include: • Aggression to people and animals • Destruction of property • Deceitfulness or theft Associated dysfunction In an individual over 18	Negatively affects school, social, and work occupations Difficulty in areas of interpersonal skills, emotional regulation Can contribute to legal difficulties which further affect performance
Pyromania	Deliberate fire setting on more than one occasion, without gain and not for political expression Tension or emotional arousal before setting the fire and/or fascination with fire Associated pleasure or relief when setting fires	Occupations typically unaffected, although work and/or legal difficulties may occur Emotional regulation is impaired Can negatively affect roles, habits, and patterns
Kleptomania	Irresistible impulse to steal objects that are not needed Sense of tension before the theft and pleasure or relief after committing the theft	Occupations typically unaffected, although work and/or legal difficulties may occur Emotional regulation is impaired Can negatively affect roles, habits and patterns

Cultural Considerations

Little has been written about the cultural issues that may relate to this category of diagnosis. It seems likely that differing expectations about childhood behavior and differing beliefs about parenting may affect the emergence and manifestation of these disorders.

Lifespan Considerations

Many of the impulse control disorders first appear during childhood. They are difficult to treat and may result in lifelong issues related to occupational engagement. For this reason, it has been hypothesized that early treatment may be vital in effort to prevent or treat these problems (Finger et al., 2012).

Among older adults, these impulse control disorders are less common, perhaps because the probability of legal and other difficulties earlier in life results in a shorter lifespan. Impulse control difficulties that emerge late in life may signal the onset of a dementing illness (Scott, Hilty, & Brook, 2004).

Internet Resources

American Academy of Child & Adolescent Psychiatry: Conduct Disorder Resource Center
http://www.aacap.org/AACAP/Families_and_Youth/Resource_Centers/Conduct_Disorder_Resource_Center/Home.aspx
Provides reliable information for both consumers and professionals.

Mental Health America
http://www.nmha.org/go/conduct-disorder
A self-help organization with information and support for consumers.

NYU Langone Medical Center, Child Study Center
http://www.aboutourkids.org/families/disorders_treatments/az_disorder_guide/conduct_disorder/support_resources
A great deal of good information about conduct disorder, as well as helpful links to other resources.

CASE STUDY

Joey Reynolds is a 7-year-old boy currently in the second grade. He has attended his current school for 6 months, having transferred in mid-year. His teacher has called Joey's mother, requesting that she attend a conference with the teacher, school psychologist, assistant principal, and occupational therapist to discuss the frequent problems the teacher has had with managing Joey's behavior in the class.

At the conference, the teacher reports that Joey has frequently hit, kicked, and bullied other children and that he shows no remorse about this behavior. His language is vulgar and inappropriate.

Mrs. Reynolds is a single parent who travels for work. Joey often stays with one or another of her extended family or neighbors while she is away. She often leaves town on short notice, and her family members are increasingly reluctant to take care of Joey. Joey's father has not seen him for 3 years. Mrs. Reynolds divorced Mr. Reynolds because he drank to excess and occasionally struck her.

Joey's mother expresses surprise, as she has never felt that Joey's behavior was problematic. She suggests that the school may be at fault, claiming that Joey has never had difficulty in his previous schools. When the assistant principal points out that his most recent prior school suspended him twice, she acknowledges that he may have had one or two episodes in the past.

The school psychologist notes that Joey has reported being at home alone frequently and that he spends the time watching television. He reported happily that he likes watching *Rambo* (Kotchef, 1982) movies and reruns of *The Sopranos* (Chase, 1999-2004).

The team requests, and Mrs. Reynolds reluctantly allows, a complete psychological evaluation, to be completed by the school psychologist. Joey is found to have average intelligence but relatively poor verbal skills and visual-spatial and sequencing deficits. In addition, he has poor understanding of social cues. The psychologist confirms the diagnosis of conduct disorder, and he also believes that Joey has a learning disorder.

THOUGHT QUESTIONS

1. What behaviors suggest that Joey has a problem?
2. What factors in Joey's social history might contribute to the problem?
3. What are some strategies that might be effective in addressing the mental disorders and improving Joey's function?

References

American Psychiatric Association. (2013). *Diagnostic and statistical manual of mental disorders* (5th ed.). Washington, DC: Author.

Baillargeon, R.H., Keenan, K., & Cao, G. (2012). The development of opposition-defiance during toddlerhood: A population-based cohort study. *Journal of Developmental and Behavioral Pediatrics, 33*(8), 608-617.

Brown University Child and Adolescent & Psychopharmacology Update. (2012). Brown University Child & Adolescent Psychopharmacology Update Study proposes new criteria for intermittent explosive disorder in DSM-5. *Brown University Child & Adolescent Psychopharmacology Update, 14*(8), 5-6.

Burke, J.D. (2012). An affective dimension within oppositional defiant disorder symptoms among boys: Personality and psychopathology outcomes into early adulthood. *Journal of Child Psychology and Psychiatry, 53*(11), 1176-1183.

Cederna-Meko, C., Koch, S.M., & Wall, J.R. (2013, March 26). Youth with oppositional defiant disorder at entry into home-based treatment, foster care, and residential treatment. *Journal of Child and Family Studies.* doi:10.1007/s10826-013-9745-y.

Chase, D. (Creator), & Van Patten, J. et al. (1999-2004). *The Sopranos* [Television series]. United States: HBO.

Dishion, T.J., Connell, A., Weaver, C., Shaw, D., Gardner, F., & Wilson, M. (2008). The family check-up with high-risk indigent families: Preventing problem behavior by increasing parents' positive behavior support in early childhood. *Child Development, 79,* 1395-1414.

Doley, R. (2003). Pyromania: Fact or fiction? *British Journal of Criminology, 43*(4), 797-807.

Fairchild, G., Passamonti, L., Hurford, G., Haben, C.C., von dem Hagen, E.A., van Goozen, S.H., . . . Calder, A.J. (2011). Brain structure abnormalities in early-onset and adolescent-onset conduct disorder. *American Journal of Psychiatry, 168*(6), 624-33.

Finger, E.C., Marsh, A., Blair, K.S., Majestic, C., Evangelou, I., Gupta, K., . . . Blair, R.J. (2012). Impaired functional but preserved structural connectivity in limbic white matter tracts in youth with conduct disorder or oppositional defiant disorder plus psychopathic traits. *Psychiatry Research: Neuroimaging, 202*(3), 239-244.

Fite, P.J., Evans, S.C., Cooley, J.L., & Rubens, S.L. (2014). Further evaluation of associations between attention-deficit/hyperactivity and oppositional defiant disorder symptoms and bullying-victimization in adolescence. *Child Psychiatry and Human Development, 45*(1), 32-41.

Freestone, M., Howard, R., Coid, J.W., & Ullrich, S. (2013). Adult antisocial syndrome co-morbid with borderline personality disorder is associated with severe conduct disorder, substance dependence and violent antisociality. *Personality & Mental Health, 7*(1), 11-21.

Grant, J.E., Odlaug, B.L., Davis, A.A., & Kim, S.W. (2009). Legal consequences of kleptomania. *Psychiatric Quarterly, 80*(4), 251-259.

Grant, J.E., Odlaug, B.L., Schreiber, L.R.N., Chamberlain, S.R., & Kim, S.W. (2013). Memantine reduces stealing behavior and impulsivity in kleptomania: A pilot study. *International Clinical Psychopharmacology, 28*(2), 106-111.

Greene, R.W., Biederman, J., Zerwas, S., Monuteaux, M.C., Goring, J.C., & Faraone, S.V. (2002). Psychiatric comorbidity, family dysfunction, and social impairment in referred youth with oppositional defiant disorder. *American Journal of Psychiatry, 159*(7), 1214-1224.

Haas, S.M., Waschbusch, D.A., Pelham, W.E., King, S., Andrade, B.F., & Carrey, N.J. (2011). Treatment response in CD/ADHD children with callous/unemotional traits. *Journal of Abnormal Child Psychology, 39,* 541-552.

Harvard Mental Health Letter (2011). Treating intermittent explosive disorder: Emerging data show medication and cognitive behavioral therapy may help some patients. *Harvard Mental Health Letter, 27*(10), 6.

Johnson, M., Östlund, S., Fransson, G., Landgren, M., Nasic, S., Kadesjö, B., . . . Fernell, E. (2012). Attention-deficit/hyperactivity disorder with oppositional defiant disorder in Swedish children—An open study of collaborative problem solving. *Acta Paediatrica, 101*(6), 624-630.

Kotcheff, T. (Director) (1982). *Rambo* [Motion picture]. United States: Columbia Pictures.

Lara, D.R. (2007). Intermittent explosive disorder is common, has an early age of onset and is associated with the development of other mental disorders in the US population. *Evidence Based Mental Health, 10*(1), 32.

Larsson, B., Fossum, S., Clifford, G., Drugli, M.B., Handegård, B.H., & Mørch, W. (2009). Treatment of oppositional defiant and conduct problems in young Norwegian children: Results of a randomized controlled trial. *European Child & Adolescent Psychiatry, 18*(1), 42-52.

Latimer, K., Wilson, P., Kemp, J., Thompson, L., Sim, F., Gillberg, C., . . . Minnis, H. (2012). Disruptive behaviour disorders: A systematic review of environmental antenatal and early years risk factors. *Child: Care, Health and Development, 38*(5), 611-628.

Lavigne, J.V., Lebailly, S.A., Gouze, K.R., Binns, H.J., Keller, J., & Pate, L. (2010). Predictors and correlates of completing behavioral parent training for the treatment of oppositional defiant disorder in pediatric primary care. *Behavior Therapy, 41*(2), 198-211.

Lindberg, N., Holi, M.M., Tani, P., & Virkkunen, M. (2005). Looking for pyromania: Characteristics of a consecutive sample of Finnish male criminals with histories of recidivist fire-setting between 1973 and 1993. *BMC Psychiatry, 5,* Article 47.

Maas, C., Mason, R., & Candler, C. (October 20, 2008). "When I get mad . . ." *OT Practice, 13*(19), 9-14.

Mandy, W., Skuse, D., Steer, C., St Pourcain, B., & Oliver, B.R. (2013). Oppositionality and socioemotional competence: Interacting risk factors in the development of childhood conduct disorder symptoms. *Journal of the American Academy of Child & Adolescent Psychiatry, 52*(7), 718-727.

Manor-Binyamini, I. (2012). Parenting children with conduct disorder in Israel: Caregiver burden and the sense of coherence. *Community Mental Health Journal, 48*(6), 781-785.

Martel, M.M., Nikolas, M., Jrenigan, K., Friderici, K., & Nigg, J.T. (2012). Diversity in pathways to common childhood disruptive behavior disorders. *Journal of Abnormal Child Psychology, 40*(8), 1223-1236.

Matthys, W., Vanderschuren, L.J.M.J., & Schutter, D.J.L.G. (2013). The neurobiology of oppositional defiant disorder and conduct disorder: Altered functioning in three mental domains. *Development and Psychopathology, 25*(1), 193-207.

Matthys, W., Vanderschuren, L.J.M.J., Schutter, D.J.L.G., & Lochman, J.E. (2012). Impaired neurocognitive functions affect social learning processes in oppositional defiant disorder and conduct disorder: Implications for interventions. *Clinical Child and Family Psychology Review, 15*(3), 234-246.

Maughan, B., & Rutter, M. (2001). Antisocial children grown up. In J. Hill & B. Maughan (Eds.), *Conduct disorders in childhood and adolescence* (pp. 507-552). Cambridge: Cambridge University Press.

McCloskey, M.S., Kleabir, K., Berman, M.E., Chen, E.Y., & Coccaro, E.F. (2010). Unhealthy aggression: Intermittent explosive disorder and adverse physical health outcomes. *Health Psychology, 29*(3), 324-32.

Moffitt, T.E. (2006). Life-course persistent versus adolescence-limited antisocial behavior. In D. Cicchetti & J. Cohen (Eds.), *Developmental psychopathology: Risk, disorder, and adaptation* (2nd ed. pp. 570-598). New York, NY: Wiley.

Montgomery, P., Bjornstad, G., & Dennis, J. (2006). Media-based behavioural treatments for behavioural problems in children. *Cochrane Database of Systematic Reviews,* Issue 1, CD002206. doi:10.1002/14651858.CD002206.pub3.

Mpofu, E., & Crystal, R. (2001). Conduct disorder in children: Challenges, and prospective cognitive behavioural treatments. *Counseling Psychology Quarterly, 14,* 21-32.

Odgers, C.L., Moffitt, T.E., Broadbent, J.M., Dickson, N., Hancox, R.J., Harrington, H., . . . Caspi, A. (2008). Female and male antisocial trajectories: From childhood origins to adult outcomes. *Development and Psychopathology, 20,* 673-716.

Pardini, D.A., Frick, P.J., & Moffitt, T.E. (2010) Building an evidence base for DSM-5 conceptualizations of oppositional defiant disorder and conduct disorder: Introduction to the special section. *Journal of Abnormal Psychology, 119*(4), 683-689.

Pardini, D. A., Stepp, S., Hipwell, A., Stouthamer-Loeber, M., & Loeber, R. (2012). The clinical utility of the proposed DSM-5 callous/unemotional subtype of conduct disorder in young girls. *Journal of the American Academy of Child and Adolescent Psychiatry, 51,* 62-73.

Parks, R.W., Green, R.D.J., Girhis, S., Hunter, M.D., Woodruff, P.W.R., & Spence, S.A. (2005). Response of pyromania to biological treatment in a homeless person. *Neuropsychiatric Disease and Treatment, 1*(3), 277-280.

Reimherr, F.W., Marchant, B.K., Olsen, J.L., Wender, P.H., & Robison, R.J. (2013). Oppositional defiant disorder in adults with ADHD. *Journal of Attention Disorders, 17*(2), 102-113.

Scott, C.L., Hilty, D.M., & Brook, M. (2004). Impulse-control disorders not elsewhere classified. In R.E. Hales & S.C. Yudofsky (Eds.), *Essentials of clinical psychiatry* (2nd ed., pp. 543-566). Arlington, VA: American Psychiatric Publishing.

Séguin, J., & Pilon, M. (2013). Conduct and oppositional defiant disorders. In L.A. Reddy, A.S. Weissman, & J.B. Hale (Eds.), *Neuropsychological assessment and intervention for youth: An evidence-based approach to emotional and behavioral disorders* (pp. 177-200). Washington, DC: American Psychological Association.

Shenk, C.E., Dorn, L.D., Kolko, D.J., Susman, E.J., Noll, J.G., & Bukstein, O.G. (2012). Predicting treatment response for oppositional defiant and conduct disorder using pre-treatment adrenal and gonadal hormones. *Journal of Child and Family Studies, 21*(6), 973-981.

Stepp, S.D., Burke, J.D., Hipwell, A.E., & Loeber, R. (2012). Trajectories of attention deficit hyperactivity disorder and oppositional defiant disorder symptoms as precursors of borderline personality disorder symptoms in adolescent girls. *Journal of Abnormal Child Psychology, 40*(1), 7-20.

Talih, F.R. (2011). Kleptomania and potential exacerbating factors: A review and case report. *Innovations in Clinical Neuroscience, 8*(10), 35-39.

Thomas, R., & Zimmer-Gembeck, M.J. (2007). Behavioral outcomes of parent-child interaction therapy and triple p-positive parenting program: A review and meta-analysis. *Journal of Abnormal Child Psychology, 35,* 475-495.

Webbink, D., Vujic, S., Koning, P., & Martin, N.G. (2012). The effects of childhood conduct disorder on human capital. *Health Economics, 21*(8), 928-45.

Webster-Stratton, C. (2000). Oppositional-defiant and conduct-disordered children. In M. Hersen & R.T. Ammerman (Eds.), *Advanced abnormal child psychology* (pp. 387-412). Mahwah, NJ: Lawrence Erlbaum Associates.

Wichstrøm, L., Berg-Nielsen, R.S., Angold, A., Egger, H.L., Solheim, E., & Sveen, T.H. (2012). Prevalence of psychiatric disorders in preschoolers. *Journal of Child Psychology and Psychiatry, 53*(6), 695-705.

Woolfenden, S.R., Williams, K., & Peat, J. (2001). Family and parenting interventions in children and adolescents with conduct disorder and delinquency aged 10-17. *Cochrane Database of Systematic Reviews,* Issue 2, CD003015. doi:10.1002/14651858.CD003015.

Substance-Related and Addictive Disorders

Learning Outcomes

By the end of this chapter, readers will be able to:
- Describe the symptoms of substance-related and addictive disorders
- Differentiate among the substance-related and addictive disorders on the basis of symptoms and onset
- Identify the causes of the substance-related and addictive disorders
- Discuss the ways in which substance-related and addictive disorders affect daily function
- Describe treatment strategies for substance-related and addictive disorders
- Discuss occupational therapy interventions for substance-related and addictive disorders

Bonder B.
Psychopathology and Function, Fifth Edition (pp 315-350).
© 2015 SLACK Incorporated.

KEY WORDS

- Substance use
- Intoxication
- Tolerance
- Withdrawal
- Addiction

- Delirium tremens
- Fetal alcohol syndrome
- 12-step program
- Gateway drug

CASE VIGNETTE

Mr. Akmanian is a 30-year-old man who worked for the United Postal Service until he sustained a back injury 3 years ago. He has been on disability since then, and he has refused offers to resume work in a less physically demanding position. He had his own apartment, but he now lives with his mother, a retired teacher.

His injury was managed with physical therapy and pain medication. Mr. Akmanian was half-hearted in his participation in physical therapy, attending sporadically and doing none of the recommended home program. Recently, his physician terminated treatment because he believed that Mr. Akmanian was showing signs of a substance use disorder. These signs included requests for early refills for his medication and complaints that the medication was not working. The physician referred him to a substance abuse clinic, but, so far, Mr. Akmanian has refused to go.

THOUGHT QUESTIONS

1. Do you feel that Mr. Akmanian has a substance-related problem?
2. What specific behaviors suggest this?
3. In what ways do you feel Mr. Akmanian's occupational performance has or might suffer?

SUBSTANCE-RELATED AND ADDICTIVE DISORDERS

SUBSTANCE/MEDICATION-INDUCED MENTAL DISORDERS
- Alcohol
  - Alcohol use disorder
  - Alcohol intoxication
  - Alcohol withdrawal
- Caffeine
  - Caffeine intoxication
  - Caffeine withdrawal

- Cannabis
  - Cannabis use disorder
  - Cannabis intoxication
  - Cannabis withdrawal
- Hallucinogens
  - Phencyclidine use disorder
  - Other hallucinogen use disorder
  - Phencyclidine intoxication
  - Other hallucinogen intoxication
  - Hallucinogen persisting perception disorder

(continued)

SUBSTANCE-RELATED AND ADDICTIVE DISORDERS

(CONTINUED)

- Inhalants
  - Inhalant use disorder
  - Inhalant intoxication
- Opioids
  - Opioid use disorder
  - Opioid intoxication
  - Opioid withdrawal
- Sedatives, hypnotics, and anxiolytics
  - Sedative, hypnotic, or anxiolytic use disorder
  - Sedative, hypnotic, or anxiolytic intoxication
  - Sedative, hypnotic, or anxiolytic withdrawal
- Stimulants
  - Stimulant use disorder
    - Amphetamine-type substance
    - Cocaine
- Stimulant intoxication
  - Amphetamine-type substance
    - Without perceptual disturbances
    - With perceptual disturbances
  - Cocaine
    - Without perceptual disturbances
    - With perceptual disturbances
- Stimulant withdrawal
- Tobacco
  - Tobacco use disorder
  - Tobacco withdrawal

NON–SUBSTANCE-RELATED

- Gambling disorder

The chapter on substance-related and addictive disorders is one of the most altered in the *Diagnostic and Statistical Manual of Mental Disorders* (DSM). It is also among the most extensive, incorporating considerable detail and specificity about substance-related disorders overall and each specific substance cluster. As is true for the fifth edition of the DSM (DSM-5; American Psychiatric Association [APA], 2013), the current chapter will be formatted somewhat differently than those that have come before. This chapter will provide an overview of substance use disorders and substance-induced disorders (i.e., intoxication, withdrawal, and other substance/medication-induced mental disorders such as psychotic disorders, bipolar, depressive disorders). This overview will be followed by a brief summary of the diagnostic listings for each substance cluster, with a description of the unique features of that cluster. Implications for occupational therapy for all substance use problems will be presented at the end of the chapter.

As shown in the Substance Abuse and Addictive Disorders box, the list of possible diagnoses in this category is a long one, and it includes a number of ways to provide detailed information about the nature of the substance use disorder in a particular situation. One challenge in this grouping of disorders is the fact that popularity of various substances ebbs and flows, and new substances appear frequently. These can include designer drugs (Dahl, 2013), use of prescription drugs traditionally thought of as serving a "bridging" function when individuals withdraw from drug use (e.g., methadone; O'Neill, 2013), and new substances, such as synthetic cannabinoids, currently being marketed as "spice" and "K2" (at least as this book went to press; they may have new names by now) (Vandrey, Dunn, Fry, & Girling, 2012).

You will notice that the term *abuse* does not appear. Rather, substance use problems are identified based on immediate use, intoxication (for those substances that can cause what is typically considered intoxication), and withdrawal. A significant number of specifiers in each category allow for still more detail about the individual circumstances. These specifiers include severity (mild, moderate, severe); the use of more than one substance; the presence of other mental disorders; combinations of use, intoxication, and withdrawal features. For some substances that may or may not cause perceptual disturbances, the presence or absence of those disturbances can also be noted.

Substance use, as the name implies, is the intake of the substance (orally, intravenously, via smoking, or inhaling). Use results in cognitive, behavioral, and physiological symptoms, with apparent changes in brain circuits that last beyond immediate intake (APA, 2013). As described in the DSM-5, substance use is diagnosed when there is a pathological pattern of behavior associated with ingesting the substance. For the 10 classes of substances included in the categorization, the following consistent criteria apply in diagnosing a substance use disorder: "impaired control, social impairment, risky use, and pharmacological criteria" (APA, 2013, p. 483). Substance use is a long-term behavior, as opposed to **intoxication,** which describes the immediate effects of the substance.

Impaired control reflects a persistent need to use the substance, with accompanying craving, increase in the frequency or amount of the substance used, substantial investment of time and effort in obtaining the substance, and the possibility that the individual wants to cut down and makes unsuccessful attempts to do so (APA, 2013). Social impairment is actually a broad descriptor for functional impairment in several or most occupations. As the individual spends more time and energy securing and using the substance, work, home life, social activities (other than those associated with substance use), and leisure diminish or become dysfunctional. Risky use, the third category of criteria, reflects the fact that many of these substances are illegal so that obtaining them is associated with risk; even those that are legal may carry health risks that the individual ignores.

Pharmacological criteria describe biological changes associated with the substance (APA, 2013). **Tolerance** is a need to increase the dose as the body accommodates to the substance. **Withdrawal** is the term used to describe the physiological symptoms that can accompany reduced use of the substance or the gradual decrease of the substance in the body as it is eliminated. Typically, when both tolerance and withdrawal symptoms are present, the substance use disorder is labeled as an **addiction**. Keep in mind, of course, that some medically necessary drugs may lead to tolerance that requires gradually increased dosage, and a number have withdrawal symptoms as well. Because such medications are needed to control a medical symptom (e.g., a cardiovascular problem), they do not fall into the substance-related disorders as conceptualized in the DSM framework. Table 17-1 shows the prevalence of the various substance-related and addictive disorders.

Substance/Medication-Induced Mental Disorders

As described in the DSM-5 (APA, 2013), these substance/medication-induced mental disorders are most often temporary, and sometimes severe central nervous system (CNS) syndromes are caused by any of a very large number of substances. These might include the 10 categories listed in the sections that follow, but they can also include a wide range of other medications. For example, some individuals have a severe reaction to diphenhydramine (Benedryl), which is a drug used most often for nasal and lung congestion (Brunton, Chabner, & Knollmann, 2011). The medication can cause a dystonic reaction that includes mental confusion and dizziness. As the drug is eliminated from the body, these effects generally resolve. Many medications have similar CNS side effects.

		TABLE 17-1	
		PREVALENCE OF SUBSTANCE ABUSE	
Disorder	Prevalence	Gender Ratio (M:F)	Source
Alcohol	82%[a]		NIDA, 2012b
Caffeine			
Cannabis	34.8%		NIDA, 2012b
Hallucinogens	0.6% to 1.7%	More males	Wu et al., 2008
Inhalants	9.7%		Wu & Ringwalt, 2006
Opioids			
Heroin	1.1%		NIDA, 2012b
Sedatives, hypnotics, anxiolytics	4.8%		NIDA, 2012b
Stimulants			
Amphetamines	5.3%		NIDA, 2012b
Cocaine	16.3%		NIDA, 2012b
Tobacco	68%		NIDA, 2012b
Non-substance: gambling	1% to 5%		Rantala & Sulkunen, 2012

[a]NIDA data are for "any use," not specifically for abuse or addiction.

Criteria for substance/medication-induced mental disorders include significant symptoms with accompanying history, examination, or laboratory findings that support the relationship between those symptoms and the use of the substance (APA, 2013).

Substance/medication-induced mental disorder is an important diagnosis for clinicians to recognize because it can occur in many medical situations. The list of medications that can cause CNS side effects is a long one, and therapists may need to monitor clients in rehabilitation, acute care, and other settings to detect these symptoms so that medication can be adjusted. The description herein of the categories of substance/medication-induced disorders will provide a more extensive discussion of this disorder, as will Chapter 20.

Intoxication Disorders

Each of the substance categories listed includes a diagnosis of intoxication that describes the symptoms of current use of the substance. The symptoms vary, depending on the effects of the substance, but overall the diagnostic criteria are common across substances, including recent intake of the substance with associated problematic behavioral or psychological changes (APA, 2013). Those behavioral or psychological changes occur during or shortly after use of the substance. The specific behaviors for the various classes of substances will be described. The key factor to keep in mind about these disorders is the fact that intoxication is a short-term diagnosis reflecting the immediate impact of the substance.

Withdrawal Disorders

Similarly, withdrawal disorders occur in the hours, days, and sometimes weeks after immediate cessation of a substance. The severity, duration, and specific symptoms vary, depending on the individual's history of use, and will be described in this chapter. In general, withdrawal disorders are characterized by physical or psychological symptoms caused by cessation of intake of a substance that has been used heavily for a prolonged period (APA, 2013). Those symptoms occurring after cessation of intake cause distress or dysfunction. The nature and extent of withdrawal symptoms, along with the response to treatment during this period immediately after stopping substance use, can determine long-term outcomes. For those substances (e.g., heroin, tobacco) where the withdrawal symptoms are prolonged and cause significant discomfort, the substance-related disorder may be more difficult to address.

Alcohol

Alcohol is a CNS depressant. Although alcohol may cause a brief sense of excitement, it ultimately has the effect of slowing responses over time. The "high" that accompanies alcohol use is actually a slowing of the CNS and autonomic function. In cases of overdose, death may occur as a result of respiratory or cardiac slowing. For alcohol use, death can occur as a result of a single episode, as is seen all too often in circumstances where young people are experimenting (e.g., fraternity parties or hazing in college). Thus, both immediate and long-term excessive alcohol use carries significant risks.

Alcohol Use Disorder

Diagnostic criteria for alcohol use disorder include a problematic pattern of alcohol use, with significant distress or impairment over a 12-month period (APA, 2013). Alcohol is taken in larger amounts over a longer period than the person had intended, and efforts to control its use are unsuccessful. A significant amount of time is spent obtaining, using, and recovering from alcohol use, and the individual experiences both cravings and difficulty with work, home, or school function. Other important activities (e.g., leisure) are given up and use is continued in hazardous situations (e.g., driving). In addition, use is continued even when the individual knows she or he has a problem, and there are signs of tolerance (need for greater amounts to achieve the same effect) and withdrawal (physical symptoms when not using the substance).

Alcohol Intoxication

For alcohol intoxication, the typical behavioral and psychological changes that occur include slurred speech, incoordination, unsteady gait, nystagmus, impairment of attention or memory, and—in very high intake situations—stupor, coma, or even death. Every year, there are reports of high school or college students who die as a result of excessive alcohol intake, often as a result of peer pressure.

Alcohol Withdrawal

Withdrawal from alcohol is characterized by autonomic hyperactivity, hand tremor, insomnia, nausea or vomiting, hallucinations, psychomotor agitation, anxiety, and—especially if use has been long-term or particularly excessive—seizures and sometimes death. Long-term users may also experience a condition known as **delirium tremens** (Eyer et al.,

2011). This condition, characterized by seizures, hallucinations, and severe tremors, occurs in approximately 5% of individuals with chronic alcohol use disorders who stop drinking. Of that group, between 5% and 15% will die, although treatment with benzodiazepines has greatly reduced mortality.

Etiology

Several theories exist about the emergence of alcohol use disorders. During the early part of the 20th century (i.e., the pre-Prohibition and Prohibition years), alcoholism was thought to be a moral failure. Since that time, it has come to be viewed as a disease, which is now the commonly held explanation. One theory holds that a genetic predisposition to alcoholism may be triggered by certain environmental factors (Hasin & Katz, 2010). A family pattern, evident even when children are raised by adoptive parents, suggests some genetic component in at least some cases (Prescott, Madden, & Stallings, 2006). Familial alcoholism seems to have an earlier onset and worse prognosis than the nonfamilial type. Although the origins of alcoholism are not entirely clear, individual and racial differences in alcohol tolerance, separate from dependence and abuse, have been noted. For example, some Black families have a gene that results in faster metabolism and less effect from alcohol consumption (Scott & Taylor, 2007). Such families have a lower rate of alcohol abuse.

Two neurological pathways seem to be involved with addiction, including alcohol addiction (APA, 2005; Clay, Allen, & Parran, 2008). The first is the mesolimbic dopamine reward pathway. This pathway is essential for survival, but it can be altered by drug abuse in a way that causes uncontrolled craving for the substance. The second is the prefrontal cortex, which is responsible for decision making. Drug abuse may change the mechanisms for controlling reward response so that "go" signals are accelerated and "stop" signals are impaired.

Women who are alcoholics have later onset and drink less, but progress more rapidly through the stages of the disorder (Kim & Hashimoto, 2012). Strong evidence exists of a link between trauma (e.g., sexual and physical abuse) and substance abuse among women (Maniglio, 2011). Female alcoholism is of particular concern because of the potential for harm to the fetus during pregnancy. Chronic alcohol abuse during pregnancy causes **fetal alcohol syndrome**, which is manifested by retardation and CNS damage in the infant (Jones & Streissguth, 2010).

As will be discussed later in this chapter, alcohol abuse is often seen in combination with other psychiatric disorders (Van Dam, Earleywine, & DiGiacomo, 2008). This "dual diagnosis" is a particular problem, as the two or more disorders affecting these individuals may reinforce each other—such as in the case of an individual who self-medicates with sedatives to reduce symptoms of an anxiety disorder—thereby complicating treatment (Hilarski & Wodarski, 2001).

Alcohol abuse is of particular concern in adolescents. According to the 2007 National Youth Risk Behavior Survey (U.S. Centers for Disease Control, 2007), 23.8% of adolescents had their first drink before the age of 13, and 26% of students had five or more drinks in the span of a couple of hours at least once in the previous 30 days.

For adolescents, as for women, a link exists between early experiences of abuse and substance abuse and from substance abuse to juvenile violence. Adverse experiences early in life lead to early onset of drinking and associated problem drinking (Rothman, Edwards, Heeren, & Hingson, 2008). Parental divorce, living with a problem drinker, sexual abuse, and living with someone with a psychiatric disorder are all associated with early onset of drinking. These problems are also associated with the probability that the individual will use substances as a way to cope.

Prognosis

Alcohol abuse is one of the more treatable substance-related disorders (Gordis, 2009). Individuals who participate in 12-step programs, cognitive behavioral interventions, or motivational enhancement therapy all show substantial reductions in drinking, and that reduction is maintained over a 12-month follow-up period. It is possible, although not fully demonstrated, that combining one or more of these approaches with pharmacological approaches may be even more effective.

Individuals with problematic use of both alcohol and drugs and who show significant dependence symptoms have a worse prognosis (Karno, Grella, Niv, Warda, & Moore, 2008).

A great deal of research exists on intervention for alcohol use, intoxication, and withdrawal (Huebner & Kantor, 2011). The best available evidence suggests that no one treatment works best for everyone, but there is an array of choices that can be effective, ranging from cognitive behavioral therapy to various forms of group therapy to **12-step programs** like Alcoholics Anonymous. Alcoholics Anonymous (Vaillant, 1999) and other 12-step programs emphasize social and spiritual support. Prognosis is good for individuals who participate actively in these programs. Vaillant (1999) used the analogy of diabetes to describe the needed course of treatment in alcohol addiction. Like diabetes, alcoholism is a chronic disease that requires careful monitoring and consistent intervention over the long term.

Alcoholism is a serious problem, with major physical and lifestyle consequences (Interdisciplinary Faculty Development Program in Substance Abuse Education, 2000). Individuals who continue to abuse may suffer liver damage, cognitive impairment, peripheral neuropathy, cardiomyopathy, chronic pancreatitis, and various cancers of the upper respiratory or gastrointestinal tract. In addition, social isolation, unemployment, and possibly homelessness or incarceration may occur for long-term chronic alcohol abusers.

Caffeine

Caffeine is the most commonly used psychoactive substance around the world (Hammond & Gold, 2008). Increasingly, some positive health benefits have been recognized and reported. Nevertheless, some individuals have an adverse reaction to excessive amounts of caffeine, and many individuals who are regular caffeine users find it difficult to reduce or eliminate their caffeine use. Note that there is no "caffeine use" diagnosis; this is due to the fact that the use of caffeine is ubiquitous, and a substantial number of people would have the diagnosis if it existed. Rather, problems emerge from excessive intake that cause symptoms of intoxication, and efforts to stop using caffeine—with associated symptoms—cause individuals distress.

Caffeine Intoxication

Caffeine intoxication is diagnosed when the intoxication criteria are met, with at least five behavioral or psychological symptoms, including restlessness, nervousness, excitement, insomnia, flushed face, diuresis, gastrointestinal disturbance, muscle twitching, rambling thought or speech, cardiac rhythm alterations, periods of excessive energy, and psychomotor agitation (APA, 2013).

Caffeine Withdrawal

Caffeine withdrawal symptoms occur within 24 hours of last caffeine use, and include headache, fatigue, depressed mood, difficulty concentrating, and sometimes flu-like symptoms.

Because caffeine is so widely used, and because of the apparent health benefits of caffeinated drinks (although it is unclear whether caffeine or some other substance in these drinks confers the benefit), it is easy to overlook the fact that there is at least moderate evidence that, for some people, caffeine use can become problematic (Ogawa & Ueki, 2007). Ogawa and Ueki (2007) reported that approximately 30% of coffee drinkers in one study indicated having had at least three symptoms of intoxication or withdrawal at some point.

Relatively little research exists about caffeine intoxication and withdrawal, although certainly some individuals seek help as a consequence of the symptoms. In such cases, an occupational therapist might get involved to assist the client in finding alternative strategies to achieve the desired outcomes. For example, if coffee drinking is a significant social activity, other social activities might be substituted instead. If caffeine is ingested largely to manage a fatigue syndrome, strategies for increasing energy through alternative means (e.g., exercise, meditation) and for energy conservation might be helpful. However, it is not common for an occupational therapist to be involved in working with these individuals.

Cannabis

This is a very interesting time in the history of the social constructions of cannabis (marijuana) use in the United States. For many years, cannabis has been illegal, and its use is strongly discouraged because of perceived problems associated with ingestion and its reputation as a **"gateway drug"** that begins a path toward use of more damaging substances (Walker, Venner, Hill, Meyers, & Miller, 2004). Cannabis is the most widely used illicit substance (Substance Abuse and Mental Health Services Administration [SAMHSA], 2011). It has resulted in significant legal difficulties for large numbers of adolescents and young adults because, in spite of its widespread use, it has been illegal. However, as of 2013, 20 states plus the District of Columbia have made cannabis legal for medicinal purposes (Boden, Gross, Babson, & Bonn-Miller, 2013), and Colorado and Washington State have legalized its recreational use. This means that—as is the case with caffeine and nicotine, both of which are legal but can be abused—the diagnostic criteria reflect the individual's lack of control for the substance and a set of problematic behaviors and emotions associated with its use.

The classic picture of cannabis use found in the popular media shows a young slacker who is lethargic and congenial, as in *Pineapple Express* (Apatow & Robertson, 2008), the Cheech and Chong movies, and *Super Troopers* (Perello, 2001). In fact, of the many illicit substances that are abused, cannabis is probably less problematic than others. Nevertheless, because the drug can cause perceptual distortions, it can be hazardous to drive while intoxicated. In addition, because cannabis is typically smoked, it can lead to lung and cardiovascular disease (PubMed Health, 2012).

Cannabis Use Disorder

The diagnostic criteria for cannabis use disorder include a problematic pattern of cannabis use, with significant impairment or distress over a 12-month period (APA, 2013). The pattern includes taking more than intended; being unsuccessful in controlling its use; spending significant time getting, using, or recovering from cannabis use; cravings; failure to meet obligations or giving up important activities; using in hazardous situations; and continued use in spite of these problems. The individual experiences signs of tolerance (need for greater amounts to achieve the same effect) and withdrawal (physical symptoms when not using the substance).

Cannabis Intoxication

Behavioral and psychological symptoms of cannabis intoxication include conjunctival irritation, increased appetite, dry mouth, and tachycardia, in addition to the symptoms of intoxication listed previously (APA, 2013).

Cannabis Withdrawal

The behavioral and psychological symptoms that accompany the general withdrawal symptoms listed previously include irritability or anger, anxiety, sleep difficulty, decreased appetite, restlessness, depressed mood, and flu-like symptoms (APA, 2013).

Cannabis-related disorders seem to be primarily socially/environmentally related. Evidence exists that use is associated with social anxiety (Buckner, Zvolensky, & Schmidt, 2012). Family environment, specifically parents' marital status, is associated as well; parental divorce is related to increased teen use (Hayatbakhsh, Williams, Bor, & Najman, 2013). Other predictors of cannabis use include living alone, coping motives for cannabis use, and recent negative life events, such as financial difficulties (van der Pol et al., 2013). The extent to which use becomes problematic is related to age at first use (Kirisci et al., 2013). However, many cannabis users do not progress to a dysfunctional level of use.

Prognosis

For most cannabis users, the activity either does not progress or ceases entirely. Several specific psychological factors may predict prolonged, heavy, and problematic use. These factors include a tendency toward what has been labeled "approach bias," as opposed to executive regulatory cognitive function (Cousijn, Goudriaan, & Wiers, 2011). This means that the substance is sufficiently attractive, and the required cognitive regulation processes are sufficiently weak for habitual users that they may find it difficult to stop. In addition, there seems to be an inverse relationship between emotional clarity and problematic cannabis use (Boden et al., 2013).

Dependence and abuse generally develop over a relatively long period of time (Walker et al., 2004). Dependence and abuse is characterized by increasing frequency of use, rather than increased amounts at a given time. Prolonged use may lead to lethargy, anhedonia, and memory and attention deficits. Some changes in perceptual skills have also been noted. However, function is not as severely impaired as in other forms of substance abuse. Prognosis is better in many cases; cannabis seems to be a drug with which many adolescents experiment but then stop using. Information about treatment strategies is limited (Copeland, 2004), although cognitive behavioral treatment seems to be effective.

Hallucinogens

Drugs in this category include d-lysergic acid diethylamide (LSD), sometimes called acid, blotter acid, or window-pane; peyote; psilocybin; and phencyclidine (PCP), also known as angel dust, super grass, and killer weed. LSD was well-known and heavily used in the 1960s, whereas PCP is a more recent and more dangerous drug. A more recent addition to the list of hallucinogens is MDMA (3, 4-methylenedioxymethamphetamine; Wu, Ringwalt, Mannelli, & Patkar, 2008) also known as Ecstasy. New hallucinogens are emerging, such as *salvia divinorum*, marketed as an "herbal high" (SAMHSA, 2008).

These hallucinogenic drugs cause hallucinations, feelings of depersonalization/derealization, and distortions of time and perception (SAMHSA, 2008). They can also cause mood swings, elevated body temperature (a particular problem with MDMA), psychotic-like effects, and seizures.

Phencyclidine Use Disorder

Phencyclidine is described separately from the other hallucinogens, perhaps because of the documented severe, potentially long-term consequences of use. It is much less frequently used than other hallucinogens, but it has significant behavioral and psychological consequences (Wu et al., 2008). PCP use is associated with inpatient referrals, significant legal history, and past-year violence (Crane, Easton, & Devine, 2013). PCP causes a schizophrenia-like psychosis by blocking certain neurotransmission processes (Javitt, Zukin, Heresco-Levy, & Umbricht, 2012). It has been reported that PCP causes unusual levels of violence and lack of emotional and behavioral control, leading to legal difficulties as a result of assault and other violent behaviors.

Diagnostic criteria for PCP use disorder include taking PCP in larger amounts of over a longer period than the person had intended, and efforts to control its use are unsuccessful (APA, 2013). Significant time is spent obtaining, using, and recovering from PCP use, and the individual experiences both cravings and difficulty with work, home, or school function as a result of use. Other important activities (e.g., leisure) are given up and use is continued in hazardous situations (e.g., driving). In addition, PCP use is continued even when the individual knows she or he has a problem, and there are signs of tolerance.

Other Hallucinogen Use Disorder

LSD has a longer history of use than PCP, and for a period of time it was a drug of choice for the counterculture in the 1960s (Stevens, 1998), although its use is not widespread at present. Peyote has been used by indigenous populations as part of religious ceremonies for generations. More recently, Ecstasy has become the most commonly used hallucinogen, with approximately half of all individuals who have used hallucinogens in the past year reporting that Ecstasy was the drug they used (Wu et al., 2008). Ecstasy is a frequent "party" drug, used by young people at bars and social gatherings as a way to heighten their experience. One notable risk is significantly increased body temperature, which is especially likely when the user is in a crowded room dancing or otherwise exerting himself or herself physically. Cases have been reported of seizures and death as a consequence of hyperthermia or excessive water consumption (Ben-Abraham, Szold, Rudick, & Weinbroum, 2003).

Diagnostic criteria for other hallucinogen use disorder include taking the hallucinogenic substance in larger amounts over a longer period than the person had intended and efforts to control its use are unsuccessful (APA, 2013). Significant time is spent obtaining, using, and recovering from hallucinogen use, and the individual experiences both cravings and difficulty with work, home, or school function as a result of use. Other important activities are given up, and use is continued in hazardous situations. Further, use is continued even when the individual knows she or he has a problem, and there are signs of tolerance.

Phencyclidine Intoxication

The signs of PCP intoxication are associated with dose (National Institute on Drug Abuse [NIDA], 2009). Low doses of PCP cause characteristic signs of intoxication (unsteady gait, slurred speech). High doses may cause seizures, paranoia, hallucinations, suicidal impulses, and aggressive behavior. Some individuals become detached, but others behave in an unpredictable and violent fashion, sometimes committing bizarre acts of violence.

Behavioral and psychological correlates of PCP intoxication include nystagmus, hypertension or tachycardia, numbness or lowered response to pain, ataxia, dysarthria, muscle rigidity, and—in severe cases—seizures or coma (APA, 2013).

Other Hallucinogen Intoxication

Other hallucinogen intoxication includes such behavioral and psychological signs as pupillary dilation, tachycardia, sweating, palpitations, blurred vision, tremors, and incoordination (APA, 2013).

Hallucinogen Persisting Perception Disorder

Long-term use of hallucinogens can lead to memory loss, difficulties with speech and thinking, depression, weight loss, and liver function abnormalities. Characteristic brain changes are found in long-term users that can result in persistent changes in perception (Ellison, Keys, & Noguchi, 1999). One college student who regularly used LSD required long-term hospitalization because his hallucinations and delusions did not resolve. Ultimately, he was diagnosed with schizophrenia. It could not be determined whether he used LSD as a result of emerging symptoms of schizophrenia or whether the LSD use led to the schizophrenia. However, he experienced severe, long-term psychological symptoms with accompanying loss of function.

Diagnostic criteria for hallucinogen persisting perception disorder include continuation of perceptual symptoms after substance use has stopped, with these symptoms causing distress or dysfunction (APA, 2013).

Etiology

Initial use of hallucinogens usually occurs as a result of experimentation with drugs. Personality disorders or adjustment problems may be predisposing factors because they might encourage such experimentation. Hallucinogens and PCP may be contaminated with or taken with other substances, particularly cannabis and alcohol. LSD, which has had periods of intense research interest about its possible medical value, has received somewhat more positive attention in recent years (Slater, 2012).

Prognosis

Users find the effects of hallucinogenic drugs unpredictable (NIDA, 2012a). For some individuals, one exposure to the negative effects, particularly during an early experience with the drug, is sufficient to end their interest in the drug. Occasionally, a pattern of long-term abuse may emerge. Heavier use has been correlated with flashbacks, possibly resulting from neurological changes caused by the drug or as a result of a hysterical reaction. There is no unanimity about the existence of this phenomenon.

Most individuals abuse these hallucinogenic drugs for relatively short periods of time before resuming previous activities or moving on to other substances. For most individuals, these drugs prompt experimentation but not usually long-term addiction. PCP is among the more dangerous of these substances, as it is easily produced in a laboratory and thus readily available. It has particularly damaging consequences, including the potential for brain damage, sometimes after very few uses (NIDA, 2012b); psychotic reactions, and violent rage. PCP users are frequently brought to emergency departments as a result of either unpleasant psychological effects or due to overdoses. These individuals can become violent or suicidal and must be watched closely.

Inhalants

Inhalable substances are readily available, making them a substance of choice for teens (Shamblen & Miller, 2012). Use of inhalable substances can have significant medical and psychological consequences, as it can lead to depression, suicide, and long-term impaired memory and learning. A particular challenge in addressing inhalant use is the fact that many ordinary substances (e.g., spray paint, glue, nail polish remover) can be targets of abuse, and restricting access can be very difficult. Users tend to be a step ahead of regulators, identifying new substances as quickly as existing ones are restricted.

Inhalant Use Disorder

Inhalant use involves volatile solvents inhaled to cause euphoria (Shamblen & Miller, 2012). Because the substances are typically toxic, they can cause significant physical damage—even on first use—and that damage can be cumulative over time.

Diagnostic criteria for inhalant use disorder include using the inhalants in larger amounts over a longer period than the person had intended, and efforts to control its use are unsuccessful (APA, 2013). Significant time is spent obtaining, using, and recovering from use, and the individual experiences both cravings and difficulty with work, home, or school function as a result of use. Other important activities are given up and use is continued in hazardous situations. Further, use is continued even when the individual knows she or he has a problem, and there are signs of tolerance.

Inhalant Intoxication

The immediate adverse effects of inhalant use include both high-risk behaviors due to disinhibition and adverse events associated with the toxic nature of the substances (Garland & Howard, 2011). Young people who use these substances frequently, and those who use inhalants to reduce other negative psychological states such as depression and anxiety, are at higher risk for these outcomes.

Behavioral correlates of inhalant intoxication include dizziness, nystagmus, incoordination, slurred speech, unsteady gait, lethargy, depressed reflexes, psychomotor retardation, tremor, generalized muscle weakness, blurred vision, and—in severe cases—stupor or coma (APA, 2013).

Etiology

Initiation to inhalant use is typically social. Young people whose friends and siblings use inhalants are more likely to do so themselves. They are also more likely to overlook any possible risks related to their use (Perron & Howard, 2008).

When an individual begins to use the substances, he or she responds to the fact that inhalants increase dopamine production in the brain, which activates the pleasure centers (Scott & Scott, 2012). This increases craving and drug consumption. Both low and high frequency users report pleasurable experiences during inhalant intoxication, with high frequency users also reporting adverse experiences such as depression and suicidal ideation. However, these high frequency users also reported more euphoria and grandiosity while intoxicated.

Prognosis

The prevalence of inhalant use is considerably lower than the use of alcohol or cannabis; however, the consequences, even for short-term use, are more severe (Shamblen & Miller, 2012). In addition, there are substantial long-term consequences, including persistent,

Figure 17-1. Heroin use causes significant health and functional problems. (©2014 Shutterstock.com.)

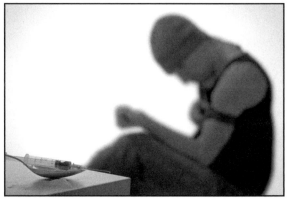

disabling neurological defects (Cairney et al., 2013). Those who begin use of inhalants before age 18 are more likely to use alcohol to excess and to be in substance abuse treatment as adults (Wu & Ringwalt, 2006). Inhalant use in adolescence is associated with suicide and criminal behavior (Shamblen & Miller, 2012).

Opioids

Abuse of opioids is a public health crisis (Pade, Cardon, Hoffman, & Beppert, 2012). This group of drugs includes some that are clearly illicit, such as heroin, and others that may be prescribed as analgesics, anesthetics, or cough suppressants. The latter group includes codeine, hydromorphone (Dilaudid), methadone, hydrocodone (Vicodin), oxycodone with aspirin or acetaminophen (Percodan, Percocet), and, more recently, oxycodone (OxyContin; National Institutes of Health [NIH], 2011). Used in properly supervised medical settings, none of the drugs in the latter group should lead to dependence; however, many of them are used without supervision or are obtained through illicit sources.

Among the illicit drugs, heroin is used with considerably less frequency than some of the drugs described in other sections of this chapter (for example, cannabis or cocaine; NIDA, 2012a). However, heroin use is a particular challenge because of its substantial impact on health and function (Figure 17-1). Methadone is a special problem. Used as a treatment for opioid addiction, it is itself addicting, which leads to abuse in some situations. Newer drugs have the same effect in minimizing withdrawal symptoms from opioids but without producing the high that is associated with methadone.

In particular, prescription misuse is a significant problem in the United States, having tripled since 1990 (Ling, Mooney, & Hillhouse, 2011). Use of marijuana, hallucinogens, cocaine, sedatives, and tranquilizers, as well as alcohol abuse, were all associated with prior nonmedical use of prescription opioids (Becker, Sullivan, Tetrault, Desai, & Fiellin, 2008). A rapid increase has been seen in the abuse of OxyContin and Vicodin (National Institute on Drug Abuse Research Report Series, 2011).

Opioid Use Disorder

Opioid use disorder is the category that is applied to sustained use of any of the opioids, including heroin, but also the nonprescription use of pain medications such as codeine. Long-term use is associated with both dysfunction and poor psychological and physical health, as will be described.

Diagnostic criteria for opioid use disorder include taking the substance in larger amounts over a longer period than the person had intended, and efforts to control its use are unsuccessful (APA, 2013). Significant time is spent obtaining, using, and recovering from use, and the individual experiences both cravings and difficulty with work, home, or school function as a result of use. Other important activities are given up, and use is continued in hazardous situations. Use is continued even when the individual knows she or he has a problem, and there are signs of tolerance and withdrawal (i.e., physical symptoms when not using the substance).

Opioid Intoxication

Use of opioids other than for pain control can lead to immediate intoxication, characterized by drowsiness, lethargy, cognitive changes, and possible hallucinations.

Behavioral correlates of opioid intoxication include constriction of pupils, slurred speech, impaired memory and attention, and drowsiness or coma (APA, 2013). A particular issue of opioid use is that, because many of these drugs (especially heroin) are illicit, there is no control over the quality of the substance. From time to time, users inadvertently overdose because the substance is of a higher concentration than usual. A single use of some of these substances can lead to death, particularly when the concentration is unexpected.

Opioid Withdrawal

Long-term use of opioids leads to increased tolerance and habituation. For that reason, withdrawal is a particular challenge. During withdrawal, the individual may have flu-like symptoms, hallucinations (especially tactile hallucinations like a sense of ants crawling under the skin), anorexia, depression, muscle aches, and numerous other physical and psychological symptoms. Depending on the duration of use and the extent of tolerance, these symptoms can be severe or even life-threatening. Although some individuals who use opioids occasionally choose to reduce or eliminate their use to regain a larger effect with a smaller amount of the substance, for many individuals who use these drugs the fear of withdrawal symptoms is a powerful incentive to continue use.

Behavioral correlates of opioid withdrawal include dysphoric mood, nausea or vomiting, muscle aches, rhinorrhea, pupillary dilation, sweating, diarrhea, yawning, fever, and insomnia (APA, 2013).

Etiology

For many individuals, dependence begins with prescription use, most often for pain control. They then transition to nonprescription use (Katz, El-Gabalawy, Keyes, Martins, & Sareen, 2013). Only a small proportion of individuals who use opioids transition to nonmedical prescription use (Ling et al., 2011). Individuals with no previous history of opioid abuse do not experience euphoria when prescribed these medications over an extended period, so they are unlikely to become addicted.

The presence of anxiety or depression increases the risk of abuse, meaning that it is particularly important to monitor opioid use in individuals with these comorbidities (Katz et al., 2013). Because abuse of opioids requires contact with illicit sources, establishment of dependence requires action on the part of the individual. It is common, for example, to find this sort of addiction in individuals with prior histories of delinquency or unstable home situations.

Prognosis

Dependence on opioid drugs is intractable (Bjornaas et al., 2008), with reports of poor outcomes as long as 20 years after initial diagnosis. The drugs cause significant tolerance effects fairly rapidly, and withdrawal symptoms are severe and unpleasant. Thus, after initial experiences with the drugs for the "high" they cause, later experiences are often attempts to avoid withdrawal symptoms. In addition, because these drugs are related to lifestyle and personality characteristics, the environment tends to support the addiction. The person's friends tend to be users, and much of the person's time is spent in pursuit of the substance, often involving illegal activity. To successfully withdraw, individuals may have to cope not only with withdrawal but also with making necessary changes in lifestyle—finding new friends, finding new, legitimate sources of income—to avoid temptation to continue abusing the substance. As has been mentioned previously, tolerance is a particular problem. As it develops, increasing amounts are required to experience the euphoria it causes.

In addition, opioid medication abuse leads to respiratory suppression with overdose, interaction with other medications, transmission of infectious diseases (specifically with intravenous administration), and involvement in other risky behaviors (Ling et al., 2011). As with other abuse, coexisting psychosis is a predictor of poor prognosis (Levin et al., 2008), and there is a relatively high rate of use-related death (Green, Grau, Carver, Kinzly, & Heimer, 2011), and an increased risk of suicide (Kuramoto, Chilcoat, Ko, & Martins, 2012).

Newer medical interventions, including use of naloxone and buprenorphine, have shown great promise as adjuncts to treatment (Tai, 2002). Naloxone immediately reverses the effects of heroin, making it useful in overdose situations.

Sedatives, Hypnotics, and Anxiolytics

Sedatives are characterized by two common patterns of abuse. In some individuals, the drug may be prescribed for a specific purpose, but tolerance develops and symptoms of dependence appear. When these drugs are prescribed for long periods of time to allow an individual to function, as in the case of severe anxiety, the situation does not qualify as substance abuse. However, in other cases, obtaining the drug becomes the primary goal, and function is negatively affected as a result. The second pattern of abuse is seen in individuals who obtain the drug through illicit means, specifically for purposes of abuse (i.e., for the "high"). In both cases, tolerance is marked.

Sedative, Hypnotic, or Anxiolytic Use Disorder

The sedative, hypnotic, or anxiolytic use disorder label describes a pattern of unhealthy use over time. Because these medications are typically prescribed for relatively chronic problems, especially anxiety disorders and insomnia, their use may be encouraged on an ongoing basis. But a number of these drugs do build tolerance in clients, meaning that the individual takes larger doses, which create the potential for physical and psychological symptoms, such as slowed respiration and drowsiness.

Symptoms of sedative, hypnotic, or anxiolytic use disorder include using the substance in larger amounts over a longer period than the person had intended, and efforts to control its use are unsuccessful (APA, 2013). Significant time is spent obtaining, using, and recovering from use, and the individual experiences both cravings and difficulty with work, home, or school function as a result of use. Other important activities are given up and use is continued in hazardous situations. Further, use is continued even when the individual knows she or he has a problem, and there are signs of tolerance and withdrawal.

Sedative, Hypnotic, or Anxiolytic Intoxication

Sedative, hypnotic, or anxiolytic intoxication is a relatively less common condition than other substance intoxication. Most often, intoxication would occur on the basis of use of increasing amounts of the substance as tolerance builds, with an eventual overdose as a possible outcome. In such a situation, the most immediate concern would be suppression of respiration. Other signs of intoxication in the diagnostic criteria include slurred speech, incoordination, unsteady gait, nystagmus, impaired cognition, and stupor or coma (APA, 2013).

Sedative, Hypnotic, or Anxiolytic Withdrawal

Withdrawal from sedative, hypnotic, or anxiolytic drugs is accompanied by a variety of physical, cognitive, and psychological symptoms. Often, these symptoms are the reverse of the intended target of the drug itself. For example, someone attempting to withdraw from an anxiolytic would experience a spike in anxiety. Other effects can include lethargy and fatigue, depersonalization, emotional lability, and memory impairment (Vikander, Koechling, Borg, Tönne, & Hiltunen, 2010). As a rule, tapering during withdrawal by gradually reducing the dose can also reduce (although not eliminate) withdrawal symptoms.

Etiology

Dependence on sedatives is less well explained than some other forms of abuse. For individuals who are exposed to the drugs as a result of some other condition, dependence probably results from the effects of the drug itself. These drugs are often prescribed for anxiety conditions, and an individual who is anxious may begin to see them as a crutch, even though they are usually recommended only for short-term use (Harris et al., 2011).

Prognosis

Sedative abuse is treatable (Gordis, 2009), although caution must be exercised in withdrawing from the substance (Bateson, 2002). Because tolerance has been built over time, there are definite withdrawal symptoms, including agitation, insomnia, and other behavioral and psychological symptoms. Cognitive behavioral intervention with gradual withdrawal can be effective.

Stimulants

Stimulant use is common, in part due to the relatively easy access to these drugs. Prescription amphetamines, such as Adderall (Shire Manufacturing), are commonly prescribed for attention-deficit/hyperactivity disorder (ADHD), and concern exists that its increasing use in this population contributes to abuse (Nelson & Galon, 2012). However, evidence suggests that with proper monitoring, this is unlikely to be a problem. Nevertheless, use of prescription amphetamines in treating ADHD means that they are present in many environments (e.g., college campuses) where they can be shared or sold (Gomes, Song, Godwin, & Toriello, 2011).

Another commonly abused stimulant is methamphetamine, an illicit substance that can be readily manufactured using available over-the-counter chemicals, such as ephedrine.

At the same time, drug users are often creative and constantly find new substances to abuse. Considerable recent attention has been paid to bath salts, which seem to be a newly popular substance for abuse. Bath salts are stimulants that can be readily abused (Winder, Stern, & Hosanagar, 2013). They are marketed as legitimate products and so have no legal controls at present. Bath salts are increasingly popular both because of their ease of access and the fact that they do not appear on standard urine screens for drug use. Even so, they represent a small percentage of illicit drug use (NIDA, 2012a).

Stimulant Use Disorder

Two major categories of stimulants exist that are most often involved in substance use disorders: amphetamines and cocaine. Patterns of onset and use tend to be different, particularly between prescription amphetamines (e.g., Adderall and other amphetamines used to treat ADHD) and methamphetamine and cocaine, both of which are always illicit. As a rule, users increase their use over time, although, as noted later, a significant number of individuals eventually self-limit (Uitermark & Cohen, 2006).

Diagnostic criteria include stimulants taken in larger amounts over a longer period than the person had intended and efforts to control its use are unsuccessful (APA, 2013). Significant time is spent obtaining, using, and recovering from use, and the individual experiences both cravings and difficulty with work, home, or school function as a result of use. Other important activities are given up and use is continued in hazardous situations. Further, use is continued even when the individual knows she or he has a problem, and there are signs of tolerance and withdrawal.

Stimulant Intoxication

As is true for other substance-related disorders, immediate, current use can cause signs of intoxication. In addition to the general criteria for intoxication, stimulants can cause tachycardia, pupillary dilation, elevated or lowered blood pressure, perspiration or chills, nausea/vomiting, weight loss, psychomotor agitation or retardation, muscle weakness, impaired respiration, chest pain or cardiac arrhythmias, confusion, seizures, and coma (APA, 2013).

Stimulant Withdrawal

During withdrawal from stimulants, many individuals experience fatigue, vivid and unpleasant dreams, insomnia (or hypersomnia), increased appetite, and psychomotor retardation or agitation (APA, 2013).

Etiology

Individuals who use stimulant drugs tend to be impulsive and compulsive and have increased sensation seeking traits (Ersche et al., 2012). They also show changes in orbitofrontal and parahippocampal volume. All of these traits suggest that there are both biological and personality qualities that encourage stimulant abuse. There is some familial vulnerability, and individuals with a family history are at greater risk for dependence, as are children exposed in utero (Berman, O'Neill, Fears, Bartzokis, & London, 2008).

Prognosis

Disagreement exists in the literature about prognosis for use of these drugs. Several reports suggest that stimulant abuse tends toward chronic use and relapsing, and that few treatments have demonstrated efficacy (Trevidi et al., 2011). These reports suggest that behavioral and pharmacological interventions have been attempted but without a great deal of evidence to delineate which are actually effective (Smith & Snow, 2012). On the other hand, other reports indicate that abuse is self-limiting for many users, with a gradual reduction and eventual elimination, even in the absence of treatment (Uitermark, & Cohen, 2006). It is probable that different research methods, focused on different populations, account for the differences in findings.

A significant issue with stimulant and cocaine use is the probability of developing medical problems over the long term. For example, there is a high rate of cardiovascular disease among amphetamine users (Westover, Nakonezny, & Haley, 2008). Other physical problems include extreme weight loss and severe dental problems.

Tobacco

The addictive substance in tobacco, nicotine, is a stimulant. It is associated with a number of pleasant effects that encourage continued use. It is also habituating for some in the sense of serving as a social crutch and in the sense that it can become linked with a variety of daily activities. For example, some individuals find that they develop a habit of smoking after their morning coffee or while consuming alcohol. Nicotine is highly habit-forming, both as a physically addictive substance and a habituating substance. Note no category exists for tobacco intoxication disorder. As a rule, tobacco is not intoxicating in the traditional sense of the word, but nicotine is toxic if taken in large doses.

Tobacco Use Disorder

Tobacco use is characterized by ingesting tobacco products in larger amounts over a longer period than the person had intended, and efforts to control its use are unsuccessful (APA, 2013). Significant time is spent obtaining, using, and recovering from use, and the individual experiences both cravings and difficulty with work, home, or school function as a result of use. Other important activities are given up and use is continued in hazardous situations. Further, use is continued even when the individual knows she or he has a problem, and there are signs of tolerance and withdrawal.

Tobacco Withdrawal

Tobacco withdrawal is accompanied by irritability or anger, anxiety, difficulty concentrating, increased appetite, restlessness, depression, and insomnia (APA, 2013). A particular difficulty of withdrawing from tobacco use is the duration of these symptoms. Some smokers report various symptoms months after their last tobacco use.

Etiology

Tobacco use most often begins in adolescence, typically involving social/peer pressure (Bruijnzeel, 2012) (Figure 17-2). Use includes various effects that are reinforcing, including increased energy, improved mood, relaxation, and improved working memory. At the same time, cessation leads to various unpleasant effects, such as depressed mood, lethargy, and irritability. For these reasons, when an individual starts tobacco use, there are significant incentives to continue.

Prognosis

Tobacco use is particularly difficult to stop (DiFranz, Wellman, & Savageau, 2012) because it is both physically addicting and habituating. In addition, the early symptoms of withdrawal can be severe and very unpleasant (Bruijnzeel, 2012), including flu-like symptoms, anxiety,

Figure 17-2. Smoking often begins in adolescence as a result of peer pressure. (©2014 Shutterstock.com.)

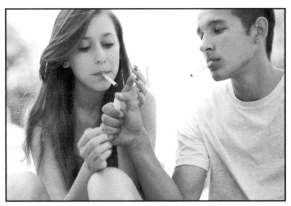

depression, and agitation. Although these symptoms are short-lived (4 days or so), the desire for nicotine tends to extend much longer. Some smokers report still craving nicotine years after they have stopped smoking.

Tobacco is associated with a number of long-term negative health consequences, including heart-disease, lung and oral cancer, and chronic obstructive pulmonary disease (Foulds, Delnevo, Ziedonis, & Steinberg, 2008). In addition, cigarette smoking is associated with increased house fires and automobile accidents (Centers for Disease Control and Prevention, 2013).

Non–Substance-Related Disorders

Gambling Disorder

Gambling first appeared as an identified mental disorder in the third edition of the DSM (DSM-III; Westphal, 2007). It is included in the substance-related and addictive disorders cluster because of the common features among the various addictive behaviors. Other behavioral addictions were considered for inclusion (e.g., shopping, sexual addiction) but were omitted because there is not sufficient research evidence about them as yet (APA, 2013). Subsequent versions of the DSM may well expand this cluster.

The rationale for including gambling disorder in this group is the research suggesting that the symptoms have more in common with substance use disorders than with obsessive-compulsive disorder (el-Guebaly, Mudry, Zohar, Tavares, & Potenza, 2012). Gambling disorder is characterized by impulsivity, as well as compulsivity, with the former being significant in the persistence of the behavior.

Diagnostic criteria for gambling disorder include persistent and recurrent gambling causing distress or dysfunction (APA, 2013). Associated behaviors include a need to gamble with increasing amounts of money, gambling to reduce feelings of distress, irritation or restlessness when attempting to control behavior, preoccupation with gambling and repeated efforts to control the behavior, efforts to recover losses and hide the extent of the problem, damage to important relationships or roles, and a need to borrow money frequently.

Etiology

Pathological gambling seems to be associated with cognitive and perceptual deficiencies (Suissa, 2011), specifically related to impulse control. In addition, cultural factors exist, including ethnic minority status and low socioeconomic status (Rantala & Sulkunen, 2012). Gambling is a common and socially sanctioned activity in our culture, as typified by office pools before important sporting events, the proliferation of casinos, and even bingo nights at churches and community centers. In this societal context, recognizing when a leisure pastime has become a serious abuse problem can be difficult, and the individual can rationalize his or her behavior for long periods of time.

Prognosis

Problem gambling tends to be persistent, although women seem to have a shorter duration of the problem than men (Jamieson, Mazmanian, Penney, Black, & Nguyen, 2011). It is not entirely clear whether this is because women typically have a later onset of the gambling disorder or a real difference in its course between genders. Gambling disorder is linked with poor physical health, stress, sleep problems, depression, and suicide (Rantala & Sulkunen, 2012).

Implications for Function and Treatment

Clearly, the substance-related and addictive disorders include a wide array of conditions with varied onset, symptoms, and outcomes. Similarly, functional implications vary widely, depending on the specific nature of the substance or behavior. At one end of the functional spectrum, caffeine and tobacco and, perhaps, cannabis, have relatively limited impact on function; their impact is largely on physical health. The main functional implication for use of these substances relates to habits and patterns, rather than specific occupations. There is even some evidence that caffeine and nicotine can improve cognitive performance.

On the other hand, many substance-related disorders have substantial negative implications for function in most occupations. These functional deficits can occur even when the substance is originally a prescribed medication. For example, work-related injuries can lead to substance use disorders as a consequence of initial pain management strategies (Parhami et al., 2012). Substance use can cause deficits in work, social, self-care, and other occupations. In addition, drug seeking behaviors, particularly for the illicit drugs, can lead to criminal behavior and resultant legal difficulties and incarceration.

In addition to functional deficits in a variety of occupations, cognitive, perceptual-motor, and other skill areas can be negatively affected. For example, research on inhalant users has found deficits in working memory, abstract reasoning, auditory and verbal working memory, processing speed, procedural memory, and visual–spatial recall (Scott & Scott, 2012).

Gambling disorder is also accompanied by functional deficits, including social and work problems. Individuals with serious gambling problems often face loneliness, financial problems, depression, and divorce (Blaszczynski, 2010).

Intervention strategies are dependent on the specific substance. For caffeine and tobacco use, behavioral therapy can be effective. In general, it is recommended that the individual withdraw from caffeine gradually to minimize the physical symptoms. Tobacco cessation can be assisted through the use of nicotine patches that gradually reduce the amount of the substance being consumed (Harmey, Griffin, & Kenny, 2012). However, regardless of the approach, most smokers will relapse several times before they succeed in stopping usage. It is important to keep in mind that tobacco use includes smokeless tobacco (e.g., chewing tobacco), which also leads to addiction (Schiller et al., 2012). For smokeless tobacco cessation, complete, rather than gradual, withdrawal seems most effective.

Because many substance-related disorders emerge in adolescence and as a result of peer pressure, strategies for managing social influences can be vital (Perron & Howard, 2008).

Management of opioid use disorders has been well described. Prescription monitoring programs focused on initially prescribed opioids can be helpful (Reifler et al., 2012). In particular, health care professionals working in primary care and pain management settings must be involved in treating opioid users (Pade et al., 2012). Opioid treatment often involves substitution or maintenance medications, typically methadone and buprenorphine (Ling et al., 2011), although evidence exists that these drugs may be abused as well, so providing them in a controlled environment, such as a methadone clinic, can be important.

Gambling disorder is often addressed through behavioral therapy focused on maladaptive behaviors and ideas (Gold & Hamond, 2007). In particular, it is important to correct inaccurate perceptions about the probability of winning and the individual's realistic potential for "beating the system." However, this alone is insufficient, as the gambler also needs behavioral strategies to manage the urge or impulse to gamble. In addition, gamblers may seek treatment because of a comorbid condition, such as depression or anxiety (Jamieson et al., 2011). This can provide an opportunity to address the gambling as well, as it is likely that the coexisting disorders interact.

In general, treatment of substance-related and addictive disorders requires careful attention to medical issues, such as the symptoms of withdrawal and the long-term health consequences of using the substance or engaging in the behavior, behavioral intervention focused on changing beliefs about both the behavior and the habits that support it, and emotional support and reinforcement for positive change. Table 17-2 summarizes the diagnostic criteria and functional implications of the various substance-related and addictive disorders.

Implications for Occupational Therapy

Occupational therapy has an important role in the management of substance-related and addictive disorders (Haertlein Sells, Stoffel, & Plach, 2011). Because the symptoms involve patterns of behavior and associated habits, it is vital to provide alternative mechanisms for addressing important personal needs. For example, an individual with a substance use problem may construct his or her daily occupational patterns around securing and using the substance. Work (or illegal activity) is focused on getting enough money to buy the substance or to gamble. Social networks are constructed around the substance or activity. Leisure interests, family interactions, and self-care fall by the wayside. If treatment is to be successful, the individual must find new ways to use the time previously devoted to the substance, and must find enough meaning in the new activities to feel that life is worthwhile and that abstinence is rewarding (Martin, Bliven, & Boisvert, 2008; Peloquin & Ciro, 2013).

The issue of time use is closely related to sociocultural considerations about work and work skills. Many substance abusers lose their jobs because of their addiction, and they must relearn job skills, as well as work-related skills, such as following directions and relating to supervisors. Time management is a particular problem related to work, as well as to other activities (Moyers & Stoffel, 2001).

More problematic is the issue of individuals who turn to substance abuse specifically because they feel hopeless about future prospects. In communities that are socioeconomically disadvantaged, substance abusers often have no job experience or skills and no hope of acquiring them. Training in work and work-related skills may mean starting with basic literacy. Although this approach can be valuable, it is time- and cost-intensive. Linkage with community services and constant follow-up is vital. All of these difficulties contribute to, or are caused by, poor self-esteem. Experiences that can provide both motivation and hope are essential.

TABLE 17-2		
DIAGNOSTIC CRITERIA AND IMPLICATIONS FOR FUNCTION: SUBSTANCE-RELATED AND ADDICTIVE DISORDERS		
DISORDER	*DIAGNOSTIC CRITERIA (APA, 2013)*	*IMPLICATIONS FOR FUNCTION*
Alcohol use disorder	A problematic pattern of alcohol use and distress or impairment for at least 1 year, that can include: • Drinking in larger amounts or over a longer period than intended • Unsuccessful attempts to control use • Substantial time spent obtaining, using, or recovering from using alcohol • Craving • Dysfunction • Important activities are given up because of alcohol use • Repeated use in situations in which it is hazardous • Tolerance • Withdrawal symptoms	Potential negative consequences for all occupations Work and self-care often ignored Social and leisure performance center on substance use Skills negatively impacted include cognitive and emotional regulation skills May negatively affect perceptual motor skills. Patterns, habits, roles center on securing and using alcohol
Cannabis use disorder	Similar to alcohol use, but with cannabis as substance being used	Potential negative consequences for all occupations Work and self-care often ignored Social and leisure performance center on substance use Skills negatively impacted include cognitive and social skills Lethargy is a typical consequence Patterns, habits, roles center on securing and using cannabis
Hallucinogen/PCP use disorder	Similar to alcohol use, but with hallucinogen/PCP	Potential negative consequences for all occupations Work and self-care often ignored

(continued)

TABLE 17-2 (CONTINUED)		
DIAGNOSTIC CRITERIA AND IMPLICATIONS FOR FUNCTION: SUBSTANCE-RELATED AND ADDICTIVE DISORDERS		
DISORDER	*DIAGNOSTIC CRITERIA (APA, 2013)*	*IMPLICATIONS FOR FUNCTION*
Hallucinogen/ PCP use disorder (continued)		Social and leisure performance center on substance use
		Skills negatively impacted include cognitive and emotional regulation skills
		Negatively affects perceptual motor skills
		Patterns, habits, roles center on securing and using PCP
Inhalant use disorder	Similar to alcohol use, but with inhalants	Potential negative consequences for all occupations
		Work and self-care often ignored
		Social and leisure performance center on substance use
		Skills negatively impacted include cognitive and emotional regulation skills
		May negatively affect perceptual motor skills.
		Patterns, habits, roles often negatively impaired due to inhalant use
Opioid use disorder	Similar to alcohol use, but with opioids	Potential negative consequences for all occupations
		Work and self-care often ignored
		Social and leisure performance center on substance use
		May encounter serious legal difficulties
		Skills negatively impacted include cognitive and emotional regulation skills, perceptual motor skills
		Patterns, habits, roles center on securing and using opioids
		(continued)

TABLE 17-2 (CONTINUED)

DIAGNOSTIC CRITERIA AND IMPLICATIONS FOR FUNCTION: SUBSTANCE-RELATED AND ADDICTIVE DISORDERS

DISORDER	DIAGNOSTIC CRITERIA (APA, 2013)	IMPLICATIONS FOR FUNCTION
Sedative, hypnotic, or anxiolytic use disorder	Similar to alcohol use, but with sedative, hypnotic, or anxiolytics	Potential negative consequences for all occupations Work and self-care often ignored Lethargy may lead to ignoring important performance Skills negatively impacted include cognitive and emotional regulation skills May negatively affect perceptual motor skills. Patterns, habits, roles impaired
Stimulant use disorder	Similar to alcohol use, but with stimulants	Potential negative consequences for all occupations Work and self-care often ignored Social and leisure performance center on substance use May encounter serious legal difficulties Skills negatively impacted include cognitive and emotional regulation skills May negatively affect perceptual motor skills. Patterns, habits, roles center on securing and using stimulants
Tobacco use disorder	Similar to alcohol use, but with tobacco Less likely to cause dysfunction	Minimal impact on occupations May compromise work if frequent breaks for nicotine are required May negatively affect social relationships Negatively affects leisure performance

(continued)

TABLE 17-2 (CONTINUED)		
DIAGNOSTIC CRITERIA AND IMPLICATIONS FOR FUNCTION: SUBSTANCE-RELATED AND ADDICTIVE DISORDERS		
DISORDER	*DIAGNOSTIC CRITERIA (APA, 2013)*	*IMPLICATIONS FOR FUNCTION*
Tobacco use disorder (continued)		Impact on performance increases as serious health impact emerges Skill deficits are minimal Patterns, habits negatively affected by need to use tobacco
Gambling disorder	Persistent gambling causing distress or dysfunction including some of the following: • Increasing need to gamble • Repeated efforts to control, with associated restlessness or irritation • Preoccupation • Gambling to reduce feeling of distress • Efforts try to recoup losses and lying to hide problem • Jeopardizing important relationships or roles • Relying on others to provide money when in debt	Work and social relationships significantly and negatively affected Self-care may be compromised depending on degree to which finances are damaged Leisure occupations negatively affected Interpersonal skills negatively affected Patterns and roles negatively affected as gambling becomes the major activity

Experiencing successes that build self-esteem and learning new methods for managing stress can assist individuals in remaining substance-free. Because loneliness is a problem for individuals who are substance abusers, group therapy can provide important social support and can help individuals establish new and more functional performance patterns.

Both family therapy and cognitive behavioral therapy can have positive impact (Liddle, Dakof, Turner, Henderson, & Greenbaum, 2008). Therapists may want to focus on interventions that strengthen parenting skills for parents and communication skills for adolescents, and on the exploration of assumptions that parents and adolescents have about occupational choices and patterns.

Physical activity seems to reduce the reinforcing effects of illicit substances (Smith, Schmidt, Iordanou, & Mustroph, 2008) and has well-supported benefits in reducing depression. Thus, activities with a significant physical component are a helpful focus of treatment.

Spiritual factors are prominent in substance-related problems, although evidence is sparse and more compelling for intervention for depression and anxiety (Miller, Forcehimes,

O'Leary, & LaNoue, 2008). Nevertheless, it seems reasonable to focus intervention on enhancing spiritual occupations. At a minimum, such interventions might ameliorate the depression and anxiety that can accompany efforts to stop using substances.

It is important for therapists to remember that individuals with substance-related and addictive disorders may present in other areas of practice. For example, an individual in a rehabilitation setting may have been injured in an accident while impaired by substance abuse. John Callahan (1990), a well-known cartoonist, became a quadriplegic as a result of an auto accident in which he was driving while intoxicated. Even after the accident, he described his main problem as substance abuse, not paralysis. Screening to identify problematic substance use is essential, regardless of the setting. Treatment for other conditions must take a client's substance use or abuse into consideration if it presents as an issue.

Occupational therapy provides a variety of options for restoring health and well-being by providing the person with meaningful alternatives to alcohol and other drugs use. Occupational therapists should be aware of the evidence in substance abuse treatment that supports four forms of intervention most strongly (Stoffel & Moyers, 2004). These treatment forms include brief intervention, motivational interviewing, cognitive behavioral therapy, and 12-step programs. Occupational therapists can help encourage readiness to change through skillful use of motivational interviewing, facilitating coping, and encouraging exploration. Use of 12-step self-help groups to build a community of support for recovery from alcohol and drug use is a potential way an occupational therapy practitioner might promote abstinence.

Screening and Brief Intervention

Research suggests that every health care provider should practice screening and, if needed, brief intervention in every practice setting (Barnett et al., 2012; Haack & Adger, 2002). Evidence exists that these brief interventions can be as effective as longer term treatment (Kaner et al., 2007). Even a 10-minute intervention can have an impact in addressing high-risk drinking among college students (Kulesza, Apperson, Larimar, & Copeland, 2010).

Screening can be performed informally or with a variety of brief interviews, including the use of the CAGE questionnaire (Ewing, 1984). The CAGE acronym reflects the four questions that are included in such assessment, specifically:

C: Has anyone ever felt you should Cut down on your drinking?

A: Have people Annoyed you by criticizing your drinking?

G: Have you ever felt Guilty about your drinking?

E: Have you ever had a drink first thing in the morning (Eye-opener) to steady your nerves or to get rid of a hangover?

A positive response to any one of these questions suggests a problem. Such individuals might benefit either from motivational interviewing that encourages efforts to reduce use or by referral to a substance abuse program (Fischer & Moyers, 2012). Brief intervention may be as straightforward as having a discussion about whether there is a problem, and encouraging realistic self-appraisal about substance use. Clinicians do not need to be experts at intervening with long-term substance abusers to have an effective positive impact on individuals in the early stages or in making sure that those who are having serious problems receive help (Bonaguro, Nalette, & Seibert, 2002).

Dual Diagnosis

Substance abuse often coexists with conduct disorder, depression, developmental disabilities, schizophrenia, manic-depressive disorder, and/or personality disorders (Chen & Biswas, 2012; Levin et al., 2008). These dual diagnoses are extremely challenging because treatment efforts are confounded by the combination of problems. Even determining which diagnosis to address first can be difficult (Chen & Biswas, 2012).

Substance abuse can lead to mood, anxiety, and psychotic disorders. Among adolescents who are substance abusers, various forms of violence are common, both with the adolescent as a victim of abuse and as a perpetrator of violent acts (Van Dalen, 2001). It is also possible that individuals abuse substances secondary to, or as a result of, another disorder. For example, alcohol abuse may emerge as a way to self-treat anxiety. It is a challenge to determine which causes which or whether substance abuse is simply associated with other psychiatric disorders, rather than a causative factor (van Dam et al., 2008). Understanding the etiology of the coexisting disorder(s) is essential to satisfactory intervention.

Treatment recommendations may vary. Recovery-oriented intervention that is focused on skill-building and behavioral management seems to be effective for some individuals (Topor, Grosso, Burt, & Falcon, 2013). Recommendations for care emphasize the need for careful assessment to ensure that the approach is tailored to the individual. A combination of psychosocial and pharmacological interventions is the most common recommendation (Murthy & Chand, 2012). However, data regarding the effectiveness of various forms of treatment are sparse, with some studies showing no increased positive effect when programs are specially planned for individuals with dual diagnoses (Cleary, Hunt, Matheson, Siegfried, & Walter, 2008). On the other hand, research also suggests that the outcomes are comparable for individuals with substance-related and other mental disorders when compared with those with only a substance-related disorder (Cridland, Deane, Hsu, & Kelly, 2012).

Dual diagnosis, as the construct relates to substance-related disorders, has been described in this chapter. However, other mental disorders can also co-occur, and those scenarios would also be referred to as dual diagnosis. For example, a young adult with an intellectual disability might also have an impulse control or eating disorder. An individual with a depressive disorder might also have a personality disorder. Any time two or more mental disorders coexist, treatment becomes more complicated and the conditions are less likely to improve. However, from the perspective of occupational therapy, the fundamentals of evaluation and treatment still apply; that is, determine the individual's occupational profile, occupations, and skills and address those issues to enhance function.

Cultural Considerations

Cultural factors play a role in the incidence, etiology, and course of all the substance abuse disorders. In the United States, some individuals from minority groups use substances as a way to cope with a sense of alienation that results from their disadvantaged status (Moloney, Hunt, & Evans, 2008). Among groups with particularly high rates of substance abuse, problems extend far beyond the individual with the disorder. Among Native Americans, the rates of substance abuse are high, perhaps because of genetic factors, and whole communities can be negatively affected (Evans-Campbell, 2008). In these communities, population-based approaches to treatment may be important, given the potential for limited access to services (Rieckmann et al., 2012). Even when such broad-based interventions are not possible, it is important to be aware that an adult's substance abuse can impact the children and others living in the household.

Different cultural and religious groups vary in their patterns of use, with some abstaining totally, others using alcohol in specific ceremonial contexts, and others using alcohol liberally (Straussner, 2001). For example, Native Americans, Hispanics, and adolescents of either White or multiple races/ethnicities have the highest rates of substance-related disorders. Blacks and Asian-Pacific Islanders had lower rates on average (Wu, Woody, Yang, Pan, & Blazer, 2011). Inhalant use is most prevalent in socially isolated and economically disadvantaged young populations, such as on Native American reservations (Shamblen & Miller, 2012). In addition, different cultural groups need treatments tailored to their needs. For example, in Native Americans, intense social support seems to improve outcomes of intervention (Spear, Crevecoeur-MacPhail, Denering, Dickerson, & Brecht, 2013).

The realities mentioned allow for identification not only of risk factors but also of protective factors that can support effective intervention. Collaboration between providers and Native American communities, for example, can improve outcomes (Whitesell, Rumbaugh Beals, Crow, Mithell, & Novins, 2012). As another example, culturally tailored prevention interventions appear to reduce tobacco use among minority adolescents (Kong, Singh, & Krishnan-Sarin, 2012).

Lifespan Considerations

Because their abuse starts early, adolescents are at risk for significant additional problems throughout life, including health consequences, disruptions in developmental tasks, and disordered interpersonal relationships (Interdisciplinary Faculty Development Program in Substance Abuse Education, 2000; Rantala & Sulkunen, 2012). In addition, alcohol is one of several gateway drugs (Walker et al., 2004). Various factors exist that encourage young people to engage in substance use. For example, college students may use stimulants in a belief that these will help them study (Gomes et al., 2011). Young people often perceive themselves as bored, and this can lead to high-risk behaviors (Wegner, 2011). Unfortunately, alcohol use in particular is often perceived as normative behavior for adolescents (Feinstein, Richter, & Foster, 2012). For those young people who are at risk of substance-related mental disorders, this can lead to ongoing problems. Health promotion and prevention programs that aid in altering normative expectations can be helpful, but they are challenging to implement effectively.

In general, rates of substance abuse are lower among older adults (Salmon & Forester, 2012). This may be because individuals with substance abuse have a higher rate of mortality at younger ages, or it may be that older adults are simply less likely to engage in excessive substance use. However, older adults are not immune from substance use disorders (Culbertson & Ziska, 2008). Older adults may develop dependence on prescription medications (Lowry, 2012) or develop or continue long-established patterns of alcohol abuse. Older men become alcoholics more often than older women. Older adults with long-standing abuse problems or who begin substance use later in life are particularly vulnerable to adverse medical consequences of their abuse (Salmon & Forester, 2012). For example, substance use disorders contribute to cognitive problems. Given the increase in cognitive deficits from various causes of dementia, individuals with substance use disorders are at an especially high risk of severe cognitive decline. Treatment for older adults with substance use is not well established, although as is true for other age groups, a multifaceted approach is likely to be most helpful.

CASE STUDY

Ms. Navratskaya is a 26-year-old divorced woman who has been living with a boyfriend, Max, for the past 6 months. Both are heroin addicts with long histories of substance abuse.

Ms. Navratskaya reports that she dropped out of high school and left home at age 16 years because her father was sexually abusing her. For a long time, she lived on the streets making money as a prostitute. She reports having been extremely depressed and using alcohol and marijuana to dull her unhappiness. At 18 year old, she met the first of a succession of boyfriends who were heroin addicts, and she was introduced to heroin through him. She often drinks heavily, smokes cigarettes, and, when her supply of heroin is low, she takes diazepam or OxyContin to "tide me over." She continues to work the streets at night as a prostitute, and she spends most of her days in a drug-induced fog.

Ms. Navratskaya recently acquired heroin that was not cut as heavily as usual; she overdosed and ended up in the emergency department. Although she indicates she does not want to stop using, she also notes that she has become increasingly depressed and has thought about taking her life. The social worker in the emergency department finally convinced her to try inpatient treatment because of concerns about her suicidal thoughts. Ms. Navratskaya stayed in the hospital for 3 days and then agreed to try methadone. She has since been attending weekly meetings at the methadone clinic.

THOUGHT QUESTIONS

1. What functional deficits would you expect Ms. Navratskaya to have?
2. Of these deficits, which are the result of her early life experiences, and which are more likely the result of her substance use? Can you make this distinction?
3. If Ms. Navratskaya is to continue her treatment, what occupational therapy strategies might be necessary?

Internet Resources

American Academy of Child & Adolescent Psychiatry Substance Use Resource Center
http://www.aacap.org/AACAP/Families_and_Youth/Resource_Centers/Substance_Abuse_Resource_Center/Home.aspx
Materials and information focused on child and adolescent substance abuse issues.

National Institute on Drug Abuse
http://www.drugabuse.gov/about-nida/other-resources
Substance abuse conditions are sufficiently prevalent and problematic to have fostered a wide array of government resources and sites. This site is one of many.

National Substance Abuse Index
http://nationalsubstanceabuseindex.org/
A National Institute of Health and Substance Abuse and Mental Health Services Administration site focused on resources for treatment.

Substance Abuse and Mental Health Services Administration
http://www.samhsa.gov/
Perhaps the main government resource for information and assistance related to substance abuse for professionals and consumers. This is a very comprehensive resource.

References

American Psychiatric Association. (2005). *Substance-related disorders conference*. Retrieved from http://www.dsm5.org/Research/Pages/Substance-RelatedDisordersConference%28February14-17,2005%29.aspx.

American Psychiatric Association. (2013). *Diagnostic and statistical manual of mental disorders* (5th ed.). Washington, DC: Author.

Apatow, J., & Robertson, S. (Producers), & Green, D.G. (Director). (2008). *Pineapple express* [Motion picture]. United States: Columbia Pictures.

Barnett, E., Spruijt-Metz, D., Unger, J.B., Sun, P., Rohrbach, L.A., & Sussman, S. (2012). Boosting a teen substance use prevention program with motivational interviewing. *Substance Use & Misuse, 47(4)*, 418-428.

Bateson, A.N. (2002). Basic pharmacologic mechanisms involved in benzodiazepine tolerance and withdrawal. *Current Pharmacy Descriptions, 8*(1), 5-21.

Becker, W.C., Sullivan, L.E., Tetrault, J.M., Desai, R.A., & Fiellin, D.A. (2008). Non-medical use, abuse and dependence on prescription opioids among U.S. adults: psychiatric, medical and substance use correlates. Drug and Alcohol Dependence, 94(1-3), 38-47.

Ben-Abraham, R., Szold, O., Rudick, V., & Weinbroum, A.A. (2003). 'Ecstasy' intoxication: Life-threatening manifestations and resuscitative measures in the intensive care setting. *European Journal of Emergency Medicine: Official Journal of the European Society for Emergency Medicine, 10*(4), 309-313.

Berman, S., O'Neill, J., Fears, S., Bartzokis, G., & London, E.D., (2008). Abuse of amphetamines and structural abnormalities in the brain. In G.R. Uhl (Ed.), *Addiction reviews 2008* (pp. 195-200). Oxford, England: Blackwell.

Bjornaas, M.A., Bekken, A.S., Ojlert, A., Haldorsen, T., Jacobsen, D., Rostrup, M., & Ekeberg, O. (2008). A 20-year prospective study of mortality and causes of death among hospitalized opioid addicts in Oslo. *BMC Psychiatry, 8*, Article 8.

Blaszczynski, A. (2010). Instrumental tool or drug: Relationship between attitudes to money and problem gambling. *Addiction Research and Theory, 18*, 681-691.

Boden, M.T., Gross, J., Babson, K.A., & Bonn-Miller, M.O. (2013). The interactive effects of emotional clarity and cognitive reappraisal on problematic cannabis use among medical cannabis users. *Addictive Behaviors, 38*(3), 1663-1668.

Bonaguro, J.A., Nalette, E., & Seibert, M.L. (2002). The role of allied health professionals in substance abuse education. In M.R. Haack & H. Adger (Eds.), *Strategic plan for interdisciplinary faculty development: Arming the nation's health professional workforce for a new approach to substance use disorders* (pp. 169-184). Providence, RI: Association for Medical Education and Research in Substance Abuse.

Bruijnzeel, A.W. (2012). Tobacco addiction and the dysregulation of brain stress systems. *Neuroscience and Biobehavioral Reviews, 36*(5), 1418-1441.

Buckner, J.D., Zvolensky, M.J., & Schmidt, N.B. (2012). Cannabis-related impairment and social anxiety: The roles of gender and cannabis use motives. *Addictive Behaviors, 37*(11), 1294-1297.

Brunton, L., Chabner, B., & Knollmann, B. (2011). Histamine, bradykinin, and their antagonists. In L. Brunton (Ed.) *Goodman & Gilman's the pharmacological basis of therapeutics* (12th ed., pp. 242-245). New York, NY: McGraw Hill.

Cairney, S., O'Connor, N., Dingwall, K.M., Maruff, P., Shafiq-Antonacci, R., Currie, J., & Currie, B. (2013). A prospective study of neurocognitive changes 15 years after chronic inhalant abuse. *Addiction, 108*(6), 1107-1114.

Callaghan, R.C., Allebeck, P., & Sidorchuk, A. (2013). Marijuana use and risk of lung cancer: A 40-year cohort study. *Cancer Causes Control, 24*(10), 1811-1820.

Callahan, J. (1990). *Don't worry, he won't get far on foot*. New York, NY: Vintage Books.

Centers for Disease Control and Prevention. (2013). *Smoking and tobacco use: Tobacco related mortality*. Retrieved from http://www.cdc.gov/tobacco/data_statistics/fact_sheets/health_effects/tobacco_related_mortality/.

Chen, S., & Biswas, B. (2012). Behavioural correlates of dual diagnosis among women in treatment for substance abuse. *Mental Health and Substance Use, 5*(3), 217-227.

Clay, S.W., Allen, J., & Parran, T. (2008). A review of addiction. *Postgraduate Medicine, 120*(2), E01-E07.

Cleary, M., Hunt, G.E., Matheson, S.L., Siegfried, N., & Walter, G. (2008). Psychosocial interventions for people with both severe mental illness and substance misuse. *Cochrane Database of Systematic Reviews, Issue 1*, CD001088. doi:10.1002/14651858.CD001088.pub.2.

Copeland, J. (2004). Developments in the treatment of cannabis use disorder. *Current Opinions in Psychiatry, 17*, 161-168.

Cousijn, J., Goudriaan, A.E., & Wiers, R.W. (2011). Reaching out towards cannabis: Approach-bias in heavy cannabis users predicts changes in cannabis use. *Addiction, 106*(9), 1667-1674.

Crane, C.A., Easton, C.J., & Devine, S. (2013). The association between phencyclidine use and partner violence: An initial examination. *Journal of Addictive Diseases, 32*(2), 150-157.

Cridland, E.K., Deane, F.P., Hsu, C., & Kelly, P.J. (2012). A comparison of treatment outcomes for individuals with substance use disorder alone and individuals with probable dual diagnosis. *International Journal of Mental Health and Addiction, 10*(5), 670-683.

Culbertson, J.W., & Ziska, M. (2008). Prescription drug misuse/abuse in the elderly. *Geriatrics, 63*(9), 22-31.

Dahl, F. (2013). Lure, variant of designer drugs is alarming: U.N. Agency. *Medscape.* Retrieved from http://www.medscape.com/viewarticle/806927.

DiFranz, J.R., Wellman, R.J., & Savageau, J.A. (2012). Does progression through the stages of physical addiction indicate increasing overall addiction to tobacco? *Psychopharmacology, 219*(3), 815-822.

el-Guebaly, N., Mudry, T., Zohar, J., Tavares, H., & Potenza, M.N. (2012). Compulsive features in behavioural addictions: The case of pathological gambling. *Addiction, 107*(10), 1726-1734.

Ellison, G., Keys, A., & Noguchi, K. (1999) Long-term changes in brain following continuous phencyclidine administration. An autoradiographic study using flunitrazepam, ketanserin, mazindol, quinuclidinyl benzilate, piperidyl-3, 4-3H(N)-TCP, and AMPA receptor ligands. *Pharmacological Toxicity, 84*(1), 9-17.

Ersche, K.D., Jones, P.S., Williams, G.B., Smith, D.G., Bullmore, E.T., & Robbins, T.W. (2012). Distinctive personality traits and neural correlates associated with stimulant drug use versus familial risk of stimulant dependence. *Biological Psychiatry, 74*(2), 137-44.

Evans-Campbell, T. (2008). Perceptions of child neglect among urban American Indian/Alaska native parents. *Child Welfare, 87*, 115-142.

Ewing, J.A. (1984). Detecting alcoholism: The CAGE questionnaire. *The Journal of the American Medical Association, 252*, 1095-1097.

Eyer, F., Schuster, T., Felgenhauer, N., Pfab, R., Strubel, T., Saugel, B., & Zilker, T. (2011). Risk assessment of moderate to severe alcohol withdrawal—Predictors for seizures and delirium tremens in the course of withdrawal. *Alcohol and Alcoholism, 46*(4), 427-433.

Feinstein, E.C., Richter, L., & Foster, S.E. (2012). Addressing the critical health problem of adolescent substance use through health care, research, and public policy. *Journal of Adolescent Health, 50*(5), 431-436.

Fischer, D.J., & Moyers, T.B. (2012). Motivational interviewing as a brief psychotherapy. In M.J. Dewan, B.N. Steenbarger, & R.P. Greenberg (Eds.), *The art and science of brief psychotherapies: An illustrated guide* (2nd ed., pp. 27-41). Arlington, VA: American Psychiatric Publishing.

Foulds, J., Delnevo, C., Ziedonis, D.M., & Steinberg, M.B. (2008). Health effects of tobacco, nicotine, and exposure to tobacco smoke pollution. In J. Brick (Ed.), *Handbook of the medical consequences of alcohol and drug abuse* (2nd ed., pp. 423-459). New York, NY: The Haworth Press/Taylor & Francis.

Garland, E.L., & Howard, M.O. (2011). Adverse consequences of acute inhalant intoxication. *Experimental and Clinical Psychopharmacology, 19*(2), 134-144.

Gold, M.S., & Hammond, C.J. (2007). Pathological gambling focused CBT: The application of addiction-based treatments provides another tool in the therapist's toolbox. *PsycCRITIQUES, 52*(42). doi:10.1037/a0008532.

Gomes, J., Song, T., Godwin, L., & Toriello, P.J. (2011). Prescription stimulant abuse on university campuses. *Journal of Human Behavior in the Social Environment, 21*(7), 822-833.

Gordis, E. (2009). Contributions of behavioral science in addiction research and treatment. In G. Alan Marlatt & K. Witkiewitz (Eds.), *Addictive behaviors: New readings on etiology, prevention, and treatment* (pp. 19-32). Washington, DC: American Psychological Association.

Green, T.C., Grau, L.E., Carver, H.W., Kinzly, M., & Heimer, R. (2011). Epidemiologic trends and geographic patterns of fatal opioid intoxications in Connecticut, USA: 1997-2007. *Drug and Alcohol Dependence, 115*(3), 221-228.

Haack, M.R., & Adger, H. (Eds.). (2002). *Strategic plan for interdisciplinary faculty development: Arming the nation's health professional workforce for a new approach to substance use disorders.* Providence, RI: Association for Medical Education and Research in Substance Abuse.

Haertlein Sells, C., Stoffel, V.C., & Plach, H. (2011). Substance-related disorders. In C. Brown & V.C. Stoffel (Eds.), *Occupational therapy in mental health: A vision for participation* (pp. 192-210). Philadelphia, PA: F.A. Davis.

Hammond, C.J., & Gold, M.S. (2008). Caffeine dependence, withdrawal, overdose and treatment: A review. *Directions in Psychiatry, 28*(3), 177-190.

Harmey, D., Griffin, P.R., & Kenny, P.J. (2012). Development of novel pharmacotherapeutics for tobacco dependence: Progress and future directions. *Nicotine & Tobacco Research, 14*(11), 1300-1318.

Harris, M.G., Burgess, P.M., Pirkis, J., Siskind, D., Slade, T., & Whiteford, H.A. (2011). Correlates of antidepressant and anxiolytic, hypnotic or sedative medication use in an Australian community sample. *Australian and New Zealand Journal of Psychiatry, 45*(3), 249-260.

Hasin, D.S., & Katz, H. (2010). Genetic and environmental factors in substance use, abuse, and dependence. In L. Scheier (Ed.), *Handbook of drug use etiology: Theory, methods, and empirical findings* (pp. 247-267). Washington, DC: American Psychological Association.

Hayatbakhsh, R., Williams, G.M., Bor, W., & Najman, J.M. (2013). Early childhood predictors of age of initiation to use of cannabis: A birth prospective study. *Drug and Alcohol Review, 32*(3), 232-240.

Hilarski, C., & Wodarski, J.S. (2001). Comorbid substance abuse and mental illness: Diagnosis and treatment. *Journal of Social Work Practice in the Addictions, 1*, 105-119.

Huebner, R.B., & Kantor, L.W. (2011). Advances in alcoholism treatment. *Alcohol Research & Health, 33*(4), 295-299.

Interdisciplinary Faculty Development Program in Substance Abuse Education (2000). *Curriculum on substance abuse screening and brief intervention.* Providence, RI: Association for Medical Education and Research in Substance Abuse.

Jamieson, J., Mazmanian, D., Penney, A., Black, N., & Nguyen, A. (2011). When problem gambling is the primary reason for seeking addiction treatment. *International Journal of Mental Health and Addiction, 9*(2), 180-192.

Javitt, D.C., Zukin, S.R., Heresco-Levy, U., & Umbricht, D. (2012). Has an angel shown the way? Etiological and therapeutic implications of the PCP/NMDA model of schizophrenia. *Schizophrenia Bulletin, 38*(5), 958-966.

Jones, K.L., & Streissguth, A.P. (2010). Fetal alcohol syndrome and fetal alcohol spectrum disorders: A brief history. *Journal of Psychiatry & Law, Special Issue: Fetal Alcohol Syndrome and Fetal Alcohol Spectrum Disorders: A Brief History, 38*(4), 373-382.

Kaner, E.F., Dickinson, H.O., Beyer, F.R., Campbell, F., Schlesinger, C., Heather, N., . . . Pienaar, E.D. (2007). Effectiveness of brief alcohol interventions in primary care populations. *Cochrane Database of Systematic Reviews, Issue 2*, CD0044148. doi:10.1002/14651585.CD004148.pub3.

Karno, M.P., Grella, C.E., Niv, N., Warda, U., & Moore, A.A. (2008). Do substance type and diagnosis make a difference? A study of remission from alcohol- versus drug-use disorders using the National Epidemiologic Survey on Alcohol and Related Conditions. *Journal of Studies on Alcohol and Drugs, 69*(4), 491-495.

Katz, C., El-Gabalawy, R., Keyes, K.M., Martins, S.S., & Sareen, J. (2013). Risk factors for incident nonmedical prescription opioid use and abuse and dependence: Results from a longitudinal nationally representative sample. *Drug and Alcohol Dependence, 132*(1-2), 107-113.

Kim, R.H., & Hashimoto, N. (2012). Women and substance abuse disorders. In P.K. Lundberg-Love, K.L. Nadal, & M.A. Paludi (Eds.), *Women and mental disorders* (Vols. 1-4, pp. 173-187). Santa Barbara, CA: Praeger/ABC-CLIO.

Kirisci, L, Tarter, R., Ridenour, T., Zhai, Z.W., Fishbein, D., Reynolds, M., & Vanyukov, M. (2013). Age of alcohol and cannabis use onset mediates the association of transmissible risk in childhood and development of alcohol and cannabis disorders: Evidence for common liability. *Experimental and Clinical Psychopharmacology, 21*(1), 38-45.

Kong, G., Singh, N., & Krishnan-Sarin, S. (2012). A review of culturally targeted/tailored tobacco prevention and cessation interventions for minority adolescents. *Nicotine & Tobacco Research, 14*(12), 1394-1406.

Kulesza, M., Apperson, M., Larimar, M.E., & Copeland, A.L. (2010). Brief alcohol intervention for college drinkers: How brief is brief? *Addictive Behaviors, 5*(7), 730-733

Kuramoto, S.J., Chilcoat, H.D., Ko, J., & Martins, S.S. (2012). Suicidal and suicide attempt across stages of nonmedical prescription opioid use and presence of prescription opioid disorders among U.S. adults. *Journal of Studies on Alcohol and Drugs, 73*(2), 178-184.

Levin, F.R., Bisanga, A., Raby, W., Aharonovich, E., Rubin, E., Mariani, J., . . . Nunes, E.V. (2008). Effects of major depressive disorder and attention-deficit disorder on the outcome of treatment for cocaine dependence. *Journal of Substance Abuse Treatment, 34*(1), 80-89.

Liddle, H.A., Dakof, G.A., Turner, R.M., Henderson, C.E., & Greenbaum, P.E. (2008). Treating adolescent drug abuse: A randomized trial comparing multidimensional family therapy and cognitive behavior therapy. *Addiction, 103*, 1660-1670.

Ling, W., Mooney, L., & Hillhouse, M. (2011). Prescription opioid abuse, pain and addiction: Clinical issues and implications. *Drug and Alcohol Review, Special Issue: Pharmaceuticals, 30*(3), 300-305.

Lowry, F. (2012). Prescription opioid abuse in the elderly an urgent concern. *Medscape.* Retrieved from http://www.medscape.com/viewarticle/776128.

Maniglio, R. (2011). The role of child sexual abuse in the etiology of substance-related disorders. *Journal of Addictive Diseases, 30*(3), 216-228.

Martin, L.M., Bliven, M., & Boisvert, R. (2008). Occupational performance, self-esteem, and quality of life in substance addictions recovery. *OTJR: Occupation, Participation & Health, 28*(2), 81-88.

Miller, W.R., Forcehimes, A., O'Leary, M.J., & LaNoue, M.D. (2008). Spiritual direction in addiction treatment: Two clinical trials. *Journal of Substance Abuse Treatment, 35,* 434-442.

Moloney, M., Hunt, G., & Evans, K. (2008). Asian American identity and drug consumption: From acculturation to normalization. *Journal of Ethnicity in Substance Abuse, 7,* 376-403.

Moyers, P.A., & Stoffel, V.C. (2001). Community-based approaches for substance use disorders. In M.E. Scaffa (Ed.), *Occupational therapy in community-based practice settings* (pp. 319-342). Philadelphia, PA: F.A. Davis.

Murthy, P., & Chand, P. (2012). Treatment of dual diagnosis disorders. *Current Opinion in Psychiatry, 25*(3), 194-200.

National Institute on Drug Abuse. (2009). *DrugFacts: Hallucinogens - LSD, Peyote, Psilocybin, and PCP.* Retrieved from http://www.drugabuse.gov/publications/drugfacts/hallucinogens-lsd-peyote-psilocybin-pcp.

National Institute on Drug Abuse. (2011). *Prescription drugs: Abuse and addictions.* Retrieved from http://www.drugabuse.gov/publications/research-reports/prescription-drugs/director.

National Institute on Drug Abuse. (2012a). *DrugFacts: Nationwide trends.* Retrieved from http://www.drugabuse.gov/publications/drugfacts/nationwide-trends.

National Institute on Drug Abuse. (2012b). *Drugs of abuse.* Retrieved from http://www.drugabuse.gov/drugs-abuse.

National Institutes of Health. (2011). *Prescription drugs: Abuse and addiction.* Retrieved from http://www.drugabuse.gov/publications/research-reports/prescription-drugs.

Nelson, A., & Galon, P. (2012). Exploring the relationship among ADHD, stimulants, and substance abuse. *Journal of Child and Adolescent Psychiatric Nursing, 25*(3), 113-118.

Ogawa, N., & Ueki, H. (2007). Clinical importance of caffeine dependence and abuse. *Psychiatry and Clinical Neurosciences, 61*(3), 263-268.

O'Neil, M.G.F. (2013). Trends in prescription drug abuse: 'Bridging medications.' *Medscape.* Retrieved from http://www.medscape.com/viewarticle/804740.

Pade, P.A., Cardon, K.E., Hoffman, R.M., & Beppert, C.M.A. (2012). Prescription opioid abuse, chronic pain, and primary care: A co-occurring disorders clinic in the chronic disease model. *Journal of Substance Abuse Treatment, 43*(4), 446-450.

Parhami, I., Hyman, M., Siani, A., Lin, S., Collard, M., Garcia, J., . . . Fong, T.W. (2012). Screening for addictive disorders within a workers' compensation clinic: An exploratory study. *Substance Use & Misuse, 47*(1), 99-107.

Peloquin, S.M., & Ciro, C.A. (2013). Self-development groups among women in recovery: Client perceptions of satisfaction and engagement. *American Journal of Occupational Therapy, 67*(1), 82-90.

Perello, R. (Producer), & Chandrasekhar, J. (Director). (2001). *Super troopers* [Motion picture]. United States: Fox Searchlight Pictures.

Perron, B.E., & Howard, M.O. (2008). Perceived risk of harm and intentions of future inhalant use among adolescent inhalant users. *Drug and Alcohol Dependence, 97*(1-2), 185-189.

Prescott, C.A., Madden, P.A.F., & Stallings, M.C. (2006). Challenges in genetic studies of the etiology of substance use and substance use disorders: Introduction to the special issue. *Behavioral Genetics, 36,* 473-482.

Rantala, V., & Sulkunen, P. (2012). Is pathological gambling just a big problem or also an addiction? *Addiction Research & Theory, 20*(1), 1-10.

Reifler, L.M., Droz, D., Bailey, J.E., Schnoll, S.H., Fant, R., Dart, R.C., & Bucher Bartelson, B. (2012). Do prescription monitoring programs impact state trends in opioid abuse/misuse? *Pain Medicine, 13*(3), 434-442.

Rieckmann, T., McCarly, D., Kovas, A., Spicer, P., Bray, J., Gilbert, S., & Mercer, J. (2012). American Indians with substance use disorders: Treatment needs and comorbid conditions. *American Journal of Drug and Alcohol Abuse, 38,* 498-504.

Rothman, E.F., Edwards, E.M., Heeren, T., & Hingson, R.W. (2008). Adverse childhood experiences predict earlier age of drinking onset: Results from a representative US sample of current and former drinkers. *Pediatrics, 122,* 298-304.

Salmon, J.M., & Forester, B.P. (2012). Substance abuse and co-occurring psychiatric disorders in older adults: A clinical case and review of the relevant literature. *Journal of Dual Diagnosis, 8*(1), 74-84.

Schiller, K.R., Luo, X., Anderson, A.J., Jenson, J.A., Allen, S.S., & Hatsukami, D.K. (2012). Comparing an immediate cessation versus reduction approach to smokeless tobacco cessation. *Nicotine & Tobacco Research, 14*(8), 902-909.

Schinke, S.P., Tepavac, L., & Cole, K.C. (2000). Preventing substance use among Native American young: Three year results. *Addiction Behavior, 25,* 387-397.

Scott, K.D., & Scott, A.A. (2012). An examination of information-processing skills among inhalant-using adolescents. *Child: Care, Health and Development, 38*(3), 412-419.

Scott, D.M., & Taylor, R.E. (2007). Health-related effects of genetic variations of alcohol-metabolizing enzymes in African Americans. *Alcohol Research & Health, 30*(1), 18-21.

Shamblen, S.R., & Miller, T. (2012). Inhalant initiation and the relationship of inhalant use to the use of other substances. *Journal of Drug Education, 42*(3), 327-346.

Slater, L. (2012, April 20). How psychedelic drugs can help patients face death. *New York Times*. Retrieved from http://www.maps.org/media/view/how_psychedelic_drugs_can_help_patients_face_death/.

Smith, M.A., Schmidt, K.T., Iordanou, J.C., & Mustroph, M.L. (2008). Aerobic exercise decreases the positive-reinforcing effects of cocaine. *Drug and Alcohol Dependence, 98*(1-2), 129-135.

Smith, J.K., & Snow, D. (2012). Stimulant abuse and dependence: Are novel treatment approaches on the horizon? *Journal of Addictions Nursing, 23*(2), 137-140.

Spear, S.E., Crevecoeur-MacPhail, D., Denering, L., Dickerson, D., & Brecht, M.L. (2013). Determinants of successful treatment outcomes among a sample of urban American Indians/Alaska Natives: The role of social environments. *Journal of Behavioral Health Services & Research, 40*(3), 330-341.

Stevens, J. (1998). *Storming heaven: LSD and the American dream*. New York, NY: Grove.

Stoffel, V.C., & Moyers, P.A. (2004). An evidence-based and occupational perspective of interventions for persons with substance-use disorders. *American Journal of Occupational Therapy, 58*, 570-586.

Straussner, S.L.A. (2001). *Ethnocultural factors in substance abuse treatment*. New York, NY: Guilford.

Substance Abuse and Mental Health Services Adminstration. (2008). *Use of Specific Hallucinogens: 2006*. Retrieved from http://www.samhsa.gov/data/2k8/hallucinogens/hallucinogens.htm.

Substance Abuse and Mental Health Services Administration. (2011). *State estimates of substance use and mental disorders from the 2008-2009 national surveys on drug use and health*. NSDUH Series H-40, HHS Publication No. (SMA) 11-4641. Rockville, MD: Author.

Suissa, A.J. (2011). Vulnerability and gambling addiction: Psychosocial benchmarks and avenues for intervention. *International Journal of Mental Health and Addiction, 9*(1), 12-23.

Tai, B. (2002, November). *US national drug abuse treatment clinical trials network*. Paper presented at the Association for Medical Education and Research in Substance Abuse Annual Meeting, Washington, DC.

Topor, D.R., Grosso, D., Burt, J., & Falcon, T. (2013). Skills for recovery: A recovery-oriented dual diagnosis group for veterans with serious mental illness and substance abuse. *Social Work with Groups: A Journal of Community and Clinical Practice, 36*(2-3), 222-235.

Trivedi, M.H., Greer, T.L., Potter, J.S., Grannemann, B.D., Nunes, E.V., Rethorst, C., . . . Somoza, E. (2011). Determining the primary endpoint for a stimulant abuse trial: Lessons learned from STRIDE (CTN 0037). *American Journal of Drug and Alcohol Abuse, 37*(5), 339-349.

Uitermark, J., & Cohen, P.D.A. (2006). Amphetamine users in Amsterdam: Patterns of use and modes of self-regulation. *Addiction Research & Theory, 14*(2), 159-188.

U.S. Centers for Disease Control. (2007). *2007 national youth risk behavior survey overview*. Retrieved June 16, 2009 from http://www.cdc.gov/yrbs.

Vaillant, G.E. (1999). The alcohol-dependent and drug-dependent person. In A.M. Nicholi (Ed.), *The Harvard guide to psychiatry* (3rd ed., pp. 672-683). Cambridge, MA: Harvard University Press.

Van Dalen, A. (2001). Juvenile violence and addiction: Tangled roots in childhood trauma. *Journal of Social Work Practice in the Addictions, 1*(1), 25-40.

Van Dam, N.T., Earleywine, M., & DiGiacomo, G. (2008). Polydrug use, cannabis, and psychosis-like symptoms. *Human Psychopharmacology, 23*, 475-485.

Van der Pol, P., Liebregts, N., de Graaf, R., Korf, D.J., van den Brink, W., & van Laar, M. (2013). Predicting the transition from frequent cannabis use to cannabis dependence: A three-year prospective study. *Drug and Alcohol Dependence, 133*(2), 352-359.

Vandrey, R., Dunn, K.E., Fry, J.A., & Girling, E.R. (2012). A survey study to characterize use of Spice products (synthetic cannabinoids). *Drug and Alcohol Dependency, 120*(1-3), 238-241.

Vikander, B., Koechling, U.M., Borg, S., Tönne, U., & Hiltunen, A.J. (2010). Benzodiazepine tapering: A prospective study. *Nordic Journal of Psychiatry, 64*(4), 273-282.

Walker, D.D., Venner, K., Hill, D.E., Meyers, R.J., & Miller, W.R. (2004). A comparison of alcohol and drug disorders: Is there evidence for a developmental sequence of drug abuse? *Addictive Behaviors, 29*(4), 817-823.

Wegner, L., (2011). Through the lens of a peer: Understanding leisure boredom and risk behaviour in adolescence. *South African Journal of Occupational Therapy, 41*(1), 18-24.

Westover, A.N., Nakonezny, P.A., & Haley, R.W. (2008). Acute myocardial infarction in young adults who abuse amphetamines. *Drug and Alcohol Dependence, 96*(1-2), 49-56.

Westphal, J. (2007). Emerging conceptual models of excessive behaviors. *International Journal of Mental Health and Addiction, 5*(2), 107-116.

Whitesell, N., Rumbaugh Beals, J., Crow, C.B., Mithell, C.M., & Novins, D.K. (2012). Epidemiology and etiology of substance use among American Indians and Alaska natives: Risk, protection, and implications for prevention. *American Journal of Drug and Alcohol Abuse, 38*(5), 376-382.

Winder, G.S., Stern, N., & Hosanagar, A. (2013). Are "bath salts" the next generation of stimulant abuse? *Journal of Substance Abuse Treatment, 44*(1), 42-45.

Wu, L., & Ringwalt, C.L. (2006). Inhalant use and disorders among adults in the United States. *Drug and Alcohol Dependence, 85*(1), 1-11.

Wu, L., Ringwalt, C.L., Mannelli, P., & Patkar, A.A. (2008). Hallucinogen use disorders among adult users of MDMA and other hallucinogens. *American Journal on Addictions, 17*(5), 354-363.

Wu, L., Woody, G.E., Yang, C., Pan, J., & Blazer, D.G. (2011). Racial/ethnic variations in substance-related disorders among adolescents in the United States. *Archives of General Psychiatry, 68*(11), 1176-1185.

Neurocognitive Disorders

Learning Outcomes

By the end of this chapter, readers will be able to:
- Describe the symptoms of neurocognitive disorders
- Differentiate among the neurocognitive disorders on the basis of symptoms and onset
- Identify the causes of the neurocognitive disorders
- Discuss the ways in which neurocognitive disorders affect daily function
- Describe treatment strategies for neurocognitive disorders
- Discuss occupational therapy interventions for neurocognitive disorders

Bonder B.
Psychopathology and Function, Fifth Edition (pp 351-374).
© 2015 SLACK Incorporated.

KEY WORDS

- Delirium
- Dementia
- Pill-rolling tremors
- Chorea

- Autosomal-dominant
- Cognitive stimulation therapy
- Procedural memory

CASE VIGNETTE

Mary Hernandez is an 87-year-old widow with three grown daughters. Mrs. Hernandez completed high school in Puerto Rico before moving to New York with her husband. She was a homemaker and has never worked outside the home. She lives on a small pension and social security earned by her husband, who was a machinist. Two of her three daughters live nearby in New York, and one has returned to Puerto Rico. Mrs. Hernandez has a close relationship with her daughters, granddaughters, and a newborn great-grandson. She likes to go to the local Hispanic Senior Center, where she plays dominoes, exchanges recipes, and watches soap operas.

In the past 2 or 3 years, Mrs. Hernandez and her daughters have noticed that she is having increasing memory difficulties. She has begun to repeat herself in conversation, telling the same stories again and again. She has also begun calling her daughters several times a day, not remembering that she already spoke with them.

Mrs. Hernandez continues to pursue her daily activities, although she recently asked one of her daughters to manage her checking account for her because she is concerned about her own ability to do so.

THOUGHT QUESTIONS

1. Do you think Mrs. Hernandez has a mental disorder?
2. What factors in the description above contribute to your conclusion?
3. Does Mrs. Hernandez have functional deficits that might cause concern?
4. What else would you like to know about Mrs. Hernandez to decide whether an occupational therapy intervention might be helpful?

NEUROCOGNITIVE DISORDER

- Delirium
- Major or mild neurocognitive disorder
  - Etiological subtype:
    - Alzheimer's disease
    - Frontotemporal lobar degeneration
    - Lewy body disease

- Vascular disease
- Traumatic brain injury
- Substance/medication induced
- HIV infection
- Prion disease
- Parkinson's disease
- Huntington's disease

This neurocognitive disorders diagnostic grouping is unusual among the mental disorders because the etiology of each condition is specific and biological. Perhaps more than any other category, it reflects the growing scientific understanding of the complex interaction between physiology and psychology. The neurocognitive disorders label represents a change from the fourth edition of the *Diagnostic and Statistical Manual of Mental Disorders* (DSM-IV; American Psychiatric Association [APA], 1994) in which this cluster was known as Delirium, Dementia, Amnestic and Other Cognitive Disorders. The change to "neurocognitive" was made because:

> the term 'neurocognitive' describes cognitive functions closely linked to the function of particular brain regions, neural pathways, or cortical/subcortical networks in the brain. In parallel with the designation '*neuro*cognitive,' neuropsychology is a subdiscipline of psychology that focuses on psychological processes and behaviors related to known structural or metabolic brain disease. (Ganguli et al., 2011, p. 205)

Thus, the cluster not only acknowledges that there is a biological/physiological basis for these disorders, but it has gone so far as to specify the nature of the biological factors in detail.

The chapter in the fifth edition of the *Diagnostic and Statistical Manual of Mental Disorders* (DSM-5; APA, 2013) begins with a table that lists and defines the various cognitive domains. This list will look familiar to occupational therapists who make regular use of the *Occupational Therapy Practice Framework* (American Occupational Therapy Association [AOTA], 2014), which includes the following (APA, 2013):

- Complex attention
- Executive function
- Learning and memory
- Language
- Perceptual-motor
- Social cognition

Subtle (and not-so-subtle) differences exist among the various conditions causing neurocognitive disorders, many of which are discussed in terms of these cognitive domains. Because for some disorders—Alzheimer's disease is a notable example—diagnosis on the basis of laboratory tests is still not feasible, the distinctions among the specific neurocognitive and functional deficits that are demonstrated by each individual are essential in making accurate diagnoses.

Similar to other diagnostic categories, the neurocognitive disorders include options for "due to another medical condition," "due to multiple etiologies," and "unspecified neurocognitive disorder" (APA, 2013). Some individuals present with symptoms that do not fit the criteria for one of the other neurocognitive disorders and, as a result, one of these temporizing diagnoses will be selected. Often, either as a result of additional testing or as the disorder unfolds over time, it is possible to identify the etiology more specifically, and the diagnosis in an undetermined case will be changed. In addition, it is not unusual for an individual to have more than one condition, such as having both Alzheimer's disease and vascular disease. In such situations, the symptoms will be a mixture of those for the two conditions. These disorders are quite common and, with the aging of the population, are expected to become increasingly prevalent over the next several decades. Table 18-1 shows the prevalence of the neurocognitive disorders.

TABLE 18-1

PREVALENCE OF NEUROCOGNITIVE DISORDERS

DISORDER	PREVALENCE	GENDER RATIO (M:F)	SOURCE
Delirium	14% to 56% of elderly hospitalized clients	Unknown, probably equal	Khurana et al., 2011
Major neurocognitive disorder	13.9%		Plassman et al., 2007
Alzheimer's disease	69.9% of all dementia cases[a]	More women	Brookmeyer et al., 2011
Frontotemporal lobar degeneration	0.00003%	More women	Knopman, Petersen, Edland, Cha, & Rocca, 2004
Lewy body disease	20% of dementia cases[a]	More women	Lewy Body Dementia Association, 2012
Vascular disease	17.4% of individuals with dementia[a]	More women	Brookmeyer et al., 2011
Traumatic brain injury	1.7 million injuries annually	Unknown	Faul, Xu, Wald, & Coronado, 2010
Substance/medication induced	12% of all dementia cases[a]	Unknown	Lisi, 2000
HIV infection	10% to 24% of HIV cases		Grant, Sacktor, & McArthur, 2005
Prion disease	0.000001		Centers for Disease Control and Prevention, 2012
Parkinson's disease	0.5%		Aarsland, Zaccai, & Brayne, 2005
Huntington's disease	0.38%		Pringsheim et al., 2012
Mild neurocognitive disorder	39.1% overall	Lowest in younger women (32.3%); similar across men and older women (41.9% to 43.6%)	APA, 2013

[a]Total exceeds 100% due to differences in reporting in different study dates and methods, and comorbidity among forms of dementia.

Delirium

It is important for occupational therapists to know and understand the nature of delirium, although, typically, the involvement of occupational therapy in the treatment of this disorder is limited. The most important defining characteristic of **delirium** is alteration in consciousness—something that is rarely present in the other neurocognitive disorders. Delirium is often misdiagnosed (Joshi et al., 2012), in part because past versions of the DSM and World Health Organization's *International Classification of Diseases* (WHO 2001) have lacked adequate specificity. In the DSM-5 (APA, 2013), the diagnostic criteria include disturbance in attention that develops over a short time period, a change from the person's normal state, and fluctuation over time. Disturbance in cognition is also evident. A large number of specifiers exist that provide detail about the nature of the disorder. These include etiological attributions as, for example, associated with intoxication or substance withdrawal, a medical condition, multiple etiologies, and whether the delirium is accompanied by hyperactivity and agitation, hypoactivity, or a mixture of alterations in activity level. It is particularly important to differentiate delirium from **dementia**—a global loss of cognitive function—to ensure adequate and accurate treatment. Among the specific differences between delirium and dementia are the rate of onset, which is rapid for delirium, compared with long-term for most forms of dementia, and altered consciousness, which is characteristic of delirium but not dementia.

Etiology, Prognosis, and Implications for Function

Delirium is most common in hospital or nursing home settings and among older adults (Khurana, Gambhir, & Kishore, 2011). It is almost always associated with a medical condition, such as high fever, head injury, or as a postsurgical syndrome. Most often, the delirium resolves as the medical condition does, with or without treatment. Early detection and intervention can shorten the course and, in the case of older adults, reduce the risk of injury (Mittal et al., 2011). However, delirium is associated with a high mortality rate, probably because it typically accompanies serious illness (LeGrand, 2012).

Delirium causes dysfunction in every occupation (Khurana et al., 2011). It disrupts habits, patterns, and roles. By definition, it impairs cognitive skill and attention. Thus, for the duration of the condition, the individual is unable to perform necessary and desired daily activities.

Major Neurocognitive Disorder

In the neurocognitive disorder cluster, the first point of distinction is whether the symptoms reflect a major or mild condition. When that distinction has been made, the specific cause of the condition is identified, assuming it is possible to do so. Symptoms of major neurocognitive disorder (major NCD) include significant cognitive decline from the previous level of performance in one or more cognitive domains based on concern of the individual, an informant, or a clinician. Substantial impairment has been documented by neuropsychological or other quantifiable assessment, and the deficits interfere with independence in daily activities (APA, 2013). In addition to the cause identified in the diagnostic label, such as Alzheimer's or vascular disease, the specifiers note whether behavioral disturbance is present and whether the disorder is mild, moderate, or severe. "Mild" reflects difficulties with instrumental activities of daily living (IADL); "moderate" reflects activities of daily living (ADL); and "severe" would indicate total dependence.

Major neurocognitive disorder will be described in greater detail in this chapter in the context of the various etiological groups.

Mild Neurocognitive Disorder

Mild neurocognitive disorder (mild NCD) is characterized by modest cognitive decline from the previous level of performance in one or more cognitive domains based on concern of the individual, an informant, or a clinician (APA, 2013). The impairment is documented by neuropsychological or other quantifiable assessment. Deficits do not interfere with independence in daily activities, but greater effort, compensatory strategies, or accommodations may be required. For mild NCD, in addition to specifying the cause, specifiers note whether behavioral disturbance is present.

The distinction between major and mild NCD is a matter of degree. The clinician must determine whether the decline is "significant" or "modest," and whether difficulties with daily activities are substantial or a matter of added effort in conjunction with the implementation of compensatory strategies. The differentiation between mild and major NCD may be applied in most of the conditions described in this chapter. For those that are progressive, it is likely that the initial diagnosis may be mild NCD, but over time, the diagnosis will shift to major NCD.

Most often, individuals present for diagnostic review based on their own or others' concerns about functional deficits. For example, one 63-year-old man had increasing difficulty at his job working as a clerk in a hardware store. He became increasingly unable to recall where stock was kept or manage the cash register. Ultimately he had to retire earlier than anticipated as a result of his inability to do the work. Although he was inclined to minimize the problem, his wife insisted that he see his physician when she noted that he put one of his shoes in the freezer. These types of ADL difficulties appear to be an early predictor of dementia, even in the absence of clear signs from neuropsychological testing (Fauth et al., 2013).

Mild NCD is a more recently described phenomenon than major neurocognitive disorder. Not long ago, it was viewed simply as a precursor to more severe dementia. However, it is now recognized as a separate entity. The majority of individuals with mild NCD will not develop a major neurocognitive disorder, although a significant subset will (Snelgrove & Hasnain, 2012). Although the DSM-5 (APA, 2013) lists the same etiological conditions for the mild disorder as for the major disorder (e.g., Alzheimer's disease, Parkinson's disease), it is likely that additional research is needed to confirm that it is accurate to assume a similar set of etiologies. Further, in spite of its inclusion in the DSM-5, there remains significant question about the validity of the mild NCD diagnosis (George, Whitehouse, & Ballenger, 2011). Because there is no clarity about what constitutes "mild" and, further, the presence of a "mild" specifier for major NCD, some argument exists about whether the diagnosis belongs in the DSM at all. It is well established that the majority of older individuals experience some degree of cognitive decline. Whether this decline constitutes a mental disorder is questionable, and new versions of the DSM have work to do in resolving this dilemma.

On the other hand, there certainly are individuals who have a notable decline in cognition but remain functional at least in ADL. One 90-year-old woman, a former teacher, was able to bathe, dress, get herself to meals, socialize with friends, and otherwise manage her self-care and social participation while residing in an assisted living facility. However, she was unable to manage her checkbook, cook, drive, take her medications unsupervised, and, if she attended a lecture or movie, recall the content and topic. Over time, her short-term memory declined so that she had increasing difficulty maintaining more than superficial social encounters, but her ADL performance remained entirely intact. Her function and cognition were certainly impaired, but she did not progress to the severe dysfunction that characterizes major NCD.

Risk factors for mild NCD include genetic factors, especially the presence of the ApoE-4 allele (Sachdev et al., 2012). In addition, high homocysteine, heart disease, slow walk, history of depression, and a lack of challenging mental activity are associated with increased risk. Lower risk is associated with better visual acuity, mental activity, and odor identification.

Major Neurocognitive Disorder Etiological Subtypes

The next section of this chapter will describe the individual disorders that are included among the neurocognitive disorders, with emphasis on etiology, prognosis, and the unique functional and other characteristics that distinguish each. Although functional implications of the various conditions vary to some extent, significant overlap exists. For this reason, consideration of functional deficits in general, in treatment, and in functional implications for occupational therapy will be presented near the end of the chapter.

Alzheimer's Disease

Alzheimer's disease (AD) is by far the most common neurocognitive disorder (George et al., 2011). It is a progressive, deteriorating condition that over the course of years eventually leads to total disability. Initially described in 1917, AD has been the focus of intense research efforts, which have provided a great deal of information about the factors contributing to the gradual decline in cognitive ability but very little information about what causes those factors to emerge or what to do to prevent or treat them.

AD seems to be the result of a combination of genetic and environmental factors (Bicalho et al., 2013). The presence of apolipoprotein E ε4 is the most important genetic risk factor. Various other genes are the focus of study (Karch et al., 2012). Sociodemographic factors, such as educational level and physical fitness, also factor into the emergence of the AD disorder. However, the most significant risk factor identified to date is aging (Leuner, Müller, & Reichert, 2012).

The AD process appears to involve excessive amounts of two proteins in the central nervous system: hyperphosphorylated tau and intracellular amyloid beta oligomers (Leuner et al., 2012). These proteins seem to initiate a cascade of pathological events, including mitochondrial dysfunction, synaptic dysfunction, oxidative stress, loss of calcium regulation, and inflammation, each of which contributes to the progressive loss of neurons. What remains unclear is the connection between the genetic and environmental risk factors and the physiological consequences; that is, what actually causes the brain proteins to go awry.

A challenge in diagnosing NCD due to AD is the absence of any definitive diagnostic test. Confirmatory diagnosis must wait until brain tissue can be examined during autopsy. Although a brain biopsy could confirm the diagnosis while the individual is still living, the procedure is so invasive that it is rarely appropriate. Therefore, the diagnosis is either possible or probable AD. The unique diagnostic criteria for major or mild NCD due to AD include insidious onset and gradual progression of impairment (APA, 2013).

For major NCD, probable AD is diagnosed if there is evidence of a causative genetic mutation and/or evidence of decline in memory, learning, and other cognitive function; progressive decline; and no evidence of another cause.

For minor NCD, probable AD is diagnosed if there is evidence of a causative genetic mutation, in addition to functional deficits. Possible AD is diagnosed if there is no evidence of a causative mutation but there is evidence of decline in cognitive function without any other obvious causation.

Several factors should be highlighted in these criteria as specific to AD. First, AD is always progressive. Although the rate of progression varies, loss of cognitive function is inexorable. Second the absence of plateaus (periods of stable function) distinguishes AD from some of the other causes of NCD. There may be occasions when the appearance of a plateau, particularly in the early stages, during which the individual is likely to retain sufficient social skills and awareness to be able to put up a good front. However, such periods tend to be brief at best, and close observation during these phases typically reveals continuing loss of function.

Frontotemporal Lobar Degeneration

Frontotemporal lobar degeneration (FTLD) is a label for a heterogeneous group of disorders that demonstrate atrophy of the frontal and temporal lobes of the brain, with no atrophy in the parietal and occipital lobes (Halliday et al., 2012). One of the disorders included in this category is Pick's disease, which is a disorder that includes the presence of distinctive Pick cells and Pick bodies (Uyama, Yokochi, Bandoh, & Mizutani, 2013). Although not included in this grouping, amyotrophic lateral sclerosis shares common genetic and clinical findings with FTLD (Hasegawa et al., 2008).

Family history is strongly suggestive of an autosomal-dominant genetic etiology for the disorder (Gilberti et al., 2012). Up to 40% of FTLD clients show this pattern. Unlike AD—which must be diagnosed by exclusion and, prior to autopsy, can only be a probable label—FTLD can be diagnosed by characteristic findings in the cerebrospinal fluid (Irwin, Trojanowski, & Grossman, 2013).

Clinical symptoms that distinguish FTLD include insidious onset and gradual progression and symptoms of either a behavioral variant or a language variant (APA, 2013). The behavioral variant includes such signs as disinhibition, apathy, loss of empathy, and decline in social cognition. The language variant is characterized by decline in language ability. FTLD generally spares learning, memory, and perceptual-motor function. The disorder may be diagnosed as probable if there is evidence of a family pattern or as possible if there is no evidence of family/genetic causality. Note that because laboratory findings require spinal fluid, a choice is often made to rely on clinical findings for the diagnosis to avoid this painful and invasive procedure.

Compared with AD, FTLD reflects social dysfunction, personality changes, and cognitive impairment in language and executive function (Gilberti et al., 2012). Memory is relatively unaffected.

Lewy Body Disease

Lewy body disease (LBD) is characterized by the presence of Lewy bodies in the brain (Bogaerts, et al., 2007). Lewy bodies are clumps of specific proteins known as alpha-synuclein and ubiquitin. Clinically, LBD is characterized by fluctuating cognition, with variation in attention and alertness from day to day and hour to hour, visual hallucinations, and Parkinson's disease-like motor symptoms (Ferman et al., 2013). Characteristic changes in rapid eye movement sleep and abnormalities can be seen on positron emission tomography or single-photon emission computed tomography scans. The presence of motor symptoms has led to speculation that LBD is closely associated with Parkinson's disease (Fereshtehnejad et al., 2013). However, Parkinson's disease tends to have earlier onset and worse dementia.

LBD can be distinguished from AD based on verbal fluency (Delbeuck, Debachy, Pasquier, & Moroni, 2013). In terms of brain changes, only AD clients display small subsets of peripheral amyloid-beta1–42-specific T-cells (Lanuti et al., 2012).

Specific symptoms of LBD include insidious, gradual onset, with fluctuating cognition, visual hallucinations, and Parkinson-like symptoms (APA, 2013). In addition, rapid eye movement sleep disorder and neuroleptic sensitivity are often present. One of the characteristics that distinguishes LBD from AD is a difference in the source of ADL dysfunction (Hamilton et al., 2013). In LBD, motor difficulty accounts for the greatest part of dysfunction. In AD, both motor and behavioral issues are pronounced in ADL dysfunction.

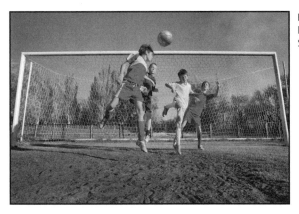

Figure 18-1. Young people may be affected by TBI sustained in sports activities. (©2014 Shutterstock.com.)

Vascular Disease

Vascular disease can affect many body systems, as interrupted blood flow inevitably results in damage to the associated system. In the case of vascular disease with impact in the central nervous system, the characteristic lesions affect cortical regions important for memory, cognition, and behavior (Jellinger, 2013). These changes result from systemic, cardiac, and local large or small vessel disease. Vascular disease is often found in conjunction with AD and other causes of dementia. Because vascular dementia can coexist with these other forms of dementia, it can be difficult to classify the cause of the observed clinical symptoms (Kling, Tojanowski, Wolk, Lee, & Arnold, 2013). Unfortunately, no clear neuropathological criteria exist for vascular and mixed dementia (Jellinger, 2013). Risk factors include high blood pressure, other vascular disease, and late-life depression (Diniz, Butters, Albert, Dew, & Reynolds, 2013).

Diagnostic criteria include presence of at least one cerebrovascular event, with decline in complex attention and frontal-executive function (APA, 2013). The diagnosis may be probable if there is a finding of cerebrovascular injury with at least some associated symptoms. A characteristic of vascular NCD is the presence of a step-wise deterioration of function. Each time a cerebrovascular event occurs, a sudden, notable decline in function occurs, which is followed by a plateau until there is another event. Of course, if the individual also has another form of NCD, this pattern may be masked.

Traumatic Brain Injury

Impact to the head, leading to cortical or other central nervous system damage, can have a wide array of consequences. Motor impairment may be the most evident sign of damage, but language, vision, hearing, or other sensory processing can also be affected. Traumatic brain injury (TBI) can lead to the classic symptoms of NCD, either mild or major. Specific cognitive and functional consequences are unpredictable because they depend on the areas of the cortex that are damaged (Sela-Kaufman, Rassovsky, Agranov, Levi, & Vakil, 2013).

Preinjury function is an important predictor of outcome following moderate TBI (Jonsson, Aaro Catroppa, Godfrey, Smedler, & Anderson, 2013; Sela-Kaufman et al., 2013). However, inflammation and white matter damage can persist for years after a single event (Johnson et al., 2013). This finding has received considerable notice in the past few years as evidence has emerged that sports-related concussions can result in symptoms of NCD (DeKosky, Ikonomovic, & Gandy, 2010; Figure 18-1).

Diagnostic criteria for TBI include evidence of an injury to the head, with loss of consciousness, posttraumatic amnesia, disorientation, and/or neurological signs (APA, 2013).

Unlike all the previous categories of NCD, no probable or possible category exists. The presence of a TBI with associated symptoms of cognitive damage makes this the most straightforward form of NCD, at least as related to diagnosis.

Substance/Medication-Induced NCD

As is true for TBI, the NCD associated with substance or medication use is fairly straightforward to identify. The diagnosis is made only if there is evidence of substance use or withdrawal. To some extent, the specific symptoms depend on the substance (Allen, Strauss, Leany, & Donahue, 2008).

Diagnostic criteria for substance/medication-induced NCD include neurocognitive symptoms that continue after intoxication and immediate withdrawal and evidence of substance use and subsequent abstinence (APA, 2013). No categories exist for probable or possible NCD for this type, as the diagnosis is made only if substance use is established.

As is true with other forms of NCD, there is the potential for multiple causes of the observed symptoms. For example, substance-related NCD can coexist with and complicate the effects of HIV induced NCD (Weber et al., 2013). Unlike the majority of the NCD diagnoses described in this chapter, substance/medication–induced NCD may improve over time, particularly if it is the result of withdrawal leading to cessation of using the substance (Allen et al., 2008). However, even in the absence of the substance, if the cortical damage has been sufficient, the symptoms may persist.

HIV Infection

It has been well-established for some time that HIV infection can lead to NCD. This has become an increasing issue, as HIV has become more treatable, and individuals who have the virus live longer (Mateen & Mills, 2012). NCD can emerge even when the individual is being successfully treated with antiretroviral medications that prevent the development of AIDS. This may be in part because these medications do not pass the blood–brain barrier. The situation is further complicated by the fact that because individuals with HIV are now living into late life, they can develop one or more of the other syndromes associated with NCD. In addition, some of these individuals may have acquired the virus through substance use that contributes to a substance/medication-induced NCD (Allen et al., 2008).

The primary criterion for diagnosing HIV infection NCD is a documented HIV infection (APA, 2013). Between one third and one half of individuals with HIV have at least mild cognitive deficits associated with the disorder, particularly in ability to plan (Cattie et al., 2012). This planning deficit impairs function in everyday activities.

Prion Disease

The most common prion disease is Creutzfeld-Jakob (Zerr, 2013). However, this cluster of diseases is generally quite rare, with no more than about one to two cases per million people worldwide. Thus, studying the diseases is as difficult as understanding the treatment. These disorders present with specific cognitive profiles, in addition to neurological abnormalities, such as ataxia, rigidity, and myoclonus.

Diagnostic criteria of prion disease include insidious onset, rapid progression, and motor features, such as ataxia, that are consistent with prion disease (APA, 2013).

Prion is an infectious disease apparently transmitted by infection from animals, such as the spongiform encephalopathy widely reported in Great Britain in the 1990s. It can be distinguished from other forms of NCD both because of its rapid course and the accompanying motor symptoms.

Parkinson's Disease

Parkinson's disease is another disorder that is clearly neurological, with observable changes that can assist in diagnosis. Although no laboratory test is available to confirm diagnosis, the characteristic motor signs, along with a trial of one of the Parkinson's medications, are confirmatory. Parkinson's disease has many symptoms in common with LBD, and some believe that the two constitute a spectrum disorder (Ballard, Kahn, & Corbett, 2011). Parkinson's is notable for motor tremors, particularly **pill-rolling tremors**, which are uncontrollable movements of the fingers that give the appearance of rolling small objects in the hand. These tremors typically appear at rest. Individuals with Parkinson's also have a characteristic shuffling gait.

Parkinson's can cause NCD, although these symptoms do not appear in every case, and their extent varies (Cronin-Golomb, 2013). NCD symptoms can include mood, sleep, and autonomic function changes, as well as impairments in cognition and perception.

The etiology of Parkinson's is as yet unclear, although genetic research suggests that at least some proportion of cases have genetic-related causes (Reichmann, 2011). Also, speculation exists that a toxin, bacterium, or virus contributes to the condition. This explanation may have emerged as a result of the outbreak of encephalitis lethargica, which followed the influenza epidemic of 1918 (Dale et al., 2003). This disorder included the typical motor changes associated with Parkinson's. Encephalitis lethargica was described by Oliver Sachs in his book *Awakenings* (1999) and in the movie of the same title, starring Robin Williams (Parkes & Lasker, 1990).

Diagnostic criteria for Parkinson's NCD include an established diagnosis of Parkinson's with insidious, gradual onset (APA, 2013).

Parkinson's disease fits the insidious onset and chronic and deteriorating pattern of many of the other NCDs. As discussed in this chapter, a larger number of medical treatments are available for this disorder than for some of the other NCDs, but there is currently no cure.

Huntington's Disease

Unlike the many disorders and syndromes contributing to NCD, the cause of Huntington's disease is well established. It is an autosomal dominant genetic disorder that affects the HTT gene (Rodrigues et al., 2011), resulting in chorea, behavioral disturbances, and dementia. It is sometimes known as Huntington's **chorea** because of the characteristic jerky and involuntary movements that are seen in the disorder.

Diagnostic criteria for Huntington's disease NCD include insidious onset, gradual progression, and established family history or genetic profile (APA, 2013).

Huntington's disease presents unique clinical challenges for treatment (Andersson, Juth, Petersén, Graff, & Edberg, 2013). The **autosomal-dominant** nature of the disease means that if an individual inherits the gene from one parent, he or she will develop the disease. Symptoms typically emerge in middle age, occurring after the age at which one generally has children. However, the presence of the gene can be assessed so that an individual can learn well before the onset of symptoms whether he or she will develop the disease. Thus, the individual must make a painful choice to be tested prior to procreating, with the potential to learn that he or she has a life and function-threatening disorder or to forego testing with another painful choice—to have children to whom you might pass the disorder along or decide not to have children—understanding that there is a 50% chance one did not inherit the gene and therefore would not pass it along. This is often a significant difficulty in working with individuals in families known to have the gene.

Implications for Function and Treatment

As discussed in the previous sections, there are differences in presentation of the various NCD, many of which are related to areas of function. Disorders that have insidious onset and a deteriorating course—including AD, frontotemporal lobar, Lewy body, prion, Parkinson's, and Huntington's—emerge with some differences. In the case of AD, early signs involve confusion about everyday activities, accompanied by deficits in short-term memory. In the case of Parkinson's, the early symptoms may be motor, rather than neurocognitive, in nature. However, in all these conditions, there is an inexorable downward spiral in function in all spheres, including occupations and skills. For some disorders (e.g., Parkinson's), skill deficits may initially be more motor focused, whereas in others (e.g., Alzheimer's) they may initially be more cognitive and perceptual. However, over time, individuals with any of these conditions will show decrements in occupations, skills, habits, patterns, and roles. For example, individuals with late-stage AD are ultimately bedridden and unable to move purposefully, swallow, talk, or otherwise function (Volicer & Simard, 2009).

Some of the other NCDs, including TBI and substance/medication-related conditions, are not necessarily progressive. Functional consequences of TBI are dependent on the location of the injury and its severity. Careful assessment is essential, as many of the signs may be quite subtle. Substance/medication-related NCD is often characterized by deficits in abstract reasoning, motor programming, and cognitive flexibility (Cuhna, Jannuzzi, de Andrade, & Guerra Bola, 2010). Distinctions among the various etiologies of NCD are summarized in Table 18-2.

An important concern around the various NCDs is the potential for excess disability resulting from comorbidity (Slaughter & Bankes, 2007). An individual may have several NCDs simultaneously (Parkinson's and Alzheimer's are frequently comorbid), or an individual with a TBI may develop Alzheimer's. In addition, individuals with NCD, particularly in the early stages, may become depressed as they recognize their own functional loss. Remediating the conditions for which there are effective treatments can improve function, even in individuals with substantial impairment. For example, increasing social interaction and meaningful activities can improve quality of life and reduce depression and by doing so improve ADL and IADL function. One woman diagnosed with Alzheimer's disease moved to a new city to live with her unmarried son. The son worked full time, and the woman, who knew no one in the new location, stayed alone in his apartment all day. Her son was dismayed that his mother's condition deteriorated rapidly and severely. Finally, he felt he had no choice but to move her to a nursing home that had a dementia care unit. He was surprised to discover when he came to visit 1 week later that his mother was much more alert and engaged—she had been lonely and depressed, but now had a social circle and activities she enjoyed. Although she still had significant cognitive impairment, the remediation of her depression resulted in improved cognition and quality of life.

Mild NCD is associated with decrements in executive function and long- and short-term memory, but, by definition, it is not accompanied by loss of ADL (Hughes, Chang, Bilt, Snitz, & Ganguli, 2012). Loss of IADL function is common. Often, social ability is well maintained, although it is increasingly superficial over time. These individuals do have some accompanying perceptual challenges; for example, mild NCD is a predictor of falls (Delbaere et al., 2012).

Treatment varies among the conditions. For some disorders, Parkinson's for example, medications are available that can slow deterioration. For others, such as Alzheimer's, effective medications remain an elusive goal, and treatment is largely focused on managing behaviors.

Substantial research has been conducted on pharmacological agents to treat AD (Misra & Medhi, 2013). Among them are cholinesterase inhibitors, memantine, and several others

TABLE 18-2

COMPARISON AND CONTRAST: CHARACTERISTICS OF DIFFERENT NEUROCOGNITIVE DISORDERS

ETIOLOGY	ONSET	PROGRESSION	SPECIFIC DEFICITS
Alzheimer's	Insidious	Gradual (variable progression)	Initial: Executive function, memory, and work Intermediate: IADL, ADL, and social Long term: All functions, including motor Spared: None
Frontotemporal lobular	Insidious	Progressive	Behavioral disinhibition (apathy, loss of empathy) Perseverative, stereotyped, or obsessive behavior Hyperorality and dietary changes Social cognition and executive function Spared: Learning, memory, and perceptual-motor
Lewy body	Insidious	Progressive	Fluctuating cognition Attention/alertness Visual hallucinations Difficulty maintaining social conventions Parkinsonian tremors and pronounced motor deficits Spared: None
Vascular	Abrupt	May or may not progress	Complex attention Executive function Other dependent on site and frequency of lesions Spared: Dependent on site
TBI	Abrupt	Not progressive	Dependent on area of damage Spared: Dependent on area of damage
Substance/medication induced	Abrupt or progressive	Progressive if substance use continues	Memory, cognition, and performance areas Motor Spared: May improve if substance use ends

(continued)

TABLE 18-2 (CONTINUED)			
COMPARISON AND CONTRAST: CHARACTERISTICS OF DIFFERENT NEUROCOGNITIVE DISORDERS			
ETIOLOGY	*ONSET*	*PROGRESSION*	*SPECIFIC DEFICITS*
HIV	Insidious	Progressive	Impaired memory, apathy, social withdrawal, and difficulty concentrating Spared: Varies
Parkinson's	Insidious	Progressive	Motor deficits may be noted first; characteristic pill-rolling, tremor, gait disturbance, and motor rigidity Anxiety, depression, and memory loss Spared: Cognitive loss is variable
Prion	Insidious	Progressive-rapid	Problems with muscular coordination Personality changes, including impaired memory, judgment, and thinking Impaired vision Insomnia and depression Spared: None
Huntington's	Insidious	Progressive	Irritability, anxiety, and depression, progresses to severe dementia Psychotic behavior Involuntary jerky movements, muscle weakness, clumsiness, and gait disturbance Spared: None

(Rountree, Atri, Lopez, & Doody, 2013). These pharmacological agents are being studied separately and in combination. Combination therapy seems to be more effective, although the impact is modest and generally reflects slower decline, rather than reversal.

For frontotemporal lobar disorder, the more effective pharmacological interventions are trazodone, fluvoxamine, and rivastigmine (Da Glória Portugal, Marinho, & Laks, 2011). Lewy body dementia and Parkinson's respond to cholinesterase inhibitors, antipsychotics, antidepressants, and levodopa (Ballard et al., 2011). Management of vascular NCD includes control of conditions, such as hypertension and diabetes, contributing to vascular damage (Brucki et al., 2011). To date, deep brain stimulation has been attempted primarily in treatment of Parkinson's, where it has been found to be effective (Ashkan, Samuel, Reddy, & Chaudhuri, 2013).

Other interventions for AD are largely focused on management, either through direct intervention with the person or through environmental modification (Gauthier et al., 2010). The goal of these kinds of interventions is managing problem behaviors, such as wandering and emotional outbursts, and on minimizing caregiver burden (Agüera-Ortiz, Frank-Garcia,

Gil, Moreno, & 5E Study Group, 2010). The issue of caregiver burden is a significant one, as the affected individual may need round-the-clock monitoring (Farran et al., 2011). Education and support may be an important component of intervention for everyone on the treatment team.

Where there are motor problems, as with Parkinson's, comprehensive multidisciplinary intervention is essential (Hindle, 2013). Such individuals may benefit from gait and balance training. Also, evidence exists that Parkinson's symptoms can be reduced to some extent through exercise, acupuncture (Zesiewica & Evatt, 2009), and dance (Hackney, Kantorovich, Levin, & Earhart, 2007).

For TBI, various neuropsychological strategies can be helpful. Interestingly, premorbid personality, particularly evidence of resilience, can make a difference in the effectiveness of these treatments (Simpson & Jones, 2013).

A number of interventions focus on efforts to prevent cognitive decline. The strongest evidence of preventive efficacy is for physical activity (Lövdén, Xu, & Wangy, 2013). Interventions in this category that have been tested include strength training, cycling, walking, playing Nintendo Wii, and *tai chi*. Cognitive interventions also seem to support good cognitive function. These strategies include use of memory tools, such as mnemonic devices and cognitive practice using the computer, or doing challenging mental activities, such as learning a new language. Table 18-3 shows the diagnostic criteria and functional implications for major and mild NCD.

Implications for Occupational Therapy

Intervention to enhance function for individuals with varying forms of NCD often involves occupational therapy. Because few effective medical treatments exist, management of behaviors and enhancement of function are frequently the focus of an individual's intervention, thus occupational therapy brings a great deal of expertise to this effort. For example, it is established that leisure activities can reduce depression in individuals with dementia and that reducing depression can enhance function (Cheng, Chow, Yu, & Chan, 2012). The effectiveness of gardening interventions, behavioral and environmental strategies (Jonveaux et al., 2013), and exercise (Grazina & Massano, 2013) have been reported. Often, intervention focuses on the management of self-care activities, such as medication management (Figure 18-2). Other interventions that can offer considerable benefit are physical activity (Langlois et al., 2012) and computer-based cognitive practice (Fazeli, Ross, Vance, & Ball, 2013).

Overall, occupational therapy supports individuals in managing self-care, participating in social and leisure activities, improving quality of life, and reducing caregiver burden (Steultjens et al., 2004). Among the specific strategies that have been examined are sensory stimulation, environmental modification, and use of functional activities (Kim, Yoo, Jung, Park, & Park, 2012). **Cognitive stimulation therapy** that encourages various cognitively challenging activities may be beneficial as well (Yuill & Hollis, 2011). Speculation exists that such activities can reduce the risk of developing some forms of dementia (Wilson et al., 2002). Enhanced task oriented training also shows promise (Ciro, Hershey, & Garrison, 2013).

Intervening with individuals with dementia requires realistic framing of goals (Chapman, Weiner, Rackley, Hynan, & Zientz, 2004; McLaren, LaMantia, & Callahan, 2013). It is unrealistic to assume that an individual will improve dramatically, but slowing or delaying functional decline can be a positive outcome and can enhance the individual's sense of enjoyment and usefulness.

When it is not possible to achieve these goals, a focus on quality of life becomes increasingly vital. A focus on familiar activities and individual strengths can enhance satisfaction.

TABLE 18-3		
DIAGNOSTIC CRITERIA AND FUNCTIONAL IMPLICATIONS: NEUROCOGNITIVE DISORDERS		
DISORDER	*DIAGNOSTIC CRITERIA (APA, 2013)*	*IMPLICATIONS FOR FUNCTION*
Delirium	Disturbed attention and cognition Develops over a brief period, is a change from the person's normal state, and fluctuates over time	Substantial impairment in all occupations, skill, and pattern areas
Major neurocognitive disorder	Significant cognitive deterioration from previous level of performance in one or more cognitive domains based on the following: • Individual or informant concern • Documented impairment in cognition Deficits interfere with independence in daily activities	Substantial impairment in all occupations, skill, and pattern areas May be specific impairments, depending on etiology of NCD
Mild neurocognitive disorder	Modest cognitive deterioration from previous level of performance in one or more cognitive domains based on the following: • Individual or informant concern • Documented modest impairment in cognition Deficits do not interfere with independence in daily activities, but greater effort or accommodations may be needed	Work, leisure, social, and self-care occupations may be negatively affected to a modest extent Greater energy required to engage in these areas Cognitive skills are negatively affected to some extent Other skill areas may be intact or moderately affected for the worse Habits, roles, patterns are negatively affected as memory declines

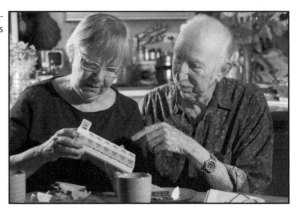

Figure 18-2. Daily living activities like managing medications can be difficult for individuals with NCD. (©2014 Shutterstock.com.)

This can be accomplished using Montessori methods (self-directed exploration of activities of interest with accompanying participation in well-learned and familiar activities) to increase individual engagement in the world and promote a sense of calm and pleasure (Elliott, 2007). These activities can also reduce depression, which will minimize excess disability.

TBI, because of its very different onset and course, requires somewhat different strategies. External memory aids may support function when short-term memory is impaired (Armstrong, Mcpherson, & Nayar, 2012). Practice of familiar and necessary activities can also improve function (Brauer, Hay, & Francisco, 2011). Computer-based practice of various memory-related tasks has been used to enhance function as well.

Various specific occupation-based programs have been developed that incorporate strategies to enhance pleasure and enjoyment, maintain health, and maximize **procedural memory**—memory for well-established habitual activities (Chabot, 2013). Among these is the Forget-Me-Not program, originated by Kim Warchol; the Tailored Activity Program, designed by Laura Gitlin; and the Montessori-based programs, initially designed by Cameron Camp (as cited by Chabot, 2013). All three programs "emphasize the importance of tailoring activities to the emotional, physical, and cognitive abilities of the client in order to reduce frustration and create a just right challenge" (Chabot, 2013, p. 3). In addition, all three draw on activities that clients enjoyed prior to developing cognitive deficits.

Although attention to caregiver needs is important for any support network coping with an individual with a severe mental disorder, caregiver support can be vital in working with individuals with NCD (Hall & Skelton, 2012). Particularly when an individual experiences an insidious onset and deteriorating course, family members and other caregivers must readjust their strategies frequently. As the individual becomes increasingly impaired, caregivers are called upon to provide greater levels of care and for more extended periods during the day. A well-known book for caregivers is called *The 36-Hour Day* (Mace & Rabins, 2012) because that is how much time caregivers might feel they are spending each day looking after loved ones. Brief occupational therapy interventions that are focused on providing management strategies can improve quality of life for both the client and the caregiver (Dooley & Hinojosa, 2004).

Cultural Considerations

The cultural beliefs and practices of the individual and caregiver have a significant impact on the nature of the intervention and the probable outcomes of care (Sun, Ong, & Burnette, 2012). Although the neurocognitive impact of the disorders is similar across cultures, the tasks needed and desired by the individual differ substantially, as do the objects and environments that support function (Hanssen, 2013). This has implications for the structuring of environments, expectations of and support for caregiving, and even written caregiver instructions. All of these must be considered with an eye toward the specific cultural factors that affect occupations and family relationships (van der Steen et al., 2013).

For example, beliefs about family harmony and filial piety can influence expectations about whether family members will assume the caregiver role (Sun et al., 2012). Likewise, help-seeking behaviors are culturally mediated, affecting whether a caregiver will seek respite or formal support. Sometimes these choices, even when the coping strategies appear to be positive ones, can result in higher levels of caregiver stress (Merritt & McCallum, 2013).

Lifespan Considerations

Dementia is much less common in children than in older adults, although when it does occur in younger people, the presentation is similar (Grover et al., 2012). The most typical form of childhood NCD is TBI (Jonsson et al., 2013). Of the various etiologies of NCD, onset of substance/medication-related is probably dispersed most broadly across the lifespan, as substance use can occur at any age. Although many of the NCDs have onset in later life, it is important to remember that they can occur in middle-aged adults as well. Alzheimer's has been diagnosed in individuals in their 40s and 50s (Alzheimer's Association, 2013). Parkinson's is not uncommon in individuals in their 40s (National Parkinson Foundation, 2013). Individuals in middle age are in their most productive work years and often have children still at home and needing their attention. These factors can make for a very challenging situation for both the individual and the family. Remember, too, that individuals with trisomy 21, described in Chapter 3, almost universally show symptoms of Alzheimer's disease by the time they reach age 40.

Internet Resources

Alzheimer's Association
http://www.alz.org/professionals_and_researchers_14899.asp
The prototypical self-help organization, the Alzheimer Association has a rich array of resources. Unlike some other self-help groups, the Association has local chapters that provide some direct services, including support groups, referrals, caregiver training, and materials for professionals.

American Parkinson Disease Association
http://www.apdaparkinson.org
A self-help organization focused on supporting individuals with Parkinson's disease and promoting research to find a cure.

National Institutes of Health. National Institute on Aging
http://www.nia.nih.gov/alzheimers/alzheimers-disease-caregiving-resource-list
Although the focus here is on Alzheimer's disease, the resources would be helpful in many situations involving NCD.

School of Social Welfare, University of Albany
http://www.albany.edu/aging/IDD/r-dementia.htm
Quite a number of universities and medical institutions have special centers focused on care of individuals with dementia. These centers tend to be more reliable resources than many of the commercial websites (some of which avoid the ".com" URL by creating what appear to be not-for-profit sites but are associated with business interests). This particular website is one example of the kinds of resources that can be found through these kinds of university centers.

U.S. National Library of Medicine. Pub Med Health
http://www.ncbi.nlm.nih.gov/pubmedhealth/PMH0001748/
This site clearly describes and discusses the various forms of dementia.

CASE STUDY

Arnold Ali Bey is a 63-year-old retired veteran with a wife and adult daughter. After putting in 20 years as a master sergeant in the army, Mr. Bey worked as a security guard at a chemical plant until his second retirement at age 60. He has long enjoyed wood-carving, fishing, and playing poker with friends with whom he served in the military. He has always been a very social person, enjoying banter with friends and family.

Mr. Bey's wife and daughter are concerned about him because of a 4-year history of deteriorating memory. He left his security job in part because he was having difficulty remembering what his responsibilities were in terms of patrolling the plant. He missed his check-in times at various stations around the plant with increasing frequency. He has also withdrawn to a large extent from his leisure activities. Although he remains very social, Mrs. Bey notes that it is difficult to have a sustained conversation with her husband and that he repeats himself frequently. Most recently, she has become concerned because Mr. Bey has started refusing to bathe, and several times in the past several weeks she has found burners left lit on the stove after Mr. Bey has been in the kitchen. Mr. Bey is otherwise healthy except for high blood pressure and a slightly enlarged prostate.

Mrs. Bey brings Mr. Bey to his primary care physician, who suspects Alzheimer's disease and refers Mr. Bey to a Geriatric Evaluation Center. At the Center, Mr. Bey is noted to have communication deficits, particularly a tendency to use vague referents such as "things" and "stuff." He could provide his name but not his current age or birth month. He did not know the current year or the name of the current U.S. president. No evidence of tremor or motor deficit was noted other than somewhat poor balance. On formal testing, he scored well below average in all cognitive domains. These tests included the Wechsler Memory Scale (2009), the Wechsler Adult Intelligence Scale (2008), digit span and similarities subtests, the Boston Naming Test (Kaplan, Goodglass, & Weintraub, 1983), the CERAD Word List Memory Test (Lamberty, Kennedy, & Flashman, 1995), and the California Proverb Test (Delis, Kramer, Kaplan, & Ober, 1983/1987). He tended to perseverate in both verbal and motor responses. All laboratory tests and blood work were normal, and there was no history of recent brain trauma. Further, Mrs. Bey confirmed that the current situation had emerged gradually over the course of several years. The neurologist diagnosed "probable" Alzheimer's disease and encouraged Mr. and Mrs. Bey to seek support and assistance from the local Alzheimer's Association.

THOUGHT QUESTIONS

1. What specific factors in the description of the medical and psychological workup characterize Alzheimer's disease?

2. Are there other forms of dementia that could be the source of Mr. Bey's difficulties? Other mental disorders?

3. What functional deficits, beyond those described, might be factors in Mr. Bey's situation?

References

Aarsland, C., Zaccai, J., & Brayne, C. (2005). A systematic review of prevalence studies of dementia in Parkinson's disease. *Movement Disorders, 20*(10), 1255-1263.

Agüera-Ortiz, F., Frank-Garcia, A., Gil, P., Moreno, A., & 5E Study Group. (2010). Clinical progression of moderate-to-severe Alzheimer's disease and caregiver burden: A 12-month multicenter prospective observational study. *International Psychogeriatrics, 22*(8), 1265-1279.

Allen D.N., Strauss, G.P.D., Leany, B., & Donahue, B. (2008). Neuropsychological assessment of individuals with substance use disorders. In A.M. Horton & D. Wedding (Eds.). *The neuropsychology handbook* (3rd ed., pp. 705-728). New York, NY: Springer.

Alzheimer's Association (2013). *Younger/early onset Alzheimer's and dementia*. Retrieved from http://www.alz.org/alzheimers_disease_early_onset.asp.

American Occupational Therapy Association. (2014) Occupational therapy practice framework: Domain & process (3rd ed.). *American Journal of Occupational Therapy, 68*(Suppl. 1), S1-S48.

American Psychiatric Association. (1994). *Diagnostic and statistical manual of mental disorders* (4th ed.). Washington, DC: Author.

American Psychiatric Association. (2013). *Diagnostic and statistical manual of mental disorders* (5th ed.). Washington, DC: Author.

Andersson, P.L., Juth, N., Petersén, A., Graff, C., & Edberg, A. (2013). Ethical aspects of undergoing a predictive genetic testing for Huntington's disease. *Nursing Ethics, 20*(2), 189-199.

Armstrong, J., Mcpherson, K., & Nayar, S. (2012). External memory aid training after traumatic brain injury: 'Making it real.' *British Journal of Occupational Therapy, 75*(12), 541-548.

Ashkan, K., Samuel, M., Reddy, P., & Chaudhuri, K.R. (2013). The impact of deep brain stimulation on the nonmotor symptoms of Parkinson's disease. *Journal of Neural Transmission, 120*(4), 639-642.

Ballard, C., Kahn, Z., & Corbett, A. (2011). Treatment of dementia with Lewy bodies and Parkinson's disease dementia. *Drugs & Aging, 28*(10), 769-777.

Bicalho, C., Pimenta, M.A., Bastos-Rodrigues, F.A., de Olivera Hanson, L., Neves, E., Melo, S.C., . . . De Marco, L. (2013). Sociodemographic characteristics, clinical factors, and genetic polymorphisms associated with Alzheimer's disease. *International Journal of Geriatric Psychiatry, 28*(6), 640-646.

Bogaerts, V., Engelborghs, S., Kumar-Singh, S., Goossens, D., Pickut, B., van der Zee, J., . . . Van Broeckhoven, C. (2007). A novel locus for dementia with Lewy bodies: A clinically and genetically heterogeneous disorder. *Brain, 130*(9), 2277-2291.

Brauer, J., Hay, C.C., & Francisco, G. (2011). A retrospective investigation of occupational therapy services received following a traumatic brain injury. *Occupational Therapy in Health Care, 25*(2/3), 119-130.

Brookmeyer, R., Evans, D.A., Hebert, L., Langa, K.M., Heeringa, S.G., Plassman, B.L., & Kukull, W.A. (2011). National estimates of the prevalence of Alzheimer's disease in the United States. *Alzheimer's Dementia, 7*(1), 61-73.

Brucki, D., Ferraz, S.M., de Freitas, A.C., Massaro, G.R., Radanovic, A.R., Schultz, M., . . . Working Group on Alzheimer's Disease and Vascular Dementia of the Brazilian Academy of Neurology. (2011). Treatment of vascular dementia: Recommendations of the Scientific Department of Cognitive Neurology and Aging of the Brazilian Academy of Neurology. *Dementia & Neuropsychologia, 5*(4), 275-287.

Cattie, J.E., Doyle, K., Weber, E., Grant, I., Woods, S.P., & HIV Neurobehavioral Research Program (HNRP) Group. (2012). Planning deficits in HIV-associated neurocognitive disorders: Component processes, cognitive correlates, and implications for everyday functioning. *Journal of Clinical and Experimental Neuropsychology, 34*(9), 906-918.

Centers for Disease Control and Prevention. (2012). *Creutzfeld-Jakob Disease*. Retrieved from http://www.cdc.gov/ncidod/dvrd/cjd/index.htm.

Chabot, M. (2013). Review of programs to support engagement of older adults with mild to moderate dementia. *American Occupational Therapy Association Special Interest Section Quarterly: Gerontology, 36*(1), 1-4.

Chapman, S., Weiner, M., Rackley, A., Hynan, L., & Zientz, J. (2004). Effects of cognitive communication stimulation for Alzheimer's disease patients treated with donepezil. *Journal of Speech, Language, and Hearing Research, 47*, 1149-1163.

Cheng, S.T., Chow, P.K., Yu, E.C., & Chan, A.C. (2012). Leisure activities alleviate depressive symptoms in nursing home residents with very mild or mild dementia. *American Journal of Geriatric Psychiatry, 20*(10), 904-908.

Ciro, C.A., Hershey, L.A., & Garrison, D. (2013). Enhanced task-oriented training in a person with dementia with Lewy bodies. *American Journal of Occupational Therapy, 67*, 556-563.

Cronin-Golomb, A. (2013). Emergence of nonmotor symptoms as the focus of research and treatment of Parkinson's disease: Introduction to the special section on nonmotor dysfunctions in Parkinson's disease. *Behavioral Neuroscience, Special Section: Non-Motor Dysfunctions in Parkinson's Disease, 127*(2), 135-138.

Cuhna, P., Jannuzzi, N., de Andrade, A., & Guerra Bolla, K.I. (2010). The frontal assessment battery (FAB) reveals neurocognitive dysfunction in substance-dependent individuals in distinct executive domains: Abstract reasoning, motor programming, and cognitive flexibility. *Addictive Behaviors, 35*(10), 875-881.

Dale, R.C., Church, A.J., Surtees, R.A.H., Lees, A.J., Adcock, J.E., Harding, B., . . . Giovannoni, G. (2003). Encephalitis lethargica syndrome: 20 new cases and evidence of basal ganglia autoimmunity. *Brain, 127*(1), 21-33.

Da Glória Portugal, M., Marinho, V., & Laks, J., (2011). Pharmacological treatment of frontotemporal lobar degeneration: Systematic review. *Revista Brasileira de Psiquiatria, 33*(1), 81-90.

DeKosky, S.T., Ikonomovic, M.D., & Gandy, S. (2010). Traumatic brain injury: Football, warfare, and long-term effects. *New England Journal of Medicine, 363*(14), 1293-1296.

Delbaere, K., Kochan, N.A., Close, J.C., Menant, J.C., Sturnieks, D.L., Brodaty, H., . . . Lord, S.R. (2012). Mild cognitive impairment as a predictor of falls in community-dwelling older people. *American Journal of Geriatric Psychiatry, 20*(10), 845-853.

Delbeuck, X., Debachy, B., Pasquier, F., & Moroni, C. (2013). Action and noun fluency testing to distinguish between Alzheimer's disease and dementia with Lewy bodies. *Journal of Clinical and Experimental Neuropsychology, 35*(3), 259-268.

Delis, D.C., Kramer, J.H., Kaplan, E., & Ober, B.A. (1983/1987). *California verbal learning test: Adult version.* San Antonio, TX: The Psychological Corporation.

Diniz, B.S., Butters, M.A., Albert, S.M., Dew, M.A., & Reynolds, C.F. (2013). Late-life depression and risk of vascular dementia and Alzheimer's disease: Systematic review and meta-analysis of community-based cohort studies. *British Journal of Psychiatry, 202*(5), 329-335.

Dooley, N.R., & Hinojosa, J. (2004). Improving quality of life for persons with Alzheimer's disease and their family caregivers: Brief occupational therapy interventions. *American Journal of Occupational Therapy, 58*, 561-569.

Elliott, G. (2007). A focus on Montessori-based dementia programming. *Canadian Nursing Home, 18*(1), 35-36, 38, 40.

Farran, C.J., Fogg, L.G., McCann, J.J., Etkin, C., Dong, X., & Barnes, L.L. (2011). Assessing family caregiver skill in managing behavioral symptoms of Alzheimer's disease. *Aging & Mental Health, 15*(4), 510-521.

Faul, M., Xu, L., Wald, M.M., & Coronado, V.G. (2010). *Traumatic brain injury in the United States: Emergency department visits, hospitalizations, and deaths.* Atlanta (GA): Centers for Disease Control and Prevention, National Center for Injury Prevention and Control. Retrieved from http://www.cdc.gov/traumaticbraininjury/pdf/blue_book.pdf.

Fauth, E.B., Schwartz, S., Tschaz, J.T., Østbye, T., Corcoran, C., & Norton, M.C. (2013). Baseline disability in activities of daily living predicts dementia risk even after controlling for baseline global cognitive ability and depressive symptoms. *International Journal of Geriatric Psychiatry, 28*(6), 597-606.

Fazeli, P.L., Ross, L.A., Vance, D.E., & Ball, K. (2013). The relationship between computer experience and computerized cognitive test performance among older adults. *Journals of Gerontology Series B: Psychological Sciences and Social Sciences, 68*, 337-346.

Fereshtehnejad, S., Religa, D., Westman, E., Aarsland, D., Lökk, J., & Eriksdotter, M. (2013). Demography, diagnostics, and medication in dementia with Lewy bodies and Parkinson's disease with dementia: Data from the Swedish Dementia Quality Registry (SveDem). *Neuropsychiatric Disease and Treatment, 9*, 927-935.

Ferman, T.J., Arvanitakis, Z., Fujishiro, H., Duara, R., Parfitt, F., Purdy, M., . . . Dickson, D.W. (2013). Pathology and temporal onset of visual hallucinations, misperceptions and family misidentification distinguishes dementia with Lewy bodies from Alzheimer's disease. *Parkinsonism & Related Disorders, 19*(2), 227-231.

Ganguli, M., Blacker, D., Blazer, D.G., Grant, I., Jest, D.V., Paulsen, J.S., Petersen, R.C. . . . Neurocognitive Disorders Work Group of the American Psychiatric Association's (APA) DSM-5 Task Force. (2011). Classification of neurocognitive disorders in DSM-5: A work in progress. *American Journal of Geriatric Psychiatry, 19*(3), 205-210.

Gauthier, S., Cummings, J., Ballard, O., Brodaty, H., Grossberg, G., Robert, P., & Lyketsos, C. (2010). Management of behavioral problems in Alzheimer's disease. *International Psychogeriatrics, 22*(3), 346-372.

George, D.R., Whitehouse, P.J., & Ballenger, J. (2011). The evolving classification of dementia: Placing the DSM-V in a meaningful historical and cultural context and pondering the future of 'Alzheimer's.' *Culture, Medicine and Psychiatry, 35*(3), 417-435.

Gilberti, N., Turla, M., Alberici, A., Bertasi, V., Civelli, P., Archetti, S., . . . Borroni, B. (2012). Prevalence of frontotemporal lobar degeneration in an isolated population: The Vallecamonica Study. *Neurological Sciences, 33*(4), 899-904.

Grant, I., Sacktor, H., & McArthur, J. (2005). HIV neurocognitive disorders. In H. E. Gendelman, I. Grant, I. Everall, S. A. Lipton, & S. Swindells (Eds.). *The neurology of AIDS* (2nd ed., pp. 357-373). London, England: Oxford University Press.

Grazina, R., & Massano, J. (2013). Physical exercise and Parkinson's disease: Influence on symptoms, disease course and prevention. *Reviews in the Neurosciences, 24*(2), 139-152.

Grover, S., Kate, N., Malhotra, S., Chakrabarti, S., Matoo, S.K., & Avashti, A. (2012). Symptom profile of delirium in children and adolescent—Does it differ from adults and elderly? *General Hospital Psychiatry, 34*(6), 626-632.

Hackney, M.E., Kantorovich, S., Levin, R., & Earhart, G.M. (2007). Effects of tango on functional mobility in Parkinson's disease: A preliminary study. *Journal of Neurological Physical Therapy, 31*(4), 173-179.

Hall, L., & Skelton, D.A. (2012). Occupational therapy for caregivers of people with dementia: A review of the United Kingdom literature. *British Journal of Occupational Therapy, 75*(6), 281-288.

Halliday, G., Bigio, E.H., Cairns, N.J., Neumann, M., Mackenzie, I.R.A., & Mann, D.M.A. (2012). Mechanisms of disease in frontotemporal lobar degeneration: Gain of function versus loss of function effects. *Acta Neuropathologica, 124*(3), 373-382.

Hamilton, J.M., Salmon, D.P., Raman, R., Hansen, L.A., Masliah, E., Peavy, G.M., & Galasko, D. (2013). Accounting for functional loss in Alzheimer's disease and dementia with Lewy bodies: Beyond cognition. *Alzheimer's & Dementia, 10*(2), 171-188, doi:10.1016/j.jalz.2013.04.003.

Hanssen, I. (2013). The influence of cultural background in intercultural dementia care: Exemplified by Sami patients. *Scandinavian Journal of Caring Sciences, 27*(2), 231-237.

Hasegawa, M., Arai, T., Nonaka, T., Kametani, F., Yoshida, M., Hasizume, Y., . . . Akiyama, H. (2008). Phosphorylated TDP-43 in frontotemporal lobar degeneration and amyotrophic lateral sclerosis. *Annals of Neurology, 64*(1), 60-70.

Hindle, J.V. (2013). The practical management of cognitive impairment and psychosis in the older Parkinson's disease patient. *Journal of Neural Transmission, 120*(4), 649-653.

Hughes, T.F., Chang, C.C., Bilt, J.V., Snitz, B.E., & Ganguli, M. (2012). Mild cognitive deficits and everyday functioning among older adults in the community: The Monongahela-Youghiogheny Healthy Aging Team Study. *American Journal of Geriatric Psychiatry, 20*(10), 836-844.

Irwin, D.J., Trojanowski, J.Q., & Grossman, M. (2013). Cerebrospinal fluid biomarkers for differentiation of frontotemporal lobar degeneration from Alzheimer's disease. *Frontiers in Aging Neuroscience, 5*, 6.

Jellinger, K.A. (2013). Pathology and pathogenesis of vascular cognitive impairment—A critical update. *Frontiers in Aging Neuroscience, 5*, 17.

Johnson, V.E., Stewart, J.E., Begbie, F.D., Trojanowski, J.Q., Smith, D.H., & Steward, W. (2013). Inflammation and white matter degeneration persist for years after a single traumatic brain injury. *Brain: A Journal of Neurology, 136*(1), 28-42.

Jonsson, C., Aaro Catroppa, C., Godfrey, C., Smedler, A., & Anderson, V. (2013). Individual profiles of predictors and their relations to 10 years outcome after childhood traumatic brain injury. *Brain Injury, 27*(7-8), 831-838.

Jonveaux, T., Rivasseau Batt, M., Fescharek, R., Benetos, A., Trognon, A., Chuzeville, S., . . . Bouvel, B. (2013). Healing gardens and cognitive behavioral units in the management of Alzheimer's disease patients: The Nancy experience. *Journal of Alzheimer's Disease, 34*(1), 325-338.

Joshi, A., Venkatesh, B., Krishnamurthy, P.H., Hollar-Wilt, L., Bixler, E., & Rapp, M. (2012). 'What's in a name?' Delirium by any other name would be as deadly. A review of the nature of delirium consultations. *Journal of Psychiatric Practice, 18*(6), 413-419.

Kaplan, E., Goodglass, H., & Weintraub, S. (1983). *Boston Naming Test*. Philadelphia, PA: Lea & Febiger.

Karch, C.M., Jeng, A.T., Nowotny, P., Cady, J., Cruchaga, C., & Goate, A.M. (2012). Expression of novel Alzheimer's disease risk genes in control and Alzheimer's disease brains. *PLoS ONE, 7*(11), e50976.

Khurana, V., Gambhir, I.S., & Kishore, D. (2011). Evaluation of delirium in elderly: A hospital-based study. *Geriatrics & Gerontology International, 11*(4), 467-473.

Kim, S., Yoo, E., Jung, M., Park, S., & Park, J. (2012). A systematic review of the effects of occupational therapy for persons with dementia: A meta-analysis of randomized controlled trials. *NeuroRehabilitation, 31*(2), 107-115.

Kling, M.A., Tojanowski, J.Q., Wolk, D.A., Lee, V.M.Y., & Arnold, S.E. (2013). Vascular disease and dementias: Paradigm shifts to drive research in new directions. *Alzheimer's & Dementia, 9*(1), 76-92.

Knopman, D.S., Petersen, R.C., Edland, S.D., Cha, R.H., & Rocca, W.A. (2004). The incidence of frontotemporal lobar degeneration in Rochester, Minnesota, 1990 through 1994. *Neurology, 62*(3), 506-508.

Lamberty, G.J., Kennedy, C.M., & Flashman, L.A. (1995). Clinical utility of the CERAD word list memory test. *Applied Neuropsychology, 2*(3-4), 170-173.

Langlois, F., Vu, T.T.M., Chasse, E., Dupuis, G., Kergoat, M.J., & Bherer, L. (2012). Benefits of physical exercise training on cognition and quality of life in frail older adults. *Journals of Gerontology: Series B: Psychological Sciences and Social Sciences, 68*, 400-404.

Lanuti, P., Ciccocioppo, F., Bonanni, L., Marchisio, M., Lachmann, R., Tabet, N., . . . Kern, F. (2012). Amyloid-specific T-cells differentiate Alzheimer's disease from Lewy body dementia. *Neurobiology of Aging, 33*(11), 2599-2611.

LeGrand, S.B. (2012). Delirium in palliative medicine: A review. *Journal of Pain and Symptom Management, 44*(4), 583-594.

Leuner, K., Müller, W.E., & Reichert, A.S. (2012). From mitochondrial dysfunction to amyloid beta formation: Novel insights into the pathogenesis of Alzheimer's disease. *Molecular Neurobiology, 46*(1), 186-193.

Lewy Body Dementia Association. (2012). *Understanding Lewy body dementias.* Retrieved from http://alzheimers.about.com/gi/o.htm?zi=1/XJ&zTi=1&sdn=alzheimers&cdn=health&tm=14&f=10&tt=2&bt=8&bts=8&zu=http%3A//www.lewybodydementia.org/.

Lisi, D.M. (2000). Definition of drug-induced cognitive impairment in the elderly. *Medscape* Pharmacotherapy. Retrieved from http://www.medscape.com/viewarticle/408593_3.

Lövdén, M., Su, W., & Wangy, H. (2013). Lifestyle change and the prevention of cognitive decline and dementia. *Current Opinions in Psychiatry, 26*(3), 239-243.

Mace, N.L., & Rabins, P.V. (2012). *The 36-hour day: A family guide to caring for people who have Alzheimer disease, related dementias, and memory loss.* New York, NY: Grand Central Life and Style.

Mateen, F.J., & Mills, E.J. (2012). Aging and HIV-related cognitive loss. *Journal of the American Medical Association, 308*(4), 349-350.

McLaren, A.N., LaMantia, M.A., & Callahan, C.M. (2013). Systematic review of non-pharmacologic interventions to delay functional decline in community-dwelling patients with dementia. *Aging & Mental Health, 17*(6), 655-666.

Merritt, M.M., & McCallum, T.J. (2013). Too much of a good thing? Positive religious coping predicts worse diurnal salivary cortisol patterns for overwhelmed African American female dementia family caregivers. *American Journal of Geriatric Psychiatry, 21*(1), 46-56.

Misra, S., & Medhi, B. (2013). Drug development status for Alzheimer's disease: Present scenario. *Neurological Sciences, 34*(6), 831-839.

Mittal, V., Muralee, S., Williamson, D., McErneny, N., Thomas, J., Cash, M., & Tampi, R.R. (2011). Delirium in the elderly: A comprehensive review. *American Journal of Alzheimer's Disease and Other Dementias, 26*(2), 97-109.

National Parkinson Foundation. (2013). *Young onset Parkinson's.* Retrieved from http://www.parkinson.org/Parkinson-s-Disease/Young-Onset-Parkinsons.

Parkes, W.F., & Lasker, L. (Producers), & Marshall, P. (Director). (1990). *Awakenings* [Motion picture]. United States: Columbia Pictures.

Plassman, B.L., Langa, K.M., Fisher, G.G., Heeringa, S.G., Weir, D.R., Ofstendal, M.B., . . . Wallace, R.B. (2007). Prevalence of dementia in the United States: The aging, demographics, and memory study. *Neuroepidemiology, 29*(1-2), 125-132.

Pringsheim, T., Wiltshire, K., Day, L., Cykeman, J., Steeves, T., & Jette, N. (2012). The incidence and prevalence of Huntington's disease: A systematic review and meta-analysis. *Movement Disorders, 27*(9), 1083-1091.

Reichmann, H. (2011). View point: Etiology in Parkinson's disease. Dual hit or spreading intoxication. *Journal of the Neurological Sciences, 310*(1-2), 9-11.

Rodrigues, G.R., Walker, R.H., Bader, B., Danek, A., Brice, A. Cazenueve, C., . . . Tumas, V. (2011). Clinical and genetic analysis of 29 Brazilian patients with Huntington's disease-like phenotype. *Arquivos de Neuro-Psiquiatria, Special Issue: Pattern of p50 Suppression Deficit in Patients with Epilepsy and Individuals with Schizophrenia, 69*(3), 419-423.

Rountree, S.D., Atri, A., Lopez, O.L., & Doody, R.S. (2013). Effectiveness of antidementia drugs in delaying Alzheimer's disease progression. *Alzheimer's & Dementia, 9*(3), 338-345.

Sachdev, P.S., Lipnicki, D.M., Crawford, J., Reppermund, S., Kochan, N.A., Troller, J.N., . . . Sydney Memory and Aging Study Team. (2012). Risk profiles of subtypes of mild cognitive impairment: The Sydney Memory and Aging Study. *American Journal of Geriatric Psychiatry, 20*(10), 854-865.

Sachs, O. (1999). *Awakenings.* New York, NY: Vintage Press.

Sela-Kaufman, M., Rassovsky, Y., Agranov, E., Levi, Y., & Vakil, E. (2013). Premorbid personality characteristics and attachment style moderate the effect of injury severity on occupational outcome in traumatic brain injury: Another aspect of reserve. *Journal of Clinical and Experimental Neuropsychology, 35*(6), 584-595.

Simpson, G., & Jones, K. (2013). How important is resilience among family members supporting relatives with traumatic brain injury or spinal cord injury? *Clinical Rehabilitation, 27*(4), 367-377.

Slaughter, S., & Bankes, J. (2007). The functional transitions model: Maximizing ability in the context of progressive disability. *Canadian Journal on Aging, 26*(1), 39-47.

Snelgrove, T.A., & Hasnain, M. (2012). A concern about the proposed DSM-V criteria reclassifying cognitive disorders. *American Journal of Geriatric Psychiatry, 20*(6), 543.

Steultjens, E.M.J., Dekker, J., Bouter, L., Jellema, S., Bakker, E.B., & Van den Ende, C.H.M. (2004). Occupational therapy for community dwelling elderly people: A systematic review. *Age* and *Ageing, 33,* 453-460.

Sun, F., Ong, R., & Burnette, D. (2012). The influence of ethnicity and culture on dementia caregiving: A review of empirical studies on Chinese Americans. *American Journal of Alzheimer's Disease & Other Dementias, 27*(1), 13-22.

Uyama, N., Yokochi, F., Bandoh, M., & Mizutani, T. (2013). Primary progressive apraxia of speech (AOS) in a patient with Pick's disease with Pick bodies: A neuropsychological and anatomical study and review of literatures. *Neurocase, 19*(1), 14-21.

Van der Steen, J.T., Hertogh, C.M., de Graas, T., Nakanishi, M., Toscani, F., & Arcand, M. (2013). Translation and cross-cultural adaptation of a family booklet on comfort care in dementia: Sensitive topics revised before implementation. *Journal of Medical Ethics, 39*(2), 104-109.

Volicer, L., & Simard, J. (2009). Management of advanced dementia. In M.F. Weiner & A.M. Lipton (2009). *The American Psychiatric Publishing textbook of Alzheimer disease and other dementias* (pp. 333-349). Arlington, VA: American Psychiatric Publishing.

Weber, E., Morgan, E.E., Iudicello, J.E., Blackstone, K., Grant, I., Ellis, R.J., . . . TMARC Group. (2013). Substance use is a risk factor for neurocognitive deficits and neuropsychiatric distress in acute and early HIV infection. *Journal of Neurovirology, 19*(1), 65-74.

Weschler Adult Intelligence Scale (4th ed.). (2008). San Antonio, TX: Pearson Education.

Weschler Memory Scale (4th ed.). (2009). San Antonio, TX: Pearson Education.

Wilson, R., Mendes de Leon, C., Barnes, L., Schneider, J., Bienias, J., Evans, D., & Bennet, D. (2002). Participation in cognitively stimulating activities and risk of incident Alzheimer disease. *Journal of the American Medical Association, 287,* 742-748.

World Health Organization. (2001). *International classification of functioning, disability and health (ICF).* Geneva, Switzerland: Author.

Yuill, N., & Hollis, V. (2011). A systematic review of cognitive stimulation therapy for older adults with mild to moderate dementia: An occupational therapy perspective. *Occupational Therapy International, 18*(4), 163-186.

Zerr, I. (2013). Human Prion diseases. *Brain, 136*(4), 996-997.

Zesiewica, T.A., & Evatt, M.L. (2009). Potential influences of complementary therapy on motor and non-motor complications in Parkinson's disease. *CNS Drugs, 23*(10), 817-835.

Personality
Disorders

Learning Outcomes

By the end of this chapter, readers will be able to:
- Describe the various personality disorders
- Differentiate among personality disorders on the basis of symptoms
- Identify the causes of personality disorders
- Describe treatment strategies for personality disorders
- Discuss the occupational perspective on personality disorders
- Discuss occupational therapy interventions for personality disorders

Bonder B.
Psychopathology and Function, Fifth Edition (pp 375-402).
© 2015 SLACK Incorporated.

KEY WORDS

- Anhedonic
- Defense mechanisms

- Milieu therapy
- Splitting

CASE VIGNETTE

Sam Morse is a 60-year-old, recently divorced insurance salesman. He lives alone in a small apartment in a large East Coast city. He has three grown daughters whom he sees very rarely. His latest ex-wife, one of four, left him after he lost his previous job as a non-profit agency director.

Mr. Morse has a long, troubled work history, having owned a small business, directed a private school, and written for a community newspaper, among many other jobs. In each case, he either failed (his business went bankrupt) or was fired, usually for non-performance and insubordination. In each case, he was engaging and confident in the interview, promising to turn the business around and do great things. In each case, when he proved unable to perform the required duties, he blamed the organization or his supervisor for their failure to recognize his greatness.

Likewise, in each of his four marriages, his now ex-wives described him as initially charming, but ultimately childish, demanding, and egocentric. They report that he took no interest in his daughters except to brag to acquaintances about how wonderful they were and how much they were like him.

THOUGHT QUESTIONS

1. What behaviors and attitudes suggest that Mr. Morse might have a mental disorder?
2. What functional deficits does Mr. Morse display that might be problematic?
3. What do you think might lead Mr. Morse to seek treatment?

PERSONALITY DISORDERS

- Cluster A
  - Paranoid personality disorder
  - Schizoid personality disorder
  - Schizotypal personality disorder
- Cluster B
  - Antisocial personality disorder
  - Borderline personality disorder

  - Histrionic personality disorder
  - Narcissistic personality disorder
- Cluster C
  - Avoidant personality disorder
  - Dependent personality disorder
  - Obsessive-compulsive personality disorder

A personality disorder is "an enduring pattern of inner experience and behavior that deviates markedly from the expectations of the individual's culture, is pervasive and inflexible, has an onset in adolescence or early adulthood, is stable over time, and leads to distress or impairment" (American Psychiatric Association [APA], 2013, p. 645). The main characteristics of personality disorders emphasize emotion and behavior instead of etiology. This is an important distinction for the diagnostic criteria for the personality disorders compared with some of the other diagnostic clusters, in particular, the neurodevelopmental disorders and neurocognitive disorders. For the neurodevelopmental disorders and neurocognitive disorders, various biological or physiological criteria are identified as factors contributing to diagnosis. For example, for neurocognitive disorders due to Alzheimer's disease, the probable diagnosis is based in part on the presence of an established familial/genetic history. No such criteria are part of the personality disorder diagnoses.

The personality disorders have been among the more controversial diagnoses for various reasons (APA, 2004):

- Some individuals who are severely disturbed meet the criteria for several personality disorders simultaneously.

- Individuals who are less severely disturbed may not meet the criteria for any of the specific disorders, resulting in a significant use of the "not otherwise specified" label.

- Individuals with the same diagnosis can be quite different from one another because they may meet different criteria within a category.

- The criteria are not always sufficiently clear to discriminate between individuals with and without the disorder.

- An inadequate scientific base exists to support the number of personality disorders in the diagnostic framework.

A high rate of comorbidity exists with other psychiatric disorders that may reflect dilemmas in making distinctions between the personality disorders and other diagnoses (Widiger & Trull, 2007). Zimmerman, Chelminski, and Young (2008) suggested that half of individuals with other psychiatric diagnoses also have personality disorders. They pointed out that this is important because these dual diagnoses are associated with significantly worse prognoses.

Also, some lack of clarity exists about whether the personality disorders are simply at the less severe end of various diagnostic spectra or whether they really do represent conceptually and symptomatically distinct entities. For example, schizotypal personality is presumably a mild, nonpsychotic relative of schizophrenia and is found in the personality disorder section. On the other hand, dysthymic disorder, which seems to be at a similar point on the affective disorder continuum—that is, a mild, nonpsychotic relative of major depression—is listed in the depressive disorders cluster, rather than with the personality disorders.

A further challenge in understanding personality disorders is that they are most often self-diagnosing (i.e., they are diagnosed only if the individual seeks help or is sent by someone else). Many individuals who meet the criteria for a diagnosis of personality disorder never feel sufficiently bad or behave peculiarly enough to enter therapy.

On the basis of these concerns, it was generally expected that there would be significant changes in the personality disorder diagnostic grouping (Skodol, 2012; Whitborne, 2013). Numerous researchers suggested a dimensional model for personality disorders, rather than the existing categorization in the fourth edition of the *Diagnostic and Statistical Manual of Mental Disorders* ([DSM-IV] APA, 2004; Huprich & Bornstein, 2007; Livesley, 2007; Widiger & Trull, 2007). These researchers reasoned that there was a presumption of hierarchy, even in the DSM-IV, that would establish a more holistic continuum (Livesley, 2007). Among the suggestions was a five-factor model based on broad domains (e.g., extraversion, agreeableness, conscientiousness, emotional instability, and openness; Widiger & Trull, 2007). Another suggestion focused on various personality and behavioral traits, such as anxiousness, egocentrism, lack of empathy, and other common problems of individuals with personality disorders, and suggested a diagnostic system based on the presence and number of these traits (Livesley, 2007). Research evidence exists that a categorical approach would improve reliability and validity of diagnosis (Tyrer et al., 2007).

In addition to proposals about the structure of the personality disorders as a group, there was consideration of whether to retain all the diagnoses in this group (Pull, 2013). An early proposal was to remove paranoid, schizoid, histrionic, dependent, and narcissistic personality disorders from the classification. Narcissistic personality disorder was reinstated in June 2011, but not the other four disorders.

Ultimately, in spite of the vigorous debate, the entire grouping was retained essentially unchanged from previous editions of the DSM (Pull, 2013). Livesley (2012) argued that tradition won out over research data. In spite of the many criticisms of the personality disorder categorization and description, all were retained in their existing clusters. As a temporizing measure, Section III of the fifth edition of the *Diagnostic and Statistical Manual of Mental Disorders* ([DSM-5] APA, 2013), which presents emerging measures and models, offers an alternative model for the personality disorders, and a recommendation that further research should focus on whether to substitute this model for the current one. The alternative model focuses on "impairments in personality *functioning* and pathological personality *traits*" (APA, 2013, p. 761). Factors identified as elements of personality functioning include identity, self-direction, empathy, and intimacy. Traits are clustered into five domains—negative affectivity, detachment, antagonism, disinhibition, and psychoticism. Within these domains are 25 specific trait facets.

The DSM-5 (APA, 2013) identifies three clusters of personality disorders, which are grouped according to common symptomatology. Paranoid, schizoid, and schizotypal personality disorders (cluster A) are characterized by odd or peculiar behavior. Cluster B—antisocial, borderline, histrionic, and narcissistic personality disorders—present with flamboyant or dramatic behavior. The third category, cluster C, is characterized primarily by anxiety or fear. Note that for all the personality disorders the first criterion is a pervasive pattern of behavior. It is the pervasive nature of the behaviors and emotions that contributes to the diagnosis. Many individuals have some element of paranoia, obsessiveness, or dependency, but the behaviors do not appear consistently or with any substantial impact on the individual's relationship.

The personality disorders are thought to result from a combination of genetic factors affecting the serotonin system and stress reactions, deficits in brain development, childhood trauma, and adverse experiences in adolescence (Buchheim, Roth, Schiepek, Pogarell, & Karch, 2013). Structural and functional deficits are noted, especially in the limbic and paralimbic brain areas and the cognitive-executive brain regions.

Family influences are evident in the emergence of these disorders. For example, parents who are **anhedonic**—that is, unable to derive pleasure from their activities—are more likely to have children with cluster A personality disorders (Cohen, Emmerson, Mann, Forbes, & Blanchard, 2010).

Personality disorders are thought to be associated with exaggerated **defense mechanisms** (Perry, Presniak, & Olsen, 2013). Defense mechanisms are psychological strategies that individuals use to protect themselves from psychic pain. Everyone uses these mechanisms; however, in personality disorders, they become maladaptive and interfere with function.

Research on the biology of personality disorders has found that, for some, deficits in function of the prefrontal cortex and/or serotonin production occur (New, Goodman, Triebwasser, & Siever, 2008). Neuroimaging studies have found differences in brain volume and function of the structures related to emotion and impulse control (Lis, Greenfield, Henry, Guilé, & Dougherty, 2007; McCloskey, Phan, & Coccaro, 2005).

Prognosis for the personality disorders appears more related to the severity of symptoms, rather than type (Crawford, Koldobsky, Mulder, & Tyre, 2011). Five years after intervention,

TABLE 19-1

PREVALENCE OF PERSONALITY DISORDERS

DIAGNOSIS	PREVALENCE	SOURCE
Cluster A		
Paranoid personality disorder	2% to 4%	Grant et al., 2004
Schizoid personality disorder	<1% of the general population	Esterberg et al., 2010
Schizotypal personality disorder	3% to 4% of the general population	Esterberg et al., 2010
Cluster B		
Antisocial	3.63%	Grant et al., 2004
Borderline	2.0%	APA, 2013
Histrionic	1.8%	Grant et al., 2008
Narcissistic personality disorder	6.2%; Gender ratio 7.7% (M), 4.8% (F)	Stinson et al 2008
Cluster C		
Avoidant personality disorder	2.4%	Grant et al., 2005
Dependent personality disorder	0.05%	Grant et al., 2005
Obsessive-compulsive personality disorder	7.9%	Grant et al., 2005

clients who started treatment with more severe symptoms of a personality disorder remained more symptomatic than those with less severe symptoms (Jansson, Hesse, & Fridell, 2008). Several types of personality disorder (avoidant, borderline, histrionic, paranoid, schizoid, and schizotypal) were strongly correlated with comorbid depression, and in these individuals, the depression was more persistent than among individuals with depression but no personality disorder (Skodol et al., 2011). In addition, individuals with personality disorders, especially paranoid, antisocial, and avoidant personality disorders, were more likely to receive public welfare than other individuals (Vaughn et al., 2010). Prognosis is worse when accompanying comorbid mental disorders are noted. Individuals with any of the personality disorders may also experience major depression, anxiety disorders, substance use disorders, and any of the medically related mental disorders. These comorbid disorders complicate treatment in what is already a complex set of symptoms. Table 19-1 shows the prevalence of the various personality disorders.

In this chapter, the personality disorders will be presented in their three clusters. Information about function and treatment will be provided for each disorder. However, as noted from the summary presented previously, some common features for all or most of these disorders and those common functional and treatment considerations will be summarized later in the chapter. Prognosis and occupational therapy intervention for all the personality disorders will be discussed at the end of the chapter.

Cluster A

The cluster A personality disorders are thought of as the most severe and most resistant to treatment (Esterberg, Goulding, & Walker, 2010). Individuals with these disorders tend to be perceived as self-centered, a factor that negatively affects their social relationships. Each of these disorders has its own unique features as well. Schizotypal personality disorder includes both cognitive-perceptual dysfunction and social and interpersonal deficits, whereas paranoid personality disorder is more associated with the interpersonal deficits. Schizoid personality disorder is associated with extreme social isolation, primarily based on lack of desire to interact, compared with paranoid personality disorder in which the individual is suspicious of others. As previously mentioned, some believe that all these disorders may actually be schizophrenia spectrum disorders.

Paranoid Personality Disorder

Paranoid personality disorder is identified by the individual's tendency to experience a sense of being threatened or persecuted (Moore & Jefferson, 2004a). Associates and coworkers will be suspected of intent to harm the individual, and jealousy and suspicion characterize most relationships. The individual is typically isolated, with few friends or close relationships. The individual relates to others in a fashion that is withdrawn, suspicious, and frequently hostile.

Paranoid personality disorder is less severe than paranoid schizophrenia and is characterized more by misinterpretation of input, rather than by outright delusions. For example, an individual who has a paranoid personality disorder may interpret a minor reprimand from a boss as "he's never liked me, he wants to fire me, and everyone here hates me." An individual with paranoid schizophrenia might interpret the same reprimand as part of a Central Intelligence Agency or Mafia plan to kill him or her.

Typically, such individuals are argumentative and withdrawn, with little sense of humor and "chips on their shoulders." They look for slights and frequently find them, tend to hold grudges, and may be litigious. These individuals are hypercritical of others, while responding poorly to any criticism of their own behavior (Esterberg et al., 2010). They tend to be excessively self-sufficient and quite egocentric. One such individual had constant trouble at work because he routinely violated company rules, reasoning that they had been instituted only to harass him.

Diagnostic criteria for paranoid personality disorder include pervasive mistrust and suspiciousness of others, reflected in suspicion that others are harming or deceiving the individual, or that others are generally untrustworthy (APA, 2013). This suspiciousness is accompanied by reluctance to confide in others and the holding of persistent grudges. Schizophrenia must be ruled out, along with other personality disorders and substance abuse.

Etiology

As with all the personality disorders, the etiology of paranoid personality disorder is believed to be some combination of biological/genetic factors and environmental factors (Livesley, 2007).

Implications for Function and Treatment

The characteristic behavior pattern of individuals with paranoid personality disorder creates considerable difficulty (Moore & Jefferson, 2004a). Work and social occupations are affected as a result of interpersonal difficulties. Individuals with paranoid personality disorder are less likely than others to have a history of competitive work (McGurk et al., 2013). The suspiciousness and irritability of these individuals, coupled with their tendency to believe that others are plotting against them, makes for troubled interactions, often resulting in lost jobs, divorce, and so on. In particular, relationships with authority figures tend to be problematic. Leisure interests may be few and often of a solitary nature. Activities/instrumental activities of daily living (ADL/IADL) and work functions, other than relationships with coworkers, are maintained at acceptable levels. One man had a job as a painter for a large corporation, moving from area to area to repaint walls. He worked mostly alone and was reported to be a good worker but hard to get along with. He ultimately lost his job, not because of poor painting skill but because of frequent fights with coworkers in the lunchroom.

Skills in these individuals remain largely intact. Motor and sensory skills, sensory integration, and cognition are, for the most part, unaffected, except for the inaccurate processing of social cues from others. Patterns are problematic because of the habitual tendency to attribute bad motives to others.

Treatment of individuals with paranoid personality disorder through behavior modification, medication, education, or psychotherapy is not notably successful (Williams, 2010). Their personality pattern tends to be intractable, although some individuals can be taught how to interact more effectively.

Schizoid Personality Disorder

Schizoid personality disorder is defined by an absence or indifference to social activity and a restricted range of emotion (Raine, 2006). These individuals are often identified as "loners" who have no interest in friendships, they appear aloof and withdrawn, and they demonstrate little emotion. They may seem self-absorbed and vague. One such woman rarely spoke to coworkers, but often had what others described as a "peculiar smile" on her face. In fact, individuals with schizoid personality disorder often seek occupations that require limited social interaction, even if they are below their skill level (Esterberg et al., 2010).

Diagnostic criteria for schizoid personality disorder include pervasive detachment from social relationships and restricted expression of emotions in interpersonal relationships, including preference for solitary activities, little interest in sexual experiences, lack of pleasure in activities, and emotional coldness, detachment, or flattened affect (APA, 2013). Schizophrenia, other personality disorders, substance abuse, and autism are among the disorders that must be ruled out.

Etiology

The cause of schizoid personality disorder is not well established. As with paranoid personality disorder, the major theories about its emergence are that it is a learned pattern of behavior or that it is due to some sort of central nervous system (CNS) dysfunction (Raine, 2006). In particular, it appears that these individuals experience early attachment difficulties that persist into adulthood (Parpottas, 2012). The persistent attachment difficulties may actually represent adaptive functioning in a difficult environment.

It is possible that there are two different trajectories of schizoid personality disorder, the first being more biological in nature and the second being more environmental. The first trajectory seems closely associated with schizophrenia and may be one end of a diagnostic spectrum (Horan, Blanchard, Clark, & Green, 2008). The more environmental etiology may reflect the individual's response to a difficult childhood, unrelated to the kinds of biological factors that characterize schizophrenia and the biological etiology of schizoid personality disorder.

Implications for Function and Treatment

As with paranoid personality disorder, the primary functional impairment is in the area of social relationships (Moore & Jefferson, 2004b). The difficulties with social relationships are thought to represent attachment avoidance (Dignam, Parry, & Burk, 2010), which affects any occupation in which social interaction is required. However, unlike those with paranoid personality disorder, these individuals tend to display little aggression, making work situations easier to maintain. They have few social relationships, and they rarely marry or have close friends. Other skills and occupations are unimpaired, meaning that these individuals are functional but lead lives restricted by the absence of meaningful friendships.

When such individuals come into treatment, it is often because they are depressed about their isolation. Social skills training may provide a mechanism for helping them to establish relationships, although their interactions tend to remain stilted, awkward, or distant. Although it is challenging to support change in such individuals, an integration of cognitive behavioral and psychodynamic therapy may be most helpful (Parpottas, 2012). In particular, gradual exposure to emotional expression and provision of safe opportunities to experience attachment may help to modify behaviors (Mallinckrodt, Daly, & Wang, 2009).

Schizotypal Personality Disorder

Individuals with schizotypal personalities have peculiar thought patterns, behaviors, and appearance (Moore & Jefferson, 2004c). This may include bizarre fantasies, beliefs about special senses or powers, or odd patterns of speaking. Neighbors and coworkers typically describe these individuals as strange and as loners. If they have friends, the friends are often described as odd as well. Typically, peculiar perceptual experiences are also present. Affect is either inappropriate or flat, and social isolation is common. Schizotypal personality disorder is differentiated from schizophrenia largely by a matter of degree—the symptoms are not severe enough to fit the criteria for schizophrenia—although the disorders are related. For this reason, it has been hypothesized that schizotypal personality disorder is a spectrum disorder at the less severe end of the range of schizophrenia (Ahmed et al., 2013). Diagnostic criteria include a pervasive pattern of interpersonal deficits characterized by discomfort with close relationships, along with cognitive or perceptual distortions, eccentric behavior, odd beliefs, unusual perceptual experiences, odd thinking and speech, and paranoia (APA, 2013). Schizophrenia and bipolar disorders must be ruled out, along with other personality disorders, neurodevelopmental disorders, and substance use disorders.

Psychological defense mechanisms that have been associated with schizotypal personality disorder include projection, passive-aggression, devaluation, rationalization, isolation, splitting, and intellectualization (Perry et al., 2013).

Etiology

As with the other personality disorders in this cluster, etiology is unclear, but it suspected to be the result of either CNS dysfunction or learning. Incidence is unknown, although the disorder is more common in family members of individuals who are schizophrenic (Ahmed et al., 2013). The schizotypal personality disorder diagnostic category is relatively new, so data are sparse.

Implications for Function and Treatment

At the level of occupations, function is distinctly impaired. Social function is particularly poor. Odd ideas held by individuals with schizotypal personality disorder make it difficult for others to understand them. The individual may avoid others because of discomfort in social situations and because they misperceive the social environment. Vocational function is impaired to the extent that social skills are required to do a job. As is true of those with schizoid personalities, these individuals may do best at jobs that require little social interaction. However, actual work performance may also be poor, lending credence to the speculation that there is some underlying CNS or cognitive dysfunction. ADL is impaired, and these individuals tend to be unkempt or to dress peculiarly. Individuals with schizotypal personality disorder are less likely than other groups to be employed and/or to live independently (McClure, Harvey, Bowie, Iacoviello, & Siever, 2013). Those who are employed tend to be underemployed (McGurk et al., 2013).

Cognitive skills are affected, as demonstrated by the fact that individuals with schizotypal personality disorder do poorly on cognitive tests (McClure et al., 2013).

Efforts at intervention are similar to those used for other disorders in this cluster and include medication, skill training, behavioral interventions, and verbal therapies (Moore & Jefferson, 2004c).

Cluster B

The cluster B personality disorders are characterized by emotional instability, disruptive and erratic interpersonal relationships, restricted affect, and lack of empathy and insight (Pankey, 2012). These characteristics are thought to be a result of deficient or abusive parenting that causes emotional dysregulation (Milne, Peel, & Greenway, 2012; Peng, Zhou, Chen, & Cai, 2011). Also, evidence exists for an inherited component of these disorders (Torgersen et al., 2012).

A significant overlap exists among the cluster B disorders, although differences can be identified if behavioral constructs are studied closely. For example, the cluster B disorders are all characterized by impulsivity. However, borderline personality disorder is associated with a lack of perseverance, whereas antisocial personality disorder is associated with lack of premeditation and sensation seeking (DeShong & Kurtz, 2013).

Antisocial Personality Disorder

Of all the personality disorders, antisocial personality disorder (APD) is most likely to be brought to the attention of health care professionals by someone other than the individual. The individual him- or herself (this diagnosis is much more common in males) tends not to be concerned about the serious issues that their behavior causes for others (Moore & Jefferson, 2004d). The associated defense mechanisms include omnipotence, denial, splitting, and acting out (Perry et al., 2013).

Diagnostic criteria include a pervasive pattern for at least 3 years of disregard for the rights of others in an individual at least 18 years old (prior to that age, a conduct disorder would be the most likely diagnosis), including failure to conform to lawful behavior, deceitfulness, impulsivity and failure to plan ahead, aggressiveness, disregard for the safety of others, irresponsibility, and lack of remorse (APA, 2013). Schizophrenia and other personality disorders must be ruled out, along with substance use disorders.

Of the psychiatric disorders, APD is among those likely to be associated with violent behavior (Fountoulakis, Leucht, & Kaprinis, 2008). This presents some difficulties in legal situations in which the violent individual might argue diminished capacity because of the psychiatric diagnosis. APD is also frequently characterized by comorbid substance abuse (Ruiz, Pincus, & Schinka, 2008), which increases the potential for violence.

It is important to distinguish antisocial personality from other disorders, especially mania, because many behaviors typical of antisocial personality also occur during manic episodes. The long-standing pattern of antisocial behavior makes it noticeably different, as does the absence of periods of remission. The tendency to engage in criminal behavior is unique to this diagnosis. A common misperception exists that individuals with psychiatric disorders are prone to criminal behavior, but for APD the data strongly support this belief (Freeston, Howard, Coid, & Ullrich, 2013).

Etiology

Individuals with APD show significant impairment in specific regions of the brain, especially those most involved in impulse control and behavior inhibition. In particular, structural differences include reduced gray matter in the prefrontal cortex and right superior temporal gyrus, as well as loss of volume in the amygdala and hippocampus (Weber, Habel, Amunts, & Schneider, 2008; Yang, Glenn, & Raine, 2008). Functional magnetic resonance images suggest poor regulation of the threat response (Crowe & Blair, 2008), and there is growing evidence of a genetic component (Viding, Larsson, & Jones, 2008).

Significant environmental factors also exist that the majority of these individuals have in common. A strong correlation exists between attachment difficulties and antisocial personality disorder (Perez, 2012). This is consistent in the belief that antisocial and violent behavior are strongly associated with poverty and childhood abuse or neglect. The ways in which parents cope and interact, in addition to the community environment, are significant risk factors for APD (Cohen, Crawford, Chen, Kasen, & Gordon, 2012).

Implications for Function and Treatment

Function in individuals with APD is impaired primarily in social and work spheres (Moore & Jefferson, 2004d). ADL are intact, with the exception of the management of finances. Typically, money is a serious problem for these individuals, and they often resort to stealing. Social relationships are impaired by the lack of depth and conscience displayed by such individuals. One man imprisoned for armed robbery and murder explained that he had to kill the security guard because the guard got in the way and, therefore, deserved to die. In work situations, the belligerence and aggressiveness of these individuals is problematic. They may be quite able to perform the tasks required, but they often cannot maintain acceptable relationships with coworkers and supervisors, as they misinterpret social situations and respond with excessive anxiety or anger. One man, during his short tenure on a construction job, routinely punched new employees just to "let them know who the real boss is!"

Some speculation has been noted that antisocial individuals have sensory and cognitive processing impairments. Deficits have been documented in cognitive flexibility (Fitzgerald & Demakis, 2007), processing of emotional cues (Frick & White, 2008), decision making (Fontaine, 2007), and facial affect recognition (Marsh & Blair, 2008).

Some research suggests that a large percentage of the prison population shows signs of learning disabilities linked to sensory processing problems, but this remains unproven (Usher, Stewart, & Wilton, 2013). Habits and patterns are problematic as the individual tends to focus energy on behaviors that are illegal and harmful to self and others.

In general, these individuals do not respond well to treatment. Psychotherapy and inpatient and outpatient **milieu therapy** have all been shown to have some value. Milieu therapy is an inpatient intervention in which the entire environment is carefully structured to ensure that actions have specific and predictable consequences, thereby, at least theoretically, remediating previous faulty learning. It is possible that parent training and collaborative problem-solving training may be helpful (Hamilton & Armando, 2008). Collaborative problem solving aims to train children to improve their frustration tolerance, increase emotional flexibility, and avoid emotional overreaction. Psychotropic medications do not seem beneficial.

The National Institute for Health and Care (2009/2013) published guidelines for treatment, management, and prevention of APD. Their recommendations include provision of group based cognitive and behavioral interventions. They recommend against the use of pharmacological interventions, except in cases where a comorbid condition would support their use.

Borderline Personality Disorder

The diagnosis of borderline personality disorder (BPD) has become increasingly common in the past decade, which is a source of dispute because some do not believe it exists as an actual mental disorder (Montandon & Feldman, 2008). Research suggests that a significant overlap with other personality disorders is noted, especially histrionic personality disorder (Crawford, Cohen, & Brook, 2001). BPD is marked by instability of mood, relationships, and self-image, usually appearing during early adulthood. Relationships and affect tend to be unstable. Affect may also be inappropriate, in particular reflected by poor control of anger. Suicidal ideation and self-mutilation may also occur, and these individuals tend to be quite impulsive. These individuals fear abandonment and have self-image problems characterized by uncertainty about sexual orientation, long-term goals, or values. Depression, posttraumatic stress disorder, and substance abuse are frequent comorbidities.

Diagnostic criteria for BPD include pervasive pattern of instability in interpersonal relationships, self-image, and affect, including impulsivity, efforts to avoid abandonment, unstable or intense interpersonal relationships characterized by alternating idealization and devaluation, frequent suicidal or self-mutilating behavior, affective instability, and inappropriate anger (APA, 2013). Depression and bipolar disorder, in addition to other personality disorders, must be ruled out.

One client with BPD had achieved a relatively stable work situation but found she had great difficulty in her social life. Her boyfriends, all short term, routinely abandoned her, and roommates moved out frequently. Much of this was due to the extreme instability of her behavior toward them. One day she would be quite enamored and invested, bringing gifts and writing long letters about how close she felt to them, but within hours or days of this behavior, she would write angry, spiteful letters; splatter their clothes with ink; and scream obscenities at them.

Etiology

It is possible that genetics contribute to occurrence of this disorder (Livesley, 2008). However, it is also possible that borderline behaviors are learned from dysfunctional relatives or are a result of childhood trauma (Sansone & Sansone, 2007). The role of CNS dysfunction in the emergence of the disorder is unclear, although there are changes in the frontolimbic regions (Rossi et al., 2013).

Associated defense mechanisms include omnipotence, idealization, devaluation, and absence of repression (Perry et al., 2013). A significant risk exists for psychotic episodes, largely in response to stress (Glaser, Van Os, Thewissen, & Myin-Germeys, 2010).

Implications for Function and Treatment

As with other personality disorders, function seems to be impaired at the level of self-care, work, and leisure occupations, as opposed to motor, sensory, and/or other skills. Work and social function are markedly impaired.

Relationships tend to be unstable, with these individuals fluctuating wildly between excessive involvement with others and devaluation of friends. A particular issue of individuals with BPD is the tendency toward **splitting**, an individual seeing him- or herself and others as either "all good" or "all bad," and to fluctuate rapidly between these poles. These rapid shifts in attitude have an impact on both self-concept and relationships with others. These relationship difficulties are the most consistent diagnostic criterion (Montandon & Feldman, 2008).

Impulsiveness and difficulty handling anger magnifies interpersonal difficulties, as does a feeling of depersonalization that arises for many individuals with BPD. Similar problems affect work; however, work problems are not solely the result of interpersonal difficulties. Because these individuals have problems identifying and maintaining a set of values and goals, they are unable to select and pursue career goals. Work history is unstable as they move from job to job or miss work because of substance abuse or suicide gestures.

ADL are unimpaired at a basic level (i.e., these individuals are able to dress, maintain hygiene, cook and eat, and so on). However, their impulsivity may lead them to ignore their ADL needs, manage money poorly, drive recklessly, and so on.

The evidence regarding impaired skills is somewhat equivocal (Bender & Skodol, 2007; Liotti, Cortina, & Farina, 2008; Rosenthal et al., 2008). Individuals with BPD show difficulties in attaching to others (Liotti et al., 2008), developing an accurate sense of self (Bender & Skodol, 2007), and interpreting and responding appropriately to emotion (Rosenthal et al., 2008). It is widely believed that some level of CNS dysfunction affects individuals with BPD. Motor skills are unaffected. Establishment and maintenance of patterns is quite problematic, as their rapid mood changes and impulsive nature impede orderly progression of activity.

Recommended treatments include long-term psychotherapy (Montandon & Feldman, 2008). In addition, a combination of short-term hospitalization, family education, and low-dose neuroleptics seem to be effective, particularly when focused on helping the individual manage feelings of rejection or abandonment (Siefert, 2012). BPD is a somewhat intractable condition, particularly when accompanied by depression, and there is a high risk for suicide attempt and completed suicide (Kolla, Eisenberg, & Links, 2008).

Histrionic Personality Disorder

Individuals with histrionic personality disorder (HPD) demonstrate excessive emotionality or theatricality and attention-seeking behavior (Crawford et al., 2001). They tend to need a great deal of approval or reassurance, which they may seek by being sexually seductive, excessively concerned with physical attractiveness, and attempting to be the center of attention in all situations. Self-centeredness is extreme, and emotions are exaggerated. At the same time, emotions shift rapidly and are quite shallow. Descriptors that are considered prototypical are "self-dramatizing" and "vain" (Shopshire & Craik, 1996). Individuals with HPD have low thresholds for frustration and are unable to delay gratification. Diagnostic criteria include pervasive pattern of excessive emotionality and attention seeking, desire to be the center of attention, inappropriate seductive or provocative behavior, rapidly shifting and shallow expression of emotion, self-dramatization, and exaggerated expression of emotion (APA, 2013). Other personality disorders and substance use disorders must be ruled out.

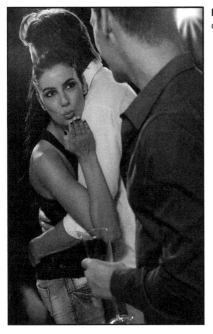

Figure 19-1. Individuals with histrionic personality disorder are often inappropriately flirtatious. (©2014 Shutterstock.com.)

Etiology

Etiology is unclear. At least some evidence exists for the possibility of a genetic link, as well as hyperresponsivity of the noradrenergic system (Widiger & Bornstein, 2001). In addition, cognitive problems, as well as problem relationships with family members, have been implicated as fostering the insecurity that is notable in these individuals.

Implications for Function and Treatment

Skills, including motor and process abilities, do not appear impaired in HPD. This disorder impairs function in a number of occupational areas, including social participation, in particular. Friendships are superficial and focus on the individual. People with HPD are unable to respond with genuine emotion to the needs of others and are frequently inappropriately flirtatious (Figure 19-1). They romanticize relationships and respond with excessive disappointment to disagreements. This leads to a very high rate of divorce among individuals with HPD (Disney, Weinstein, & Oltmanns, 2012). One young woman arrived at work to announce loudly and tearfully that she would have to "end it all" because her boyfriend had to cancel a date because he had the flu.

Individuals with HPD are often inappropriately flirtatious. Such individuals are unpleasant to be around, but they are typically able to function at work (U.S. National Library of Medicine, 2008). However, they may have problems with coworkers or supervisors and are prone to quit unpredictably in fits of pique or when they become bored. ADL are usually not impaired; in fact, such individuals may spend a great deal of time on hygiene and grooming to be attractive to others. They often dress quite seductively, then act puzzled when others respond to the apparent seduction.

Therapeutic efforts should focus on the skills required to increase connection with others and to deal with obstacles to personality growth (Horowitz & Lerner, 2010). However, making changes tends to be quite difficult for people with HPD. Most often, when these individuals seek treatment, they want a "quick fix" for an immediate crisis, rather than any major change in their attitudes or behaviors. One woman came into therapy because her father had "disowned" her and she was "now an orphan." It turned out he had stopped her allowance when she got her first job at age 25. She came to therapy to instruct the counselor to call her father and tell him to resume the allowance.

Narcissistic Personality Disorder

Grandiosity is a defining feature of narcissistic personality disorder (NPD). This is accompanied by a lack of empathy for others and excessive need for attention. Individuals with NPD identify themselves as special, exaggerate accomplishments, and feel entitled to recognition and special attention. However, these feelings fluctuate with feelings of insecurity and unworthiness (Vater et al., 2013). Diagnostic criteria include a pervasive pattern of grandiosity, a need for admiration, and lack of empathy, including a grandiose sense of self-importance, preoccupation with fantasies of unlimited success, belief that he or she is special, the need for excessive admiration, a sense of entitlement, and exploitativeness in relationships with others (APA, 2013). The disorder must be distinguished from other personality disorders, mania or hypomania, and substance use disorders.

Etiology

NPD is not well-researched, perhaps because it was added to the diagnostic list only in the third edition of the *Diagnostic and Statistical Manual of Mental Disorders* (DSM-III; Young, 2008). In fact, NPD was very nearly eliminated from the DSM-5 (Morey & Stagner, 2012) because there seemed to be poor diagnostic specificity. In addition, there was some evidence that the core defining characteristics can be seen in all the personality disorders. Ultimately, a decision was made to retain the diagnosis.

Like HPD, NPD may be a learned pattern of adaptation, perhaps the result of disordered family life (Widiger & Bornstein, 2001). These individuals may get conflicting messages from parents, feel undervalued, and, as a result, come to undervalue themselves. At the same time, their grandiosity is an attempt to win approval that may not have been forthcoming in their homes.

The core defense mechanisms include omnipotence, idealization, devaluation, denial, and fantasy (Perry et al., 2013). Individuals with NPD are also likely to show the splitting that characterizes BPD.

Implications for Function and Treatment

NPD does not appear to cause dysfunction at the skill level. Sensory perceptual skills and motor and praxis skills are intact. Primary dysfunction is noted in social participation (Young, 2008). These individuals are self-centered and are unable to display empathy for others, making friendships difficult. They charm others briefly until their disregard for others' feelings becomes obvious; therefore, relationships tend to be brief and often contentious. This pattern of relationships is also problematic in work situations where interactions with supervisors may be difficult. In some situations, vocational performance may be unusually good as the individual strives for great success, whereas, in others, performance is poor as the individual becomes resentful of expectations of others. Good performance rarely lasts. One man had a work history of more than a dozen jobs, each of which lasted no more than 6 months. As each new job began, he had "great new plans to save the company." As each job ended, he excoriated

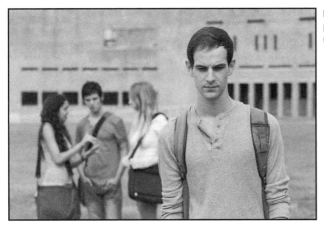

Figure 19-2. Individuals with avoidant personality disorder often feel isolated. (©2014 Shutterstock.com.)

his coworkers for failing to recognize his "genius." ADL are usually unimpaired, although money management may become an issue. In an attempt to impress others, these individuals may spend to excess. Patterns can also be problematic as the individual's social interactions are extremely unstable, reducing the ability to arrange consistent work and social habits.

When individuals with NPD present for treatment, it is usually for depression as a result of their social isolation (Young, 2008). It is rare that they are able to develop insight or to change behaviors, as they tend to blame others for their problems and to be impatient with the therapeutic process. In most instances, the depression, rather than the personality disorder, is the focus of treatment. In addition, individuals with NPD have higher rates of suicidal behavior, and their attempts have higher than expected lethality, compared with other individuals who have suicidal impulses (Blasco-Fontecilla et al., 2009).

Cluster C

This cluster includes the personality disorders reflective of anxiety and fear (Oleski, Cox, Robinson, & Grant, 2012). Obsessive-compulsive personality disorder is the most common of the personality disorders, and the cluster C disorders as a group are highly correlated with major depressive disorder and the anxiety disorders.

An array of theories exist for the development of these disorders, including speculation about attachment difficulties, traumatic life events, and psychological stress and dysfunction (Birgenheir & Pepper, 2011). However, the evidence is conflicting and inconclusive.

Avoidant Personality Disorder

Social discomfort and avoidance of interpersonal relationships is the primary characteristic of avoidant personality disorder (APA, 2013). Individuals with avoidant personality disorder fear that others will disapprove of them. As a result, they avoid interaction and often experience significant loneliness (Figure 19-2). Diagnostic criteria include a pervasive pattern of social inhibition, feelings of inadequacy and sensitivity as characterized by avoidance of activities that require social interaction, restraint in intimate relationships, fear of criticism or rejection, and self-perception of social inadequacy (APA, 2013). The disorder must be distinguished from anxiety disorders, other personality disorders, and substance use disorders.

Etiology

Some evidence exists that avoidant personality disorder is inherited (Gjerde, 2012), although it is challenging to discern what is genetic and what is environmental. It is likely that early environment and learning are contributing factors (Alden, Laposa, Taylor, & Ryder, 2002).

Implications for Function and Treatment

Individuals with avoidant personality disorder engage in many occupations without difficulty but can be affected by the inability to form relationships. These individuals work and care for themselves, but they have emotionally and socially restricted lives. Skills are unimpaired, with the exception of social skills. Superficial relationships may be adequate. One client was a university professor who managed brief casual interactions with students, as well as the more formalized classroom relationships. However, his personal life was barren of friends or close family ties, and four marriages had ended in divorce because of his inability to manage intimacy.

As with NPD, these individuals often seek treatment as a result of depression (Gilbert & Gordon, 2013). Treatment may focus on insight, behavior change, or a combination of the two. Unlike individuals with NPD, these individuals may be able to make a commitment to treatment and to benefit from it.

Dependent Personality Disorder

Individuals with avoidant personality disorder avoid relationships, whereas individuals with dependent personality disorder feel they cannot survive without them. They are dependent and submissive, have difficulty making decisions, and look to others to tell them what to do. As a result, they are unable to successfully initiate activity. They fear being alone. Diagnostic criteria include a pervasive and excessive need to be taken care of, resulting in submissive and clinging behavior and fear of separation demonstrated by difficulty making independent decisions, excessive need for reassurance, unwillingness to assume responsibility, difficulty expressing differences of opinion, and a feeling of helplessness when alone (APA, 2013). The disorder must be distinguished from other personality disorders and substance use disorders.

Etiology

Recent research suggests a genetic component exists in the development of dependent personality disorder (Gjerde et al., 2012). As with other disorders in this cluster, there is very likely a strong element of learning (Young, 2008).

Implications for Function and Treatment

It is unclear whether any dysfunction at the skill level is noted. It is possible that CNS function is impaired, particularly the ability to accurately process sensory input.

Function is distinctly impaired in a number of occupations, as measured by the Global Assessment of Function (Bornstein, 2012). Social function is particularly poor. Social support ameliorates some of the functional deficits found in individuals with dependent personality disorder, whereas stress can exacerbate dependency.

Individuals with dependent personality disorder are more likely to experience physical illness and to make use of the health care system than is true for the general population (Bornstein, 2012). They also have an increased risk of self-harm, and are more likely to be abused by significant others in their lives (Loas, Cormier, & Perez-Diaz, 2011).

Efforts at intervention are similar to those used for other disorders in this cluster, including medication, skill training, behavioral interventions, and verbal therapies (Young, 2008).

Obsessive-Compulsive Personality Disorder

Obsessive-compulsive personality disorder (OCPD) is potentially the most disabling of the cluster C personality disorders, as these individuals are obsessive and rigid and engage in ritualistic behavior. Defining descriptors are "perfectionistic," "methodical," and "serious" (Mancebo, Eisen, Grant, & Rasmussen, 2005). These individuals never feel that they have done well enough, and they focus on minor details, wasting time that could be better spent elsewhere. Decision making is difficult because these individuals are unable to evaluate choices and act. They are judgmental and moralistic, often quite stingy, and have difficulty expressing warmth. Diagnostic criteria include a pervasive pattern of preoccupation with order and perfectionism, lack of flexibility, preoccupation with details, overconscientiousness, miserliness, rigidity, and stubbornness (APA, 2013). The disorder must be distinguished from obsessive-compulsive disorder (OCD), hoarding disorder, and other personality disorders.

OCPD is difficult to diagnose because it overlaps significantly with other psychiatric disorders (Fineberg, Saxena, Zohar, & Craig, 2007). In particular, OCPD is strongly correlated with OCD (Gordon, Salkovskis, Oldenfield, & Carter, 2013), and some consider it to be at the mild end of a spectrum disorder.

Etiology

OCPD has both genetic and environmental origins (Taylor, Asmundson, & Jang, 2011). There is certainly a learned component, and, in fact, many young children display obsessive-compulsive behavior (e.g., "step on a crack, break your mother's back" leads to careful avoidance of sidewalk irregularities for many 8 year olds). Although this behavior is most often outgrown, it clearly persists for some individuals.

Implications for Function and Intervention

Primary impairments resulting from OCPD are social and work (Ettner, Maclean, & French, 2011). The rigidity and moralistic nature of these individuals makes it difficult for them to form warm relationships. Their perfectionism, difficulty making decisions, and inability to use time well make work performance less than optimal. Task completion, in particular, is problematic. One individual, a bookkeeper, was unable to complete any page that had an erasure and, as a result, was frequently unable to complete assigned tasks.

Treatment of OCPD is difficult. Intervention most often focuses on depression. These individuals tend to be aware of their behavior and the problems it causes, leading to considerable depression or anxiety. Cognitively-based interventions may focus on facilitating a reconfiguration of self-esteem (Cummings, Hayes, Cardaciotto, & Newman, 2012). Among the cognitive therapies that have shown positive outcomes is dialectical behavior therapy (Lynch & Cheavens, 2008). Supportive and expressive psychotherapies have demonstrated some success (Vinnars & Barber, 2008).

Prognosis for Personality Disorders

On the whole, the prognosis for the various personality disorders is not good. The behaviors associated with all personality disorders tend to be fairly ingrained and pervasive—ways of being in the world as opposed to discrete symptoms. In addition, individuals with personality disorders often externalize their problems, blaming others when life does not go as they wish. However, there is certainly some evidence that individuals with personality disorders can change. For example, it has long been thought that APD is particularly unresponsive to treatment, and, certainly, there is evidence that a significant number of individuals with the disorder have long criminal histories or otherwise dysfunctional life trajectories (Shaw & Porter, 2012). However, evidence also exists that APD can be treated and that good outcomes are possible.

Symptoms of BPD can be improved, although treatment is challenging and typically long term. In one study focused on dialectical behavioral therapy (a variant of cognitive behavioral therapy), 31% of participants remained unchanged, 11% deteriorated, and approximately 15% showed a symptom level equivalent to that of the general population. Ten percent of participants dropped out (Kröger, Harbeck, Armbrust, & Kliem, 2013).

Avoidant personality disorder is difficult to treat. In addition, such individuals may not seek treatment because intervention would require establishing a relationship with a therapist.

OCPD is a relatively stable, long-term disorder. Of the adolescents with OCPD, 32% still had the diagnosis 2 years later (Mancebo et al., 2005). Particularly when there is a comorbid OCD, the individual is likely to continue to be symptomatic, even after treatment (Eisen et al., 2013).

In some sense, dependent personality disorder appears amenable to treatment. Certainly, these individuals are more likely than others with personality disorders to seek treatment (Bornstein, 2012). However, outcomes may be poor because of a tendency for the client to become dependent on the therapist.

For each of the personality disorders, there is evidence that change is possible. Also, substantial evidence exists that change is difficult, and successful intervention is likely to require sustained, and probably repeated, efforts.

Implications for Occupational Therapy

Although the manifestations of various personality disorders differ, according to Ward (1999) the following underlying issues are similar:
- Inaccurate perceptions of self and others
- Inadequate social skills
- Poorly developed personal values and goals
- Poor self-esteem

For some, particularly the cluster A disorders, inaccurate perceptions extend to many situations. This cluster may also be characterized by subtle neurological deficits, in addition to the learning of maladaptive behavioral patterns that has been implicated as an etiological factor for all the personality disorders. Although some individuals with personality disorder have relatively poor insight, these individuals may recognize the functional limitations that characterize their performance (Falklof & Haglund, 2010). A particular contribution of occupational therapy is the provision of specific skills training (Michael & Tilly, 2012).

Occupational therapists are likely to be involved in treatment teams working with individuals with personality disorders, and these integrative approaches seem to be helpful (De Groot, Verheul, & Trijsburg, 2008). Psychotherapy is a common intervention (Bartak, Soeteman, Verheul, & Busschbach, 2007; McMain, 2007; Paris, 2007; Verheul & Hebrink, 2007). Biological treatments are focused primarily on psychotropic medications (Herpetz et al., 2007), although only weak evidence exists about the value of medications (Paris, 2008). In particular, cognitive behavioral methods may be more effective when implemented in a coordinated way. Regardless of modality, treatment of personality disorders tends to be protracted and difficult (Wright, Haigh, & McKeown, 2007).

Because of the commonality of issues, a similar approach to occupational therapy intervention may be suitable for all the personality disorders. Opportunities for group interaction with clear, consistent feedback may be quite valuable. A variety of group/cooperative activities may be helpful, and include activities ranging from planning a social event to social skills training. A particular goal is interpreting accurately what others say and developing empathy, along with consistent, clear, and nonjudgmental feedback from the therapist and from other group members may assist in accomplishing this goal. Such behavioral strategies can be quite effective (Lee & Harris, 2010).

It is fairly characteristic that individuals with personality disorders show little regard for, or understanding of, the feelings of others, and they must learn to make an active effort to do so. One histrionic client, a young female college student, was quite astonished to learn that other women resented her tendency to flirt with their boyfriends. It had never occurred to her to consider their feelings, even though she expressed unhappiness about her lack of girlfriends. Providing these interventions in community settings allows for practice of skills in daily life (Clark, Ball, & Baltby, 2006; Lima, 2008).

Realistic appraisal of self is similarly problematic. Providing a range of opportunities, including leisure, social, and work-related activities, may be useful as a mechanism for exploration and for learning strengths and weaknesses. Both successes and failures must be analyzed. This not only enhances self-awareness, but is also provides a way to explore values and goals.

Activities that build self-esteem through experiences of success and the appreciation of others may help to convince these individuals of their worth. However, the insecurity tends to be so deep that it is quite problematic to provide them with all the reassurance they need. In addition, their behaviors often alienate others to the point that structuring activities in which they can experience appropriate and genuine feedback can be a challenge.

The three clusters present with somewhat differing characteristics that must also be addressed. Cluster A personality disorders may respond to sensory integrative/sensorimotor interventions because of the suspected neurological component. Cluster B may benefit from behavioral approaches because of the probability that they reflect deficits in early learning. For example, a work experience might be structured in the clinic, with reinforcement for desired behaviors. Individuals with cluster C personality disorders may be particularly amenable to social skills training because this is the predominant deficit for them. Behavior modification may be helpful in reducing anxiety for these individuals as well. Table 19-2 shows the symptoms and functional consequences of the personality disorders.

	TABLE 19-2	
DIAGNOSTIC CRITERIA AND FUNCTIONAL IMPLICATIONS: PERSONALITY DISORDERS		
DISORDER	*DIAGNOSTIC CRITERIA (APA, 2013)*	*IMPLICATIONS FOR FUNCTION*
Cluster A		
Paranoid	Tendency to suspect others and to interpret their actions as hostile	Work, leisure, social, and all patterns are negatively affected Process and communication skills are impaired
Schizoid	Lack of interest in social relationships Restricted emotional range	Work, leisure, social, and all patterns are negatively affected Process and possibly communication skills are impaired
Schizotypal	Poor relationships Restricted emotional range Odd perceptual experiences Odd appearance and speech Inappropriate affect	Work, leisure, social, and ADL/IADL patterns negatively are affected Process skills are impaired
Cluster B		
Antisocial	At least 18 years old Previous conduct disorder At least four types of antisocial behavior (e.g., theft, lying, child abuse) that occur in a persistent pattern Lacks remorse/guilt Inability to sustain relationships	Work, leisure, social, and IADL (especially financial) patterns are negatively affected Process and motor skills are not affected Habits/roles emphasize illegal behaviors
Borderline	Relationships fluctuate between intense involvement and devaluation Impulsiveness and instability Lack of control of anger Suicide gestures or self-mutilation	Work, leisure, social, and ADL/IADL patterns are negatively affected Process/communication skills are impaired, as are roles, habits, and routines
Histrionic	Excessive concern with appearance, seduction Excessive need for praise and reassurance Self-centered, lack of empathy for others	Work, leisure, social, and communication skills are negatively affected Patterns may or may not be impaired
		(continued)

TABLE 19-2 (CONTINUED)		
DIAGNOSTIC CRITERIA AND FUNCTIONAL IMPLICATIONS: PERSONALITY DISORDERS		
DISORDER	DIAGNOSTIC CRITERIA (APA, 2013)	IMPLICATIONS FOR FUNCTION
Histrionic (continued)	Exaggerated expressions of emotion, with rapid mood shifts and shallow emotion Need for constant attention	
Narcissistic	Sense of self-importance Preoccupied by fantasies of success Belief that he or she is special, arrogance Sense of entitlement, exploits others, requires admiration Lacks empathy	Social, work, and sometimes leisure roles are impaired by grandiosity
Cluster C		
Avoidant	Discomfort with social relationships Avoidance of social relationships and activities	Social, possibly work, and leisure skills are not impaired, although communication may be poor Patterns are not severely negatively affected in most cases
Dependent	Excessively dependent and submissive Fear of abandonment Easily hurt by criticism	Social, possibly work, and leisure performance are impaired Process and communication skills are impaired
Obsessive-compulsive	Perfectionistic Indecisiveness Preoccupation with detail Lack of generosity Excessively moralistic, conscientious	Work, leisure, and social skills are impaired Excessively patterned and rigid Skills are not severely negatively affected

Cultural Considerations

Clear cultural differences exist in the behavioral expectations that confound personality disorder diagnoses (Kianpoor & Rhoades, 2005; Millon, 2000). In some cases, these differences are reflected in the somewhat different presentations of an identified syndrome (Kianpoor & Rhoades, 2005). In others, cultural groups demonstrate behavioral clusters that might be recognizable as personality disorders but are not included in the DSM structure. One example is *Djinnati*, a syndrome found in Iran that is characterized by trance states and a sense of being possessed. However, there is also evidence that, at least among cultural groups somewhat acculturated to the United States, signs of personality disorder are consistent across groups (Matsunaga et al., 2000).

Culture affects how one describes oneself, and whether one is likely to acquiesce to others (Allik, 2005). There are also cultures in which what Westerners would consider excessive deference and dependence might be expected (Widiger & Bornstein, 2001).

Remember, culture is not something that only other groups have. U.S. culture has its own set of beliefs and values, many of which affect perceptions of mental disorders. A clear and recent example is the debate about how to conceptualize narcissistic personality disorder (Campbell, Miller, & Buffardi, 2010). Some believe that the United States has created a "culture of narcissism," as evidenced by enthusiastic postings on Facebook, Twitter, and publication of frequent "selfies" that display the most minor thoughts and activities as if there is a huge audience waiting for such information. Although none of this is the exclusive domain of the United States, there certainly are cultures that do not participate in this self-revelation to such a great (and often enthusiastic) extent.

Lifespan Considerations

Personality disorders typically emerge early in life (Cohen, 2008). A challenging aspect of identifying personality disorders is the fact that adolescence, when most are diagnosed, is a time of significant behavioral change, and it is possible to misdiagnose normal behavior as disturbed (Miller, Muehlenkamp, & Jacobson, 2008). Nevertheless, personality disorders seem rooted in childhood and adolescence, particularly as related to faulty learning and childhood trauma.

Because they are relatively intractable, personality disorders are also not uncommon in late life. The more flamboyant characteristics may diminish; therefore, diagnostic criteria for older adults may be more accurate if greater weight is given to the less observable but more stable internal psychological factors of personality disorders (van Alphen, Derksen, Sadavoy, & Rosowsky, 2012). Personality disorders can be complicated in later life by the onset of neurocognitive disorders that impose dementia on top of personality disorders behaviors.

Resources

American Psychological Association Online
http://www.apa.org/topics/topicperson.html
This page focuses on personality and includes links to information about personality development and personality disorders. Also lists other mental health topics covered for the public by the APA.

Mayo Clinic
http://www.mayoclinic.com/health/personality-disorders/ds00562
Information from the Mayo Clinic with regard to all the personality disorders, including overview, treatment suggestions, and links.

MedlinePlus
http://www.nlm.nih.gov/medlineplus/personalitydisorders.html
Provides a brief, but comprehensive, overview of each of the personality disorders, along with references, resources, and links.

CASE STUDY

Wendy Arthur is a 39-year-old, single, White woman. She lives alone in an apartment in a blue collar neighborhood in Chicago. She is rarely in touch with her family. Her parents live in Santa Fe, as do her two sisters. Wendy's parents provided her with a small trust fund, which enables her to live through her frequent periods of unemployment. She briefly had two roommates as a way to make ends meet, but they both moved out as soon as their lease allowed. Wendy never felt particularly close to them, but was angry that they deserted her and left her to handle the rent. She felt certain that they talked about her behind her back, and had formed a "cabal" to "get back at me."

Wendy worked as a secretary for a large appliance company, but she lost her job about the time her roommates moved out. Her boss told her they were "right-sizing," but Wendy suspects that one of her coworkers complained about her. Wendy believes that she was a particularly effective employee and that her coworker was jealous. She is now spending most of her time in her apartment drinking and surfing the Web, making hostile comments on various blogs.

Wendy dates from time to time, but she has not been able to sustain a long-term relationship. In fact, she rarely gets beyond a first date. She is disappointed that there are no men interesting and sexy enough to suit her. She has few other social relationships; her neighbors seem to avoid her and she rarely reaches out to anyone in other ways. On the rare occasions that she is included in social gatherings, she is awkward, withdrawn, and feels that others are intentionally shunning her.

Wendy reluctantly decides to enter therapy at the urging of her parents, who are concerned about her drinking and inability to find a new job. She tells the therapist that others don't understand her and that there is a conspiracy among employers to keep her out of work.

THOUGHT QUESTIONS

1. What are the characteristics of Wendy's behavior that might be causing her difficulties?
2. Do these characteristics fit any of the personality disorder clusters? If so, which one?
3. Is there a particular personality disorder that seems to fit best with Wendy's characteristics?
4. What might an occupational therapist consider in trying to help Wendy address her dilemma?

References

Ahmed, A.O., Green, B.A., Goodrum, N.M., Doane, N.J., Birgenheir, D., & Buckley, P.F. (2013). Does a latent class underlie schizotypal personality disorder? Implications for schizophrenia. *Journal of Abnormal Psychology, 122*(2), 475-491.

Alden, L.E., Laposa, J.M., Taylor, C.T., & Ryder, A.G. (2002). Avoidant personality disorder: Current status and future directions. *Journal of Personality disorders, 16*, 1-29.

Allik, J. (2005). Personality dimensions across cultures. *Personality Disorders, 19*, 212-232.

American Psychiatric Association. (2004). *Personality disorders conference.* Retrieved from http://www.dsm5.org/Research/Pages/PersonalityDisordersConference%28December1-3,2004%29.aspx.

American Psychiatric Association. (2013). *Diagnostic and statistical manual of mental disorders* (5th ed.). Washington, DC: Author.

Bartak, A., Soeteman, D.I., Verheul, R., & Busschbach, J.J. (2007). Strengthening the status of psychotherapy for personality disorders: An integrated perspective on effects and costs. *Canadian Journal of Psychiatry, 52,* 803-810.

Bender, D.S., & Skodol, A.E. (2007). Borderline personality disorder as a self-other representational disturbance. *Journal of Personality disorders, 21,* 500-517.

Birgenheir, D.G., & Pepper, C.M. (2011). Negative life experiences and the development of cluster C personality disorders: A cognitive perspective. *Cognitive Behaviour Therapy, 40*(3), 190-205.

Blasco-Fontecilla, H., Baca-Garcia, E., Dervic, K., Perez-Rodriguez, M.M., Lopez-Castroman, J., Saiz-Ruiz, J., & Oquendo, M.A. (2009). Specific features of suicidal behavior in patients with narcissistic personality disorder. *Journal of Clinical Psychiatry, 70*(11), 1583-1587.

Bornstein, R.F. (2012). Illuminating a neglected clinical issue: Societal costs of interpersonal dependency and dependent personality disorder. *Journal of Clinical Psychology, 68*(7), 766-781.

Buchheim, A., Roth, G., Schiepek, G., Pogarell, O., & Karch, S. (2013). Neurobiology of borderline personality disorder (BPD) and antisocial personality disorder (APD). *Schweizer Archiv für Neurologie und Psychiatrie, 164*(4), 115-122.

Campbell, W.K., Miller, J.D., & Buffardi, L.E. (2010). The United States and the "culture of narcissism": An examination of perceptions of national character. *Social Psychological and Personality Science, 1*(3), 222-229.

Clark, E.L., Ball, A., & Baltby, S. (2006). How a successful course developing community living skills was designed, facilitated and evaluated with female clients, the majority of whom have been diagnosed with borderline personality disorder and previously described as difficult to engage. *Mental Health Occupational Therapy, 11*(1), 31-34.

Cohen, P. (2008). Child development and personality disorder. *Psychiatric Clinics of North America, 31*(3), 477-493.

Cohen, A.S., Emmerson, L.C., Mann, M.C., Forbes, C.B., & Blanchard, J.J. (2010). Schizotypal, schizoid and paranoid characteristics in the biological parents of social anhedonics. *Psychiatry Research, 178*(1), 79-83.

Cohen, P., Crawford, T., Chen, H., Kasen, S., & Gordon, K. (2012). Predictors, correlates, and consequences of trajectories of antisocial personality disorder symptoms from early adolescence to mid-30s. In C.S. Widom (Ed.), *Trauma, psychopathology, and violence: Causes, consequences, or correlates?* (pp. 109-129). New York, NY: Oxford University Press.

Crawford, M.J., Koldobsky, N., Mulder, R., & Tyre, P. (2011) Classifying personality disorder according to severity. *Journal of Personality Disorders, 25,* 321-330.

Crawford, T.N., Cohen, P., & Brook, J.S. (2001). Dramatic-erratic personality disorder symptoms: I. Continuity from early adolescence into adulthood. *Journal of Personality disorders, 15,* 319-335.

Crowe, S.L., & Blair, R.J. (2008). The development of antisocial behavior: What can we learn from neuroimaging studies? *Development and Psychopathology, 20,* 1145-1159.

Cummings, J.A., Hayes, A.M., Cardaciotto, L., & Newman, C.F. (2012). The dynamics of self-esteem in cognitive therapy for avoidant and obsessive-compulsive personality disorders: An adaptive role of self-esteem variability? *Cognitive Therapy and Research, 36*(4), 272-281.

De Groot, E.R., Verheul, R., & Trijsburg, R.W. (2008). An integrative perspective on psychotherapeutic treatments for borderline personality disorder. *Journal of Personality Disorders, 22,* 332-352.

DeShong, H.L., & Kurtz, J.E. (2013). Four factors of impulsivity differentiate antisocial and borderline personality disorders. *Journal of Personality Disorders, 27*(2), 144-156.

Dignam, P., Parry, P., & Berk, M. (2010). Detached from attachment: Neurobiology and phenomenology have a human face. *Acta Neuropsychiatrica, 22,* 202-206.

Disney, K.L., Weinstein, Y., & Oltmanns, T.F. (2012). Personality disorder symptoms are differentially related to divorce frequency. *Journal of Family Psychology, 26*(6), 959-965.

Eisen, J.L., Sibrava, N.J., Boisseau, C.L., Mancebo, M.C., Stout, R.L., Pinto, A., . . . Rasmussen, S.A. (2013). Five-year course of obsessive-compulsive disorder: Predictors of remission and relapse. *Journal of Clinical Psychiatry, 74*(3), 233-239.

Esterberg, M.L., Goulding, S.M., & Walker, E.F. (2010). Cluster A personality disorders: Schizotypal, schizoid and paranoid personality disorders in childhood and adolescence. *Journal of Psychopathology and Behavioral Assessment, 32*(4), 515-528.

Ettner, S.L., Maclean, J.C., & French, M.T. (2011). Does having a dysfunctional personality hurt your career? Axis II personality disorders and labor market outcomes. *Industrial Relations, 50*(1), 149-173.

Falklof, I., & Haglund, L. (2010). Daily occupations and adaptation to daily life described by women suffering from borderline personality disorder. *Occupational Therapy in Mental Health, 26*(4), 354-374.

Fineberg, N.A., Saxena, S., Zohar, J., & Craig, K.J. (2007). Obsessive-compulsive disorder: Boundary issues. *CNS Spectrums, 12,* 359-364.

Fitzgerald, K.L., & Demakis, G.J. (2007). The neuropsychology of antisocial personality disorder. *Disease-a-Month: DM, 53,* 177-183.

Fontaine, R.G. (2007). Toward a conceptual framework of instrumental antisocial decisions-making and behavior in youth. *Clinical Psychology Review, 27,* 655-675.

Fountoulakis, K.N., Leucht, S., & Kaprinis, G.S. (2008). Personality disorders and violence. *Current Opinion in Psychiatry, 21,* 84-92.

Freeston, M., Howard, R., Coid, J.W., & Ullrich, S. (2013). Adult antisocial syndrome co-morbid with borderline personality disorder is associated with severe conduct disorder, substance dependence and violent antisociality. *Personality and Mental Health, 7*(1), 11-21.

Frick, P.J., & White, S.F. (2008). Research review: The importance of callous-unemotional traits for developmental models of aggressive and antisocial behavior. *Journal of Child Psychology, Psychiatry, and Allied Disciplines, 49,* 359-375.

Gilbert, S.E., & Gordon, K.C. (2013). Interpersonal psychotherapy informed treatment for avoidant personality disorder with subsequent depression. *Clinical Case Studies, 12*(2), 111-127.

Gjerde, L.C., Czajkowski. N., Røysamb, E., Ørstavik, R. E., Knudsen, G. P., Østby, K., . . . Reichborn-Kjennerud, T. (2012). The heritability of avoidant and dependent personality disorder assessed by personal interview and questionnaire. *Acta Psychiatrica Scandinavica, 126*(6), 448-457.

Glaser, J.P., Van Os, J., Thewissen, V., & Myin-Germeys, I. (2010). Psychotic reactivity in borderline personality disorder. *Acta Psychiatrica Scandinavica, 121*(2), 125-134.

Gordon, O.M., Salkovskis, P.M., Oldenfield, V.B., & Carter, N. (2013). The association between obsessive compulsive disorder and obsessive compulsive personality disorder: Prevalence and clinical presentation. *British Journal of Clinical Psychology, 52*(3), 300-315.

Grant, B.F., Chou, S.P., Goldstein, R.B., Huang, B., Stinson, F.S., Saha, T.D., . . . Ruan, W.J. (2008). Prevalence, correlates, disability, and comorbidity of DSM-IV borderline personality disorder: Results from the Wave 2 national epidemiologic survey on alcohol and related conditions. *Journal of Clinical Psychiatry, 69,* 533-545.

Grant, B.F., Hasin, D.S., Stinson, F.S., Dawson, D.A., Chou, P., Ruan, J., & Huang, B. (2005). Co-occurrence of 12-month mood and anxiety disorders and personality disorders in the US: Results from the national epidemiologic survey on alcohol and related conditions. *Journal of Psychiatric Research, 39*(1), 1-9.

Grant, B.F., Hasin, D.S., Stinson, F.S., Dawson, D.A., Chou, S.P., Ruan, W.J., & Pickering, R.P. (2004). Prevalence, correlates, and disability of personality disorders in the United States: Results from the national epidemiologic survey on alcohol and related conditions. *Journal of Clinical Psychiatry, 65,* 948-958.

Hamilton, S.S., & Armando, J. (2008). Oppositional defiant disorder. *American Family Physician, 78,* 861-866.

Herpetz, S.C., Zanarini, M., Schultz, C.S., Siever, L., Lieb, K., & Möller, H.J. (2007). World Federation of Societies of Biological Psychiatry (WFSBP) guidelines for biological treatment of personality disorders. *World Journal of Biological Psychiatry, 8,* 212-244.

Horan, W.P., Blanchard, J.J., Clark, L.A., & Green, M.F. (2008). Affective traits in schizophrenia and schizotypy. *Schizophrenia Bulletin, 34,* 856-874.

Horowitz, M.J., & Lerner, U. (2010). Treatment of histrionic personality disorder. In J.F. Clarkin, P. Fonagy, & G.O. Gabbard (Eds.) *Psychodynamic psychotherapy for personality disorders: A clinical handbook* (pp. 289-309). Arlington, VA: American Psychiatric Publishing.

Huprich, S.K., & Bornstein, R.F. (2007). An overview of issues related to categorical and dimensional models of personality disorder assessment. *Journal of Personality Assessment, 89,* 3-15.

Jansson, I., Hesse, M., & Fridell, M. (2008). Personality disorder features as predictors of symptoms five years post-treatment. *American Journal on Addictions, 17*(3), 172-175.

Kianpoor, M., & Rhoades, G.F., Jr. (2005). "Djinnati," a possession state in Baloochistan, Iran. *Journal of Trauma Practice, 4*(1/2), 147-155.

Kolla, N.J., Eisenberg, H., & Links, P.S. (2008). Epidemiology, risk factors, and psychopharmacological management of suicidal behavior in borderline personality disorder. *Archives of Suicide Research, 12,* 1-19.

Kröger, C., Harbeck, S., Armbrust, M., & Kliem, S. (2013). Effectiveness, response, and dropout of dialectical behavior therapy for borderline personality disorder in an inpatient setting. *Behaviour Research and Therapy, 51*(8), 411-416.

Lee, S., & Harris, M. (2010). The development of an effective occupational therapy assessment and treatment pathway for women with a diagnosis of borderline personality disorder in an inpatient setting: Implementing the model of human occupation. *British Journal of Occupational Therapy, 73*(11), 559-563.

Lima, A. (2008). "The colours of my being"—A community intervention for a person with borderline personality disorder and comorbid minor depression. *Mental Health Occupational Therapy, 13,* 109-112.

Liotti, G., Cortina, M., & Farina, B. (2008). Attachment theory and multiple integrated treatments of borderline patients. *Journal of the American Academy of Psychoanalysis and Dynamic Psychiatry, 36,* 295-315.

Lis, E., Greenfield, B., Henry, M., Guilé, J.M., & Dougherty, G. (2007). Neuroimaging and genetics of borderline personality disorder: A review. *Journal of Psychiatry & Neuroscience, 32,* 162-173.

Livesley, W.J. (2007). A framework for integrating dimensional and categorical classifications of personality disorder. *Journal of Personality disorders, 21,* 199-224.

Livesley, W.J. (2008). Toward a genetically-informed model of borderline personality disorder. *Journal of Personality disorders, 22,* 42-71.

Livesley, J. (2012). Tradition versus empiricism in the current DSM-5 proposal for revising the classification of personality disorders. *Criminal Behaviour and Mental Health, 22*(2), 81-90.

Loas, G., Cormier, J., & Perez-Diaz, F. (2011). Dependent personality disorder and physical abuse. *Psychiatry Research, 185*(1-2), 167-170.

Lynch, T.R., & Cheavens, J.S. (2008). Dialectical behavior therapy for comorbid personality disorders. *Journal of Clinical Psychology, 64*(2), 154-167.

Mallinckrodt, B., Daly, K., & Wang, C.-C. (2009). An attachment approach to adult psychotherapy. In J.H. Obegi & E. Berant (Eds.), *Attachment theory and research in clinical work with adults* (pp. 234-268). New York, NY: Guilford.

Mancebo, M.C., Eisen, J.L., Grant, J.E., & Rasmussen, S.A. (2005). Obsessive compulsive personality disorder and obsessive compulsive disorder: Clinical characteristics, diagnostic difficulties, and treatment. *Annals of Clinical Psychiatry, 14,* 197-204.

Marsh, A.A., & Blair, R.J. (2008). Deficits in facial affect recognition among antisocial populations: A meta-analysis. *Neuroscience and Biobehavioral Reviews, 31,* 454-465.

Matsunaga, H., Kiriike, N., Iwasaki, Y., Miyata, A., Matsui, T., Nagata, T., . . . Kave, W.H. (2000). Multi-impulsivity among bulimic patients in Japan. *International Journal of Eating Disorders, 27,* 348-352.

McCloskey, M.S., Phan, K.L., & Coccaro, E.F. (2005). Neuroimaging and personality disorders. *Current Psychiatry Reports, 7,* 65-72.

McClure, M.M., Harvey, P.D., Bowie, C.R., Iacoviello, B., & Siever, L.J. (2013). Functional outcomes, functional capacity, and cognitive impairment in schizotypal personality disorder. *Schizophrenia Research, 144*(1-3), 146-150.

McGurk, S.R., Mueser, K.T., Mischel, R., Adams, R., Harvey, P.D., McClure, M.M., . . . Siever, L.J. (2013). Vocational functioning in schizotypal and paranoid personality disorders. *Psychiatry Research, 210*(2), 498-504.

McMain, S. (2007). Effectiveness of psychosocial treatments on suicidality in personality disorders. *Canadian Journal of Psychiatry, 52*(6, Suppl. 1), 103S-114S.

Michael, S., & Tilly, C. (2012). STEPPS-practical training program for borderline sufferers. *Ergotherapie & Rehabilitation, 51*(2), 17-21.

Miller, A.L., Muehlenkamp, J.J., & Jacobson, C.M. (2008). Fact or fiction: Diagnosing borderline personality disorder in adolescents. *Clinical Psychology Review, 28,* 969-981.

Millon, T. (2000). Sociocultural conceptions of the borderline personality. *Psychiatric Clinics of North America, 23,* 123-136.

Milne, L., Peel, K., & Greenway, P. (2012). The role of parental disciple and family environment during childhood and in cluster B personality symptoms in adulthood. In A.M. Columbus (Ed.), *Advances in psychology research* (Vol. 88, pp. 95-115). Hauppauge, NY: Nova Science.

Montandon, M., & Feldman, M.D. (2008). Borderline personality disorder. In F.F. Ferri (Ed.), *Ferri's clinical advisor 2008: Instant diagnosis and treatment.* Philadelphia, PA: Mosby Elsevier. Retrieved from http://www.mdconsult.com/das/book/body/127763362-2/0/1701/92.html?tocnode=56562675&fromURL=92.html#4-u1.0-B978-0-323-04134-8..50005-7--subchapter18_1838.

Moore, D.P., & Jefferson, J.W. (2004a). Paranoid personality disorder. In D.P. Moore & J.W. Jefferson (Eds.), *Handbook of medical psychiatry* (2nd ed.). Philadelphia, PA: Mosby Elsevier.

Moore, D.P., & Jefferson, J.W. (2004b). Schizoid personality disorder. In D.P. Moore & J.W. Jefferson (Eds.), *Handbook of medical psychiatry* (2nd ed.). Philadelphia, PA: Mosby Elsevier. Moore, D.P., & Jefferson, J.W. (2004c). Schizotypal personality disorder. In D.P. Moore & J.W. Jefferson (Eds.), *Handbook of medical psychiatry* (2nd ed.). Philadelphia, PA: Mosby Elsevier. Moore, D.P., & Jefferson, J.W. (2004d). Antisocial personality disorder. In D.P. Moore & J.W. Jefferson (Eds.), Handbook of medical psychiatry (2nd ed.). Philadelphia, PA: Mosby Elsevier.

Morey, L.C., & Stagner, B.H. (2012). Narcissistic pathology as core personality dysfunction: Comparing the DSM-IV and the DSM-5 proposal for narcissistic personality disorder. *Journal of Clinical Psychology, 68*(8), 908-921.

National Institute for Health and Care Excellence. (2009/2013). *Antisocial personality disorder: Guidelines for treatment, management, and prevention.* Retrieved from http://www.guidance.nice.org.uk/cg77.

New, A.S., Goodman, M., Triebwasser, J., & Siever, L.J. (2008). Recent advances in the biological study of personality disorders. *Psychiatric Clinics of North America, 13,* 441-461.

Oleski, J. Cox, B.J., Robinson, J., & Grant, B. (2012). The predictive validity of cluster C personality disorders on the persistence of major depression in the national epidemiologic survey on alcohol and related conditions. *Journal of Personality Disorders, 26*(3), 322-333.

Pankey, J. (2012). Functional analytic psychotherapy (FAP) for cluster B personality disorders: Creating meaning, mattering, and skills. *International Journal of Behavioral Consultation and Therapy, Special Issue: Functional Analytic Psychotherapy, 7*(2-3), 117-124.

Paris, J. (2007). Intermittent psychotherapy: An alternative to continuous long-term treatment for patients with personality disorders. *Journal of Psychiatric Practice, 13,* 153-158.

Paris, J. (2008). Clinical trials of treatment for personality disorders. *Psychiatric Clinics of North America, 31,* 517-526.

Parpottas, P. (2012). A critique on the use of standard psychopathological classifications in understanding human distress: The example of 'schizoid personality disorder'. *Counseling Psychology Review, 27*(1), 44-52.

Peng, Y., Zhou, S., Chen, Z., & Cai, R. (2011). Childhood abuse, attachment, and adolescent cluster-B personality disorder tendency. *Chinese Journal of Clinical Psychology, 19*(1), 63-65.

Perez, P.R. (2012). The etiology of psychopathy: A neuropsychological perspective. *Aggression and Violent Behavior, 17*(6), 519-522.

Perry, J.C., Presniak, M.D., & Olson, T.R. (2013). Defense mechanisms in schizotypal, borderline, antisocial, and narcissistic personality disorders. *Psychiatry: Interpersonal and Biological Processes, 76*(1), 32-52.

Pull, C.B. (2013). Too few or too many? Reactions to removing versus retaining specific personality disorders in DSM-5. *Current Opinion in Psychiatry, 26*(1), 73-78.

Raine, A. (2006). Schizotypal personality: Neurodevelopmental and psychosocial trajectories. *Annual Review of Clinical Psychology, 2,* 291-326.

Rosenthal, M.Z., Gratz, K.L., Kosson, D.S., Cheavens, J.S., Lejuez, W., & Lynch, T.R. (2008). Borderline personality disorder and emotional responding: A review of the research literature. *Clinical Psychology Review, 21,* 75-91.

Rossi, R., Pievani, M., Lorenzi, M., Boccardi, M., Beneduce, R., Bignotti, S., . . . Frisoni, G.B. (2013). Structural brain features of borderline personality and bipolar disorders. *Psychiatry Research: Neuroimaging, 213*(2), 83-91.

Ruiz, M.A., Pincus, A.L., & Schinka, J.A. (2008). Externalizing pathology and the five-factor model: A meta-analysis of personality traits associated with antisocial personality disorder, substance use disorder, and their co-occurrence. *Journal of Personality Disorder, 22,* 365-388.

Sansone, R.A., & Sansone, L.A. (2007). Childhood trauma, borderline personality, and eating disorders: A developmental cascade. *Eating Disorders, 15,* 333-346.

Shaw, J., & Porter, S. (2012). Forever a psychopath? Psychopathy and the criminal career trajectory. In H. Häkkänen-Nyholm & J. Nyholm (Eds.), *Psychopathy and law: A practitioner's guide* (pp. 201-221). New York, NY: Wiley-Blackwell.

Shopshire, M.S., & Craik, K.H. (1996). An act-based conceptual analysis of the obsessive-compulsive, paranoid, and histrionic personality disorders. *Journal of Personality Disorders, 10,* 203-218.

Siefert, C.J. (2012). A goal-oriented limited-duration approach for borderline personality disorder during brief inpatient hospitalizations. *Psychotherapy, 49*(4), 502-518.

Skodol, A.E. (2012). Personality disorders in DSM-5. *Annual Review of Clinical Psychology, 8,* 317-344.

Skodol, A.E., Grillo, C.M., Keyes, K.M., Geier, T., Grant, B.F., & Hasin, D.S. (2011). Relationship of personality disorders to the course of major depressive disorder in a nationally representative sample. *American Journal of Psychiatry, 168*(3), 257-264.

Stinson, F.S., Dawson, D.A., Goldstein, R.B., Chou, S.P., Huang, B., Smith, S.M.,. . . Grant, B.F. (2008). Prevalence, correlates, disability, and comorbidity of DSM-IV narcissistic personality disorder: Results from the wave 2 national epidemiologic survey on alcohol and related conditions. *Journal of Clinical Psychiatry, 69*(7), 1033-1045.

Taylor, S., Asmundson, G.J.G., & Jang, K.L. (2011). Etiology of obsessive-compulsive symptoms and obsessive-compulsive personality traits: Common genes, mostly different environments. *Depression and Anxiety, 28*(10), 863-869.

Torgersen, S., Myers, J., Reichborn-Kjennerud, T., Røysamb, E., Kubarych, T.S., & Kendler, K.S. (2012). The heritability of cluster B personality disorders assessed both by personal interview and questionnaire. *Journal of Personality Disorders, 26*(6), 848-866.

Tyrer, P., Coombs, N., Ibrahimi, F., Mathilakath, A., Bajaj, P., Ranger, M.,. . . Din, R. (2007). Critical developments in the assessment of personality disorder. *British Journal of Psychiatry, 49*(Suppl.), S51-S59.

U.S. National Library of Medicine. (2008). *Histrionic personality disorder.* Retrieved from http://www.nlm.nih.gov/medlineplus/ency/article/001531.htm.

Usher, A.M., Stewart, L.A., & Wilton, G. (2013). Attention deficit hyperactivity disorder in a Canadian prison population. *International Journal of Law and Psychiatry, 36*(3-4), 311-315.

van Alphen, S.P.J., Derksen, J.J.L., Sadavoy, J., & Rosowsky, E. (2012). Features and challenges of personality disorders in late life. *Aging & Mental Health, 16*(7), 805-810.

Vater, A., Ritter, K., Schröder-Abé, M., Schütz, A., Lammers, C., Bosson, J.K., & Roepka, S. (2013). When grandiosity and vulnerability collide: Implicit and explicit self-esteem in patients with narcissistic personality disorder. *Journal of Behavior Therapy and Experimental Psychiatry, 44*(1), 37-47.

Vaughn, M.F., Fu, Q., Beaver, D., Delisi, M., Perron, B., & Howard, M. (2010). Are personality disorders associated with social welfare burden in the United States? *Journal of Personality Disorders, 24*(6), 709-720.

Verheul, R., & Hebrink, M. (2007). The efficacy of various modalities of psychotherapy for personality disorders: A systematic review of the evidence and clinical recommendations. *International Review of Psychiatry, 19*, 25-38.

Viding, E., Larsson, H., & Jones, A.P. (2008). Quantitative genetic studies of antisocial behavior. *Philosophical Transactions of the Royal Society of London. Series B, Biological Sciences, 363*, 1519-1527.

Vinnars, B., & Barber, J.P. (2008). Supportive-expressive psychotherapy for comorbid personality disorders: A case study. *Journal of Clinical Psychology, 64*(2), 195-206.

Ward, J.D. (1999). Psychosocial dysfunction in adults. In M.E. Neistadt & E.B. Crepeau (Eds.), *Willard and Spackman's occupational therapy* (9th ed., pp. 716-740). Philadelphia, PA: Lippincott, Williams, & Wilkins.

Weber, S., Habel, U., Amunts, K., & Schneider, F. (2008). Structural brain abnormalities in psychopaths—A review. *Behavioral Science and Law, 26*(1), 7-28.

Whitborne, S.K. (2013). What's new (and old) in the DSM-5 personality disorders. *Psychology Today.* Retrieved from http://www.psychologytoday.com/blog/fulfillment-any-age/201303/whats-new-and-old-in-the-dsm-5-personality-disorders.

Widiger, T.A., & Bornstein, R.F. (2001). Histrionic, narcissistic, and dependent personality disorders. In H.E. Adams & P. Sutker (Eds.), *Comprehensive handbook of psychopathology* (3rd ed., pp. 507-529). New York, NY: Plenum.

Widiger, T.A., & Trull, T.J. (2007). Plate tectonics in the classification of personality disorder: Shifting to a dimensional model. *American Psychologist, 62*(2), 71-82.

Williams, P. (2010). Psychotherapeutic treatment of cluster A personality disorders. In J.F. Clarkin, P. Fonagy, & G.O. Gabbard, (Eds.), *Psychodynamic psychotherapy for personality disorders: A clinical handbook* (pp. 165-185). Arlington, VA: American Psychiatric Publishing.

Wright, K., Haigh, K., & McKeown, M. (2007). Reclaiming the humanity in personality disorder. *International Journal of Mental Health Nursing, 16*(4), 236-246.

Yang, Y., Glenn, A.L., & Raine, A. (2008). Brain abnormalities in antisocial individuals: Implications for the law. *Behavioral Science and Law, 26*(1), 65-71.

Young, J.Q. (2008). Narcissistic personality disorder. In F.F. Ferri (Ed.), *Ferri's clinical advisor 2008: Instant diagnosis and treatment.* Philadelphia, PA: Mosby Elsevier.

Zimmerman, M., Chelminski, I., & Young, D. (2008). The frequency of personality disorders in *psychiatric patients. Psychiatric Clinics of North America, 31*, 405-420.

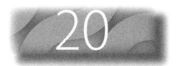

Other
Conditions

Learning Outcomes

By the end of this chapter, readers will be able to:

- Describe the medication-induced and other conditions that may be a focus of clinical attention
- Differentiate among medication-induced and other conditions that may be a focus of clinical attention on the basis of symptoms
- Identify the causes of medication-induced and other conditions that may be a focus of clinical attention
- Describe treatment strategies for medication-induced and other conditions
- Discuss the occupational perspective on medication-induced and other conditions that may be a focus of clinical attention
- Discuss occupational therapy interventions for medication-induced and other conditions that may be a focus of clinical attention

Bonder B.
Psychopathology and Function, Fifth Edition (pp 403-411).
© 2015 SLACK Incorporated.

Key Words

- Dystonia
- Akathisia
- Tardive dyskinesia

Case Vignette

A school psychologist has been asked by the second grade teacher to meet with one of her students, a girl who came to school that morning with a vivid red mark on her face. When the teacher asked what had happened, the student told her that she fell off her bike. The teacher was concerned for several reasons: first, the student did not lift her gaze from the floor throughout the conversation and was very withdrawn and subdued; second, the mark looked very much like a handprint; and third, the student had, in the past 3 months, come to class with a large bruise on her leg, an odd looking burn on the back of one of her hands, and sprained a wrist.

Thought Questions

1. Why might the teacher have asked the psychologist to consult with her student?
2. If you, as the occupational therapist, had seen the child this morning, what do you think your responsibility might be?
3. What is the mental health aspect of this situation?

Medication-Induced Disorders and Other Conditions That May be a Focus of Clinical Attention

- Medication-induced disorders
  - Medication-induced movement disorders and other adverse effects of medication
  - Other conditions that may be a focus of clinical attention
- Other conditions that may be a focus of clinical attention
  - Relational problems
  - Problems related to family upbringing
  - Other problems related to primary support group
- Abuse and neglect
  - Child maltreatment and neglect problems
  - Child physical abuse
  - Child sexual abuse
  - Child psychological abuse
  - Adult maltreatment and neglect problems
  - Spouse or partner violence, sexual
  - Spouse or partner neglect
  - Spouse or partner abuse, psychological
  - Adult abuse by nonspouse or nonpartner
- Educational and occupational problems
  - Educational problems
  - Occupational problems
- Housing and economic problems
  - Housing problems
  - Economic problems

In spite of the voluminous and detailed delineation of mental disorders described in previous chapters, a large number of conditions exist that might bring an individual into treatment that are not consistent with the diagnoses we have considered so far. There are several reasons this might be so. First, clinicians are encouraged to adhere quite strictly to the diagnostic criteria for both clinical and research reasons. The criteria were carefully established with an eye toward consistency, although, as you have seen throughout this text, many are worded in a way that gives clinicians considerable latitude. As we have seen, it is important to select treatments based on available evidence and to record and document treatment to improve future outcomes. This requires caution in addressing circumstances of individuals whose symptoms do not fit the established categories. Many individuals who seek help are themselves well aware that they are dealing with problems of life as opposed to mental disorders. Individuals who have lost their jobs, broken up with partners, or who are living in abusive relationships may meet the criteria for depression, or they may simply be distressed and need help coping.

Another important function of the "other conditions" list is to allow for greater clarity about the personal and environmental circumstances that may contribute to the onset or severity of the mental disorders covered in previous chapters. People who are struggling with economic issues, such as job loss, can experience an accompanying depressive or anxiety disorder. Many individuals who have been or are currently dealing with abuse can also have a related posttraumatic stress disorder. Identifying and addressing the social circumstances associated with the mental disorder can enhance treatment outcomes.

This chapter covers two chapters from the fifth edition of the *Diagnostic and Statistical Manual of Mental Disorders* (DSM-5; American Psychiatric Association [APA], 2013). For the first time, the DSM includes a chapter focused on the problems that can result from use of medications. In addition, as in the past, a chapter addresses the many problems of daily life that might result in an individual seeking help, even in the absence of a specific mental disorder.

Medication-Induced Movement Disorders

The disorders in this cluster will be addressed in greater detail in the next chapter. They are distinct from the substance-related disorders because they typically emerge as a consequence of use of psychotropic and other medications used as prescribed. Although progress in psychopharmacology has been an important contributing factor in enabling individuals with mental disorders to function effectively in daily life, they are not without dilemmas (Goldberg & Ernst, 2012). Such medications can cause Parkinson-like symptoms, **dystonia** (i.e., prolonged contraction of the muscles), **akathisia** (i.e., restlessness and fidgeting), and postural tremor. **Tardive dyskinesia** is severe movement disorder associated with several of the antipsychotic medications. Tardive dyskinesia is characterized by involuntary athetoid or choreiform movements, usually of the tongue, face, and limbs (Mihanović, Bodor, Kezić, Restek-Petrović, & Silić, 2009). It contributes to the challenges faced by individuals with psychotic disorders both because of the movement disorder itself and because of the peculiar and often stigmatizing appearance it creates.

Movement disorders and other side effects of medication can certainly be managed (Goldberg & Ernst, 2012). A change in medication or an altered dose may help in some situations, although discontinuation of a medication can also cause movement symptoms and other side effects. A careful balance is required to ensure maximum benefit and minimum harm whenever a psychotropic medication is part of treatment.

From the perspective of occupational therapy, there are two main considerations. The first relates to the need for caution in providing some interventions and helping the client to manage symptoms related to the medications. An individual with a severe hand tremor would not be a good candidate for a woodworking project that involves the use of sharp implements or requires precise measuring. A person with peculiar facial movements resulting from medication might find it helpful to role play, explaining the behavior to minimize its interference with social encounters.

A second consideration is that some occupational therapy interventions might reduce at least some of the symptoms related to the medications. Good evidence exists that rhythmic movement can help to minimize the tremors associated with Parkinson's disease and increase participation in other activities (Foster, Golden, Duncan, & Earhart, 2013). It is possible that these kinds of activities might also be helpful for individuals with other kinds of dystonia, although there is no firm evidence of this.

Other Conditions That May Be a Focus of Clinical Attention

Other conditions that may be a focus of clinical attention are grouped into the following several clusters (APA, 2013):

- Relational problems
- Abuse and neglect
- Educational and occupational problems
- Housing and economic problems
- Other problems related to the social environment
- Other circumstances of personal history

Several of these condition groups emphasize function, particularly those focused on relational problems and educational and occupational problems.

Relational Problems

Relational problems are among the most common reasons that individuals seek therapy. Difficulties in important relationships can affect quality of life, as well as physical health and economic productivity (Steenwyk, Doeden, Furrow, & Atkins, 2012). Couples may struggle to communicate effectively, to manage empathic interactions, and to meet each other's emotional and instrumental needs. These kinds of relationship difficulties may be more pronounced in lesbian, gay, bisexual, and transgender couples because of the added challenges of being in relationships perceived as nontraditional (Lingiardi & Nardelli, 2012). Relationship problems can also occur between parents and children.

A number of possible interventions exist, from couples' and family therapy to individual and group treatment (Litt, 2010). Parent training can improve parenting skills, which has a direct impact on children's interpersonal competence (Mintz, Hamre, & Hatfield, 2011). In addition, training can improve awareness of affect, improving individuals' effective and supportive communication (Lech, Andersson, & Holmqvist, 2012).

Abuse and Neglect

Abuse and neglect are common and serious societal concerns. They can affect individuals of any age and in any socioeconomic group. Abuse and neglect occur worldwide and often result in symptoms of posttraumatic stress disorder (Mbagaya, Oburu, Bakermans-Kranenburg, 2013). Childhood sexual abuse alone has been reported to have occurred in approximately

20% of the population, with estimates that childhood physical abuse occurs in 11% to 26% of the population under age 18 (Shi, 2013).

Child abuse and neglect have serious immediate and long-term consequences. Children who experience abuse or neglect are at high risk of mental health problems in adolescence and beyond (Mills et al., 2013). Prevention and early intervention are essential and can minimize the long-term consequences (Fallon et al., 2013).

Abuse and neglect occur all too frequently in spousal, partner, and dating relationships, as well as in relationships between children and adults (Greenlees, 2012). Difficulty with anger management is a core feature in these situations (Donohue, Tracy, & Gorney, 2009). Spousal abuse is strongly correlated with comorbid disorders, including impulse-control and personality disorders in the abuser (Dutton, 2007).

Life stressors, such as military deployment and return of a spouse, may contribute to the problem (Rabenhorst et al., 2012). Also, speculation exists that spousal abuse reflects a troubled dynamic between a dependent wife (Loas, Cormier, & Perez-Diaz, 2011) and a husband who struggles with expression of his own emotions (Borochowitz, 2008). It is important to keep in mind, of course, that wives may also be the abusers in the relationship. It is important to avoid a "blame the victim" mentality (Loas et al., 2011). Although it is the case that many abused adults struggle to leave the abusive relationship, this is rarely because they are willing to be abused. Rather, they may feel they have no options, may lack the self-confidence that would enable them to move forward independently, or may be fearful about the consequences of a departure. The latter is a serious concern, as a decision to leave can trigger a significant escalation of abuse.

As the proportion of older adults in the population has increased, and as awareness has grown, the dilemma of elder abuse has also grown (Naughton, Drennan, Lyons, & Lafferty, 2013). As is true for all forms of abuse, this is a problem worldwide, and it has significant personal and societal costs. Contributing factors are both personal and environmental (Mysyuk, Westendorp, & Lindenberg, 2013). For example, an older adult who has a cognitive impairment may be at high risk for financial abuse. Although a large proportion of abuse cases occur within families (Anetzberger, 2009), abuse can also occur in institutional settings (Castle & Beach, 2013).

Health care providers, including occupational therapists, must be alert to signs that suggest abuse (Figure 20-1). Health care providers are required to report suspected child abuse and neglect (Pietrantonio et al., 2013), as well as elder abuse and neglect (Anetzberger, 2009). It is not required or necessarily desirable that the reporting individual do an investigation to confirm the abuse. Ideally, this is the role of protective services, where trained social workers can undertake an evaluation of the situation and make sure that steps are taken to ameliorate the problem.

Educational and Occupational Problems

Educational and occupational problems are frequent consequences of mental disorders. For example, children with autism or attention-deficit/hyperactivity disorder (ADHD) may struggle in school, as was described in Chapter 3. Likewise, individuals with schizophrenia may struggle to maintain employment, as discussed in Chapter 4.

At the same time, educational and occupational problems can contribute to the occurrence of a mental disorder. The financial downturn of the early 21st century caused a significant increase in unemployment. Given that individuals who are involuntarily unemployed experience high rates of depression and anxiety (Howe, Hornberger, Weihs, Moreno, & Neiderhiser, 2012), it is reasonable to assume that there was an increase in anxiety and depression accompanying the increase in unemployment.

Figure 20-1. Therapists must be alert to signs of abuse and aware of their reporting responsibilities. (©2014 Shutterstock.com.)

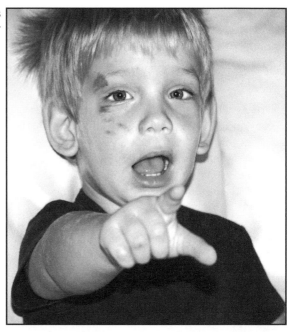

Figure 20-2. Individuals with mental disorders are more likely than others to be homeless. (©2014 Shutterstock.com.)

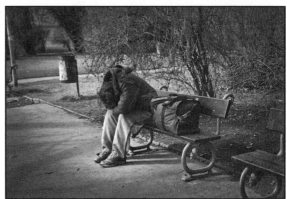

Housing and Economic Problems

Occupational problems are often associated with economic problems, including the potential for homelessness (Figure 20-2), and homelessness is strongly correlated with a variety of mental disorders (Strehlau, Torchall, Li, Schuetz, & Kraus, 2012). It can be difficult to know whether the mental disorder precedes the homelessness, whether homelessness contributes to mental disorders, or, as is most likely, some combination of the two.

Implications for Occupational Therapy

In this chapter, the ways in which circumstantial events are associated with mental disorders and distress are demonstrated. Difficulty with a variety of occupations and environmental stressors, such as homelessness and abuse, contribute to a variety of mental disorders and can be caused, in some measure, by those same disorders.

CASE STUDY

D'Andrea is a 16-year-old tenth grader who has been living with various friends for the past year. She is now 4 months pregnant (it is unclear who the father is) and recently has been unable to find any friends who will allow her to stay with them. Her mother and her mother's boyfriend live in another town. D'Andrea left home because the boyfriend attempted to abuse her sexually and her mother refused to believe there was a problem. Her father died several years ago, and her mother uses all of the social security funds intended for D'Andrea for herself. D'Andrea tried to get the check for herself by using a friend's address and asking to have the checks sent there. This failed when it was discovered by the mother, and the mother tried to force D'Andrea to return home, but she refused.

D'Andrea misses a great deal of school, in part because she is exhausted and has severe morning sickness as a result of her pregnancy. She also dislikes coming to school on days she has slept on the street because she feels she looks disheveled and dislikes being made fun of. She frequently goes without meals. At the moment, she is failing all of her courses. D'Andrea's mother has now called the school, insisting that they force her to withdraw and return home. D'Andrea is insistent she does not want to return to her mother. However, she has no place to live and is equally insistent that she does not want to enter foster care.

THOUGHT QUESTIONS

1. Does D'Andrea meet the definition of homeless? Why or why not?
2. What legal issues might be involved in this situation?
3. What resources might be helpful to D'Andrea?
4. Assuming that the various legal issues could be sorted out, what might occupational therapy have to contribute to this situation to improve D'Andrea's prospects?

When one considers the occupational performance correlates of mental disorders, the contributions of occupational therapy become evident. For example, children who have experienced abuse benefit from opportunities to express and examine the trauma, and to experience pleasurable and successful activities (Precin & Precin, 2011). Life skills training can improve performance and quality of life for individuals who are homeless (Helfrich, Peters, & Chan, 2011). Thus, while the psychiatrist and psychologist may focus on emotional symptoms and social workers focus on identifying social and economic resources, occupational therapy has a vital role to play in addressing the skills that contribute to successful and meaningful accomplishment of daily activities. Throughout this book you have seen these considerations addressed. Chapters 22 and 23 will consider in greater detail the occupational therapy assessment and intervention for individuals with mental disorders.

Resources

HelpGuide.org
http://www.helpguide.org/index.htm
A wide array of self-help resources focused on mental health issues. These include resources for domestic violence, housing, work, relationships, and specific mental disorders.

Homelessness Resource Guide
http://homeless.samhsa.gov/

Given the frequency with which homelessness is associated with substance abuse or other mental disorders, the Substance Abuse and Mental Health Services Administration maintains a website that addresses these issues. It includes resources appropriate for helping homeless individuals deal with their situations.

Mental Health America
http://www.nmha.org/go/about-us

An alliance of mental health professionals, clients, and family members focused on expanding programming for mental health promotion. Includes a long list of educational materials.

National Children's Alliance
http://www.nationalchildrensalliance.org/index.php?s=100

Resources for issues related to child abuse and neglect. The Alliance has resources for many other issues relevant to children, as well as funding opportunities.

References

American Psychiatric Association. (APA; 2013). *Diagnostic and statistical manual of mental disorders* (5th ed.). Washington, DC: Author.

Anetzberger, G. (2009). Elder abuse. In B. R. Bonder & V. dal Bello-Haas (Eds.), *Functional performance in older adults* (3rd ed., pp. 609-632). Philadelphia, PA: F.A. Davis.

Borochowitz, D.Y. (2008). The taming of the shrew: Batterers' constructions of their wives' narratives. *Violence Against Women, 14*(10), 1166-1180.

Castle, N., & Beach, S. (2013). Elder abuse in assisted living. *Journal of Applied Gerontology, 32*(2), 248-267.

Donohue, B., Tracy, K., & Gorney, S. (2009). Anger (negative impulse) control. In W.T. O'Donohue & J.E. Fisher (Eds.), *General principles and empirically supported techniques of cognitive behavior therapy* (pp. 115-123). Hoboken, NJ: John Wiley & Sons.

Dutton, D.G. (2007). *The abusive personality: Violence and control in intimate relations* (2nd ed.). New York, NY: Guilford.

Fallon, B., Ma, J., Allan, K., Pillhofer, M., Trocmé, N., & Jud, A. (2013). Opportunities for prevention and intervention with young children: Lessons from the Canadian incidence study of reported child abuse and neglect. *Child and Adolescent Psychiatry and Mental Health, 7*(1), 4-13.

Foster, E.R., Golden, L., Duncan, R.P., & Earhart, G.M. (2013). Community-based Argentine Tango dance program is associated with increased activity participation among individuals with Parkinson's disease. *Archives of Physical Medicine & Rehabilitation, 94*(2), 240-249.

Goldberg, J.F., & Ernst, C.L. (2012). *Managing the side effects of psychotropic medications.* Arlington, VA: American Psychiatric Publishing.

Greenlees, G.T. (2012). Drawing the necessary line: A review of dating domestic violence statutes around the United States. *Family Court Review, 50*(4), 679-692.

Helfrich, C.A., Peters, C.Y., & Chan, D.V. (2011). Trauma symptoms of individuals with mental illness at risk for homelessness participating in a life skills intervention. *Occupational Therapy International, 18*(3), 115-123.

Howe, G.W., Hornberger, A.P. Weihs, K., Moreno, F., & Neiderhiser, J.M. (2012). Higher-order structure in the trajectories of depression and anxiety following sudden involuntary unemployment. *Journal of Abnormal Psychology, 121*(2), 325-338.

Lech, B., Andersson, G., & Holmqvist, R. (2012). Affect consciousness and adult attachment. *Psychology, 3*(9), 675-680.

Lingiardi, V., & Nardelli, N. (2012). Partner relational problem: Listening beyond homo-ignorance and homo-prejudice. In P. Levounis, J. Drescher, & M.E. Barber (Eds.), *The LGBT casebook* (pp. 223-230). Arlington, VA: American Psychiatric Publishing.

Litt, B. (2010). From relational problems to psychological solutions: EMDR in couples therapy. In M. Luber (Ed.), *Eye movement desensitization and reprocessing (EMDR) scripted protocols: Special populations* (pp. 139-149). New York, NY: Springer.

Loas, G., Cormier, J., & Perez-Diaz, F. (2011). Dependent personality disorder and physical abuse. *Psychiatry Research, 185*(1-2), 167-170.

Mbagaya, C., Oburu, P., & Bakermans-Kranenburg, M.J. (2013). Child physical abuse and neglect in Kenya, Zambia and the Netherlands: A cross-cultural comparison of prevalence, psychopathological sequelae and mediation by PTSS. *International Journal of Psychology, 48*(2), 95-107.

Mihanović, M., Bodor, D., Kezić, S., Restek-Petrović, B., & Silić, A. (2009). Differential diagnosis of psychotropic side effects and symptoms and signs of psychiatric disorders. *Psychiatria Danubina, 21*(4), 570-574.

Mills, R., Scott, J., Alati, R., O'Callaghan, M., Najman, J.M., & Strathearn, L. (2013). Child maltreatment and adolescent mental health problems in a large birth cohort. *Child Abuse & Neglect, 37*(5), 292-302.

Mintz, T.M., Hamre, B.K., & Hatfield, B.E. (2011). The role of effortful control in mediating the association between maternal sensitivity and children's social and relational competence and problems in first grade. *Early Education and Development, 22*(3), 360-387.

Mysyuk, Y., Westendorp, R.G.J., & Lindenberg J. (2013). Framing abuse: Explaining the incidence, perpetuation, and intervention in elder abuse. *International Psychogeriatrics, Special Issue: Elder Abuse in an International Perspective, 25*(8), 1267-1274.

Naughton, C., Drennan, J., Lyons, I., & Lafferty, A. (2013). The relationship between older people's awareness of the term elder abuse and actual experiences of elder abuse. *International Psychogeriatrics, 25*(8), 1257-1266.

Pietrantonio, A.M., Wright, E., Gibson, K.N., Alldred, T., Jacobson, D., & Niec, A. (2013). Mandatory reporting of child abuse and neglect: Crafting a positive process for health professionals and caregivers. *Child Abuse & Neglect, 37*(2-3), 102-109.

Precin, P.J., & Precin, P. (2011). Occupation as therapy for trauma recovery: A case study. *Work, 38*(1), 77-81.

Rabenhorst, M.M., Thomsen, C.J., Milner, J.S., Foster, R.E., Linkh, D.J., & Copeland, C.W. (2012). Spouse abuse and combat-related deployments in active duty Air Force couples. *Psychology of Violence, 2*(3), 273-284.

Shi, L., (2013). Childhood abuse and neglect in an outpatient clinical sample: Prevalence and impact. *American Journal of Family Therapy, 41*(3), 198-211.

Steenwyk, S.A.M., Doeden, M.A., Furrow, J.L., & Atkins, D.C. (2012). Relational problems. In P. Sturmey & M. Hersen (Eds.), *Handbook of evidence-based practice in clinical psychology, Vol. 2: Adult disorders* (pp. 549-568). Hoboken, NJ: John Wiley & Sons.

Strehlau, V., Torchall, I., Li, K., Schuetz, C., & Kraus, M.J. (2012). Mental health, concurrent disorders, and health care utilization in homeless women. *Journal of Psychiatric Practice, 18*(5), 349-360.

Psychopharmacology

Chris Paxos, PharmD and Sara E. Dugan, PharmD

Learning Outcomes

By the end of this chapter, readers will be able to:
- Identify common medications and pharmacologic classes used to treat psychiatric disorders
- Identify which pharmacologic classes are used most frequently to treat regularly encountered psychiatric disorders
- Describe the mechanism of action of common medications and pharmacologic classes
- List recommended monitoring parameters for each pharmacologic class
- Discuss individual factors, such as pharmacokinetics, pharmacodynamics, and pharmacogenomics, that may alter a client's response to therapy (compared with both other clients and clients as they age)
- Describe the role that occupational therapists and certified occupational therapy assistants can play in optimizing client outcomes related to the use of psychiatric medications

Bonder B.
Psychopathology and Function, Fifth Edition (pp 413-455).
© 2015 SLACK Incorporated.

KEY WORDS

- Agranulocytosis
- Neurons
- Dendrites
- Soma
- Axon
- Agonists
- Antagonists
- Pharmacodynamics
- Pharmacokinetics
- Pharmacogenetics
- Pharmacogenomics
- First-generation antipsychotics
- Second-generation antipsychotics

- Extrapyramidal symptoms
- Neuroleptics
- Acute dystonic reaction
- Pseudoparkinsonism
- Akathisia
- Tardive dyskinesia
- Neuroleptic malignant syndrome
- Hyponatremia
- Enantiomers
- Serotonin syndrome
- Controlled substances
- Pro-drug

History of Psychopharmacology

The use of psychoactive substances can be traced back over a millennium. Hallucinogens, opiates, cocaine, and cannabis were used in parts of the world as diverse as Greece, Egypt, China, and South America. The multiform uses of psychoactive substances in these cultures ranged from religious and ceremonial to medicinal and recreational. Modern psychopharmacology for the treatment of mental illnesses is a relatively young medical field, sparked by a number of serendipitous findings (Moriarty, Alagna, & Lake, 1984).

The 1950s ignited the psychopharmacology revolution with a number of important discoveries, including antipsychotic, antidepressant, and benzodiazepine medications. A French surgeon noted the calming effects of chlorpromazine and suggested its use to his colleagues in psychiatry. By 1954, chlorpromazine was approved in the United States as the first antipsychotic medication for the treatment of schizophrenia. It played a pivotal role in the deinstitutionalization of a large number of clients from the nation's state psychiatric hospitals (Moriarty et al., 1984).

The 1950s also delivered the first antidepressant medications, monoamine oxidase inhibitors (MAOIs) and tricyclic antidepressants (TCAs). An MAOI was found to possess mood elevating properties while used for the treatment of tuberculosis. Similarly, the antidepressant properties of the first TCA, imipramine, were discovered by chance in clients with schizophrenia (Krishnan, 2006). Chlordiazepoxide, the first commercially available benzodiazepine, an anxiolytic (antianxiety medication), was synthesized in the 1950s and approved for use in 1960, marking the end of a decade with significant achievements in the field of psychopharmacology (López-Muñoz, Álamo, & García-García, 2011).

Psychopharmacology is still evolving, as the advances of the 1980s continue to shape and influence the field today. Fluoxetine, the first selective serotonin reuptake inhibitor (SSRI), was released in 1987. With improved tolerability and decreased lethality in the case of overdose compared with TCAs, fluoxetine spurred the development of an entirely new generation of antidepressants that current manufacturers continue to attempt to improve (Prozac, 2013). Clozapine was first synthesized in the 1950s; however, it was not released in the United States due to concerns of **agranulocytosis** (a dangerously low white blood cell count that affects the body's ability to fight infection) and death reported with its use in Europe. Renewed interest in its use and strict monitoring parameters eventually led to its release in the United States in 1989. Clozapine was touted as a second-generation antipsychotic (SGA), and it was found to be more effective than other currently available antipsychotics. Interest in creating other SGAs quickly developed and persists to the present day. Although newer SGAs have successfully lessened much of the agranulocytosis risk, developing an antipsychotic medication that matches the superior efficacy of clozapine has remained elusive (Marder & Wirshing, 2006).

Role of Medications in Mental Illness

With all of the new psychopharmacologic drug discoveries over the past 50 years, it seems reasonable to consider why all these medications are necessary. Approximately 25% of adults in the United States report having a mental illness (Reeves et al., 2011). Data from the 2012 National Health Interview survey show that approximately 5.3% of children aged 4 to 17 years have emotional and behavioral difficulties, according to their parents.

Pediatric-focused settings typically include a large number of clients on psychostimulants and related medications for the treatment of attention-deficit/hyperactivity disorder (ADHD), along with antidepressants and anxiolytics for treating depression and anxiety, respectively. Antipsychotic medications are seen less commonly and most often in the context of children with autism who are taking them to treat irritability and aggression.

Environments with an adult population will likely include a mix of most types of psychotropic medications. Depression and anxiety disorders continue to be frequently encountered (Reeves et al., 2011). Sedative-hypnotic medications are used to treat sleep disturbances, which often plague adults. Bipolar disorder and schizophrenia often develop in young adulthood, requiring the use of mood stabilizers or antipsychotics.

Many mental disorders are chronic conditions that can remain problematic and can come and go throughout the client's life, meaning usage of all the medication classes mentioned may be continued into the later years of life. In addition, dementia becomes more prevalent as clients age; therefore, dementia medications will be used most commonly in this client group.

As demonstrated, there are large numbers of individuals experiencing mental disorders, so very few practice settings exists where you will not encounter medications. Acutely, the goals of treatment are to alleviate the symptoms or behaviors that interfere with the client's life, such as depression, sleep disturbance, hallucinations, inattention, or other symptoms. Long-term goals for medication use are to maintain the improvement in symptoms that help the client to move toward recovery and optimal functioning. Unfortunately, both the mental disorders and the medications used to treat them can impact how well the client is able to participate in activities of daily life. By having a solid understanding of why medications are being used and what to monitor for (adverse effects and toxicity), occupational therapists and certified occupational therapist assistants (COTAs) can contribute to the overall evaluation of the client status, ultimately moving clients toward the achievement of optimal outcomes (recovery) and their highest level of functioning. In the sections that follow, a review will include how medications work (both in improving symptoms and in causing adverse effects) and what needs to be monitored when clients receive these medications.

Drug Development Process

In the late 1950s, thalidomide was utilized in countries outside of the United States for the treatment of morning sickness in pregnancy. Unfortunately, it was soon discovered

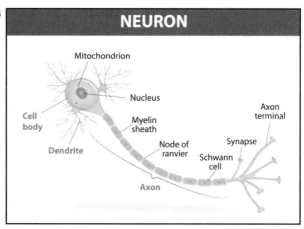

Figure 21-1. Neuron. (©2014 Shutterstock.com.)

NEURON

Mitochondrion

Nucleus

Cell body

Myelin sheath

Axon terminal

Dendrite

Node of ranvier

Schwann cell

Synapse

Axon

that thalidomide was associated with thousands of birth defects in children whose mothers had taken the medication while pregnant. In response to the thalidomide tragedy, the U.S. Congress passed the Kefauver-Harris Amendment in 1962, which granted the U.S. Food and Drug Administration (FDA) the authority to monitor the safety and efficacy of medications (Cowan, 2002). A new drug can take many years and billions of dollars to develop and involves multiple stages of study to ensure safety and efficacy. Unanticipated adverse effects that are not discovered during clinical trials may become apparent following approval; therefore, postmarketing surveillance is used to continue tracking the safety of commercially available products (Katzung, 2012).

Neurotransmission

As demonstrated in previous chapters, many mental disorders are thought to be a result of a change or alteration in brain functioning due to changes in the way the brain interprets the signals that are sent to it or in how the brain responds to these signals.

The brain is composed of millions of cells called **neurons**, which use sophisticated electrical and chemical signals to "talk" to each other to enable body functions (Sadock & Sadock, 2007a). Each nerve cell has different areas that help it to receive information, process that information, and send messages or responses to the information it has received. These areas are called the **dendrites**, the **soma**, and the **axon** (Figure 21-1). Neurons may have a number of dendrites, which are projections or branches of the cell that reach out to receive signals from other neurons (Sadock & Sadock, 2007a). Dendrites transmit the information they have received to the soma, or cell body, which contains the nucleus of the neuron that regulates the functions of the neuron. The soma then processes the signals received and directs a neuronal response (Sadock & Sadock, 2007a). The neuronal response may require activity in the axon—an extension of the neuron that can connect to a number of other neurons—and this activity sends messages or signals to other neurons (Sadock & Sadock, 2007a).

The connections between neurons occur between the dendrites of one neuron and what is called the axon terminal of another neuron. Axon terminals contain enzymes that can make or break down chemicals called neurotransmitters (Sadock & Sadock, 2007a). Neurotransmitters are the chemicals that are released into the synapse, the small space between the neurons, when a neuron fires or is activated to transmit a message to other neurons (Sadock & Sadock, 2007a; Figure 21-2). After the neurotransmitters have sent the message to the postsynaptic

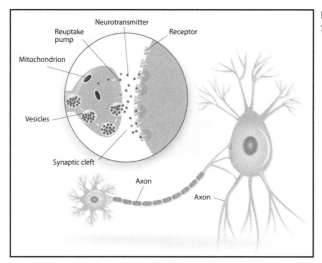

Figure 21-2. Synapse. (©2014 Shutterstock.com.)

receptors, they need to be cleared out of the synapse so that the system can be reset in preparation for the next communication. This is accomplished by a couple of different mechanisms. Either the neurotransmitters are broken down by enzymes that are in the synapse itself, or the neurotransmitters are pumped back into the presynaptic neuron—the one they were released from—and either broken down by an enzyme or repackaged in preparation for the next message (Sadock & Sadock, 2007a; Stahl, 2013).

Neurotransmitters play a vital role in the function of the brain and, as you might imagine, there are many different neurotransmitters. Neurotransmitters with particular importance in causing or preventing symptoms of mental disorders include acetylcholine (ACh), dopamine (DA), γ-aminobutyric acid (GABA), glutamate, norepinephrine (NE), and 5-hydroxytryptamine or serotonin (5HT) (Stahl, 2013). All of these neurotransmitters are involved in various bodily functions relevant to symptoms of mental disorders.

Each neurotransmitter may have a number of different receptors that it stimulates. For example, DA activates at least five receptors, called D_1, D_2, D_3, D_4, and D_5. Each of the receptors may work just a little differently. The placement of the receptors may also be important, as the exact same receptor may have different actions, depending on whether it is on a presynaptic or a postsynaptic neuron. Finally, medications that work on receptors are often called **agonists**, partial agonists, or **antagonists**. Agonists are medications that combine with a receptor and can cause the same effects that a neurotransmitter would cause; partial agonists are medications that combine with a receptor and cause the same effects as a neurotransmitter but to a smaller degree. Antagonists are the last group; these medications block the receptor and prevent a neurotransmitter from causing its intended effect.

Pharmacodynamics, Pharmacokinetics, and Pharmacogenomics

When an individual takes a medication, two considerations exist. First, what does the medication do to the body? This effect is referred to as **pharmacodynamics**. Second, what does the body do to the medication? This effect is referred to as **pharmacokinetics**. For example, you are having trouble sleeping, and you want to take a medication that will help you to fall asleep. Your expectation is that the medication will be effective and cause you to fall asleep. This is the pharmacodynamic action of the medication. The pharmacokinetics, or what your body does to the medication, can be divided into the following four sections: absorption (A), distribution (D), metabolism (M), and elimination (E). For the first two sections, your body dissolves a tablet and absorbs it, moving the medication from your stomach into your blood stream (A); in the blood stream, the medication is distributed to all parts of your body, including your brain where it needs to be to work (D). The way some of these body systems work will change over a client's lifespan. An infant is often able to absorb medications from a patch or cream more readily than an adult. Older adults often have declining kidney function. All of these factors need to be taken into account when thinking about the best medication–client match. This also means that clients who have been taking a medication with no problem may start having adverse effects or develop a tolerance and receive little effect from a previously effective medication; thus, it is important to monitor clients for any changes so modifications can be made as their needs alter.

As one tries to predict how a client will respond to medications, he or she will need to consider the roles that age and genes play in this process. Two terms are often referred to when evaluating an individual's genetic make-up and its impact on response to medications: pharmacogenetics and pharmacogenomics. Although these two terms are related, they are not interchangeable. **Pharmacogenetics** involves the study of variations in an *individual* gene and that particular gene's impact in the response to medication (Cavallari & Lam, 2011). **Pharmacogenomics** involves the study of a number of genes and their impact on the response to medication (Cavallari & Lam, 2011). Initial pharmacogenetic studies often focused on one aspect of medication treatment, such as metabolism or elimination, to determine whether genetic differences were noted in how clients metabolized and eliminated certain medications (Liou, Stringer, & Hirayama, 2012). As a result, a number of polymorphisms, or different genetic variations, have been identified that help determine how well a client can metabolize or eliminate a medication, ultimately encouraging the use of higher or lower doses of particular medications to compensate for this (Liou et al., 2012).

Although occupational therapists do not prescribe medications, they have a key role in providing the education and monitoring to help clients understand and achieve optimal treatment outcomes. With this in mind, the remainder of the chapter will provide a clearer understanding of how the medications work, what adverse effects are commonly experienced, and any screening or monitoring that is recommended for these medications.

Antipsychotics

The underlying causes of schizophrenia have yet to be elucidated; however, it is likely that multiple etiologies are responsible for producing the varying clinical presentations of the disorder (Crismon, Argo, & Buckley, 2008; Freedman, 2003). The DA hypothesis of schizophrenia suggests that alterations in DA neurotransmission are responsible for the signs and symptoms of schizophrenia. Hyperdopaminergia, or excessive DA neurotransmission, is thought to cause the positive symptoms of schizophrenia, such as hallucinations and delusions. Hypodopaminergia, or deficient DA neurotransmission, may be responsible for the negative symptoms of schizophrenia. Therefore, medications that correct these dopamine abnormalities, such as antipsychotics, can treat the symptoms of schizophrenia. Antipsychotics are categorized as either **first-generation antipsychotics** (FGAs) or **second-generation antipsychotics** (SGAs) (Crismon et al., 2008; Stahl, 2013).

FGAs are commonly referred to as typical, classical, conventional, or traditional. They are potent antagonists of the dopamine-2 (D_2) receptor. When antipsychotics block D_2 receptors, they alleviate the positive symptoms of schizophrenia. Prominent hallucinations and delusions may lessen or completely resolve over time. Unfortunately, potent DA receptor blockade in other areas of the brain produces adverse neurological effects, including a number of movement disorders termed **extrapyramidal symptoms** (EPS) (Kane & Correll, 2010).

Second generation antipsychotics, also referred to as atypical antipsychotics, assert their therapeutic effects in the treatment of schizophrenia through a combination of DA and 5HT receptor antagonism. While no SGAs share the exact same pharmacology, all are thought to block the D_2 and 5HT-2A ($5HT_{2A}$) receptors (Lexi-Comp, 2013). This combination of receptor blocking provides SGAs with several advantages over FGAs, including significantly less EPS, as well as possibly greater efficacy in treating the negative and cognitive symptoms of schizophrenia (Stahl, 2013). Nevertheless, only one antipsychotic, clozapine, has demonstrated superior efficacy over all others. Unfortunately, clozapine also causes agranulocytosis. Other antipsychotic medications are less likely to cause agranulocytosis, but are also less effective in relieving symptoms of psychosis (Crismon et al., 2008; Freedman, 2003; TEVA Pharmaceuticals, 2011a).

Antipsychotics are available in diverse dosage formulations. All agents are available as oral formulations, such as tablets, capsules, or oral solutions. Asenapine is unique in that it is available as a sublingual tablet. Four SGAs are available as orally dissolving tablets. This form of the medication is beneficial in clients who have difficulty swallowing. In addition, orally dissolving tablets may be appropriate to confirm ingestion of the medication in settings with supervised medication administration. Long-acting injectable medications, administered every 2 or 4 weeks, depending on the agent, are available for nonadherent clients or for clients preferring injections versus daily medication administration (Kane & Garcia-Ribera, 2009; Lexi-Comp, 2013).

Contraindications vary among individual agents. In general, all antipsychotics are contraindicated in clients who have experienced a hypersensitivity reaction to that particular agent. Haloperidol, due to its high risk of EPS, is contraindicated in Parkinson's disease. Unfortunately, adverse effects are common with antipsychotic therapy. Many FGAs and SGAs cause the following to varying degrees: sedation, orthostatic hypotension, and anticholinergic effects. Both sedation and orthostatic hypotension increase the risk of falls, especially in the older adult population. Anticholinergic effects include dry mouth, blurred vision, constipation, urinary retention, and memory impairment. Older adult clients are particularly susceptible to confusion caused by anticholinergic effects; thus, the medications that cause these effects should be avoided in clients with dementia (Crismon et al., 2008; Muench & Hamer, 2010). Table 21-1 shows the adverse effects associated with receptor antagonism.

EPS, caused by DA receptor blockade in the central nervous system (CNS), earned antipsychotics the moniker "**neuroleptics**" (to seize the nerve). FGAs are significantly more likely to produce EPS than SGAs. Early-onset EPS includes dystonia, pseudoparkinsonism, and akathisia. An **acute dystonic reaction** is a contraction of muscle groups, usually of the head or neck. Acute dystonia generally appears within hours to days of initiating an antipsychotic or dosage increases. **Pseudoparkinsonism** resembles idiopathic Parkinson's disease, with symptoms of tremor, mask-like facies, cogwheel rigidity, and festinating gait. **Akathisia**, an inner sensation of restlessness or inability to sit still, may present as pacing, shuffling back and forth, or tapping of the feet. Finally, **tardive dyskinesia**, a form of late-onset EPS, typically occurs with months to years of antipsychotic exposure. It manifests as rhythmic, involuntary movements of the tongue, face, mouth, or jaw. Early signs may be reversible; however, continued treatment may result in irreversible symptoms, despite antipsychotic discontinuation. All clients receiving extended antipsychotic therapy should be periodically screened for tardive dyskinesia. To minimize the risk of any of these adverse effects, clients should receive the lowest feasible dose for the shortest amount of time possible (Caroff, Miller, Dhopesh, & Campbell, 2011). Table 21-2 summarizes the considerations associated with EPS.

TABLE 21-1	
RECEPTORS AND RECEPTOR ANTAGONISM	
RECEPTOR	*ADVERSE EFFECTS INDUCED BY RECEPTOR ANTAGONISM*
Histamine-1	Sedation Weight gain
Muscarinic (various Subtypes)	Anticholinergic effects, which include the following: • Dry mouth • Blurred vision • Constipation • Urinary retention • Memory impairment
Alpha-1	Orthostatic hypotension

Although EPS has traditionally been the primary concern of long-term antipsychotic therapy, antipsychotic drugs can also lead to weight gain, high cholesterol, and glucose intolerance or diabetes mellitus. Current guidelines recommend that all clients should be monitored throughout therapy for changes in personal and family medical history, weight and body mass index, waist circumference, blood pressure, fasting plasma glucose, and fasting plasma lipids (American Diabetes Association, 2004).

In addition to the substantial risks of inducing EPS and diabetes mellitus, antipsychotic medications are responsible for a host of miscellaneous adverse effects as well, including **neuroleptic malignant syndrome**. Neuroleptic malignant syndrome is a rare, potentially life-threatening, syndrome causing altered mental status, hyperthermia, muscle rigidity, autonomic dysfunction (Gillman, 2010). Other miscellaneous adverse effects include seizures (Crismon et al., 2008), cardiac irregularities, sudden death (Doyle & Rosenthal, 2013), and sexual dysfunction (Henderson & Doraiswamy, 2008).

Overall, clients should be educated about the adverse effects of medication, as most can be managed. For example, sedation is common with many antipsychotic medications, but it tends to decrease over time due to the development of tolerance to the sedating effects. Occasional constipation may be managed by increasing fluid intake, exercise, and fiber. Strategies for dry mouth include increasing water intake, using over-the-counter remedies, or sucking on sugarless candy. Clients should also be educated about the more serious adverse effects that should be reported immediately. Counsel the client to report rashes, blurred vision, and movement disorders. These adverse effects, among many others, may necessitate a dose reduction, change in the antipsychotic medication, or use of additional medications (Muench & Hamer, 2010).

Despite the potential benefits, antipsychotic medication use requires a great deal of monitoring to ensure proper and safe use. It is important for therapists to be aware that it may take upwards of 6 to 8 weeks to achieve near-maximal response at a given dose and to assess for the presence of positive and negative symptoms. As the client's condition improves, he or she may experience less prominent hallucinations or delusions, decreased suspiciousness, increased interest in activities and hobbies, or improvement in hygiene or self-care. In addition to target symptom management, medication effectiveness should be gauged by the client's functional status, making the occupational therapy evaluation an important contribution to medication management. Routine monitoring is also essential for the early detection

TABLE 21-2			
EXTRAPYRAMIDAL SYMPTOMS			
	TIME OF ONSET	*CLINICAL PRESENTATION*	*MANAGEMENT STRATEGIES*
Early-Onset EPS			
Acute dystonia	Hours to days	Prolonged contraction of muscle groups, usually of the head or neck Potential swallowing or breathing difficulties	Parenteral anticholinergics, such as benztropine (Cogentin) and diphenhydramine (Benadryl)
Akathisia	Weeks to months	Motor restlessness, such as pacing and inability to sit still	Antipsychotic dose reduction Switch to an antipsychotic with lower EPS liability Beta-blockers, such as propranolol (Inderal)
Pseudoparkinsonism	Weeks to months	Mask-like facies, tremor, pill rolling hand motion, cogwheel rigidity, and shuffling gait	Antipsychotic dose reduction Switch to an antipsychotic with lower EPS liability Oral anticholinergics, such as benztropine (Cogentin), trihexyphenidyl (Artane), and diphenhydramine (Benadryl) Amantadine (Symmetrel)
Late-Onset EPS			
Tardive dyskinesia	Months to years	Rhythmic, involuntary movements of the tongue, face, mouth, or jaw (e.g., protrusion of tongue, puckering of mouth, chewing movements)	Prevention is critical Consider antipsychotic discontinuation Consider switching from a first-generation antipsychotic to a second-generation antipsychotic (e.g., quetiapine or clozapine), if applicable

CLINICAL PEARL: ANTIPSYCHOTICS AND THE HEART

Antipsychotics have the potential to cause abnormal electrocardiographic changes, including the widening of the QT interval. Clients complaining of symptoms of dizziness, syncope, or palpitations should receive an immediate electrocardiogram (Doyle & Rosenthal, 2013). The occupational therapist should promptly report these symptoms to the physician.

CLINICAL PEARL: ANTIPSYCHOTICS AND TARDIVE DYSKINESIA

Tardive dyskinesia (TD) is a late-onset form of extrapyramidal symptoms that may occur months to years after antipsychotic therapy. TD is potentially irreversible and may persist even after antipsychotic discontinuation, meaning that TD prevention is of the utmost importance. Clinicians should monitor for TD using the Abnormal Involuntary Movement Scale (AIMS). Frequency of AIMS assessments may vary, depending on client risk factors (Caroff et al., 2011).

of adverse effects. Clients receiving any antipsychotic medication, particularly the FGAs, should be monitored for the development of EPS (Crismon et al., 2008). Overall, the ideal agent blends tolerability with a robust therapeutic response (American Psychiatric Association [APA], 2004; Freedman, 2003; Lexi-Comp, 2013). The Clinical Pearls boxes describe specific clinical considerations with use of antipsychotic medications. The Case Vignette box is focused on the role of occupational therapy in supporting medication management in a client with schizophrenia.

Mood Stabilizers

Mood stabilizers are a diverse class of medications that work in a number of different ways. Many of the medication classes covered in this chapter contain medications that are different but generally work in the same way, which is analogous to different varieties of apples—Red Delicious, Granny Smith, Rome, and Ida Red—they are slightly different but all are apples. The mood stabilizer class is more like a fruit salad with bananas, apples, oranges, and grapes—they are all fruit but each is unique.

The family of medications called mood stabilizers is so named because these agents are designed to keep a client's mood "stable," very literally preventing the extreme manic events and the extreme low depressed episodes. Note, this does not mean that a client's mood will not change—good days and bad days are natural—but these medications help prevent the extremes in both directions. Clients who use these medications are most often diagnosed with schizoaffective disorder or bipolar disorder. Antipsychotic medications are also used to treat these conditions and are technically mood stabilizing medications. They have been described in the previous section. The medications typically included in the class of mood stabilizers are lithium, valproic acid derivatives, carbamazepine, oxcarbazepine, and lamotrigine. Aside from lithium, the remainder of these medications are also used to treat seizure disorders or epilepsy, in addition to other indications, such as preventing migraines (valproic acid derivatives) and treating trigeminal neuralgia (carbamazepine and oxcarbazepine).

CASE VIGNETTE: ANTIPSYCHOTICS

John, a 28-year-old, White man, was diagnosed with schizophrenia 10 years ago. He has tried multiple antipsychotics medications, many with good response, but he is consistently medication nonadherent. Quetiapine and asenapine have both provided remission of his psychotic symptoms in the past; however, the client discontinues medications when his symptoms subside. At his current appointment, John appears to be in distress as a result of the return of psychotic symptoms. The psychiatrist recommends initiating a long-acting intramuscular antipsychotic. John agrees with the psychiatrist's recommendation.

THOUGHT QUESTIONS

1. Why might John be a good candidate for antipsychotic therapy via long-acting intramuscular injection?
2. Prior to prescribing a long-acting intramuscular injection, what must the psychiatrist consider?
3. What might be the occupational therapist's role in helping John manage his situation?

As discussed in Chapter 5, the most current thinking is that the bipolar disorders are along a spectrum between schizophrenia and depressive disorders. It is not entirely known what causes bipolar disorder, but it is thought that some of the neurons in the brain are functioning abnormally. In very general terms, the mood stabilizers tend to decrease neuronal firing; thus, the neurons are not sending out as many signals to other areas of the brain that result in mood symptoms. Lithium has been used since the mid-1900s and is considered one of the most effective long-term medications for bipolar disorder (Drayton, 2011). It has been shown to assist in controlling the symptoms of mania and depression, delay the recurrence of these symptoms, and be protective of neurons thought to be involved in causing the symptoms of bipolar disorder (Drayton, 2011; McKnight et al., 2012). The full effects of lithium are not usually seen with the first dose but develop over time, which is why it is often used in combination with other medications, including antipsychotics, to treat acutely manic clients (Drayton, 2011; McKnight et al., 2012). The exact mechanism of action of lithium is not known. Lithium also seems to reduce the risk of suicide (Malhi, Tanious, Das, Coulston, & Berk, 2013; Meyer, 2011).

Lithium has a significant number of adverse effects, with reports indicating that one-third to more than 90% of clients taking lithium experience some of these effects (Drayton, 2011). Initially, lithium therapy may cause nausea, vomiting, diarrhea, muscle weakness, and lethargy. These adverse effects often subside as the client becomes accustomed to the medication (Drayton, 2011; Roxane Laboratories, Inc., 2012b). Headache, confusion, memory problems, trouble concentrating, or trouble with motor functions, including tremor, are adverse effects that can affect the client's functional abilities (Drayton, 2011; Roxane Laboratories, Inc., 2012b).

Long-term use of lithium may be associated with kidney damage in some clients; however, this risk appears to be attenuated by staying hydrated, using lower doses, and avoiding toxicity (Drayton, 2011). Drying or thinning of the hair, skin conditions, weight gain, heart arrhythmias, and hypothyroidism have also been reported with lithium use (Roxane Laboratories, Inc., 2012b). Skin conditions such as acne or rashes, diminished sexual functioning, and neurological effects, such as slurred speech, lack of coordination, and extrapyramidal movements have also been reported with chronic lithium use (Drayton, 2011; Roxane Laboratories, Inc., 2012b).

Lithium is quickly absorbed when taken orally, and it is filtered by the kidneys for elimination in the urine (Drayton, 2011). Due to the close proximity of the effective and the toxic blood concentrations, it is important to closely monitor lithium levels, especially in older clients whose kidneys may not be as efficient at eliminating the drug (Drayton, 2011). Lithium toxicity may initially cause coarse tremor, impairment in coordination or gait, vomiting, diarrhea, drowsiness, or confusion (Drayton, 2011; Roxane Laboratories, Inc., 2012b). Higher lithium levels may present with seizures, cardiac arrhythmias, lack of coordination, altered mental status, and kidney damage (Drayton, 2011; Roxane Laboratories, Inc., 2012b). Clients with suspected lithium toxicity need to seek medical care. Therapists should be alert to these symptoms and report them promptly.

Drug interactions are problematic with lithium. Medicines used to treat blood pressure, including diuretics, all have some impact on the kidneys and reducing the amount of lithium that is eliminated, thus increasing lithium levels (Roxane Laboratories, Inc., 2012b). Nonsteroidal anti-inflammatory drugs, such as aspirin or ibuprofen that can be obtained with or without a prescription, can also cause the body to retain sodium, lithium, and water, resulting in higher lithium levels and possible toxicity (Roxane Laboratories, Inc., 2012b). Caffeine can result in a greater elimination of lithium and lower blood levels (Drayton, 2011). This does not mean clients cannot have a cup of coffee in the morning, but it is important that they stay well hydrated and do not dramatically change the amount of caffeine they are eating or drinking.

Monitoring clients on lithium includes tracking the symptoms of bipolar disorder and the adverse effects mentioned above. New-onset diarrhea, vomiting, the exacerbation of tremor, and mental status changes, such as sedation, confusion, or dizziness, may suggest lithium levels are too high and should be investigated (Drayton, 2011; Roxane Laboratories, Inc., 2012b). Blood work, including, on occasion, complete blood counts, and electrocardiogram monitoring may be required (Drayton, 2011).

Next in the mood stabilizers are the valproic acid derivatives. The exact mechanism of valproic acid is not completely understood. It has been observed that valproic acid alters electrolyte channels, specifically sodium and calcium channels on neuronal cells (McNamara, 2011). Sodium and, to a lesser extent, calcium channels are involved in creating action potentials, which is the electrical communication within a nerve cell (Barrett, Boitano, Barman, Brooks, 2012). Use of valproic acid derivatives may provide neuroprotection and possibly neurogenesis, or the development of new neurons, in some brain areas (Atmaca, 2009).

Valproic acid is a first-line option for acute manic or mixed episodes and for maintenance therapy to prevent new mood episodes, and it is a second-line option for bipolar depression (Connolly & Thase, 2011). Outside of bipolar disorder, valproic acid products are also used for the treatment of epilepsy and the prevention of migraines (AbbVie, Inc., 2013). A significant risk of birth defects exists, specifically neural tube defects; therefore, valproic acid products should not be used by women who are pregnant or may become pregnant (AbbVie, Inc., 2013).

Clients may experience loss of appetite, nausea, vomiting, or diarrhea, but these will abate and can be minimized if the medication is taken with food or if the extended-release tablet is used (AbbVie, Inc., 2013; Drayton, 2011). Sedation, dizziness, headache, weakness, and tremor are also common, and these may interfere with daily activities or increase the risk of falls. Weight gain, which is common with valproic acid, is experienced by up to half of clients, making this an important piece of information to share with clients, and it should be monitored throughout therapy (AbbVie, Inc., 2013; Drayton, 2011). Some potentially serious adverse effects exist, including hyperammonemia (elevated ammonia levels), which may cause disorientation and loss of coordination; decreased platelets, which may increase the risk of bleeding; liver toxicity; and pancreatitis (AbbVie, Inc., 2013; Drayton, 2011). Similar to other medications that are used for seizure disorders, valproic acid products may increase the risk of suicidal thoughts or behavior; clients and family members should be encouraged to report any worsening of depression, suicidal thoughts or behavior, or unusual changes in behavior or mood (AbbVie, Inc., 2013). Monitoring clients taking valproic acid products includes watching for improvement in symptoms and the development of any adverse effects.

Lamotrigine has developed a bit of a different role in that it is used for maintenance treatment of clients with bipolar disorder, as well as for those with depressive symptoms (GlaxoSmithKline, 2011; Stahl, 2013). The exact mechanism of action for lamotrigine is not known (GlaxoSmithKline, 2011; McNamara, 2011). Theories of how lamotrigine works includes that it may inhibit sodium channels, which would then keep sodium from entering the neuron, preventing depolarization, and stabilizing the neuron (GlaxoSmithKline, 2011; McNamara, 2011). Lamotrigine is also associated with actions on the presynaptic release of excitatory amino acids glutamate and aspartate, which are thought to cause other neurons to fire (GlaxoSmithKline, 2011; McNamara, 2011). It is thought that reducing neuronal firing and decreasing the excitatory neurotransmission may establish equilibrium in the brain and alleviate any mood symptoms.

When clients begin lamotrigine therapy, they are prescribed low doses, and then the doses are slowly titrated up to effective levels to help with their moods. This is done to reduce the risk of the client developing a potentially fatal condition called Stevens Johnson syndrome, which often starts with a rash and can progress to multiorgan system failure (GlaxoSmithKline, 2011; McNamara, 2011). Other rare, but serious, concerns with lamotrigine include increase in suicidal thoughts or behaviors and the development of aseptic meningitis, or inflammation of the brain and spinal cord, which may cause clients to be confused, report headache and neck pain, or experience nausea, vomiting, or sedation (GlaxoSmithKline, 2011).

Other less severe and more common adverse effects that clients may experience include dizziness, sedation, double vision, and the loss of coordination (GlaxoSmithKline, 2011). Each of these side effects may be a concern if the client is having difficulty walking or is on other medications that also may cause some of these effects, as the combination of symptoms contributes to increased risk of falls. Nausea and headache are also common but lessen as the client becomes more accustomed to the medication (GlaxoSmithKline, 2011; McNamara, 2011).

Monitoring parameters for clients on lamotrigine include looking for a rash when the medication is initiated to prevent the development of potentially fatal dermatologic conditions (GlaxoSmithKline, 2011). Symptom improvement should occur in the first few months of treatment, not within the first few doses (GlaxoSmithKline, 2011; McNamara, 2011).

Carbamazepine is considered a second-line treatment option for manic and mixed episodes of bipolar disorder, as it is less effective than lithium or valproate (Connolly & Thase, 2011; Drayton, 2011). Although carbamazepine is used in clients with bipolar depression and for maintenance treatment of bipolar disorder, its efficacy in these areas is not well documented (Drayton, 2011). Carbamazepine is approved for the treatment of epilepsy and nerve pain or pain associated with trigeminal neuralgia (Taro Pharmaceuticals U.S.A., Inc., 2013). The exact mechanism of action is not known, but it is thought to have an effect on neuronal sodium channels (Taro Pharmaceuticals U.S.A., Inc., 2013; McNamara, 2011).

Carbamazepine is one medication that may require clients to have genetic testing performed prior to starting therapy. Clients of Asian ancestry have been found to have up to a 10-time higher likelihood of developing Stevens Johnson syndrome or toxic epidermal necrolysis, which are potentially fatal skin conditions if they have the HLA-B*1502 gene. These potentially fatal conditions may occur in other ethnic populations as well. Any new rash when starting carbamazepine should be immediately reported to the physician (Taro Pharmaceuticals U.S.A., Inc., 2013).

Other serious adverse effects associated with carbamazepine include the development of a hypersensitivity reaction, significantly decreased red and white blood cells, and possible increase in suicidal behavior or thoughts (Taro Pharmaceuticals U.S.A., Inc., 2013). Dizziness, drowsiness, and unsteadiness are common (Taro Pharmaceuticals U.S.A., Inc., 2013). These effects should resolve as the client becomes accustomed to the medication. Clients should not abruptly stop taking carbamazepine, as this could cause health problems, including seizures, even if the client does not have a seizure disorder.

Carbamazepine increases the activity of liver enzymes, which results in a number of drug interactions and can affect liver function. The full effect on liver enzymes is usually seen after the client has been on the medication for 1 month (McNamara, 2011).

Carbamazepine is a complicated medication; therefore, it is not surprising that a significant amount of monitoring is needed. Monitoring the client for adverse effects, especially those affecting the brain, such as drowsiness, dizziness, confusion, blurred vision, and unsteadiness, can help identify those clients who are receiving too much medication. Individuals who have used carbamazepine long term have been reported to have lower vitamin D levels, which may make them more likely to develop osteoporosis and potential bone fracture if they were to fall.

Oxcarbazepine is related to carbamazepine, and it has been used in clients who have not responded to treatment with other mood stabilizers. This drug is FDA approved for the treatment of seizures and not for bipolar disorder. However, as noted, it is sometimes used in bipolar disorder when other medications have failed (Connolly & Thase, 2011). The exact mechanism of the action is unknown, but it, too, is thought to bind to sodium channels, resulting in less neuronal firing (McNamara, 2011; Novartis Pharmaceuticals Corporation, 2011; Stahl, 2013).

Factors to be aware of for clients using oxcarbazepine include the potential for low sodium levels, or **hyponatremia**; hypersensitivity reactions; rashes, including Stevens Johnson syndrome; and suicidal behavior (Novartis Pharmaceuticals Corporation, 2011). Of these, the hyponatremia is the main unique concern. This occurs most commonly during the first 3 months of treatment, and most clients do not have any symptoms; however, if hyponatremia becomes severe, nausea, malaise, headache, confusion, lethargy and seizures may occur (Novartis Pharmaceuticals Corporation, 2011). Other less severe and more frequently seen adverse effects include fatigue, headache, nausea, vomiting, abdominal pain, dizziness, drowsiness, and double vision (Novartis Pharmaceuticals Corporation, 2011). Clients using oxcarbazepine may also experience negative consequences from drug interactions.

Antidepressants

The class of antidepressants contains a large number of medications that are not all alike. The use of antidepressants has increased dramatically over the past few decades, and there is an increasing push to truly test their efficacy. Some of these medications, although designed to help treat depression, have been found to be effective at treating anxiety disorders and are used as a first-line for these conditions as well. Generally, this class will focus on three of the neurotransmitters: 5HT, NE, and DA. Although diversity exists in how the various subcategories of antidepressants work, there has not been consistent evidence suggesting that one medication or category of antidepressants is more effective than another. They all result in the resolution of symptoms in approximately two-thirds of clients.

For all of the medications in this class, the FDA has issued a warning regarding the risk of an increase in suicidal thoughts and behaviors in children, adolescents, and young adults. This is most commonly seen in the early months of treatment. All clients should be watched for changes in mood, thoughts, or behaviors, and these changes should be reported to their physician.

Selective 5HT Reuptake Inhibitors

The SSRI class was introduced to the U.S. public in the late 1980s, and its launch was greatly anticipated. Mental health providers were pleased to see these medications come to the market because they were found to be as effective as the traditional antidepressants, but they did not have as severe adverse effects and were safer if taken in overdose. Just as the name states, this category of medications is very selective, preventing the neurons from taking up 5HT. This keeps a greater amount of 5HT in the synapses to work on the receptors of the next neuron to pass on its signal. The way in which this action reduces depression is not well understood.

Six medications are included in the SSRI category; they are citalopram, escitalopram, fluoxetine, fluvoxamine, paroxetine, and sertraline. These medications are not interchangeable, as some clients will respond to one SSRI but not to another. The most closely related of these medications are citalopram and escitalopram, both of which are **enantiomers**. Enantiomers are mirror images of each other, meaning they are very similar but not identical. Think of your hands—they are alike, but if you put them on top of each other, they would not line up. Each of the SSRI antidepressants may have slightly different secondary activities. Fluoxetine and paroxetine, for example, have a little activity on the NE reuptake pump, but generally their main actions are on the 5HT reuptake pump.

Adverse effects associated with the SSRIs include sleep changes (insomnia or sedation), headache, nausea, diarrhea, and/or dry mouth (Lexi-Comp, 2013). Most of these adverse effects will abate as the client grows accustomed to the medication. Clients can also take the medication with a small snack at bedtime to help manage these adverse effects. If the client experiences insomnia, then the antidepressant would be best taken in the morning (with food to help with the nausea). For individuals who have anxiety, these medications may cause an initial increase in anxiety or restlessness, which also will go away after the first couple of weeks' use (Lexi-Comp, 2013; Stahl, 2013). Another concern with initiating any antidepressants, including the SSRIs, is the possibility for an increased risk of suicidal thoughts and behavior in children, adolescents, and young adults (Lexi-Comp, 2013). It is important that family and caregivers are watching and checking in with this client population for at least the first few months when they start these medications.

In clients who have been on SSRIs for some time, sexual dysfunction may become a problem. Sexual dysfunction can include decreased libido or sex drive, lack of desire, or orgasm problems. These adverse effects may not go away and may become more evident later in treatment. Decreasing the dosage may help, but often switching the SSRI to a different antidepressant is required. SSRIs have also been associated with an increased risk of bleeding, especially in clients who are using medications to thin their blood to prevent blood clots (Lexi-Comp, 2013). Finally, in clients who are discontinuing treatment with SSRIs, a documented withdrawal syndrome has been documented, where clients experience flu-like symptoms, such as headache, dizziness, and fatigue. Some clients develop agitation, dizziness, shock-like sensations, and sleeping problems (Lexi-Comp, 2013). These withdrawal effects can include seizures; however, overall, withdrawal is not dangerous for the client, although it will likely make them uncomfortable (Lexi-Comp). For this reason, it is recommended that clients speak with their pharmacist or physician prior to discontinuing SSRI therapy so the dose can be reduced slowly.

Drug interactions are a concern with the use of SSRIs. Medications such as fluoxetine, paroxetine, and fluvoxamine all act as enzyme inhibitors, meaning they block the enzymes from metabolizing other medications, resulting in higher concentrations and potential toxicity (Lexi-Comp, 2013). The SSRIs also may interact with other medications that impact 5HT levels. The greatest concern lies around medications that also increase 5HT levels, which, in combination with SSRIs, can lead to **serotonin syndrome**. Symptoms of serotonin syndrome include the following three primary areas: altered mental status, neuromuscular hyperactivity, and autonomic instability (Iqbal, Basil, Kaplan, & Iqbal, 2012). Altered mental status can range from irritability and hyperactivity to restlessness, anxiety, and confusion to drowsiness, hallucinations, or coma (Iqbal et al., 2012). Neuromuscular hyperactivity refers to muscular rigidity or sustained muscle contractions, teeth grinding, lack of balance, and/or tremor (Iqbal et al., 2012). Finally, the autonomic instability includes dilated (large) pupils, increased heart rate and breathing rates, fever, sweating, and changes in blood pressure (Iqbal et al., 2012). Monitoring with clients taking SSRIs focuses on the improvement of symptoms and identifying adverse effects, including bruising and bleeding (Lexi-Comp, 2013).

Serotonin Norepinephrine Reuptake Inhibitors

In the treatment of depression, the next class of medications that is often used after the SSRIs is the serotonin norepinephrine reuptake inhibitors (SNRIs). As the name implies, these medications inhibit the reuptake of 5HT and NE (Stahl, 2013). By increasing the concentrations of these two neurotransmitters, symptoms of depression and anxiety are likely improved through changes in complex messaging. The improvement in depression and anxiety symptoms often does not become fully apparent until a few weeks into therapy (Stahl, 2013). The SNRI class includes three medications that will be discussed: venlafaxine, desvenlafaxine, and duloxetine. A fourth agent, levomilnacipran, was recently approved by the FDA and more information will be available about it in late 2013 (Lexi-Comp, 2013).

Venlafaxine was the first SNRI developed. Its actions change slightly, depending on the dose administered. 5HT reuptake inhibition occurs at lower doses, and NE reuptake inhibition occurs at higher doses. Weak DA reuptake inhibition is noted at the higher doses (Stahl, 2013). Both venlafaxine and desvenlafaxine interact with other medications that have actions on NE and 5HT, including other antidepressants such as the MAOIs (Lexi-Comp, 2013).

Duloxetine is the other agent currently available in this class of medications. Duloxetine appears to have balanced activity of inhibition of 5HT and NE at all doses (Stahl, 2013). These effects can help treat anxiety and depression symptoms, but there has also been a fair amount of research performed to support its use in treating pain. Duloxetine is one of the first medications that is efficacious for depression and pain but which also successfully treats each condition independently. For this reason, there is a large group of clients that may use this medication for reasons other than depression or anxiety. Duloxetine acts as an inhibitor of a metabolic enzyme and can result in increased concentrations of other medications, again, emphasizing the importance of having an accurate, updated medication list so that preventable interactions and adverse consequences can be avoided.

Similar to the SSRIs, the SNRIs may also cause an increased risk of bleeding in clients who take blood thinning medications due to the increased 5HT, which prevents clot formation (Stahl, 2013). Common adverse effects seen with venlafaxine and desvenlafaxine include dizziness, insomnia, sweating, nausea, and dry mouth (Lexi-Comp, 2013), as well as sexual dysfunction and high blood pressure. Monitoring for clients on SNRI medications includes watching for symptom improvement and identifying adverse effects, including bleeding and bruising, high blood pressure, and heart rate changes (Lexi-Comp, 2013).

Norepinephrine Dopamine Reuptake Inhibitor

Another reuptake inhibitor is bupropion, an "activating" medication that does not commonly make clients who take it sleepy. In addition to helping alleviate symptoms of depression, it has also been used as a common treatment in tobacco cessation treatment plans (Lexi-Comp, 2013; Stahl, 2013). The actions most relevant for assisting with cravings and withdrawal symptoms are most likely related to the boost in DA, which can help alleviate the cravings and uncomfortable symptoms that result from ending tobacco use (Stahl, 2013).

Bupropion acts as an inhibitor of an enzyme that is responsible for metabolizing a number of other medications, including opiates; other antidepressants, such as amitriptyline; and some antipsychotics, such as aripiprazole and iloperidone (Lexi-Comp, 2013). This enzyme inhibition means that these medications will not be metabolized as well, resulting in higher concentrations and potentially more adverse effects (Lexi-Comp, 2013). Other drug interaction considerations with bupropion include risk of significantly elevated blood pressure or hypertensive crisis if bupropion is used with an MAOI (Lexi-Comp, 2013). Bupropion increases the risk of clients having a seizure, so use of any other medications that increases the chances of a client having a seizure are of concern (Lexi-Comp, 2013).

The risk of seizure associated with bupropion is also a concern for clients who have other risk factors for having a seizure, including alcohol or benzodiazepine use, eating disorders, seizure history, and head injuries. In clients who do not have risk factors for seizures, there is a low likelihood that they will have a seizure on this medication. Other more common adverse effects that clients experience include tachycardia or elevated heart rate, headache, insomnia, dizziness, dry mouth, weight loss, and nausea (Lexi-Comp, 2013). Most of these effects tend to be mild and may diminish as the client continues taking the medication. Little reported sexual dysfunction with bupropion is noted, possibly due to its lack of effect on the levels of 5HT, which makes bupropion a good choice for clients who develop sexual dysfunction with other antidepressants. Monitoring for clients taking bupropion includes symptom improvement, adverse effects, and increased weight and blood pressure (Lexi-Comp, 2013).

Alpha-2 Antagonists

We will now shift focus slightly and talk about a drug with a different mechanism of action—alpha-2 (α_2) antagonism. Mirtazapine, an α_2 antagonist, also has other actions that impact its effects and adverse events. Mirtazapine is noted to block $5HT_{2A}$, $5HT_{2C}$, and $5HT_3$ receptors (Stahl, 2013). Mirtazapine is well absorbed and is available as an orally dissolving tablet, which can be used for individuals who may not be adherent or cannot swallow a tablet. The medication is metabolized by liver enzymes and is susceptible to a number of drug interactions. Other considerations for drug interactions include medications that impact blood pressure, as mirtazapine is associated with changes in blood pressure. It is also important to exercise caution regarding drug interactions with other medications that cause increases in NE and 5HT, as it is possible that serotonin syndrome or elevated blood pressure may occur due to these interactions, and MAOI medications in particular should not be used with mirtazapine.

Mirtazapine is associated with a different adverse effect profile than that of the SSRIs or SNRIs. The most common adverse effects experienced by clients include somnolence, dry mouth, increased appetite, constipation, weight gain, and changes in blood pressure (Lexi-Comp, 2013). Clients are encouraged to take mirtazapine at bedtime so the sedation does not disrupt their daily activities, although the sedative effect can be helpful for individuals experiencing insomnia. The changes in blood pressure include orthostasis or dizziness upon standing quickly. It is important that the client be mindful of this and rise slowly so as not to get dizzy and fall (Lexi-Comp, 2013). Conversely, there have been reports of increases in blood pressure with the use of mirtazapine as a result of the increase in NE (Lexi-Comp). Monitoring for clients on mirtazapine includes watching for symptom improvement, adverse effects, and changes in weight and blood pressure.

5HT Antagonist/Reuptake Inhibitors

Another group of antidepressants are referred to as 5HT antagonist/reuptake inhibitors. These include nefazodone and trazodone. These medications are grouped together because they work similarly, but they do have some important differences. The 5HT antagonist reuptake inhibitors are thought to block the $5HT_{2A}$ and $5HT_{2C}$ receptors and the 5HT reuptake pump (Stahl, 2013).

The use of these medications for the treatment of depression is limited. Nefazodone's use is restricted due to its risk of severe liver toxicity. Trazodone is most often used at lower doses to treat insomnia. Drug interactions are of concern with both medications. Changes in heart rhythms have been reported, so other medications that also may change heart rhythms, such as antipsychotics, should be used with caution or avoided if possible to prevent the development of an abnormal heart beat (Lexi-Comp, 2013). Trazodone also has various anticholinergic effects, such as sedation, dry mouth, constipation, and blurred vision (Lexi-Comp, 2013). Any other medications that have these effects, including antihistamines such as hydroxyzine, may produce worsening of these adverse effects and may result in delirium in older adults (Lexi-Comp, 2013).

When thinking about adverse effects for nefazodone, liver toxicity is one of the most significant. It is not a common effect but it can be severe when it occurs, so any elevations in liver function tests should be addressed promptly (Lexi-Comp, 2013). Other common adverse effects reported with nefazodone use include headache, drowsiness, insomnia, agitation, dizziness, dry mouth, nausea, constipation, and weakness (Lexi-Comp, 2013). Trazodone, on the other hand, is most commonly associated with sedation, dizziness, and dry mouth. Blurred vision, nausea, headache, and constipation are reported less frequently (Lexi-Comp, 2013). Common to nefazodone and trazodone, and many of the agents previously discussed, is the warning about increased risk of suicidal thoughts or behaviors in children, adolescents, and young adults (Lexi-Comp, 2013). These medications increase 5HT levels and have been reported to increase bleeding and bruising, especially if used in clients who are taking medications, such as aspirin or warfarin, to prevent clots (Lexi-Comp, 2013). Some of these medications carry a number of considerations in terms of the many potential adverse effects that need to be considered by the client prior to starting therapy.

Monitoring clients taking either nefazodone or trazodone includes watching for efficacy, adverse effects, and changes in blood pressure and heart rate. Any new bleeding or bruising in clients using either of these medications should be reported. Nefazodone requires routine monitoring of liver function. Clients taking trazodone may need electrocardiograms if they have a history of heart problems or are taking other medications that can affect heart rhythm. Both of these medications can cause withdrawal effects if stopped abruptly, so any changes the client wants to make to treatment should be discussed with the pharmacist and physician prior to adjusting therapy.

Vilazodone is one of the more recent additions to the antidepressant class. It can be used early in the treatment of depression, although SSRIs and SNRIs still tend to be treatment options of first choice. Vilazodone works by the now familiar inhibition of 5HT reuptake, and this blockade of the 5HT reuptake pump results in an increase in 5HT (Lexi-Comp, 2013). In addition to this stand-by, vilazodone has a mechanism of action that has not yet been discussed in the antidepressant section: a partial agonist of the $5HT_{1A}$ receptor (Lexi-Comp, 2013). Partial agonists are compounds that "activate" the receptor but do not cause as much of a response as a full agonist. By having partial agonist activity at the $5HT_{1A}$ receptors, vilazodone allows some 5HT to be released, more than if 5HT itself were binding to the receptor. This results in some DA being released by that multistep process. These actions are thought to result in an overall increase in the amount of 5HT and DA, which can help to alleviate the symptoms of depression.

Vilazodone is well absorbed and is metabolized by liver enzymes but does have a number of drug interaction considerations (Lexi-Comp, 2013). Other medications, including many antidepressants that increase 5HT concentrations, may increase the risk of developing serotonin syndrome (Lexi-Comp).

Adverse effects common to antidepressants that increase 5HT, such as increased risk of bleeding (especially in clients who are on blood thinning medications), and sexual dysfunction are present (Lexi-Comp, 2013). Other common adverse effects include nausea and diarrhea that tend to abate when the client has become used to taking the medication. Monitoring for clients on vilazodone includes watching for symptom improvement and adverse effects.

Tricyclic Antidepressants and Monoamine Oxidase Inhibitors

The remaining two classes of antidepressant medications include medications that have been used for the longest period of time to treat depression: TCAs and MAOIs. These medications have fallen out of favor for a few reasons. TCAs are associated with a number of adverse effects that make them difficult for clients to tolerate, and they can be fatal when taken in overdose. MAOIs have been discussed briefly in other sections, and these carry a significant number of serious drug and food interactions that could result in serotonin syndrome or a hypertensive crisis (i.e., high blood pressure emergency), either of which has the potential to be fatal. Although these medications may not be the most common, there are a number of significant considerations that you should be aware of when you do encounter them.

TCAs generally work by inhibiting the reuptake of the 5HT and NE, resulting in higher concentrations of 5HT and NE (Stahl, 2013). The SNRI class was likely derived from the TCA class. The other actions that many TCAs have are inhibition of the sodium channels, histamine (H1) receptors, alpha-1 NE receptors, and muscarinic (M1) ACh receptors (Stahl, 2013). Adverse effects that are cause for concern include abnormal heart rate, weight gain, drowsiness, dry mouth, blurred vision, and dizziness with an associated increased risk of falls.

Numerous considerations exist for who should be using these medications. Older adults and clients with kidney, liver, or heart disease should be closely monitored. Dangerous interactions with these medications include other antidepressants that increase NE or 5HT; those medications that have anticholinergic effects, such as constipation, dry mouth, or blurred vision; any other sedating medications; and medications that can also lower blood pressure.

The last class discussed in this section is the MAOI medications. These medications are reserved for clients who are refractory or do not respond to other antidepressants. The main reasons for the limited use of MAOIs are the drug interactions and food interactions that can occur with these medications, which have the potential to be fatal. Monoamines are the neurotransmitters 5HT, NE and DA. Monoamine oxidase is a set of two enzymes (MAO-A and MAO-B) that break down 5HT, NE and DA. The MAOIs are phenelzine, tranylcypromine, isocarboxazid and selegiline. When combined with medications that can increase concentrations of 5HT, such as other antidepressants (SSRI, SNRI), opiate pain medications, or migraine medications, a risk exists that the client will develop serotonin syndrome. In addition, medications that increase NE and DA, such as SNRIs, mirtazapine, and over-the-counter medications, such as decongestants (e.g., pseudoephedrine) used for colds, can increase the risk that the client will develop a high blood pressure emergency, which can result in a heart attack, stroke, or even death. Clients with severely elevated blood pressure may experience a headache, a change in heart beat or palpitations, nausea, vomiting, sweating, and neck stiffness (Stahl, 2013). Many medications interact with the MAOIs, so it is vitally

CLINICAL PEARL: ANTIDEPRESSANTS

All antidepressants carry a warning regarding increased risk for clients developing suicidal thoughts and behaviors (Lexi-Comp, 2013). This risk has been seen mainly in children, adolescents, and young adults under the age of 25. Such changes were most often seen within the first few months of therapy, so it is important that clients are aware of the increased risk and that their family and caregivers help to monitor for changes in thoughts or behaviors that may signal an increased risk of suicidal tendencies. This information should be communicated back to the client's physicians.

important that a full medication list be reviewed prior to starting these medications. Usually, it is recommended that clients spend at least 2 weeks drug free to ensure that all medication is out of their body before switching to or off of an MAOI.

In addition to all of these concerns regarding other medications, the MAOIs also restrict the foods that clients can eat. Specifically, clients need to be mindful of the amount of tyramine in their diet. Tyramine taken in from food causes the body to release more NE, which cannot be broken down by clients taking MAOIs (Stahl, 2013). Foods that contain tyramine that should be avoided by clients on MAOIs include dried, aged, or smoked meats (sausage, pepperoni, salami); aged cheese (blue cheese, aged cheddar); broad bean pods (fava beans); sauerkraut; soy sauce; tap beer; and red wine (e.g., Chianti). Although this list may not be incredibly restrictive, it does require the client to be mindful and pay attention to what he or she is eating and drinking, something that can be challenging for someone experiencing symptoms of depression. Clients who use the MAOI medications need to have their medication lists closely watched to prevent any unintentional interaction that could have significant implications. The Clinical Pearl box and Evidence in Practice box provide brief summary information relevant to antidepressants.

Anxiolytics

The armamentarium of anxiolytic agents encompasses a diverse group of medications, including antidepressants, benzodiazepines, buspirone, anticonvulsants, antipsychotics, and other miscellaneous agents. Some medications display efficacy across several indications, whereas others have much narrower uses. For example, antidepressant medications demonstrate substantial efficacy in generalized anxiety disorder (GAD), social anxiety disorder, obsessive compulsive disorder (OCD), posttraumatic stress disorder (PTSD), and panic disorder, whereas buspirone is indicated only for the treatment of GAD (Ravindran & Stein, 2010). Certain medications have the potential for abuse, whereas others are non–habit forming. For instance, benzodiazepines and pregabalin are considered **controlled substances** (i.e., possess abuse potential), whereas other medications, such as antidepressants, are non–habit forming (Lexi-Comp, 2013; Melton & Kirkwood, 2008). Some medications produce anxiolytic effects with the first dose, whereas others have delayed onsets of action. For example, benzodiazepines and hydroxyzine produce anxiolysis almost immediately, but buspirone requires several weeks for the onset of therapeutic effects (Melton & Kirkwood, 2008). Finally, some medications are effective as monotherapy (the use of a single drug), whereas others are considered adjunctive treatments. Antidepressants, for instance, are effective as monotherapy; however, antipsychotics are predominantly used as adjuncts to antidepressant therapy. Overall,

EVIDENCE IN PRACTICE: ANTIDEPRESSANTS

Uncovering the differences between antidepressant medications in terms of efficacy has been a large focus of the depression literature. The Sequenced Treatment Alternatives to Relieve Depression (STAR*D) trial was conducted with adults with depression to determine the effectiveness of numerous antidepressants and serves as one of the largest depression trials ever conducted (Fava et al., 2003). This trial helped to confirm that the antidepressants appear to be generally similar in efficacy; however, the more options clients tried, the less likely they were to respond to subsequent medications (Fava et al., 2003; Stahl, 2013). A more recent meta-analysis suggested that there may be some differences in efficacy and tolerability between the antidepressant medications, but definitive results are not yet available (Capriani, et al., 2009).

anxiolytic medications share little in common other than their anxiolytic-producing effects (Ravindran & Stein, 2010).

Antidepressants are effective anxiolytic medications. A wealth of evidence supports their use for GAD, social anxiety disorder, PTSD, OCD, and panic disorder. Treatment guidelines typically regard antidepressants as first-line, or the treatment of choice, for anxiety disorders. In addition to anxiolysis, antidepressants effectively treat comorbid depression in clients with anxiety disorders. Furthermore, they are non–habit forming, an important characteristic when managing clients with comorbid substance-related disorders. Unfortunately, antidepressants take several weeks to exert maximal therapeutic effects. Consequently, clinicians often initiate other anxiolytic medications simultaneously to provide more immediate symptom relief while awaiting the onset of antidepressant effects (Melton & Kirkwood, 2008; Ravindran & Stein, 2010). A more in-depth review of antidepressants can be found in the antidepressant medication section.

GABA is the major inhibitory neurotransmitter of the CNS. GABA binds to both GABA-A and GABA-B receptors; however, GABA-A receptors are of particular importance in the pharmacology of anxiolytic medications. Two common medication classes enhance GABAergic neurotransmission via interactions with the GABA-A receptor—barbiturates and benzodiazepines (Longo & Johnson, 2000; Melton & Kirkwood, 2008).

Barbiturates, such as phenobarbital, were once widely used sedative-hypnotic medications. Similar to other GABAergic medications, barbiturates are controlled substances because of their abuse potential. Barbiturates are more likely than benzodiazepines to depress respiratory drive and to be lethal in overdose. Therefore, they have been largely replaced by the safer benzodiazepines (Melton & Kirkwood, 2008).

Benzodiazepines are among the most commonly used sedative-hypnotic medications. Benzodiazepines produce anxiolytic, hypnotic, myorelaxant, and anticonvulsant effects (Longo & Johnson, 2000; Melton & Kirkwood, 2008). Benzodiazepines predominately differ in pharmacokinetic parameters, such as onset and duration of effects. Although most benzodiazepines reach peak concentrations quickly (1 to 2 hours), half-life elimination varies dramatically (5 to 120 hours). Benzodiazepines are used for a number of FDA-approved and off-label indications, including GAD, panic disorder, insomnia, seizures, and acute alcohol withdrawal (Lexi-Comp, 2013). Unlike antidepressants, benzodiazepines produce anxiolytic effects almost immediately and can be prescribed on a scheduled or as-needed basis. Unfortunately, benzodiazepines are effective only for the treatment of anxiety, whereas antidepressants treat both anxiety and depression (Melton & Kirkwood, 2008).

Although all benzodiazepines are available orally, some can be administered intramuscularly or intravenously, and this flexibility of administration allows for their use in settings ranging from outpatient to intensive care (Lexi-Comp, 2013). However, there are substantial concerns with benzodiazepine therapy. Sedation is the most common benzodiazepine adverse effect, and tolerance develops with continued use. Clients should be counseled to avoid operating machinery or performing activities that require mental alertness until they understand how the medication will affect them. Benzodiazepines are also associated with psychomotor retardation, such as ataxia, muscle weakness, and motor incoordination. Along with sedation, psychomotor retardation greatly increases the risk of falls and accidents, particularly in the elderly. At times, benzodiazepines may cause the opposite of what is expected. Paradoxical reactions, including increased excitement, irritability, or aggression, have been reported. Although rare, paradoxical disinhibition appears to be more common in older adults, children, and individuals with developmental disabilities (Mancuso, Tanzi, & Gabay, 2004).

Clients should be advised not to abruptly discontinue benzodiazepine therapy without their physician's supervision. Benzodiazepine withdrawal—characterized by anxiety, agitation, tension, dysphoria, insomnia, sweating, and, of particular concern, seizures—can occur with abrupt withdrawal. Discontinuing benzodiazepines requires careful tapering of the dose over weeks or months to prevent withdrawal effects (Chouinard, 2004; Rickels, DeMartinis, Rynn, & Mandos, 1999). Problematic interactions with other drugs include reactions to other CNS depressants, which will produce additive CNS depression in combination with benzodiazepines. All clients must be counseled to abstain from alcohol consumption throughout therapy (Lexi-Comp, 2013). All clients should have any symptoms of anxiety monitored throughout therapy. Also, adverse effects, particularly on cognition and motor skills, should be monitored to ensure that concentration, balance, and ability to function are not impaired. Finally, clients should be monitored for drug-seeking behavior. Overall, benzodiazepines have an important role in the short-term relief of anxiety. Their major advantage includes the quick onset of action. The disadvantages of benzodiazepine use include the lack of ability to treat depressive symptoms, the risk of dependency, and the potential withdrawal symptoms upon discontinuation (Longo & Johnson, 2000; Melton & Kirkwood, 2008).

Buspirone is a miscellaneous anxiolytic medication, and the only member of its drug class. It is a non–habit-forming anxiolytic that acts as a partial agonist at $5HT_{1A}$ receptors. Buspirone is only FDA approved for the treatment of GAD; however, it has been studied for other uses, such as augmenting antidepressants for the treatment of major depressive disorder. Buspirone is generally well tolerated but is associated with the following adverse effects: dizziness, sedation, headaches, and restlessness. Various medications can interact with buspirone, including antidepressants, placing the client at risk for serotonin syndrome. Furthermore, grapefruit juice inhibits the metabolism of buspirone. Efficacy is monitored by assessing anxiety symptoms, noting that the onset of therapeutic effects is delayed for several weeks after initiating buspirone therapy. Furthermore, the client should be monitored and counseled to follow instructions about use, as buspirone is typically dosed two or three times daily. In addition, adverse effects require monitoring to ensure that dizziness does not provoke falls and excessive sedation does not cause accidents (Lexi-Comp, 2013; Loane & Politis, 2012).

Hydroxyzine is an antihistamine, also known as a histamine-1 (H_1) receptor antagonist, and is commonly used in the treatment of anxiety, particularly GAD. Hydroxyzine is FDA approved for the treatment of anxiety and is available as both a hydrochloride (Atarax) and pamoate salt (Vistaril). Sedation is a common adverse effect, but tolerance develops to the sedating effects with continued use. Similar to other antihistamines, the anticholinergic effects—dry mouth, blurred vision, constipation, urinary retention, and confusion—are common with hydroxyzine therapy; therefore, caution is warranted in clients with comorbid glaucoma, benign prostatic hyperplasia, or dementia (Lexi-Comp, 2013). Symptoms of anxiety should be monitored in all clients receiving hydroxyzine therapy. Sedation may contribute to falls and accidents, whereas anticholinergic effects may contribute to, among other things, confusion and memory impairment in older adults (Lexi-Comp, 2013).

Gabapentin and pregabalin, somewhat related compounds, are classified as anticonvulsants and are used in the treatment of anxiety disorders, notably GAD. Pregabalin is a controlled substance, whereas gabapentin is not controlled. Both medications are FDA approved as adjunctive therapy for partial seizures and pain associated with postherpetic neuralgia, whereas pregabalin carries additional FDA approvals for fibromyalgia and neuropathic pain associated with diabetes mellitus (Frampton & Foster, 2006; Lexi-Comp, 2013). Neither agent is approved for the treatment of anxiety; however, robust data support pregabalin as an effective treatment for the management of GAD (Frampton & Foster, 2006). Common adverse effects of both medications include sedation, dizziness, peripheral edema (swelling in the extremities), and tremor. As mandated by the FDA, all anticonvulsant medications carry a warning regarding the risk of suicidal ideation while receiving therapy. Clients should be monitored for improvements in anxiety symptoms, as well as the emergence of suicidal thoughts or behaviors. Clients should also be monitored for adverse effects, such as troublesome sedation or dizziness, tremulousness, exacerbation of comorbid congestive heart failure secondary to edema, and signs and symptoms of hypersensitivity reactions. Finally, both gabapentin and pregabalin are predominantly excreted via the kidneys; therefore, renal function tests are required because dose adjustments are necessary in clients with renal impairment (Frampton & Foster, 2006; Lexi-Comp, 2013).

The beta-blocker propranolol is commonly used in psychiatric medicine. As the most lipophilic, or "lipid loving," beta-blocker available, propranolol readily crosses the blood-brain barrier, penetrates the CNS, and exerts its therapeutic effects. All FDA-approved indications for propranolol are either cardiovascular (e.g., hypertension) or neurologic (e.g., migraine prophylaxis) in nature, whereas all psychiatric indications constitute off-label usage. With regard to anxiety disorders, propranolol is most commonly used for the treatment of social anxiety disorder, particularly nongeneralized or performance-related anxiety. For example, administration of propranolol at least 30 minutes before a performance (e.g., public speaking) may decrease physical manifestations of anxiety, such as tremor, palpitations, and blushing. Common adverse effects include bradycardia, or slow heart rate, and fatigue. Beta-blockers are associated with a host of contraindications, mostly related to cardiovascular function, and clients should not receive these medications if uncompensated congestive heart failure, severe bradycardia, or severe respiratory disease, among other conditions, are present. Drug interactions are numerous; however, medications contributing to bradycardia are most problematic and should be minimized if possible (Schneier, 2006).

Several alpha-blocking medications are available, yet prazosin is the most commonly used in psychiatric medicine. Although formally FDA approved to treat hypertension, prazosin has garnered extensive data for its off-label use in PTSD. When administered at bedtime, prazosin decreases the severity of PTSD-related nightmares and sleep disruption (Raskind et al., 2007). Most adverse effects are related to the vasodilation, or dilation of blood vessels, induced by prazosin. Common adverse effects include dizziness, headache, and orthostatic hypotension. In addition to other high blood pressure medications, prazosin interacts negatively with common erectile dysfunction medications, such as sildenafil (Viagra, Pfizer, Inc.). A precipitously low drop in blood pressure may occur with concurrent use. Monitoring parameters include documenting the frequency and severity of nightmares, as well as documenting sitting and standing blood pressures (Lexi-Comp, 2013; Pfizer, Inc., 2009).

SGAs are increasingly used in the realm of anxiety disorders. Currently, no SGA has garnered FDA approval in any anxiety disorder. Most clinical trials in the PTSD, GAD, and OCD literature have investigated SGAs as adjuncts to antidepressant therapy. Olanzapine,

EVIDENCE IN PRACTICE: ANXIOLYTICS

A review of the 200 most frequently prescribed medications in 2000 found that 9.5% of medications reported falls as an adverse effect, and 93% had an adverse effect that could lead to falls (Smith, 2003). The evidence linking benzodiazepines to falls is particularly convincing. A meta-analysis exploring the risk of medication-induced falls revealed a significant association between benzodiazepines and falls in older adults (Woolcott et al., 2009). Benzodiazepines should be regarded as a high risk of fall drug class.

risperidone, quetiapine, and aripiprazole are the most robustly studied of the SGA agents (Ravindran & Stein, 2010). Data for their use in panic disorder, as well as for the other six SGAs, are less robust and their use is not recommended at this time (Ravindran & Stein, 2010).

Treatment guidelines generally recommend antidepressant pharmacotherapy as first-line treatment options for GAD, OCD, social anxiety disorder, PTSD, and panic disorder; however, individual agents vary widely with regard to safety profiles, tolerability, and the clinical evidence available. Antidepressants are not habit-forming, although they do have a delayed onset of action (Melton & Kirkwood, 2008; Ravindran & Stein, 2010). Benzodiazepines are typically used as adjuncts to antidepressants or when there is an urgent need to quell anxiety; nevertheless, it is widely thought that the duration of benzodiazepine therapy should be minimized and that monotherapy should be avoided for most clients. Furthermore, benzodiazepines have numerous disadvantages, including abuse potential. In addition to abuse potential, the therapeutic benefits of benzodiazepines in certain anxiety disorders, such as PTSD, are largely unproven (Braun, Greenberg, Dasberg, & Lerer, 1990; Cates, Bishop, Davis, Lowe, & Woolley, 2004). Buspirone, which is FDA approved only for GAD, is considered a second-line option after antidepressant therapy because antidepressants also treat comorbid depression (Loane & Politis, 2012; Melton & Kirkwood, 2008). The role of antipsychotic medications appears to be the augmentation of antidepressant agents, but their considerable adverse effect burden discourages their first-line and widespread use (Ravindran & Stein, 2010). The choice of anxiolytic is determined by a number of factors, including support for use in the literature, adverse effect profiles, safety profiles, and, to some degree, trial and error. Furthermore, combining anxiolytics is common in clinical practice. The Evidence in Practice box provides some added information about anxiolytic use.

Hypnotics

Sleep–wake disorders encompass a diverse group of conditions, including insomnia, restless legs syndrome, and narcolepsy. An assorted group of medications is used for the treatment of each disorder. Insomnia utilizes numerous sedative-hypnotic medications, such as benzodiazepines, as well as a host of miscellaneous agents, such as melatonin agonists and sedating antihistamines (Schutte-Rodin, Broch, Buysse, Dorsey, & Sateia, 2008). Restless legs syndrome is often treated with iron supplementation, dopamine agonists, benzodiazepines, or even opioid medications (Earley, 2003). Narcolepsy treatment involves the use of psychostimulants, sodium oxybate, and antidepressants (Roth, 2007). A thorough understanding of each condition will enable the clinician to confidently counsel and monitor the pharmacotherapy used in the treatment of sleep–wake disorders.

The treatment of insomnia should include the aggressive treatment of any underlying causes. Numerous psychiatric and medical conditions, such as depression or pain, among others, may contribute to insomnia (Silber, 2005). Together with the treatment of underlying conditions, counseling on caffeine intake, alcohol intake, and sleep hygiene is necessary for all clients with sleep onset or sleep maintenance difficulties. Common medications for the treatment of insomnia include benzodiazepines, benzodiazepine receptor agonists, ramelteon, antidepressants, antihistamines, antipsychotics, and herbal medications (Schutte-Rodin et al., 2008).

Five benzodiazepines—triazolam, quazepam, temazepam, flurazepam, and estazolam—are FDA approved for the treatment of insomnia, and each agent differs in its pharmacokinetics. For example, triazolam has a very short half-life (1.5 to 5.5 hours) and may be helpful for sleep onset but not sleep maintenance. In contrast, flurazepam has an exceedingly long half-life (greater than 100 hours), which is useful for sleep maintenance, although it will contribute to morning grogginess (Lexi-Comp, 2013). As discussed previously, benzodiazepines are associated with motor incoordination and falls, making these agents particularly inappropriate for older adults. Rebound insomnia may occur after the abrupt discontinuation of the benzodiazepines, particularly with triazolam therapy. Furthermore, tolerance and dependence occurs with prolonged use (Schutte-Rodin et al., 2008; Silber, 2005). For a complete discussion on benzodiazepines, please review the anxiolytics section.

Benzodiazepine receptor agonists bind to the same receptor as benzodiazepines, the GABA-A receptor, but have different affinities for various subtypes within this receptor family. A major difference from benzodiazepines is that benzodiazepine receptor agonists appear to provide only hypnotic, or sleep-inducing, properties. The three currently available agents, zolpidem, zaleplon, and eszopiclone, have relatively short half-lives and no active metabolites, making their pharmacokinetics more desirable than that of most benzodiazepines. Similar to benzodiazepines, the benzodiazepine receptor agonists are controlled substances due to abuse potential, and caution is warranted in clients with substance-related disorders. The benzodiazepine receptor agonists possess multiple advantages over traditional benzodiazepines, such as lower risk of rebound insomnia, tolerance, and withdrawal upon discontinuation (Schutte-Rodin et al., 2008; Silber, 2005). The FDA has recently lowered the maximum dose of zolpidem in women due to their slower metabolism and elimination of the medication; however, both men and women should continue to be counseled on next-day sedation, cognitive impairment, and fall risk (U.S. FDA, 2013). Clients should be monitored for effects on sleep, as well as for possible adverse effects (Lexi-Comp, 2013).

Ramelteon is a non–habit-forming option for the treatment of insomnia. Ramelteon stimulates melatonin receptors (i.e., MT1 and MT2 receptors) in the CNS, and it is useful for clients with sleep onset difficulties. As a non–habit-forming medication, it is appropriate to consider ramelteon in clients with comorbid insomnia and substance-related disorders. Ramelteon is generally well-tolerated, with common adverse effects of headache, fatigue, nausea, and dizziness. Clients should be monitored for effects on sleep (Cada, Levien, & Baker, 2006; Lexi-Comp, 2013).

Sedating antihistamines, antidepressants, and antipsychotic medications are frequently prescribed for the treatment of insomnia. Although all of these agents are non–habit forming, each class has potential disadvantages. Sedating antihistamines, such as diphenhydramine, are available over-the-counter. Unfortunately, adverse effects limit their usefulness. Diphenhydramine is profoundly anticholinergic, causing dry mouth, constipation, and confusion, so it should be avoided in older adults. Furthermore, significant next-day impairment has been reported with its use. Finally, tolerance to the sedating effects of all antihistamines occurs quickly (Silber, 2005).

Sedating antipsychotic medications, such as quetiapine, are used off-label for the treatment of insomnia. The potential risks of EPS and weight gain discourage the use of these agents, unless the client has comorbid disorders, such as schizophrenia or bipolar disorder. Sedating antidepressants, such as mirtazapine and trazodone, are commonly used for the treatment of insomnia as well. Interestingly, sedation with mirtazapine lessens as the dose increases. Appetite stimulation and weight gain are common adverse effects. Trazodone is commonly used for insomnia; however, sedation and orthostatic hypotension are common side effects. Similar to antipsychotic medications, antidepressant use is recommended only in clients with comorbid disorders, such as depression, as the data for their use solely in primary insomnia are lacking (Lexi-Comp, 2013; Schutte-Rodin et al., 2008).

The use of herbal medications is common in clinical practice, and many herbals are used for the treatment of insomnia. Valerian is thought to exert its effects via GABA, although the mechanism is not fully understood. Kava has been associated with case reports of liver toxicity and should be avoided. The use of melatonin has been associated with benefits in sleep onset, although no benefits were observed in total sleep time. Overall, herbal medications lack the systematic evaluation required before they can be routinely recommended for the treatment of insomnia (Lexi-Comp, 2013; Schutte-Rodin et al., 2008).

The pharmacotherapy of restless legs syndrome utilizes a diverse group of medications. Restless legs syndrome is typically characterized by an urge to move the legs, with uncomfortable, but usually not painful, sensations in the legs. Restless legs syndrome predominantly occurs at bedtime, and symptoms appear to improve with movement of the legs. Restless legs syndrome may be a symptom of iron deficiency; thus, clients should have their iron levels examined.

Medications that stimulate DA receptors, such as the DA agonists ropinirole and pramipexole, are common first-line agents. Ropinirole and pramipexole are commonly associated with stomach upset, orthostatic hypotension, and may exacerbate symptoms of psychosis, such as hallucinations. Rarely, impulse control disorders, such as gambling, manifest after the initiation of a DA agonist. The DA agonist, levodopa, is less commonly used than ropinirole and pramipexole due to the risk of augmentation, where symptoms begin to occur progressively earlier in the day. Benzodiazepines, discussed in depth in the anxiolytics section, can be used. A last-line approach for the treatment of restless legs syndrome involves the use of opioid medications, such as oxycodone, tramadol, or hydrocodone. Opioids are controlled substances and carry a potential for abuse. Furthermore, constipation, nausea, sedation, and confusion are the common adverse effects. Regardless of the medications chosen, clients should continue to have their symptoms of restless legs syndrome monitored throughout therapy. Adverse effects should be monitored and minimized if possible (Earley, 2003; Lexi-Comp, 2013).

The pharmacotherapy for narcolepsy typically involves the following two areas: excessive daytime sleepiness and cataplexy. Excessive daytime sleepiness is often managed with psychostimulants, such as methylphenidate and amphetamines, which will be discussed in detail in the psychostimulants section of this chapter. Extended-release psychostimulants may be taken in the morning, or immediate-release doses can be given prior to tasks requiring mental alertness. Other stimulants, including modafinil and armodafinil, are also utilized. Cataplexy, the sudden loss of muscle tone following a strong emotional stimulus (e.g., anger, laughter), can be treated with antidepressant medications. Antidepressants, discussed in detail in the antidepressants section, have demonstrated anticataplectic effects. A unique compound, sodium oxybate, has been shown to improve both daytime sleepiness and cataplexy. Clients are required to measure out and drink two cups of medication throughout the night. Clients must possess the capability, including eye sight and the ability to measure, to properly use the medication, as well as dosing cups to avoid over- or underdosing. Because sodium oxybate is

---

CLINICAL PEARL: HYPNOTICS

Hypnotic medications have been associated with complex sleep-related behaviors. Examples of these behaviors include driving, preparing and eating food, and making phone calls while asleep, with the individual having no memory of the event the following morning. Although considered rare, the seriousness of such behaviors warrants discontinuation of the offending medication. The U.S. Food and Drug Administration (FDA) requires complex sleep behavior warnings for all hypnotic medications (FDA, 2007).

---

a powerful sedative-hypnotic medication, it is contraindicated with the concomitant use of alcohol or other sedative-hypnotics. Common adverse effects include dizziness, nausea, and involuntarily urinating at nighttime, termed *enuresis*. Sodium oxybate can be prescribed only by specially registered prescribers and is available only through a centralized pharmacy program (Lexi-Comp, 2013; Roth, 2007). The Clinical Pearl box provides added information on hypnotics.

Dementia Medications

Alzheimer's disease, the most common cause of dementia, is a progressive neurodegenerative disorder affecting more five million adults in the United States. The prevalence of Alzheimer's disease is expected to double by 2050 (Slattum, Swerdlow, & Massey Hill, 2008). Characteristic symptoms and hypothesized causes have been described in Chapter 18. No commercially available pharmacotherapeutic agents affect the formation or deposition of β-amyloid plaques; however, two classes of medications have been developed based on the cholinergic hypothesis and glutamate-induced excitotoxicity.

Acetylcholinesterase inhibitors (AChE-Is) improve cognition and may indirectly aid with function in clients with Alzheimer's disease. They enhance cholinergic neurotransmission in the CNS by inhibiting the enzyme acetylcholinesterase, which is responsible for the degradation of ACh. By inhibiting this enzyme, more ACh is available to exert its effects in the CNS. Unfortunately, AChE-Is do not reverse the progression of Alzheimer's disease, rather they slow the progression (Cummings, 2004; Lexi-Comp, 2013). The first AChE-I, tacrine, is rarely used in clinical practice due to hepatotoxicity concerns, as well as a cumbersome dose schedule that requires clients to take the AChE-I four times per day (Sedky, Nazir, Joshi, Kaur, & Lippmann, 2012).

Currently, the following three AChE-Is are commercially available: donepezil, galantamine, and rivastigmine. All are FDA approved for the treatment of Alzheimer's disease. All agents are available only in oral dosage formulations, with the exception of rivastigmine, which is also available as a once-daily transdermal patch (Cummings, 2004; Lexi-Comp, 2013).

The AChE-Is are associated with several adverse effects, precautions, interactions, and monitoring parameters that are important for their safe and effective use. Adverse effects common to all agents in this class include gastrointestinal complaints, such as nausea, vomiting, and diarrhea; potential weight loss; insomnia; and bradycardia (Cummings, 2004; Lexi-Comp, 2013). Bradycardia, an abnormally slow heart rate, is caused by enhanced cholinergic neurotransmission in the peripheral nervous system and may contribute to syncopal episodes or falls (Park-Wyllie et al., 2009). Cognitive and general functioning should be routinely assessed, and weight, gastrointestinal symptoms, and heart rate should be monitored periodically (Lexi-Comp, 2013).

Along with the AChE-Is, memantine is the only other FDA-approved medication for the treatment of Alzheimer's disease. Memantine is an antagonist at the N-methyl-D-aspartate receptor. Memantine is indicated for the treatment of moderate-to-severe Alzheimer's disease. It is available as immediate-release tablets, taken twice daily, or as extended-release tablets, taken once daily. Memantine is well tolerated with adverse effects consisting of constipation, dizziness, and headache. Less commonly reported adverse effects, such as hallucinations, have been associated with memantine use.

With only two classes of FDA-approved medications for the treatment of Alzheimer's disease, most clients will be considered for either AChE-I or N-methyl-D-aspartate receptor antagonist therapy at some point in time. Initially, clinicians should ensure that the physical causes of cognitive impairment, such as hypothyroidism, vitamin B12 deficiency, and folate deficiency, are monitored and corrected if needed (Slattum, Swerdlow, & Massey Hill, 2008). Acetylcholinesterase inhibitors, with the exception of tacrine, should be the initial pharmacotherapy interventions. Intolerable adverse effects to one agent do not preclude the use of other agents in the class. Similarly, if one agent is ineffective, switching to another AChE-I may be beneficial. Memantine is often added to AChE-I therapy in moderate-to-severe disease, and the concomitant use of both medications is common and well tolerated in clinical practice (Jones, 2010). Acetylcholinesterase inhibitors and memantine are neither disease modifying nor reverse disease progression; nevertheless, clinicians should ensure that dosages are maximized to achieve full therapeutic potential (Cummings, 2004). Other medications are used adjunctively, such as antipsychotics, for behavioral and psychological symptoms associated with Alzheimer's disease. Antipsychotic use in this client population constitutes off-label use and is associated with increased mortality; therefore, the judicious use of antipsychotics, as well as monitoring for adverse effects, is imperative (Rochon et al., 2008; Schneider, Dagerman, & Insel, 2005).

With so few pharmacotherapeutic options available, many clients or caregivers turn to complementary or alternative medicine to prevent or treat forms of dementia. Two of the most common and widely studied alternative therapy agents are vitamin E and Ginkgo biloba. Ginkgo biloba is the seventh most commonly used natural product in the United States (Barnes & Bloom, 2008). Multiple clinical trials have failed to show benefit with Ginkgo biloba in preventing or delaying cognitive decline (DeKosky et al., 2008; Dodge, Zitzelberger, Oken, Howieson, & Kaye, 2008; Snitz et al., 2009); furthermore, in one study, twice as many hemorrhagic strokes occurred with the use of Ginkgo biloba (DeKosky et al., 2008). Although this adverse effect was not clinically significant, more research is needed to investigate the safety of this approach to treatment. Vitamin E is a lipid-soluble vitamin and free radical scavenger. A large trial failed to show benefit with vitamin E therapy in clients with mild cognitive impairment (Petersen et al., 2005), although research is ongoing. In addition, a meta-analysis concluded that vitamin E supplementation greater than or equal to 400 IU/day for at least 1 year increased all-cause mortality (Miller et al., 2005). Due to the lack of established efficacy and potential safety concerns with both agents, neither Ginkgo biloba nor vitamin E can be recommended for preventing or treating Alzheimer's disease.

Pharmacotherapy for the treatment of Alzheimer's disease is an area of intense research. New medication classes that affect β-amyloid, such as secretase inhibitors, are currently under investigation (Ballard et al., 2011). Florbetapir F18, a radiopharmaceutical, was recently approved by the FDA. Florbetapir aids in the evaluation of cognitive decline by binding to β-amyloid plaques and estimating plaque density during positron emission tomography

EVIDENCE IN PRACTICE: DEMENTIA MEDICATIONS

Older people with dementia often display behavioral and psychological symptoms. Although nonpharmacologic strategies are the preferred method of treatment, antipsychotic medications are often used to manage aggression, agitation, hallucinations, and delusions. The evidence suggests that antipsychotic medications increase the risk of death when used to treat dementia-related psychosis; therefore, the lowest dose possible should be used for the shortest amount of time possible. The most common causes of death are cardiovascular (e.g., stroke) and infectious (e.g., pneumonia) in nature (Schneider, Dagerman, & Insel, 2005).

(Eli Lilly and Company, 2012). Currently, its use is not widespread in clinical practice. As more of the pathophysiology of Alzheimer's disease is discovered, medications with more specific targets of action and disease-modifying capabilities can be developed (Ballard et al.). The Evidence in Practice box provides added facts about medication for dementia.

Psychostimulants

Psychostimulants, or stimulant medications, are medications that are just that—stimulating. Psychostimulants will be discussed here, mainly for their role in treating ADHD. However, these medications may also be used to treat narcolepsy and depression. The focus in this chapter will be on two main classes of stimulants: mixed amphetamine salts and methylphenidate. In addition, this section will cover the following three nonstimulant medications: atomoxetine, clonidine, and guanfacine. Atomoxetine, clonidine, and guanfacine all work on the same neurotransmitter, NE, as psychostimulants; therefore, all three are also used for the treatment of ADHD.

Researchers who study ADHD have not yet uncovered a cause for the condition, but they have identified a few areas of the brain in which lack of attention, impulsivity, and hyperactivity appear to be involved (Sadock & Sadock, 2007b; Stahl, 2013). These areas of the brain utilize NE and DA, and the actions of these two chemicals appear to be involved in inattention, impulsivity, and hyperactivity. Genetics appear to play a role in the development of ADHD and its response to treatment, although specifics are not currently available and this information has not yet been helpful in selecting the best treatment option (Hodgkins, Shaw, Coghill, & Hechtman, 2012). Each of the medications that will be discussed have some action on NE, DA, or both (Sadock & Sadock, 2007b; Stahl, 2013). Slight differences exist between the methylphenidate and amphetamine classes of stimulants, so they will be discussed individually.

Methylphenidate is a stimulant that is believed to function by increasing the amount of NE and DA in synapses (Hodgkins et al., 2012; Stahl, 2013). This is accomplished by preventing the reuptake pumps from moving the NE or DA back into the neuron after they have been released (Hodgkins et al., 2012; Stahl, 2013). By increasing the NE and DA in the synapse, methylphenidate is able to act on the receptors and bring the neurons back into balance. This helps to prevent symptoms such as, among others, fidgeting, restlessness, lack of attention, and inability to finish tasks (Hodgkins et al, 2012; Stahl, 2013).

Various methylphenidate preparations are available. These contain the same active medication, but they differ in how long they take to start working and how long the effects of the medication last. Immediate-release tablets are available, which begin to dissolve when taken and take effect within the first 30 minutes and last for approximately 3 to 6 hours. Clients often need to take the medication two to three times daily to provide symptom control throughout the day (Lexi-Comp, 2013). The effects of Ritalin (methylphenidate) may last up to 8 hours, although it also usually requires two doses each day (Lexi-Comp, 2013). Extended-release capsules include Metadate CD (methylphenidate hydrochloride) and Ritalin LA, and their effects last up to 8 to 12 hours. Concerta (methylphenidate) is a delayed-release product whose effects can last up to 12 hours (Lexi-Comp, 2013). Quillivant XR (methylphenidate hydrochloride) is an extended-release suspension whose effects can last more than 15 hours (Tris Pharma, Inc., 2013). Daytrana (methylphenidate) is a patch that is recommended to be left on the skin for 9 hours.

When the patch is removed, the medication will continue to be active for a short time. If adverse effects, such as insomnia, are problematic, the patch can be removed sooner (Lexi-Comp, 2013). Because most of these preparations are extended or delayed-release, meaning the medication is not released and absorbed right away, it is important that the clients do not crush or chew the tablets or capsules and that the patch is not cut (Lexi-Comp, 2013). If any of these were to happen, a large amount of methylphenidate would be available and be absorbed by the client, likely resulting in high blood levels and adverse effects. The dosage form that is selected is individualized for each client, and no evidence that extended-release preparations are superior to immediate-release preparations are noted at this time (Hodgkins et al., 2012). The goal for some clients using extended-release or longer-acting preparations is to have methylphenidate in the body to last throughout the day to control symptoms during school or work, so the client can accomplish the tasks that are required of them.

Amphetamine salts are the other class of stimulant medications. This class has fewer agents than the methylphenidate class, but these agents have some other interesting differences. The amphetamine salts have been reported to block the reuptake of NE, DA, and 5HT (similar to methylphenidate), which increases the concentration of these chemicals in the synapse to continue to deliver their message to the next neuron (Hodgkins et al., 2012). The general effect is that there is an increase in NE and DA in the neurons to assist in controlling inattention, impulsivity, and hyperactivity (Hodgkins et al., 2012).

The amphetamine salt preparations that are available include dextroamphetamine and mixed amphetamine salt preparations. Another related product, lisdexamfetamine, is a **pro-drug** of dextroamphetamine. A pro-drug is one where the medication itself is not active but needs to be activated or converted to an active form by the body.

Medications in both the amphetamine and methylphenidate classes are controlled substances and have the potential to be addictive (Lexi-Comp, 2013). With their actions of increasing the available DA, it is possible that some of the DA is free to work on the reward pathway that may result in the misuse of the medication (Stahl, 2013). Studies have not shown that treatment with these stimulants increases the risk for children to develop a substance use disorder, and they actually seem to reduce the risk of developing a substance use disorder, compared with individuals with ADHD who did not receive treatment (Cortese et al., 2013). Abuse of these medications is a concern, but reports suggest that less than 15% of clients, and as low as 5% for school-aged children being treated, abuse their medications (Cortese et al., 2013). The immediate-release preparations are the most likely dosage form to be abused; therefore, use of some of the longer-acting agents may deter some of this misuse. Use of an agent such as lisdexamfetamine requires activation, and it is not active if injected or snorted, which can also help to further reduce these numbers. As a reminder, if the long-acting dosage forms are crushed or chewed, higher doses of stimulant may be ingested, potentially resulting in significant toxicity.

Increased blood pressure and heart rate are potential concerns with stimulant medication use (Cortese et al., 2013; Lexi-Comp, 2013). This increase in blood pressure is due to the blood vessels being constricted or the tightening of smooth muscle around the blood vessel tube, causing the tube to become smaller. Think about the blood vessels like a garden hose; if there is water going through a large hose, the water comes out but not with an incredible amount of force. If you put the same amount of water through a smaller hose, it will come out at a much higher pressure. With this higher pressure in the blood vessels, the heart often needs to work harder and faster, which can put stress on the heart itself. Linked to these effects are rare cases of heart attack, stroke, and sudden death, outcomes that have been seen mainly in individuals using stimulant medications who had heart problems (Lexi-Comp, 2013). However, in most clients, the increase in blood pressure and heart rate is minor and does not cause problems (Cortese et al., 2013).

Loss of appetite has been reported in up to 30% of children on stimulants and is a common concern of parents. Most trials are of short duration, so it is difficult to determine whether this attenuation of appetite is lost over time, but notably, this effect appeared to occur even at relatively small doses (Cortese et al., 2013). To assist with the lack of appetite, it is recommended that stimulants be given after a meal, and it is suggested to have a later evening meal when the effects of the medication may be lower, compared with concentrations throughout the rest of the day (Cortese et al., 2013). No clear evidence exists of whether lowering the dose of the medication, changing to another medication, or providing drug holidays (days on the weekends where the client does not take the stimulant) can help with the adverse effects of loss of appetite, and decisions should be made on an individual basis regarding how to proceed (Cortese et al., 2013).

Growth delays have also been associated with the use of stimulant medications. A review of 18 studies of stimulants found there were deficits in the height and weight of clients who were taking stimulants. Within 2 years following discontinuation of the stimulant medication, studies further indicated that the height and weight deficits were no longer apparent (Cortese et al. 2013).

By increasing NE and DA, the goal is to help the client to be more attentive, which may also result in being more awake and alert. Therefore, it should not be a surprise that these medications can cause insomnia or difficulty sleeping, and more than 10% of clients taking stimulants have reported difficulty sleeping as an adverse effect (Cortese et al., 2013; Lexi-Comp, 2013). Many clients also report that they have difficulty falling asleep. Lowering the dose of the client's stimulant or changing to a preparation that does not last as long may help to alleviate this problem (Cortese et al., 2013). Counseling the client about good sleep habits or sleep hygiene is also recommended for all clients on stimulants (Cortese et al., 2013).

Another common concern of the use of stimulants is the possibility of worsening a tic disorder. A variety of different tics may occur. During childhood, tics may develop and then improve. Often, they are influenced by other factors, including emotions or stress, so the relationship of tics with stimulants is difficult to clearly measure. Current evidence suggests that stimulant use is not associated with the new development of a tic disorder (Cortese et al., 2013). Information for clients with a preexisting tic disorder is a little more muddled. It does not appear that use of stimulants, especially methylphenidate, worsen tics for these clients, but there have been reports of high-dose amphetamine preparations worsening tics in some clients; therefore, further investigation is needed to more solidly understand this relationship (Bloch, Panza, Landeros-Weisenberger, & Leckman, 2009; Cortese et al., 2013). Should a client with a tic disorder experience a worsening of their tics, decreasing the dose of the stimulant or potentially changing the stimulant to methylphenidate is suggested (Bloch et al., 2009; Cortese et al., 2013).

Three other agents that are not stimulants but are used to treat ADHD and seem to fit best into this section will be discussed. These medications include atomoxetine, and the alpha agonists, clonidine and guanfacine.

Atomoxetine is FDA approved for the treatment of ADHD and is often used as a first-line option for adults who have ADHD. It works by blocking the reuptake of NE, resulting in higher concentrations of NE to act on the receptors (Lexi-Comp, 2013; Stahl, 2013). With limited actions on the DA reward system (the nucleus accumbens), the potential for abusing atomoxetine is quite low (Stahl, 2013). The lack of abuse potential is an advantage of atomoxetine, but a disadvantage of its use is that the benefits of improving ADHD symptoms are usually not seen for 2 to 4 weeks after starting treatment. Because ADHD is a condition that may be problematic for many years, clients may be on atomoxetine for an extended period of time.

Atomoxetine is well absorbed, so it is easy to get into the body. Common adverse effects experienced by clients taking atomoxetine include headache, insomnia, drowsiness, dry mouth, nausea, abdominal pain, decreased appetite, and vomiting (Lexi-Comp, 2013). Most of these adverse effects subside within the first few weeks of treatment. An overlap of the symptoms of liver toxicity, such as headache, abdominal pain, and vomiting, may be noted; therefore, if any of these adverse effects are severe, the client should be encouraged to contact his or her physician. Norepinephrine plays a role in moods and thinking. Although not a common side effect, if clients develop any significant changes in mood or thoughts, including thoughts about suicide, they should contact their physician. This is most likely to occur during the first months of therapy.

The last class of medications discussed in this section is the alpha agonists, specifically clonidine and guanfacine. Alpha agonists are not used as first-line treatment for ADHD. They are typically reserved for clients who are not able to take other medications for ADHD or who have not responded to other treatments, such as stimulants, atomoxetine, or antidepressants (Pliszka et al., 2006). These alpha agonists specifically work on α_2 receptors. Two medications are included in this class: clonidine and guanfacine. It is thought that clonidine is more likely to sit on the receptors that are responsible for blood pressure and sedation changes, which is why adverse effects seem to be more likely with clonidine than with guanfacine.

Both clonidine and guanfacine are available as immediate-release and extended-release preparations. The immediate-release preparations are sometimes used in addition to stimulants in clients who may have symptoms after their stimulant wears off but cannot use higher doses of stimulant or longer-acting agents due to insomnia concerns (Pliszka et al., 2006). Clonidine and guanfacine are well absorbed and metabolized. The main concern is in regard to drug interactions in clients using another medication that may lower blood pressure, resulting in dizziness when they stand up quickly, increasing the risk of falling (Lexi-Comp, 2013).

Adverse effects seen with the alpha agonists include sedation, dizziness, low blood pressure, headache, constipation, dry mouth, and fatigue (Lexi-Comp, 2013). Changes in heart rate or heart rhythms may occur; therefore, it is important to be cautious when using these products in individuals with heart problems (Lexi-Comp, 2013). Clients who take clonidine or guanfacine may develop a tolerance to the blood pressure lowering effects of these medications, meaning that the clients' bodies can become used to having the medication, and they no longer experience low blood pressure. Although this sounds like a good thing, it is something to be mindful of because the body compensates by increasing the pressure of the blood vessels to offset the effects of the medication. Should the clonidine or guanfacine be abruptly stopped, the client may develop significantly elevated blood pressure. This is true even of the clonidine patch, which is applied once weekly. Therefore, these clients should be reminded to ensure they take their medications regularly and, if they plan on stopping their medications,

CASE VIGNETTE: PSYCHOSTIMULANTS

Marvin is an 8-year-old boy who has been diagnosed with attention-deficit/hyperactivity disorder—hyperactive type. He is described as an active child who has a difficult time staying engaged in any task, waiting his turn, or sitting still. This has caused significant problems with his teachers and his parents, as testing has shown that he is able to cognitively perform the school work required of him, but he cannot control himself enough to sit still and complete any of the assignments. Despite having an individualized education plan and contingency chart, Marvin continues to demonstrate symptoms that are disruptive, which have left him with few friends and struggling academically. His parents reluctantly agree to start medication, and he is placed on Concerta (methylphenidate). Both his parents and teachers see a change immediately in his ability to concentrate, socialize, and complete his school work. At their 2 month follow-up appointment, Marvin's mother is pleased with his progress, but, unfortunately, he has difficulty settling down in the evening to go to sleep, and often his parents will find him up after 11 o'clock as they go to bed.

THOUGHT QUESTIONS

1. Please name at least five adverse effects that are associated with the use of methylphenidate.
2. What are three options that can help Marvin with his insomnia?
3. How might this medication assist Marvin in his school and home life?

to speak with the pharmacist and physician so this may be accomplished safely. Monitoring of the alpha agonists includes watching blood pressure and heart rate, as well as the client's adherence with medications. The Case Vignette discusses the use of psychostimulants.

Substance-Related Disorder Medications

As is discussed in Chapter 17, occasionally the use of alternative medications is needed to help clients who are suffering from substance-related disorders. The focus of this section will be on medications that are predominantly used for the treatment of substance-related disorders, specifically alcohol-related disorders, opiate-related disorders, and tobacco-related disorders. A common theme seen in this section is that the treatments for these disorders often compete with the abused substance (i.e., alcohol, heroin, or tobacco) to block or diminish its effects.

The discussion will begin with the treatment of alcohol addiction and specifically the use of acamprosate, disulfiram, and naltrexone. These are not all of the medications that may be used to treat alcohol addiction, but they are three unique classes that are commonly utilized. Each of these treatments is used to help clients remain abstinent from alcohol. However, these are not medications used as a client is withdrawing from alcohol, and it should be noted that abrupt discontinuation of alcohol in a client who has been regularly ingesting it in large amounts may be dangerous. Some of the most significant and potentially fatal effects of withdrawal are seizures or neurological damage as a result of nutritional deficiencies, mainly folic acid and thiamine (O'Brien, 2011).

Acamprosate is often used in clients who are not currently using alcohol to assist with cravings for alcohol. The full extent of its efficacy is unclear, and further research is being performed to determine how effective acamprosate is in helping clients to abstain.

Acamprosate is given as two tablets three times daily, so clients take a large number of tablets for this regimen (Forest Laboratories, Inc., 2013). Clients may take this medication for extended periods of time. Adverse effects most often occur when clients are starting the medication and include diarrhea, nausea, depression, and anxiety (Forest Laboratories, Inc., 2013). Data from the trials of acamprosate and a placebo showed that clients seemed to tolerate acamprosate quite well, and the number of clients who stopped taking acamprosate or the placebo were similar (Forest Laboratories, Inc., 2013). Compared with placebo pills, a greater number of clients taking acamprosate experienced suicidal thoughts, attempted suicide, or completed suicide, so any changes in behaviors should be monitored for and reported back to the client's health care team (Forest Laboratories, Inc., 2013).

Disulfiram is often helpful for clients who require a deterrent to alcohol use. It irreversibly inhibits an enzyme, aldehyde dehydrogenase, which plays a role in the metabolism of alcohol (Stahl, 2013; TEVA Pharmaceuticals, 2011b). Clients who take disulfiram and then drink alcohol feel warm or flushed; they often have nausea and vomiting, develop a headache, and experience low blood pressure and dizziness or unsteadiness on their feet (Stahl, 2013; TEVA Pharmaceuticals, 2011b). Severe reactions with disulfiram have resulted in slowed breathing; heart problems, including arrhythmias or a heart attack; seizures; loss of consciousness; and death (TEVA Pharmaceuticals, 2011b). The mild-to-moderate effects are designed to provide the client with a negative experience as a result of drinking alcohol, thus helping them to refrain from using alcohol, and effects may occur as long as there is medication in the client's bloodstream (TEVA Pharmaceuticals, 2011b). One obvious catch is that the client needs to take the medication for it to be effective, and adherence is often a problem. Clients can be continued on disulfiram for months or years until they are able to abstain from alcohol use without the assistance of disulfiram (TEVA Pharmaceuticals, 2011b).

Clients who are started on disulfiram should not have alcohol in their system to avoid the development of the adverse effects, as they may be associated with taking the medication instead of being associated with the ingestion of alcohol (TEVA Pharmaceuticals, 2011b). Serious adverse effects that have been reported with the use of disulfiram include inflammation of nerves, which may result in visual changes, pain, tingling, or numbness, and any new sensations a client develops should be reported to his or her physician for further investigation (TEVA Pharmaceuticals, 2011b). It is worth reminding clients that alcohol may be present in some over-the-counter cough and cold products, which may result in an unintentional reaction.

Naltrexone is the last medication to be discussed in regard to the treatment of alcohol use. This medication works differently from the first two mentioned in this section. A client taking naltrexone will not feel the full pleasurable effect or high of alcohol. It is recommended that clients who may be using opiates be given a test dose before starting treatment. If treatment is for alcohol with no opiate use, a test dose is not required (Mallinckrodt, Inc., 2011).

Clients may use this medication for an extended period of time to assist with abstaining from substance use. Naltrexone tablets have been shown to decrease heavy drinking, but it may be a struggle for clients to make the decision every day to take the naltrexone. The long-acting naltrexone injection may be more helpful in these situations. The injection of naltrexone is given once monthly. It has been shown to improve drinking outcomes in clients who were trying to abstain and were well tolerated by clients (Mannelli, Peindl, Masand, Patkar, 2007; Roozen, de Waart, & van den Brink, 2007).

Adverse effects associated with naltrexone are thought to be mild, and they subside with continued use. Most commonly reported adverse effects include headache; nausea; dizziness;

nervousness; fatigue; sleep changes, with both insomnia or sedation occurring; anxiety; and vomiting (Mallinckrodt, Inc., 2011). Liver damage has also been reported to occur in conjunction with high doses of naltrexone. The monthly naltrexone injection has also been associated with injection site pain and a decrease in platelets, which may result in some clients bruising or bleeding more easily (Alkermes, Inc., 2013). The use of naltrexone tablets or injection with other medications is generally safe, with the exception of opiate pain medications, which act on the same receptor as naltrexone and will not be as effective (Mallinckrodt, Inc., 2011). Clients who are using naltrexone and planning to undergo a surgery that will require strong pain medication use, such as an opiate, will need to let their health care providers know so that a plan for tapering or discontinuing naltrexone can be developed.

Naltrexone is a good pivot point to direct the discussion from alcohol addiction to opiate addiction, although there is overlap with the treatments of some of these conditions. Specific treatments for opiate addiction include methadone, buprenorphine, and naloxone. Unlike the treatments for alcohol addiction, these medications for opiate addiction are more closely related in the way they work, with each having activity on the opiate receptors.

Methadone is a commonly used medication for the treatment of opiate addiction. Methadone is an opiate that binds to opiate receptors (Stahl, 2013). It may seem curious that a client would use an opiate to treat opiate addiction. Methadone can compete with other opiates to occupy the opiate receptors, so even if a client takes another opiate, such as heroin or morphine, they will likely not experience the pleasurable sensations they were anticipating. However, pain relief as a result of taking the methadone may still occur (Bart, 2012). A restriction on the use of methadone for clients with opiate addiction is the fact that clients need to attend a clinic or treatment facility every day to receive their methadone dose, a strategy required to minimize abuse of the methadone itself. Although clients may by maintained on the medication for months or years, they will need to continue to visit these facilities to continue therapy, which may be problematic for some clients.

Safety concerns are significant with the use of methadone. Cardiac arrhythmias; low blood pressure, including dizziness; decreased breathing frequency; and concerns regarding decreased movement in the gastrointestinal tract are all potential adverse effects (Roxane Laboratories, Inc., 2013). The most common adverse effects experienced by clients taking methadone include lightheadedness, dizziness, sedation, nausea, vomiting, and sweating (Roxane Laboratories, Inc., 2013). A number of interactions with other medications and methadone have been documented (Lexi-Comp Online, 2013). Medications that change the metabolism of methadone are concerning, as are other medications that are sedating, which may decrease the breathing frequency of clients, especially individuals with lung disorders, and medications that change the heart rhythms (Roxane Laboratories, Inc., 2013).

Buprenorphine is available as two related but slightly different products that are used for the treatment of opiate addiction: buprenorphine alone and a buprenorphine/naloxone combination. Buprenorphine is an opiate with activity at the opiate receptors (Roxane Laboratories, Inc., 2012a; Stahl, 2013). By binding to the receptors, buprenorphine can keep the abused substances from working, while also keeping withdrawal symptoms from occurring in the client (Bart, 2012). The potential exists that clients will try to misuse the buprenorphine to get a rush or high from it. To accomplish this, clients may consider crushing and injecting the buprenorphine to get a faster effect. To keep this from occurring, a combination product has been developed that includes buprenorphine and naloxone. Naloxone is an opiate receptor antagonist or blocker, meaning it will keep any opiate from acting on the opiate receptor (Bart, 2012). The combination tablets contain a low dose of naloxone, and if the tablet is taken by mouth the body then gets rid of the naloxone before it can block the actions of buprenorphine (Bart, 2012).

Buprenorphine is available as tablets for use under the tongue (called sublingual tablets), as an injectable solution, or as a patch. Sublingual tablets are the main preparation used for maintenance therapy in clients with opiate addiction. Injectable solution and patches are approved for the treatment of pain and are not often used in treatment regimens for opiate addiction. The tablets are dissolved under the client's tongue, and the medication is absorbed through the mouth. It is important that the clients do not swallow the tablets because although the medication would be absorbed, it would be metabolized so quickly that the client would not have much effect from the tablet (Bart, 2012).

Adverse effects most commonly experienced by clients include headache, pain, diarrhea, insomnia, and rhinitis (Roxane Laboratories, Inc., 2012a). Other serious adverse effects with buprenorphine include liver damage. The recommended monitoring of clients taking buprenorphine includes watching for symptoms of withdrawal and adverse effects and getting blood work done to monitor liver function (Roxane Laboratories, Inc., 2012a).

Agents used to treat tobacco or nicotine addiction are the last class of medications discussed in the substance-related disorders section. Tobacco use continues to be a major concern, and the obstacles clients face when attempting to quit tobacco use often result in their turning to pharmacologic treatment to help them succeed. Nicotine, which is an addicting substance found in tobacco products, has been found to enter the body and work on ACh receptors (Stahl, 2013). Medications that will be covered in this section include varenicline and nicotine replacement products. Bupropion is also used as a tobacco cessation agent.

Varenicline is a common option for clients who are trying to quit smoking. It is a prescription medication. The specifics of how varenicline work are still unclear. It appears to diminish the pleasure that clients receive from smoking cigarettes and decreases the cravings for nicotine, while diminishing the withdrawal symptoms associated with smoking cessation (Smith Connery & Kleber, 2007).

Nausea is one of the most common adverse effects of varenicline, so clients are started on low doses and slowly titrated up to their full dose of 1 mg twice daily over the first week (Pfizer, Inc., 2013). Over the first few days when a client takes varenicline, he or she may want to take the medication at bedtime or with food to minimize the nausea. Other common adverse effects reported include constipation, flatulence, and vomiting, which may subside as the client becomes used to the medication (Pfizer, Inc., 2013). Abnormal dreams or dreams that are strange or vivid and sleep disturbances have also been reported with varenicline (Pfizer, Inc., 2013). Clients who experience changes in mood, such as agitation, hostility, or depressed mood or thoughts, should contact their health care providers (Pfizer, Inc., 2013). Allergic reactions, such as swelling of the lips or face and rash, have been reported, although rarely, shortly after a client starts taking the medication (Pfizer, Inc., 2013).

Clients who opt not to use varenicline may turn to nicotine replacement therapy. This group of medications refers to a number of different products that are available for purchase over-the-counter without a prescription and that provide for the delivery of nicotine to the body (Stahl, 2013). The nicotine from these products is able to activate the ACh receptors, resulting in DA release that is thought to assist with curbing the cravings and withdrawal symptoms (Stahl, 2013). The amount of nicotine delivered by these products is designed to be lower than that provided by smoking cigarettes, and it can be slowly titrated down until the client has no nicotine in his or her system and no longer experiences the discomfort of cravings or withdrawals (Stahl, 2013). Numerous different nicotine replacement products are available that can be used, including patches, gum, lozenges, nasal sprays, and inhalers. All of these preparations deliver nicotine directly and begin to work with the first dose of the medication (GlaxoSmithKline Consumer Healthcare, 2011, 2012; Pharmacia & Upjohn Company, 2008, 2010; Stahl, 2013).

CLINICAL PEARL: SUBSTANCE-RELATED DISORDERS

Opiate medications, such as methadone and buprenorphine, can be used to treat opiate addiction. They also can be used to treat pain and may be addicting themselves. If a client decides to ingest additional opiates, such as heroin or morphine, with the methadone or buprenorphine, he or she may experience significant adverse effects, including sedation and slowed breathing, which can be life threatening.

Nicotine patches are used to deliver nicotine throughout the day in a consistent manner, whereas gum, lozenges, nasal spray, and inhalers have more intermittent delivery (Benowitz, 2009). This plays a role, as the patch is applied once daily, whereas the other products need to be utilized on a scheduled basis to ensure that they are helpful in assisting with the cravings and withdrawal symptoms that clients may experience (Benowitz, 2009; Stahl, 2013). It is important that clients are clear on what to expect from these products to achieve the greatest amount of success (Benowitz, 2009). It is not uncommon for clients to use more than one type of nicotine replacement product, such as a daily patch in conjunction with the gum if they need an extra boost for a craving throughout the day (Benowitz, 2009).

Proper use of these products is important to ensure the greatest benefit. For example, nicotine gum should be chewed until a peppery or tingly taste is detected, then the gum should be 'parked' or placed between the cheek and the gum so the nicotine can be absorbed by the tissue in the mouth (GlaxoSmithKline Consumer Healthcare, 2012). Also, it is recommended that clients do not eat or drink for 15 minutes before chewing the gum (GlaxoSmithKline Consumer Healthcare, 2012). The duration of use of any of the products is dependent on how long the client needs extra assistance in remaining abstinent from tobacco products.

Adverse effects of the patches include skin irritation, whereas gum and lozenges may cause abnormal tastes. Nicotine itself may result in increases in blood pressure or heart rate, so clients with heart problems should use the lowest possible dose and be monitored for any changes. The Clinical Pearls box provides added information about medications for substance-related disorders.

Summary: Psychopharmacology and Occupational Therapy

This chapter has described a wide range of psychotropic medications. The list continues to grow as research offers new substances that may improve symptomatic outcomes or reduce some of the many side effects that characterize these drugs. One important message to take away is that, to some extent, identifying the most helpful medication for a given individual may be as much art as science. Much remains to be learned about how these drugs work, why one might be more effective for an individual as compared to another, possibly very similar, medication, and how to ameliorate the side effects that reduce a client's motivation to sustain a medication plan (see Appendix A).

On the basis of this discussion, a number of clear roles are apparent for occupational therapists and COTAs. Like every member of the treatment team, the occupational therapist must be alert to emerging side effects (e.g., noticing jaundice that might signify a liver ailment) and to a client's ability (or lack of ability) to manage the prescribed medication regimen. Some clients with mental disorders may not be able to report these factors accurately, so much of the responsibility falls on the caregivers who see the client more frequently than might the physician. The occupational therapist might also be involved in helping clients manage their medication schedules. In addition, all members of the team must be alert to the signs of suicidal ideation, a side effect seen with numerous psychotropic medications. Chapter 6 describes strategies for managing suicidal ideation and behavior.

Second, occupational therapists and COTAs must be alert to side effects that might affect the intervention. Unsteady balance or tremors that might contribute to falls must be monitored and considered in the activity choices. Clients who experience sleepiness or fuzzy cognition as a result of medication might not be ideal candidates for activities that require use of sharp implements.

A unique role for the occupational therapist is in assessing the impact of the medications in addressing symptoms, especially functional symptoms. As demonstrated throughout the discussion of the various mental disorders, dysfunction is a common symptom. The occupational therapist is best prepared to evaluate function and to note changes in the individual as medication begins to have impact. Chapters 22 and 23 will describe this role in greater detail. As noted throughout this chapter, improvement in functional ability is one of the most important signs to indicate that the chosen medications are having the desired effect. Hence, the occupational therapist and COTA become important informants as the physician and client work together to identify a successful medication plan.

Internet Resources

American Psychiatric Association
http://www.psych.org

As the primary organization for psychiatrists who bear responsibility for prescribing psychotropic medications, the American Psychiatric Association provides a great deal of information about medications, including continuing education offerings and news items about medications.

Centers for Disease Control and Prevention (CDC)
http://www.cdc.gov

The CDC receives reports of adverse effects of medications and maintains databases on an array of information about mental disorders and their treatment.

U.S. Food and Drug Administration (FDA)
http://www.fda.gov

The FDA is responsible for approving new medications, and monitoring those in use for adverse effects, manufacturing defects, and other concerns regarding use. The FDA website provides helpful information about the drug approval process and their strategies for protecting consumers.

CASE STUDY

L.T. is a 37-year-old White man who was diagnosed with schizophrenia approximately 17 years ago. He has required multiple inpatient psychiatric hospitalizations in the past, and has undergone trials of numerous antipsychotic medications, including haloperidol, quetiapine, and the long-acting paliperidone injection. L.T.'s medical records indicate that each trial of an antipsychotic medication was adequately dosed and was of sufficient duration. Pharmacy records indicate the client routinely refills his prescriptions every month. Despite three trials, the client continues to have persistent negative symptoms, including apathy, social withdrawal, and emotional blunting. L.T. has not worked since he was first diagnosed with a mental illness. Recently, his mother, who is his main support system, was placed in a nursing home following a stroke. His father has type 2 diabetes mellitus, which has led to end-stage renal disease. L.T. has two older sisters who are busy with their teenage children and adjusting to their mother's illness.

L.T. comes to his psychiatric appointment accompanied by a mental health case manager. His appearance is noted as disheveled. His case manager reports that L.T. smokes approximately one pack of cigarettes per day. He denies alcohol and illicit substance use. He is generally cooperative with the examination, but verbal and motor responses are slow. At the time of the visit, his physical examination and laboratory findings are all within normal limits. Due to his incomplete response to earlier trials of several antipsychotic medications, the psychiatrist initiates clozapine therapy.

One year later, L.T. comes to his psychiatric appointment, again accompanied by his mental health case manager. The clozapine has been titrated to 300 mg twice per day. Due to the risk of agranulocytosis, L.T. continues to have his blood drawn every week, and all blood cell count values are normal. The psychiatrist notes L.T.'s excellent response to treatment. He is no longer apathetic and is much more communicative. He is able to use public transportation and visits his mother weekly in the nursing home. His sisters have noticed a significant difference in his behavior, and the three of them have lunch together once per month. His volunteer position at a local library evolved into a part-time paid position. He takes great pride in his job and is very pleased with the additional freedom his earned income has provided.

Despite the robust response to clozapine therapy, he is unhappy with the considerable adverse effects caused by the medication. He experiences substantial sedation, orthostatic hypotension (which resulted in a fall one night while going to the lavatory), and constipation. He reports the sedation and orthostatic hypotension have somewhat lessened with time, but he requires occasional laxatives for the constipation. Finally, although considerably more active since starting the clozapine, he is not happy with the weight he has gained since starting the medication. He reports that he does not exercise regularly, and he eats mostly fast food and frozen, pre-prepared meals. After 1 year of clozapine therapy, his physical examination and laboratory findings show his blood pressure has increased, as has his fasting blood glucose levels. He has gained approximately 25 pounds. L.T. presents to his psychiatric appointment with a request to change his antipsychotic medication, because he states, "I do not want to be fat."

(continued)

CASE STUDY (CONTINUED)

THOUGHT QUESTIONS

1. What nonpharmacologic strategies may be useful for managing the side effects of these medications?
2. What is the role of the occupational therapist in helping the client and his physician manage his medications?
3. Are there strategies the occupational therapist might suggest that would address the client's concern about increased weight gain?
4. How might these medications affect the client's function?
5. How might these medications affect the treatment plan developed by the therapist and client?

References

AbbVie, Inc. (2013, May). Depakote [package insert]. North Chicago, IL: Author.

Alkermes, Inc. (2013, July). Vivitrol [package insert]. Waltham, MA: Author.

American Diabetes Association. (2004). Consensus development conference on antipsychotic drugs and obesity and diabetes. *Journal of Clinical Psychiatry, 65*, 267-272.

American Psychiatric Association. (2004). Practice guideline for the treatment of patient with schizophrenia. *American Journal of Psychiatry, 161*, 1-56.

Atmaca, M. (2009). Valproate and neuroprotecetive effects for bipolar disorder. *International Review of Psychiatry, 21*, 410-413.

Ballard, C., Gauthier, S., Corbett, A., Brayne, C., Aarsland, D., & Jones, E. (2011). Alzheimer's disease. *Lancet, 377*, 1019-1031.

Barnes, P. M., & Bloom, B. (2008). Complementary and alternative medicine use among adults and children: United States, 2007, 12, 1-23. http://www.cdc.gov/nchs/data/nhsr/nhsr012.pdf

Barrett, K.E., Boitano, S., Barman, S.M., & Brooks, H.L. (Eds.) (2012). *Ganong's review of medical physiology* (24th ed.). New York, NY: McGraw-Hill. Retrieved from http://accessmedicine.mhmedical.com/book.aspx?bookid=393.

Bart, G. (2012). Maintenance medication for opiate addiction: The foundation of recovery. *Journal of Addictive Disorders, 31*, 207-225.

Benowitz, N.L. (2009). Pharmacology of nicotine: Addiction, smoking-induced disease and therapeutics. *Annual Review of Pharmacology and Toxicology, 49*, 57-71.

Bloch, M.H., Panza, K.E., Landeros-Weisenberger, A., & Leckman, J.F. (2009) Meta-analysis: Treatment of attention-deficit/hyperactivity disorder in children with comorbid tic disorders. *Journal of the American Academy of Child and Adolescent Psychiatry, 48*, 884-893.

Braun, P., Greenberg, D., Dasberg, H., & Lerer, B. (1990). Core symptoms of posttraumatic stress disorder unimproved by alprazolam treatment. *Journal of Clinical Psychiatry, 51*, 236-238.

Cada, D.J., Levien, T., & Baker, D.E. (2006). Ramelteon. *Hospital Pharmacy, 41*, 59-69.

Capriani, A., Furukawa, T.A., Salanti, G., Geddes, J.R., Higgins, J.P.T., Churchill, R., . . . Barbui, C. (2009). Comparative efficacy and acceptability of 12 new-generation antidepressants: A multiple-treatments meta-analysis. *Lancet, 373*, 746-758.

Caroff, S.N., Miller, D.D., Dhopesh, V., & Campbell, E.C. (2011). Is there a rational management strategy for tardive dyskinesia? *Current Psychiatry, 10*, 23-32.

Cates, M.E., Bishop, M.H., Davis, L.L., Lowe, J.S., & Woolley, T.W. (2004). Clonazepam for treatment of sleep disturbances associated with combat-related posttraumatic stress disorder. *The Annals of Pharmacotherapy, 38*, 1395-1399.

Cavallari, L.H., & Lam, W.F. (2011). Chapter 9: Pharmacogenetics. In J.T. DiPiro, R.L. Talbert, G.C. Yee, G.R. Matzke, B.G. Wells, & L.M. Posey (Eds.), *Pharmacotherapy: A pathophysiologic approach* (8th ed.). New York, NY: McGraw-Hill.

Chouinard, G. (2004). Issues in the clinical use of benzodiazepines: Potency, withdrawal, and rebound. *Journal of Clinical Psychiatry, 65*(Suppl. 5), S7-S12.

Connolly, K.R., & Thase, M.E. (2011). The clinical management of bipolar disorder: A review of evidence-based guidelines. *Primary Care Companion for CNS Disorders, 13*(4), pii. doi:10.4088/PCC.10r01097.

Cortese, S., Holtmann, M., Banaschewski, T., Buitelaar, J., Coghill, D., Danckaerts, M., . . . Sergeant, J. (2013). Practitioner review: Current best practice in the management of adverse events during treatment with ADHD medications in children and adolescents. *Journal of Child Psychology and Psychiatry, 54*, 227-246.

Cowan, C.C. (2002). The process of evaluating and regulating a new drug: Phases of a drug study. *Journal of the American Association of Nurse Anesthetists, 70*, 385-390.

Crismon, M.L., Argo, T.R., & Buckley, P.F. (2008). Schizophrenia. In J.T. DiPiro, R.L. Talbert, G.C. Yee, G.R. Matzke, B.G. Wells, & L.M. Posey (Eds.), *Pharmacotherapy: A pathophysiologic approach* (pp. 1099-1122). New York, NY: McGraw-Hill.

Cummings, J.L. (2004). Alzheimer's disease. *New England Journal of Medicine, 351*, 56-67.

DeKosky, S.T., Williamson, J.D., Fitzpatrick, A.L., Kronmal, R.A., Ives, D.G., Saxton, J.A., . . . Furberg, C.D. (2008). Ginkgo biloba for prevention of dementia: A randomized controlled trial. *JAMA, 300*, 2253-2262.

Dodge, H.H., Zitzelberger, T., Oken, B.S., Howieson, D., & Kaye, J. (2008). A randomized placebo-controlled trial of Ginkgo biloba for the prevention of cognitive decline. *Neurology, 70*, 1809-1817.

Doyle, M., & Rosenthal, L.J. (2013). Psychotropic medications, associated QTc prolongation, and sudden cardiac death: A review for clinicians. *Psychiatric Annals, 43*, 58-65.

Drayton, S.J. (2011). Chapter 78: Bipolar disorder. In J.T. DiPiro, R.L. Talbert, G.C. Yee, G.R. Matzke, B.G. Wells, & L.M. Posey (Eds.), *Pharmacotherapy: A pathophysiologic approach* (8th ed.). New York, NY: McGraw-Hill.

Earley, C.J. (2003). Restless legs syndrome. *New England Journal of Medicine, 348*, 2103-2109.

Eli Lilly and Company. (2012, April). Amyvid [package insert]. Indianapolis, IN: Author.

Eli Lilly and Company. (2013, July). Prozac [package insert]. Indianapolis, IN: Author.

Fava, M., Rush, A.,J., Trivedi, M.H., Nierenberg, A.A., Thase, M.E., Sackeim, H.A., . . . Kupfer, D.J. (2003). Background and rationale for the sequenced treatment alternatives to relieve depression (STAR*D) study. *The Psychiatric Clinics of North America, 26*(2), 457-494.

Forest Laboratories, Inc. (2013, August). Acamprosate [package insert]. Inwood, NY: Author.

Frampton, J.E., & Foster, R.H. (2006). Pregabalin in the treatment of generalised anxiety disorder. *CNS Drugs, 20*, 685-693.

Freedman, R. (2003). Schizophrenia. *New England Journal of Medicine, 349*, 1738-1749.

Gillman, P.K. (2010). Neuroleptic malignant syndrome: Mechanisms, interactions, and causality. *Movement Disorders, 25*, 1780-1790.

GlaxoSmithKline. (2011, December). Lamictal [package insert]. Research Triangle Park, NC: Author.

GlaxoSmithKline Consumer Health. (2011). Nicoderm CQ [package insert]. Moon Township, PA: Author.

GlaxoSmithKline Consumer Health. (2012). Nicorette [package insert]. Moon Township, PA: Author.

Henderson, D.C., & Doraiswamy, P.M. (2008). Prolactin-related and metabolic adverse effects of atypical antipsychotic agents. *Journal of Clinical Psychiatry, 69*(Suppl. 1), 32-44.

Hodgkins, P., Shaw, M., Coghill, D., & Hechtman, L. (2012). Amfetamine and methylphenidate medications for attention-deficit/hyperactivity disorder: Complementary treatment options. *European Child and Adolescent Psychiatry, 21*, 477-492.

Iqbal, M.M., Basil, M.J., Kaplan, J., & Iqbal, T. (2012). Overview of 5HT syndrome. *Annals of Clinical Psychiatry, 24*, 310-318.

Jones, R.W. (2010). A review of comparing the safety and tolerability of memantine with the acetylcholinesterase inhibitors. *International Journal of Geriatric Psychiatry, 24*, 547-553.

Kane, J.M., & Correll, C.U. (2010). Past and present progress in the pharmacologic treatment of schizophrenia. *Journal of Clinical Psychiatry, 71*, 1115-1124.

Kane, J.M., & Garcia-Ribera, C. (2009). Clinical guideline recommendations for antipsychotic long-acting injections. *British Journal of Psychiatry, 52*, 63-67.

Katzung, B.G. (2012). Development & regulation of drugs. In B.G. Katzung, S.B. Masters, & A.J. Trevor (Eds.), *Basic and clinical pharmacology* (pp. 69-77). New York, NY: McGraw-Hill.

Krishnan, K.R. (2006). Monoamine oxidase inhibitors. In A.F. Schatzberg & C.B. Nemeroff (Eds.), *Essentials of clinical psychopharmacology* (pp. 113-126). Washington, DC: American Psychiatric.

Lexi-Comp Online. (2013, August 1). *Lexi-Drugs Online™*. Hudson, Ohio: Author.

Liou, S.Y., Stringer, F., & Hirayama, M. (2012). The impact of pharmacogenomics research on drug development. *Drug Metabolism and Pharmacokinetics, 27*, 2-8.

Loane, C., & Politis, M. (2012). Buspirone: What is it all about? *Brain Research, 1461*, 111-118.

Longo, L.P., & Johnson, B. (2000). Addiction: Part I. Benzodiazepines—Side effects, abuse risk and alternatives. *American Family Physician, 61*, 2121-2128.

López-Muñoz, F., Álamo, C., & García-García, P. (2011). The discovery of chlordiazepoxide and the clinical introduction of benzodiazepines: Half a century of anxiolytic drugs. *Journal of Anxiety Disorders, 25,* 554-562.

Malhi, G.S., Tanious, M., Das, P., Coulston, C.M., & Berk, M. (2013). Potential mechanisms of action of lithium in bipolar disorder. *CNS Drugs, 27,* 135-153.

Mallinckrodt, Inc. (2011, April). Naltrexone [package insert]. Hazelwood, MO: Author.

Mancuso, C.E., Tanzi, M.G., & Gabay, M. (2004). Paradoxical reactions to benzodiazepines: Literature review and treatment options. *Pharmacotherapy, 24,* 1177-1185.

Mannelli, P., Peindl, K., Masand, P.S., & Patkar, A.A. (2007). Long-acting injectable naltrexone for the treatment of alcohol dependence. *Expert Review of Neurotherapeutics, 7,* 1265-1277.

Marder, S.R., & Wirshing, D.A. (2006). Clozapine. In A.F. Schatzberg & C.B. Nemeroff (Eds.), *Essentials of clinical psychopharmacology* (pp. 229-244). Washington, DC: American Psychiatric.

McKnight, R.F., Adida, M., Budge, K., Stockton, S., Goodwin, G.M., & Geddes, J.R. (2012). Lithium toxicity profile: A systematic review and meta-analysis. *Lancet, 379,* 721-728.

McNamara, J.O. (2011). Chapter 21. Pharmacotherapy of the epilepsies. In L.L. Brunton, D.K. Blumenthal, N. Murri, R. Hilal-Dandan, & B.C. Knollmann (Eds.), *Goodman & Gilman's the pharmacological basis of therapeutics* (12th ed.). New York, NY: McGraw-Hill.

Melton, S.T., & Kirkwood, C.K. (2008). Anxiety disorders I: Generalized anxiety, panic, and social anxiety disorder. In J.T. DiPiro, R.L. Talbert, G.C. Yee, G.R. Matzke, B.G. Wells, & L.M. Posey (Eds.), *Pharmacotherapy: A pathophysiologic approach* (pp. 1209-1228). New York, NY: McGraw-Hill.

Meyer, J.M. (2011). Chapter 16: Pharmacotherapy of psychosis and mania. In L.L. Brunton, D.K. Blumenthal, N. Murri, R. Hilal-Dandan, & B.C. Knollmann (Eds.), *Goodman & Gilman's the pharmacological basis of therapeutics* (12th ed.). New York, NY: McGraw-Hill.

Miller, E.R., Pastor-Barriuso, R., Dalal, D., Riemersma, R.A., Appel, L.J., & Guallar, E. (2005). Meta-analysis: High-dosage vitamin E supplementation may increase all-cause mortality. *Annals of Internal Medicine, 142,* 37-46.

Moriarty, K.M., Alagna, S.W., & Lake, C.R. (1984). Psychopharmacology: A historical perspective. *Psychiatric Clinics of North America, 7,* 411-433.

Muench, J., & Hamer, A.M. (2010). Adverse effects of antipsychotic medications. *American Family Physician, 81,* 617-622.

National Health Interview Survey. (2012). *Health 3.A. Emotional and behavioral difficulties: percentage of children ages 4 – 17 reported by a parent to have serious or minor difficulties with emotions, concentration, behavior, or getting along with other people by selected characteristics, 2001-2011* [Data file]. Retrieved from http://www.childstats.gov/americaschildren/tables/health3a.asp.

Novartis Pharmaceuticals Corporation. (2011, March). Oxcarbazepine [package insert]. East Hanover, NJ: Author.

O'Brien, C.P. (2011). Chapter 24: Drug addiction. In L.L. Brunton, D.K. Blumenthal, N. Murri, R. Hilal-Dandan, & B.C. Knollmann (Eds.), *Goodman & Gilman's the pharmacological basis of therapeutics* (12th ed.). New York, NY: McGraw-Hill.

Park-Wyllie, L., Mamdani, M.M., Li, P., Gill, S.S., Laupacis, A., & Juurlink, D.N. (2009). Cholinesterase inhibitors and hospitalization for bradycardia: A population-based study. *PLoS Medicine, 6,* 1-9.

Petersen, R.C., Thomas, R.G., Grundman, M., Bennett, D., Doody, R., Ferris, S., . . . Thal, L.J. (2005). Vitamin E and donepezil for the treatment of mild cognitive impairment. *New England Journal of Medicine, 352,* 2379-2388.

Pfizer, Inc. (2013, February). Chantix [package insert]. New York, NY: Author.

Pfizer, Inc. (2009, July). Minipress [package insert]. New York, NY: Author.

Pharmacia & Upjohn Company. (2008, December). Nicotrol inhalant [package insert]. New York, NY: Author.

Pharmacia & Upjohn Company. (2010, June). Nicotrol NS [package insert]. New York, NY: Author.

Pliszka, S.R., Crismon, M.L., Hughes, C.W., Conners, C.K., Emslie, G.J., Jensen, P.S., . . . Lopez, M. (2006). The Texas children's medication algorithm project: Revision of the algorithm for pharmacotherapy of attention-deficit/hyperactivity disorder. *Journal of the American Academy of Child and Adolescent Psychiatry, 45,* 642-657.

Raskind, M.A., Peskind, E.R., Hoff, D.J., Hart, K.L., Holmes, H.A., Warren, D., . . . McFall, M.E. (2007). A parallel group placebo controlled study of prazosin for trauma nightmares and sleep disturbances in combat veterans with post-traumatic stress disorder. *Biological Psychiatry, 61,* 928-934.

Ravindran, L.N., & Stein, M.B. (2010). The pharmacologic treatment of anxiety disorders: A review of progress. *Journal of Clinical Psychiatry, 71,* 839-854.

Reeves, W.C., Strine, T.W., Pratt, L.A., Thompson, W., Ahluwalia, I., Dhingra, S.S., . . . Safran, M.A. (2011). Mental illness surveillance among adults in the United States. *Morbidity and Mortality Weekly Report, 60,* 1-32. Retrieved from http://www.cdc.gov/mmwr/pdf/other/su6003.pdf.

Rickels, K., DeMartinis, N., Rynn, M., & Mandos, L. (1999). Pharmacologic strategies for discontinuing benzo-diazepine treatment. *Journal of Clinical Psychopharmacology, 19*(Suppl. 2), S12-S16.

Rochon, P.A., Normand, S.L., Gomes, T., Gill, S.S., Anderson, G.M., Melo, M., . . . Gurwitz, J.H. (2008). Antipsychotic therapy and short-term serious events in older adults with dementia. *Archives of Internal Medicine, 168*, 1090-1096.

Roth, T. (2007). Narcolepsy: Treatment issues. *Journal of Clinical Psychiatry, 10*(Suppl. 13), 16-19.

Roozen, H.G., de Waart, R., & van den Brink, W. (2007) Efficacy and tolerability of naltrexone in the treatment of alcohol dependence: Oral versus injectable delivery. *European Addiction Research, 13*, 201-206.

Roxane Laboratories, Inc. (2012a, September). Buprenorphine [package insert]. Columbus, OH: Author.

Roxane Laboratories, Inc. (2012b, October). Lithium carbonate [package insert]. Columbus, OH: Author.

Roxane Laboratories, Inc. (2013, April). Methadone [package insert]. Columbus, OH: Author.

Sadock, B.J., & Sadock, V.A. (2007a). Chapter 3: The brain and behavior. In B.J. Saddock, V.A. Saddock, & P. Ruiz (Eds.), *Kaplan & Sadock's synopsis of psychiatry: Behavioral sciences/clinical psychiatry* (10th ed.). Philadelphia, PA: Lippincott Williams & Wilkins.

Sadock, B.J., & Sadock, V.A. (2007b). Chapter 43: Attention-deficit disorder. In B.J. Saddock, V.A. Saddock, & P. Ruiz (Eds.), *Kaplan & Sadock's synopsis of psychiatry: Behavioral sciences/clinical psychiatry* (10th ed.). Philadelphia, PA: Lippincott Williams & Wilkins.

Schneier, F.R. (2006). Social anxiety disorder. *New England Journal of Medicine, 355*, 1029-1036.

Schneider, L.S., Dagerman, K.S., & Insel, P. (2005). Risk of death with atypical antipsychotic drug treatment for dementia: Meta-analysis of randomized placebo-controlled trials. *JAMA, 294*, 1934-1943.

Schutte-Rodin, S., Broch, L., Buysse, D., Dorsey, C., & Sateia, M. (2008). Clinical guideline for the evaluation and management of chronic insomnia in adults. *Journal of Clinical Sleep Medicine, 4*, 487-504.

Sedky, K., Nazir, R., Joshi, A., Kaur, G., & Lippmann, S. (2012). Which psychotropic medications induce hepatotoxicity? *General Hospital Psychiatry, 34*, 53-61.

Silber, M.H. (2005). Chronic insomnia. *New England Journal of Medicine, 353*, 803-810.

Slattum, P.W., Swerdlow, R.H., & Massey Hill, A. (2008). Alzheimer's disease. In J.T. DiPiro, R.L. Talbert, G.C. Yee, G.R. Matzke, B.G. Wells, & L.M. Posey (Eds.), *Pharmacotherapy: A pathophysiologic approach* (pp. 947-962). New York, NY: McGraw-Hill.

Smith, R.G. (2003). Fall-contributing adverse effects of the most frequently prescribed drugs. *Journal of the American Podiatric Medical Association, 93*, 42-50.

Smith Connery, H., & Kleber, H.D. (2007). Guideline Watch: Practice guideline for the treatment of patients with substance use disorders, 2nd edition. In *American Psychiatric Association Practice Guidelines for the Treatment of Psychiatric Disorders*. Arlington, VA: American Psychiatric Association.

Snitz, B.E., O'Meara, E.S., Carlson, M.C., Arnold, A.M., Ives, D.G., Rapp, S.R., . . . DeKosky, S.T. (2009). Ginkgo biloba for preventing cognitive decline in older adults: A randomized trial. *JAMA, 302*, 2663-2670.

Stahl, S.M. (2013). *Stahl's Essential Psychopharmacology: Neuroscientific Basis and Practical Applications.* New York, NY: Cambridge University Press.

Taro Pharmaceuticals U.S.A., Inc. (2013, April). Carbamazepine [package insert]. Hawthorne, NY: Author.

TEVA Pharmaceuticals. (2011a, November). Clozapine [package insert]. Sellersville, PA: Author.

TEVA Pharmaceuticals. (2011b, March). Disulfiram [package insert]. Sellersville, PA: Author.

Tris Pharma, Inc. for Pfizer Inc. (2013, February). Quillivant XR [package insert]. Monmouth Junction, NJ: Author.

U.S. Food and Drug Administration. (2007). *FDA requests label change for all sleep disorder drug products* [Data file]. Retrieved from http://www.fda.gov/newsevents/newsroom/pressannouncements/2007/ucm108868.htm.

U.S. Food and Drug Administration. (2013). *Drug safety communication—FDA requires lower recommended doses* [Data file]. Retrieved from http://www.fda.gov/safety/medwatch/safetyinformation/safetyalerts-forhumanmedicalproducts/ucm334738.htm.

Woolcott, J.C., Richardson, K.J., Wiens, M.O., Patel, B., Marin, J., Khan, K.M., & Marra, C.A. (2009). Meta-analysis of the impact of 9 medication classes on falls in elderly patients. *Archives of Internal Medicine, 169*, 1952-1960.

Evaluation of Occupational Performance Deficits in Mental Health

Learning Outcomes

By the end of this chapter, readers will be able to:

- Describe the steps in the occupational therapy process

- Define evaluation

- Describe steps in the occupational therapy evaluation process

- Discuss the factors involved in establishing adequate psychometric properties in standardized assessments

- Discuss the purpose of screening

- Describe mechanisms for evaluating the various elements of occupational performance for individual clients

- Describe mechanisms for evaluating environmental factors that relate to occupational performance

Bonder B.
Psychopathology and Function, Fifth Edition (pp 457-480).
© 2015 SLACK Incorporated.

KEY WORDS

- Function
- Evaluation
- Assessment
- Goal attainment scaling
- Occupational profile
- Screening
- Psychometric properties
- Reliable
- Valid

- Norm-referenced
- Criterion referenced
- Floor effect
- Ceiling effect
- Habits
- Routines
- Roles
- Rituals

CASE VIGNETTE, MR. SHIMBIR (PART 1)

Abdi Shimbir is a 34-year-old Somali immigrant to the United States. Mr. Shimbir relocated from Somalia in 2010, following his uncle, who arrived in the United States one decade earlier as a refugee from the Somali civil war. Both have settled in Minneapolis, Minnesota, one of the communities with a significant number of Somali refugees. Mr. Shimbir, like his uncle before him, wanted to leave behind the instability of the political and economic unrest that continued to plague his home country. In Somalia, Mr. Shimbir was a farmer. He arrived in the United States knowing no English and with very few possessions. He was allowed into the country only because of his uncle's presence and promise to help him.

Mr. Shimbir had a difficult time in Somalia before being able to leave. He spent time in refugee camps, often without enough to eat and with little to occupy his time. He was under pressure to join one or another of the warring factions in the camps. When he arrived in the United States, he was anxious and had frequent nightmares, which have continued during his time in the United States. He sometimes becomes agitated when leaving his apartment.

The Somali community in Minneapolis has been welcoming, but Mr. Shimbir's adjustment has been difficult. He has struggled to learn the English language. He has been unable to find work, in part because of his struggles with learning English and in part because of his limited skills and education.

THOUGHT QUESTIONS

1. What do you think a psychiatrist might focus on in the above description to assist Mr. Shimbir with his adjustment?
2. Do you think Mr. Shimbir might have an identifiable mental disorder? If so, what might it be?
3. What do you think an occupational therapist might want to know about Mr. Shimbir and his situation to determine whether occupational therapy intervention would be helpful? How does this differ from the psychiatrist's focus?

The previous chapters have detailed the diagnosis of mental disorders from a medical perspective, or, more specifically, a psychiatric perspective. As presented, the emphasis for diagnoses in the *Diagnostic and Statistical Manual of Mental Disorders* (DSM) is on disordered thought, emotion, and behavior. Functional difficulties, on the other hand, are stated in the most general terms (usually, difficulty with function, with particular attention to social and occupational performance; American Psychiatric Association [APA], 2013). It is not typical for a psychiatric or psychological evaluation to emphasize detailed understanding of activities in the workplace or at home. Occupational therapists play a vital role in helping individuals diagnosed with mental disorders to address those essential—but sometimes overlooked—areas of their lives. Improvement in the ability to perform home and workplace activities can lead to the individual's better overall function, as well as improving general mental health.

Occupational therapists focus on "the therapeutic use of everyday life activities (occupations) with individuals or groups for the purpose of enhancing or enabling participation in roles, habits, and routines in home, school, workplace, community, and other settings" (American Occupational Therapy Association [AOTA], 2014, p. S1). To do this, occupational therapists must have a clear picture of the precise nature of the occupations in which the individual needs and wants to participate, as well as the strengths of that individual and the challenges he or she face to participate successfully. Occupational therapists evaluate and treat **function**, defined as "a person's ability to perform a specific daily life activity" (Doucet & Gutman, 2013, p. 7). This definition of function is quite different from the medical definition, which focuses on cellular and organ-level activity of the body, and for this reason, the occupational therapy evaluation has a very different structure.

It is helpful to be aware of the terminology that describes the process of gathering information. **Evaluation** is the overall process of gathering and analyzing information in preparation for development of an intervention strategy (AOTA, 2010). **Assessment** refers to the specific instruments or tools, usually standardized, that contribute information to the evaluation. The evaluation process is typically a combination of interview and discussion with the client; administration of standardized evaluations; and use of other strategies, such as goal attainment scaling and observation of performance.

It is important not only to gather initial information but to identify strategies for reevaluating the individual's performance periodically; first, to alter an intervention as needed and second, to assess the extent to which the intervention has ultimately been successful. Some instruments lend themselves to repeated administration and are sufficiently sensitive to provide such information, but other measurement strategies may also be required.

Strategies other than the administration of standardized instruments may also be helpful. For example, **goal attainment scaling** is a method that focuses on the measurement of individual goals (Doig, Fleming, Kuipers, & Cornwell, 2010). The client and therapist together identify a behavioral statement as a goal. Then, after a period of intervention, they determine whether the outcome is much better, better, the same, worse, or much worse than expected. A score is attached to each of these outcomes so that an overall assessment of progress can be made.

However, some difference of opinion exists in the profession about whether the evaluation should start with the occupational profile ("top down") or with understanding of body impairments ("bottom up"; Doucet & Gutman, 2013). This discussion has been ongoing for decades. However, according to Doucet and Gutman (2013), the most essential factor in evaluation is meeting the client's needs. It can be argued that the *Occupational Therapy Practice Framework: Domain and Process* (AOTA, 2014) has weighed in on the value of a top down approach by emphasizing the importance of the **occupational profile**.

The occupational profile clarifies characteristics of the client and his or her activities. As described in the *Practice Framework* (AOTA, 2014, p. S13), the occupational profile is designed to address the following questions:

- Why is the client seeking service, and what are the client's current concerns relative to engaging in occupations and in daily life activities?

- In what occupations does the client feel successful, and what barriers are affecting his or her success?
- What aspects of his or her environments or contexts does the client see as supporting engagement in desired occupations, and what aspects are inhibiting engagement?
- What is the client's occupational history (i.e., life experiences)?
- What are the client's values and interests?
- What are the client's daily life roles?
- What are the client's patterns of engagement in occupations, and how have they changed over time?
- What are the client's priorities and desired targeted outcomes related to occupational performance, prevention, participation, role competence, health and wellness, quality of life, well-being, and occupational justice?

When the broad parameters of the client's needs have been identified, an analysis of occupational performance follows, exploring occupations, client factors, performance skills, performance patterns, and contexts and environments (AOTA, 2014). Note that this process is identical regardless of the medical (including psychiatric) diagnosis of the client. Although knowing the medical diagnosis may give the therapist some clues about the kinds of performance problems to expect, occupational performance is often only loosely associated with diagnosis. For example, if a referral is made to an occupational therapist for intervention with a child who has an intellectual disability, the therapist would expect some limitations in cognitive skills, possibly some delay in the development of motor skills, and the potential for difficulties with communication and social skills. However, the diagnosis would not provide information about the child's abilities, interests, and current activities.

Individuals with severe psychiatric disorders may lead lives that are both satisfying and filled with occupational accomplishments. Some examples of such accomplishments are as follows:

- An individual with schizophrenia is also an accomplished psychiatrist and founding member of an advocacy organization for individuals with mental health problems
- A well-known actress must be hospitalized from time to time for treatment of her bipolar disorder
- An individual with a chronic substance abuse problem is a noted country western singer
- A NASA astronaut has clinical depression
- A billionaire businessman has dyslexia

These are a few examples from a long list that demonstrates the importance of emphasizing strengths as well as deficits. In each of these situations, having only the psychiatric diagnosis could lead a therapist to anticipate a very different set of outcomes for these individuals, all of whom are well-known, well-regarded, and very accomplished. For this reason and for many others, a comprehensive occupational therapy evaluation is central to positive outcomes for the client.

Selecting Assessments

Occupational therapists utilize numerous measurement strategies. These should be selected for a given client based on what information is needed to create a helpful plan for intervention and the best strategies for obtaining the needed information.

An initial step is **screening**, a process that identifies whether a given individual needs more extensive evaluation and what areas might need to be examined most closely. For example, because a significant number of older adults have some degree of cognitive impairment that can affect self-care and other performance, a therapist might administer one of the many brief screening instruments for cognitive impairment (e.g., the Mini-Mental State Examination; Folstein, Folstein, & McHugh, 1975). If the individual shows significant deficits on the screening instrument, a more extensive evaluation might be implemented to provide more information about the degree of cognitive impairment and the specific nature of the deficits. On the other hand, if the individual shows no significant problems on the screening, it may be possible to move on to evaluate other important aspects of function.

A detailed evaluation process may involve both less formal mechanisms, such as the interview and observation of a client (Shotwell, 2014), and conversation with family members, employers, and others who may have helpful information (assuming the client agrees to these contacts). Such strategies tend to be nonstandardized in the sense that their administration is unique to the particular situation, no standard scoring system is applied, and their psychometric properties have not been measured. However, these strategies are often structured, such as in the case of lists of relevant factors for discussion with the client or specific areas of performance to be observed. Also, a growing number of standardized instruments are available that focus on informant or proxy evaluation through verbal report from those close to the client. Among these is the Family/Collateral Interview (Mundt, Freed, & Griest, 2000), which asks family members to identify changes in occupations and behaviors of individuals suspected of having Alzheimer's disease.

Standardized instruments can provide much, if not all, of the information needed to construct an occupational profile and to determine the skills, client factors, and contextual factors that can contribute to successful occupational performance. These assessments have the advantage of providing a structured method for gathering the relevant information, as they have been developed over time with attention to **psychometric properties** (Classen & Velozo, 2014). This means that the instruments have been designed so that the results are **reliable** (consistent across time and raters) and **valid** (measure what they purport to measure; Lorch & Herge, 2007). Selection of an instrument will depend on the precise nature of the information needed.

In some situations, occupational therapists may want to be able to compare a client's performance with that of a broader population. This would require an instrument that is **norm-referenced** (e.g., Bayley Scales of Infant and Toddler Development, third edition; Bayley, 2005). Norm-referenced instruments provide information about comparable groups of people and the range of their scores. On the other hand, it may be more important to be able to compare the client's performance with a needed level of performance, regardless of how others might perform. In this case, the appropriate instrument would be one that is **criterion referenced** (e.g., Assessment of Motor and Process Skills [AMPS]; Fisher & Bray Jones, 2012, and its companion for school aged clients [Munkholm, Berg, Löfgren, & Fisher, 2010]). These instruments provide information about scores as they relate to task performance, rather than to other individuals. It is important to know how sensitive the instrument is to change, as it is easy to misunderstand a client's characteristics if the instrument is a relatively insensitive one. It is also important to know whether the instrument has a **floor** or **ceiling effect**; that is, measures accurately only to a particular level of ability. For example, a test might be able to measure a particular kind of performance in an average range but not for people who are exceptionally able (ceiling effect) or have particularly significant deficits (floor effect).

The following section is a description of the evaluation process as it relates to occupational performance. Most often—although not always—the client comes to occupational therapy because of a physician referral; thus, some medical or psychiatric diagnosis has already been

ANALYZING PSYCHOMETRIC PROPERTIES OF AN INSTRUMENT

Charlie Adams is an 8-year-old boy who has been diagnosed with autism. His parents have chosen to have him attend a regular school where he has a personal aide in the classroom. Charlie has good math skills, although reading is challenging for him. He struggles with social interactions as well. Knowing that participation in recreational activities is an important aspect of occupational participation, the occupational therapist working with Charlie decides that assessment of this aspect of occupation is essential. He examines a number of instruments for this purpose and decides on the Children's Assessment or Participation and Enjoyment/Preference for Activities of Children (CAPE/PAC; King et al., 2004).

The therapist thought this might be a useful instrument because it appeared to be an effective mechanism for exploring the aspect of occupation that he felt needed assessment and because it was neither norm nor criterion referenced. Instead, it appeared to be designed to gather the kind of individualized information he wanted to obtain about Charlie's interests.

A careful review of the literature reveals that the CAPE/PAC was originally developed for children with physical disabilities. This causes the occupational therapist some concern because an instrument that has been designed for one population may not automatically measure other populations effectively, and its measurement properties will not apply to Charlie's assessment. Further exploration reveals that the CAPE/PAC has been studied for use with individuals with high functioning autism after its initial development (Potvin, Snider, Prelock, Kehayia, & Wood-Dauphinee, 2013).

Potvin et al. (2013) found that for children with high functioning autism, test–retest reliability was in the 0.7 range (of a possible 1.0). The children who participated in the study were able to respond to the questions, and there was reasonably good agreement between parents' ratings and children's self-ratings of enjoyment. This last finding was supportive of the content validity of the instrument.

The therapist concluded that the instrument was satisfactory for purposes of his evaluation with Charlie.

THOUGHT QUESTIONS

1. Test–retest reliability in the 0.7 range is considered moderate. Do you agree that this was adequate in this situation? Why or why not?
2. What areas of occupation do you think will need to be assessed in other ways, given the nature of Charlie's situation?
3. Why might it be problematic to use an instrument developed for another population?

made. The therapist must use that information, along with her or his understanding of human occupation, to determine the client's current occupational profile and to help the client establish an occupational profile that is meaningful, satisfying, and meets his or her basic needs (Schindler, 2010). Each area of occupational performance listed in the *Practice Framework* (AOTA, 2014) will be discussed, with emphasis on how the occupational therapy evaluation complements and supplements the psychiatric diagnostic process.

A listing of some of the instruments used for an occupational therapy evaluation can be found in Appendix B. For additional information about the many instruments that are applicable to various aspects of occupational performance, please see the resources list at the end of this chapter.

Occupational Profile

Many therapists complete occupational profiles largely through discussion with clients (Shotwell, 2014). Structured interviewing can yield a picture of the client's activities, preferences, and concerns; however, there are several limitations to the approach. The first is the possibility that some critical information will be overlooked. Another is that the quality of the information obtained relies heavily on the therapist's interviewing and recording skills. In addition, this method requires that the client is able and willing to be responsive and that he or she has the insight and awareness to respond accurately. In settings where the presenting symptoms are related to cognition and emotion, these conditions may not be met. Cultural differences and/or language differences can contribute to misunderstanding or can limit the therapist's ability to obtain sufficiently detailed information.

Numerous structured or standardized instruments are available that can help to address these concerns and allow the therapist to obtain a comprehensive assessment. One of these is the Canadian Occupational Performance Measure ([COPM] Law et al., 2005). An advantage of the COPM for use in clinical practice is that it yields both descriptive information and a numerical score. The former is helpful to the therapist and client in designing the intervention and the latter can provide a concrete measure of progress—evidence that is often important to third-party payers.

As has been demonstrated throughout this text, family interactions contribute significantly to mental health and mental disorders. Thus, when it is feasible, understanding the individual's occupations in the context of the family can be helpful. An instrument like the Family Routines Inventory (Jensen, James, Boyce, & Hartnett, 1983) can provide both general information about family-related occupations and a sense of the routines that are important to the family.

In some situations where the individual is not able to provide such information, family members may be able to assist (e.g., by using the Alzheimer's Disease-Related Quality of Life assessment instrument; Kasper, Black, Shore, & Rabins, 2009). If this proxy strategy is used, it must be completed with considerable caution because family members may have different perceptions of the issues around the client and from each other, they may not know the client well, and because family members may themselves have psychological or emotional difficulties.

Occupations

A comprehensive occupational profile will provide information that directs analysis of occupational performance (AOTA, 2014). The analysis examines occupations, client factors, activity demands, performance patterns, performance skills, and contexts and environments. Each of these factors contributes to one's overall ability to participate in occupations. Both the client's strengths and deficits in each area must be explored. Examining the client's strengths can help to direct the intervention toward a focus on those occupations that he or she both enjoys and does well. Understanding of performance challenges can identify areas for intervention to remediate client factors, alter activity demands, or modify the context in which the occupation occurs.

Figure 22-1. Performance and skills are most helpfully evaluated in the client's environment. (©2014 Shutterstock.com.)

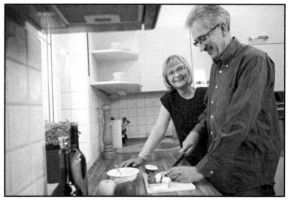

Occupations include necessary activities, such as self-care, sleep, and work, as well as activities that are more self-selected and directed, such as play and leisure. Understanding a client's occupations may begin with an open-ended interview that asks the client to elaborate on aspects of the occupational profile to provide details about what he or she does currently, how this differs from some previous point in life, and what he or she needs and wants to do. For individuals with psychiatric disorders, their changes from past to present (and those desired in the future) can be particularly significant. As noted, a variety of psychiatric conditions interfere with the expanding of performance skills (e.g., intellectual disorders) and many interfere with current performance (e.g., depression, schizophrenia, anxiety disorders, among others). Instruments such as the COPM (Law et al., 2005) can be used to guide the conversation for a less formal, but still structured, interview.

Among the questions that need to be addressed is which of these occupations are essential to a particular individual. Almost all individuals need to accomplish at least some activities of daily living (ADL), although, depending on the situation, support from someone else may be needed. For example, an individual with Alzheimer's disease may ultimately be unable to manage bathing, dressing, and perhaps even eating. In such a case, it would be important to first establish what the individual is still capable of and, second, what areas will require caregiver assistance. It can be particularly helpful to observe the client's occupational performance in his or her environment (Figure 22-1). Evaluation of ADL using the AMPS has shown that deficits occur similarly across disorders, which is further evidence of the differences between DSM diagnoses and occupational therapists consideration of functional performance (Moore, Merritt, & Doble, 2010).

Performance and skills are most helpfully evaluated in the client's environment. Some individuals may have sufficient limitations to make some instrumental activities of daily living (IADL) difficult. A young adult with serious developmental delay may not be able to acquire the skills to manage finances. Education as a major occupation often ends in adolescence and young adulthood, meaning that it may not be a part of the occupational profile for older individuals. In addition, some situations exist in which an individual with a mental disorder may be unable or unwilling to work. If she or he has some other means of financial support, work may be an optional activity for him or her. For example, an individual with schizophrenia may have sufficient deficits that make managing a job impossible, and financial support may be available through Social Security Disability (Social Security Disability Help, 2013) or other governmental support programs. Keep in mind that an individual who is not able to work must establish other occupational interests to support a meaningful life.

On the other hand, rest and sleep are never optional. Everyone needs to participate in these occupations, and difficulties in doing so may actually make various mental disorders worse

(Kållestad et al., 2012) by increasing lethargy, anxiety, and cognitive problems. Likewise, everyone needs to participate, to at least some extent, in play, leisure, and social occupations. Failure to do so contributes to depression and anxiety while greatly diminishing quality of life (Iwasaki, Coyle, & Shank, 2010).

Although education must be considered in children and adolescents, work will be an important area of focus for some adolescents and for many adults. Difficulties in work performance may not be strictly within the control of the individual. Individuals with mental disorders may be excluded from full participation as a result of social stigma, not incapacity (Pescosolido, Medina, Martin, & Long, 2013). This can contribute to the individual's stress level, causing performance to deteriorate further.

Boredom is a significant factor in mental disorders (Carriere, Cheyne, & Smilek, 2008). In particular, there is an association between boredom and depression, although it is not clear which precedes which. This finding supports the importance of understanding work, play, and leisure as vital areas of occupation. Careful evaluation to determine the extent of which individuals are engaged or isolated can make a difference in terms of both the structure of intervention and its success.

To fully understand the individual's participation in various occupations, evaluation needs to focus not only on what the individual needs and wants to do but also on the factors that interfere with participation. During the evaluation of performance areas, it is important to begin to assess the reasons for which participation is challenging. Is it the individual's mental disorder's associated cognitive symptoms that make concentration at work difficult? If so, further evaluation of cognitive skills will be useful. Do the client's paranoid delusions lead to social difficulties? If so, social skills will require additional evaluation. Have the medications being taken to reduce hallucinations caused tardive dyskinesia or other motor problems? In this case, careful evaluation of motor skills would be necessary. Are there situational issues— lack of social support, difficult employer—that contribute to performance deficits? If so, evaluation of the environment is essential.

Numerous occupational therapy evaluation instruments can examine the aspects of occupational performance. Instruments such as the Children's Leisure Assessment Scale (Rosenblum, Sachs, & Schreuer, 2010), the Child Occupational Self Assessment (Kramer, Kielhofner, & Smith, 2010), the Practical Skills Test (Chang, Helfrich, & Coster, 2013), and the Health Enhancement Lifestyle Profile (Hwang, 2009) evaluate aspects of performance that may be overlooked by other disciplines but are central to the creation of satisfying occupational profiles. Appendix B lists some of these instruments. The Sample Evaluation Plan box provides an example of how a therapist might plan an evaluation of areas of occupation.

Client Factors

Values, Beliefs, Spirituality

A focus on values when working with clients is essential (Erlandsson, Eklund, & Persson, 2011) and represents a central concern for occupational therapy evaluation. Evaluation of values, beliefs, and spirituality can be done through interview. There are also a variety of value orientation instruments and instruments that gather information about spirituality. Therapists need to know how clients feel about particular areas of occupation, those they value most highly, and what values contribute to those perceptions. For example, an individual who values independence might be more inclined toward a work occupation that does not involve routine, such as a creative career like writing or painting.

SAMPLE EVALUATION PLAN: AREAS OF OCCUPATION

Ms. Mason is a 27-year-old accountant who was diagnosed with obsessive-compulsive disorder (OCD) 10 years ago. During her years of education, she found strategies for managing her disorder through a combination of cognitive–behavioral therapy and medication. Ms. Mason recently passed the certified public accountant examination and has just been hired by a large accounting firm. On her first day of work, she stood at the door to the office suite, stepping in and out of the door repeatedly. When she was finally able to enter, she made her way to her office where she spent the remainder of her first day filing and refiling two memos from human resources about her benefits. On her second day, she never reached the office because she was unable to finish dressing due to changing her clothing multiple times and putting each discarded garment in the washing machine.

Ms. Mason has returned to her psychiatrist for assistance in managing her exacerbated symptoms as she makes this life transition to a new job. The psychiatrist prescribes sertraline (Zoloft), and makes a referral to an occupational therapist.

The therapist administers the following instruments to assess Ms. Mason's status and needs:

Occupational Profile:
- Canadian Occupational Performance Measure (Law et al., 2005)
- Interview

Occupations:
- ADL: Executive Function Performance Test (Baum et al., 2008)
- IADL: Modified Assessment of Living Skills and Resources: Revised 2 (Clemson, Bundy, Unsworth, & Singh, 2009).
- Rest and sleep: Occupational Profile of Sleep (Pierce & Summers, 2011)
- Work: Interview
- Play and leisure: Interest checklist (Matsutsuyu, 1969, in Rogers, Weinstein, & Figone, 1978)
- Social participation: Interview

During the course of the evaluation, the therapist finds that Ms. Mason is able to identify a constellation of activities that she enjoys and values. In general, she is able to support her ADL and IADL, although she occasionally takes a long time to complete cleaning tasks. She enjoys accounting and was initially excited about her new job. However, through their conversation and her completion of the standardized instruments, a significant distance was identified between her usual and effective work activities and her current status.

The therapist concludes, with Ms. Mason's agreement, that she has an occupational profile that reflects satisfying engagement in meaningful occupations and that she has many strengths in areas of occupation. However, she is currently struggling in the area of work, and further evaluation is required to ascertain how to best address this concern. We will return to this case later to examine what other factors were evaluated and how the deficits that were identified contribute to Ms. Mason's current situation.

Beliefs may be personal or more culturally mediated. In the *Practice Framework* (AOTA, 2014), cultural factors are incorporated into the contexts category. However, it is worthwhile to point out that every aspect of a client's occupational performance has at least some cultural influences (see Bonder & Martin, 2013 for elaboration on this issue). Personal beliefs may come from family influences, life experience, or inherent personality traits. As has been demonstrated in previous chapters, some beliefs may be a direct consequence of a psychiatric condition. For example, individuals with paranoid personality disorder or paranoid schizo-phrenia have very firm, but dysfunctional, beliefs about their relationships with others.

Evaluation of spirituality and interventions focused on these occupations has received increasing emphasis in occupational therapy (Bonder, 2010). Participation in religious activities can have a positive impact on some aspects of mental health (Cornah, 2006; Royal College of Psychiatry, 2010). For example, regular attendees at religious institutions have lower rates of depression and stress (Cornah, 2006). On the other hand, some mental disorders have a negative relationship with religion, as in the case of individuals with schizophrenia or bipolar disorder with religious delusions (Barber, 2013). Both helpful and damaging involvement with spiritual occupations must be evaluated and considered in framing intervention strategies. For an older man struggling with depression, strategies to facilitate his return to previous religious involve-ment may be a source of great comfort, whereas in an individual dealing with religious delu-sions associated with paranoid schizophrenia, identifying other activities that can provide social support without reinforcing those delusions may be essential. It is helpful to keep in mind that spirituality may be expressed in ways that do not involve participation in formal religious occu-pations. Understanding a client's spirituality and spiritual/religious preferences can be obtained through interview or through standardized assessments such as the COPM (Law et al., 2005).

Body Functions

Physicians, physical therapists, physician assistants, and nurses typically begin their evaluation processes with a focus on body functions. For instance, in a mental health context, evaluation might include a blood test to measure thyroid disorders that might contribute to depression (American Academy of Child & Adolescent Psychiatry, 2012). However, for occupational therapists, these body functions are relevant only as they affect the client's abil-ity to accomplish occupations. Therefore, an occupational therapy evaluation might focus on specific mental functions, such as attention, memory, and perception (AOTA, 2014). These affect the client's ability to dress, cook, or perform a job.

Consider a young woman who presents with severely restricted food intake and an intense fear of gaining weight. These are among the symptoms of anorexia nervosa, as described in Chapter 12. The physician will be concerned with identifying and addressing malnutrition-related consequences of the near-starvation diets that characterize anorexia. Gastrointestinal problems, anemia, and osteoporosis are all common consequences of anorexia and must be addressed, as well as the identification of the physical and psychological factors that have led to the anorexic behavior. The physical therapist is likely to focus on the potential for decon-ditioning in such a situation and the accompanying loss of functional mobility.

From the perspective of occupational therapy, the focus of evaluation will be on the client's occupational performance; that is, the ways in which her food-related behaviors prevent her from participating fully in other, potentially more meaningful and healthful activities. The therapist will certainly need to be aware of the physical functions that might prevent this participation, such as low energy that reduces endurance or poor thyroid function that contributes to cognitive difficulties, but the therapist will undertake a detailed evaluation of physical functions only to the extent that these impair occupational performance (Abeyderra, Willis, & Forsyth, 2006).

Body Structures

What is true for the evaluation of body functions is equally true for the evaluation of body structures. In mental health settings, body structures are often, although not always, unimpaired. However, as we have seen, some physical illnesses (e.g., cerebrovascular accident [CVA]) are closely associated with mental disorders (depression, in the case of CVA) and can cause physical manifestations that affect body structures (hemiplegia, again in CVA).

Performance Skills

Performance skills are "goal-directed actions that are observable as small units of engagement in daily-life occupations" (AOTA, 2014, p. S7). Individuals who have mental disorders frequently experience challenges in several of these areas. The preceding chapters have provided an overview of some of those challenges, and it is often up to the occupational therapist to evaluate these skills in detail. Identification of the skills that may be impaired or inadequate can be done in the process of completing an occupational profile and an exploration of occupations as described previously.

Sensory Perceptual Skills

As noted in previous chapters, many mental disorders are associated with difficulties in sensory processing. It seems likely that the hallucinations that characterize schizophrenia are the result of sensory processing difficulties (Javitt, 2009). Individuals with intellectual disabilities, autism, and eating disorders also may struggle to process and interpret sensory input. One example of an instrument to evaluate sensory perceptual skills is the Adolescent/Adult Sensory Profile (Brown & Dunn, 2002).

Motor and Praxis Skills

Motor and praxis skills are perhaps somewhat less likely than other skill areas to be affected by mental disorders. However, there are a number of notable exceptions, such as motor coordination disorder and Parkinson's disease. Unfortunately, some of the treatments for mental disorders can have profound consequences for motor and praxis skills. In particular, as described in previous chapters, individuals with schizophrenia may develop tardive dyskinesia as a consequence of antipsychotic medication use (Tenback, van Harten, Slooff, & van Os, 2010). The AMPS (Fisher & Bray Jones, 2012) is helpful in measuring these skills.

Emotional Regulation Skills

For individuals with mental disorders, emotional regulation skills are likely to be poorly developed, dysfunctional, or otherwise impaired (Leahy, 2012). For example, an individual diagnosed with borderline personality disorder will almost certainly have difficulty responding to others' feelings, an individual with bipolar disorder may have very poor anger management, and an individual with posttraumatic stress disorder will have difficulty managing anxiety. From the perspective of the psychiatrist or psychologist, these issues would be a focus of evaluation to determine how to facilitate more effective, emotional control to reduce distress.

From the perspective of an occupational therapist, difficulty with emotional regulation would be of concern, particularly as it affects social participation. Social participation is an important area of occupation (AOTA, 2014) and is one that has been linked to overall health and mental well-being (Carolan, Onaga, Pernice-Duca, & Jimenez, 2011). Thus, for the individual with borderline personality disorder, the focus of evaluation might be on identifying specific behaviors that lead others to avoid the person. For the individual with bipolar disorder, monitoring the impact of medications in reducing outbursts might be important, particularly in the context of engagement with activities. For an individual with posttraumatic stress disorder, the occupational therapy evaluation might explore the specific situations that increase anxiety, as well as those that the person finds soothing or distracting. In each of these situations, it is the impact of emotional regulation—or lack thereof—on the ability to engage in meaningful occupations that is the focus of occupational therapy.

Numerous instruments can measure various aspects of emotional regulation, including instruments such as the Adult Manifest Anxiety Scale (Reynolds, Richmond, & Lowe, 2003). Instruments can measure depression, anger, and coping mechanisms (see Appendix B for additional examples).

Cognitive Skills

Cognitive skills tend to be problematic in individuals with mental disorders. Some diagnoses quite specifically include cognitive deficits as a criterion (for example, the neurodevelopmental and neurocognitive disorders). Other disorders are hypothesized to have at least some cognitive component. For example, depression is thought to be in part characterized by negative memory (Phillips, Hine, & Bhullar, 2012), a disorder of cognitive interpretation of phenomena. The specific characteristics of the cognitive deficits differ among the various diagnoses (Vance, Dodson, Watkins, Kennedy, & Keltner, 2013), but the presence of some cognitive deficit is common. Instruments, such as the Loewenstein Occupational Therapy Cognitive Assessment, examine cognition as related to occupational performance (Su, Chen, Tsai, Tsai, & Su, 2007). Some measures of executive function also assess other skills, performance areas, or patterns. For example, the Weekly Calendar Planning Activity (Weiner, Toglia, & Berg, 2012) focuses primarily on executive function, but it can also assist clients in examining their occupational patterns and use of time.

Occupational therapists emphasize cognitive skills because many occupations rely, to some extent, on cognition. In a systematic review of occupational therapy interventions, Arbesman and Logsdon (2011) focused on education and work and noted that cognitive skills can have a profound impact on one's ability to engage in these activities. The therapist must understand the individual's cognitive status and abilities, as well as the probability that those functions can change, either based on improvement through treatment or because the nature of a condition causes decline. In the case of a child with a severe intellectual disability, there may be limits on the extent to which cognition can be improved (although it is never wise to assume that a child or other client cannot improve at all), whereas cognition may improve in an individual who is experiencing a depressive episode as the depression lifts. In the former case, evaluation will need to ascertain what intervention might best match tasks to cognitive skills, whereas in the latter case, it would be better to focus evaluation on the valued occupations that might contribute to improved life satisfaction.

Communication and Social Skills

Communication and social deficits are found in disparate mental disorders such as anorexia nervosa (Morris, 2012), substance abuse (Lai et al., 2013), and autism (Tani et al., 2012). In fact, one of the challenges of traditional approaches to psychotherapy is that they rely heavily on verbal interaction, and many individuals with mental disorders struggle with communication. Occupational therapy offers an important alternative by providing other strategies for emotional expression.

However, deficits in social and communication skills can compromise community integration and ability to participate in normal social roles (Gibson, DaAmico, Jaffe, & Arbesman, 2011). For example, maintaining employment requires, at a minimum, the ability to comprehend verbal and often written instructions, and to interact appropriately with coworkers. Individuals who do not have at least a minimal level of skills in these areas will struggle to enter or remain in the workplace. Many other aspects of occupational performance also require effective communication and social skills. Thus, careful evaluation is essential. Among the instruments that can provide helpful information is the Assessment of Communication and Interaction Skills (Forsyth, Salamy, Simon, & Kielhofner, 1998).

Performance Patterns

It is important to identify the activities that are part of a client's life, and it is also important to know the pattern of these activities. Individuals with mental disorders often struggle with these patterns, either lacking the organization that creates comfortable habits and roles (e.g., in the case of schizophrenia) or having habits and rituals that interfere with ordinary daily activities (as with someone who has an obsessive-compulsive anxiety disorder). Patterns are often evaluated through interview, and some of the instruments available may help to evaluate specific areas of interest. In addition, it can be helpful for individuals to keep a diary of their daily activities to help to identify important patterns, both positive and negative.

Habits

Habits are automatic behaviors that are undertaken regularly (AOTA, 2014), and they are often helpful. For example, most of us have habits around dressing, grooming, and other daily activities. Having specific habits can relieve us of the need to constantly make choices about every move we make. For instance, flossing one's teeth every night may be habitual. The activity is important to dental health (and, by extension, to positive nutritional status). The fact that this behavior is a habit means that the individual does not need to have intense focus each time he or she flosses.

However, habits can also be unhelpful if they are misdirected. An individual with obsessive-compulsive disorder may have habits such as stepping over a threshold repeatedly, washing hands for 1 hour at a time, or chewing every bite of food 100 times, which interfere with achievement of other meaningful occupations. The absence of habits can also be problematic in occupational performance. Someone who has to reconsider the steps of getting dressed every time he or she changes clothing will use time and energy that could be better devoted to other activities. It is useful to identify any habits that may interfere with performance as well as those that might be developed to enhance health and well-being (Hilton, Ackermann, & Smith, 2011). A student who habitually waits until the night before an examination to read the class materials is unlikely to be as successful as one whose study habits keep him or her current with class work.

Numerous standardized instruments are available to assess habits. For example, the Assessment of Life Habits (Fougeyrollas & Noreau, 2003) evaluates habits related to self-care, mobility, employment, and other areas of performance.

Routines

Routines are sequences of habits, or clusters of behavior that (at least ideally) accomplish an occupation. As is true for habits, routines can be helpful or problematic. Most people have morning rituals that enable them to prepare for school or work with minimum cognitive and emotional investment, allowing them to reduce the energy needed to start the day. However, if the ritual becomes so elaborate and complex that it takes time from other occupations—perhaps making the individual late for work regularly—the routine no longer serves a useful purpose. For children with autism and their families, routines can reduce the sensory overload that many of these children find difficult (Dunn, Cox, Foster, Mische-Lawson, & Tanquary 2012). At the same time, children with autism may have routines associated with self-stimulation (hand flapping, rocking) that interfere with positive occupations. Evaluation of routines can be performed through interview or journaling or keeping a diary.

Roles

Roles are behaviors that are associated with societally dictated expectations (AOTA, 2014). Worker, student, parent, and friend are all roles. Although individuals in a particular role will enact some aspects of the role differently, some characteristics are generally expected. A friend is someone who spends time with others, shares some interests, and, perhaps, provides emotional support. For individuals with psychiatric disorders, some expected roles may be absent (perhaps an adult with bipolar disorder is unable to manage a work environment) and some may be enacted in ways that are not helpful or positive (an individual with borderline personality disorder might be excessively demanding in the role of friend). Individuals who do not have a set of expected roles often experience poor quality of life (Prusti & Bränholm, 2000).

Among the standardized instruments used to evaluate roles is the Life Balance Inventory (Matuska, 2012), which focuses on examining the interaction of roles that lead to a satisfying occupational profile.

Rituals

Rituals are routines that incorporate symbolic actions to reflect spiritual, cultural, or social meanings (AOTA, 2014). Attendance at worship services is a typical form of ritual, and participation in religious activities can contribute to positive mental health (Brown, Carney, Parrish, & Klem, 2013). Athletes tend to have rituals that they believe contribute to positive performance (using a specific piece of equipment or wearing a specific garment). As is true for other aspects of performance patterns, some rituals can be detrimental to occupational performance. Many of the anxiety disorders incorporate rituals that are intended to reduce stress, but they may also simultaneously impair function. For example, an individual who has to wash his or her hands in a particular pattern may be unable to function while traveling.

Routines, roles, and rituals can all be performed individually or in groups (AOTA, 2014). Spiritual rituals might include one's personal prayers but also may include participation in a worship service at a religious facility.

Numerous standardized instruments are available for evaluating spirituality, including the Spiritual Well-Being Scale (Ellison & Paloutzian, 1991). Other rituals may be more personally developed (e.g., a family's Thanksgiving dinner), in which case interview and observation are more helpful evaluation mechanisms.

Context and Environment

As described in the *Practice Framework* (AOTA, 2014), contexts include the following:
- Cultural
- Personal
- Temporal
- Virtual
- Environment
  - Physical
  - Social

Some contextual and environmental factors must be assessed through interview and observation because they will, of necessity, be highly personal. For example, a person's cultural identity can best be determined by asking. To understand the cultural context in which the individual lives, observation can yield helpful information, assuming that there is time for

Sample Evaluation Plan for Ms. Mason

The therapist and Ms. Mason establish that she has an occupational profile that satisfies and meets her needs when she is fully able to engage in the activities that constitute that profile. However, her self-report makes it clear that she is, at the time of the referral, far from her ideal occupational participation in her work role. At this point, Ms. Mason and the therapist agree that additional information is needed and focused on her performance skills and patterns. In addition to asking a series of questions designed to elicit information about factors that are causing Ms. Mason difficulty, the occupational therapist selects several additional evaluation instruments focused on the skills and patterns that are the most probable causes of her difficulties.

The additional instruments administered include the following:

- To understand Ms. Mason's cognitive processing: the Assessment of Motor & Process Skills (Fisher & Bray Jones, 2012)
- To discern how Ms. Mason handles relationships: the Assessment of Communication and Interaction Skills (Forsyth, Salamy, Simon, & Kielhofner, 1998)
- To explore Ms. Mason's current level of anxiety: the Adult Manifest Anxiety Scale (Reynolds, Richmond, & Lowe, 2003)
- To explore habits, routines, and rituals: the Assessment of Life Habits (Fougeyrollas & Noreau, 2003) and the Life Balance Inventory (Matuska, 2012)

The evaluation provides helpful insights about Ms. Mason's difficulties. It is clear from the Assessment of Motor & Process Skills instrument that Ms. Mason's process skills are deficient, probably because her anxiety interferes with her ability to focus on the task at hand. In addition, she shows considerable difficulty terminating tasks, returning over and over to "perfect" the product. The Assessment of Communication and Interaction Skills instrument shows that she is particularly reticent in her communication style, again mostly because of the anxiety that interferes with her ability to interact with others. Her score on the Adult Manifest Anxiety Scale shows extremely high anxiety, and the evaluation of her habits and routines by the Assessment of Life Habits shows substantial difficulties in these areas. She clearly uses routines repeatedly in an attempt to reduce her anxiety; however, the result of her actions is increased anxiety because of her failure to complete each task in a reasonable time frame. Her occupations emphasize ADL, IADL, and work, with little leisure or relaxation, as assessed by the Life Balance Inventory.

As the therapist and Ms. Mason look at the results of the evaluation, they agree that the likely trigger for the current exacerbation of her psychiatric symptoms is the change in routine resulting from her new job. Ms. Mason notes that she is worried about her ability to perform effectively at work and to relate to a new set of people on the job.

Thought Questions

1. Has the therapist measured all the relevant factors needed to frame a treatment plan for Ms. Mason? If not, what other areas do you feel should be evaluated?
2. What goals might be appropriate for intervention based on the information provided?

this. In many clinical settings, time is a significant factor, and the therapist may have to rely on the client, family and friends, and available demographic databases to determine what cultural, social, and physical factors might support or impede occupational performance.

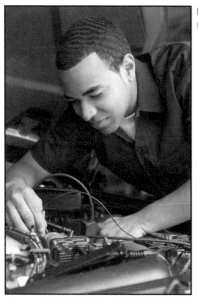

Figure 22-2. Observing a person's work can assist in identifying the needed skills. (©2014 Shutterstock.com.)

Other contextual and environmental factors can be measured through standardized instruments. In particular, the home environment can be evaluated using such instruments as the Home Environment Assessment Protocol (Gitlin et al., 2002). Some of these instruments focus on home safety, which is certainly a significant issue for many individuals (especially for older adults with dementia), but other considerations about the home environment—Is it clean and organized or in disarray? Is it a welcoming space or dingy and unappealing?—can be measured most effectively through conversation and observation. Similarly, it can be helpful to observe the specific nature of a job or school task to understand the skills and patterns required to perform it (Figure 22-2).

Although the home is a central component of an individual's physical (and often social) environment, there are many other locations in which individuals participate in occupations. It is important to know what resources are available in the community. Does it have a library? Does it have a community center? Is there easy access to transportation? Is it safe? For some individuals, having a mental disorder is compounded by environmental deprivation that makes life stressful. Increasingly, instruments such as the School Setting Interview (Hemmingsson, Egilson, Hoffman, & Kielhofner, 2012) provide standardized methods for evaluating the community context more broadly.

Likewise, numerous measures of social environment are available. One such tool is the Family Environment Scale (Moos & Moos, 1994), which measures interactions among family members and perceptions about relationships. Another is the Life Stressor and Social Resources Inventory (Moos, 1995). These assessments can supplement information gleaned from the interview.

Activity Demands

The occupational therapy process is essentially focused on matching client needs, skills, and interests with the requirements of the specific activities in which they participate. Thus, therapists must not only analyze the client's occupational performance but also his or her activity demands, as noted by Crepeau, Schell, Gillen, and Scaffa (2014):

Occupational analysis attends carefully to the specific details of the client's occupations within a specific context. Indeed, it is the customized approach that differentiates the occupational therapy perspective from that of many other professions who do activity analysis, such as vocational educators and industrial engineers. (p. 235)

As described in the *Practice Framework* (AOTA, 2014), aspects of the activity that must be considered include the following:

- Objects used and their properties
- Space demands
- Social demands
- Sequencing and timing
- Required actions
- Required body functions
- Required body structures

Therapists must be alert to those factors that are essential—that cannot be modified—and those that it may be possible to alter. Those factors that cannot be changed would require that the client's skills are adequate to perform the task, and those that can be modified can be adjusted to fit the client's skills. For example, consider Ms. Mason, whose situation is described in the Sample Evaluation boxes. Her work role as an accountant undoubtedly relies heavily on the ability to work through each project in a particular sequence. Thus, the anxiety that prevents Ms. Mason from moving through tasks in sequence, causing her to get "stuck," would be an issue, as sequencing is not a modifiable characteristic of the task. On the other hand, most work places include social interactions both for accomplishment of projects and as a mechanism for enhancing satisfaction with work. In Ms. Mason's case, her work projects do not require the involvement of anyone else, so she can complete them independently. Therefore, if her anxiety interferes with interpersonal interactions in the workplace, it does not compromise her ability to do the job.

Therefore, the sequencing required for the task is not modifiable, and the therapist and Ms. Mason will have to work on her skill deficit in that regard. The social demands of the task are modifiable, and, although in time Ms. Mason might learn to manage social interactions more comfortably, this deficit does not eliminate the possibility of her continuing in her job.

Activity analysis often involves observation, which is best accomplished with the list of performance areas, skills, and patterns used as a guide to the specific tasks and components to be evaluated. Just as the individual's motor and praxis skills need to be considered, the degree to which particular motor and praxis skills are required for the activity in question must also be determined.

Cultural Considerations

We have repeatedly examined the impact of culture on the understanding of mental disorder and occupational performance, and its influence is central to the strategies used for evaluating clients. Think about just one aspect of an occupation: cooking. In completing an occupational profile, a therapist may discover that the client has primary responsibility for cooking meals in the home. This finding, by itself, provides limited information about the specific skills needed for the activity (e.g., bread-making or tortilla preparation), the patterns and rituals involved (e.g., breakfast on the go or bacon and eggs every morning), and the specific cultural context (e.g., at home or at a church-sponsored meal). Evaluating a client's ability to prepare a simple lunch by making a peanut butter and jelly sandwich would be irrelevant if the client eats traditional Japanese or Turkish meals. These cultural variables appear in every aspect of occupational performance.

Another culturally mediated factor in evaluation of a client is the use of translated assessments. It cannot be assumed that a translated instrument maintains equivalent measurement properties, although in some instances it might (Siedlecki et al., 2010). In addition, not all of the constructs being measured translate, even if the language use is identical. For example, in a study of positive aging in a small Maya village in Guatemala, Bonder, Bazyk, Reilly, and Toyota (2005) used the Life Satisfaction Inventory (Neugarten, Havighurst, & Tobin, 1961) as a measure. The instrument was translated into Guatemalan Spanish by a fluent speaker of that language and then back-translated into English by another Guatemalan Spanish speaker to ensure accuracy. However, the participants in the study seemed perplexed by the questions, some of which asked the respondents to compare themselves to others or to themselves at other times in their lives. Lengthy discussion among researchers and participants revealed that Mayan culture actively discourages such comparisons because they can result in jealousy and unhappiness. Thus, although the words translated, the constructs did not.

Lifespan Considerations

A large number of instruments are designed specifically to assess important areas of occupational performance and the skills that support function. Many instruments were designed to focus on a particular age group; thus, instruments such as the Bayley Scales of Infant and Toddler Development (Bayley, 2005) addresses early life motor and skill development and the Modified Assessment of Living Skills and Resources (Clemson, Bundy, Unsworth, & Singh, 2009) examines IADL performance of older adults. Some instruments, such as the AMPS (Fisher & Bray Jones, 2012), have been studied in multiple age groups and can be implemented across the lifespan, but caution must be exercised with other instruments that are associated with specific ages.

Additional Factors

Evaluation occurs within a context. For some therapists working in mental health settings, that context is an inpatient facility, which most often provides acute care and means that client length-of-stay is quite limited. In this situation, evaluation time will be limited. Other therapists work in one of the many forms of community-based care for individuals with mental disorders, ranging from community mental health clinics to schools to sheltered workshops (AOTA, 2000). Increasingly, population-based and wellness programs are a focus of mental health practice in occupational therapy (Bazyk, 2011; Fazio, 2010). Each setting has its own culture, constraints, and areas of emphasis that will guide evaluation and intervention choices.

Therapists' time is a major consideration. In this era of rapidly rising health care costs and constrained resources, therapists must use their time to the greatest effect (Lloyd & Williams, 2010). This is particularly true in acute care, but effective time use is vital in every setting. For this reason, instruments such as the COPM (Law et al., 2005) that address more than one aspect of performance can be most helpful. Thus, therapists should use their findings from these global instruments to carefully identify the areas, skills, and patterns requiring more detailed assessment. Likewise, certified occupational therapy assistants can provide helpful assistance by offering their observations about client performance and needs. Given their active involvement in direct intervention, they often obtain information during interaction with the individual, and they typically have important observational data about performance, skills, and needs.

In Chapter 2, we discussed the impact of the movement toward evidence-based practice. Schell, Scarffa, Gilbert, and Cohn (2014) noted that practitioners must be "willing to examine evaluation and intervention practices to see if they are effective" (p. 55), and to modify their practices based on the evidence. This means that selection of instruments must be (a) guided by evidence-based theories and strategies and (b) implemented using well-supported instruments.

It is also important to keep in mind the ethical principles that guide every aspect of occupational therapy practice. These include acknowledging one's areas of competence and limitation. Some instruments (e.g., the AMPS [Fisher & Bray Jones, 2012]) require training. They cannot be appropriately administered by one who has not had that training. Many instruments are copyrighted, and cannot be used unless they are purchased. Also, appropriate interpretation of results is vital. This includes representing findings accurately in reports and also providing careful explanation of the meaning of the findings to the clients.

Finally, the ability to present and explain the occupational therapy evaluation process and the specifics of a client's assessment to both that individual and to an interdisciplinary treatment team is increasingly important to ensure positive outcomes for the client and to clearly establish the contributions made by occupational therapy to the well-being of the client. For decades, advocacy for the value of occupational therapy has been important, and in today's health care environment it is more essential than ever (AOTA, n.d.). In mental health, where achieving insurance parity with other kinds of physical health conditions has been a hard-fought process, it is particularly important to help clients and other professionals understand how vital the occupational therapy perspective is in helping clients lead meaningful and satisfying lives.

Internet and Other Resources

Center on Human Development and Disability, Clinical Training Unit, University of Washington, Assessment Tools

http://depts.washington.edu/lend/seminars/modules/ot/otpractice_tools.htm
A list of tools used in the Child Development Clinic at Washington University.

Model of Human Occupation Assessment Selection Tool

http://www.cade.uic.edu/moho/resources/findTheAssessment/home.aspx
Provides a lengthy list of instruments focused on aspects of the Model of Human Occupation (MOHO), including their psychometric properties and other information.

Asher, I.E. (2007). *Occupational therapy assessment tools: An annotated bibliography* (3rd ed.). Bethesda, MD: American Occupational Therapy Association.

Hemphill-Pearson, B. (2007). *Assessments in occupational therapy mental health: An integrative approach* (2nd ed.). Thorofare, NJ: Slack Incorporated.

Scaffa, M.E., Reitz, S.M., & Pizzi, M.A. (Eds.). (2010). *Occupational therapy in the promotion of health and wellness*. Philadelphia, PA: F.A. Davis.

Schell, B.A.B., Gillen, G., & Scaffa, M.E. (Eds.). (2014). *Willard & Spackman's occupational therapy* (12th ed.). Philadelphia, PA: Wolters Kluwer/Lippincott Williams & Wilkins.

References

Abeyderra, K., Willis, S., & Forsyth, K. (2006). Occupation focused assessment and intervention for clients with anorexia. *International Journal of Therapy & Rehabilitation, 13*(7), 296.

American Academy of Child & Adolescent Psychiatry. (2012). *Comprehensive psychiatric evaluation. Facts for Families, No. 52.* Retrieved from http://www.aacap.org/AACAP/Families_and_Youth/Facts_for_Families/Facts_for_Families_Pages/Comprehensive_Psychiatric_Evaluation_52.aspx.

American Occupational Therapy Association. (n.d.) *Advocacy & policy.* Retrieved from http://www.aota.org/Advocacy-Policy.aspx.

American Occupational Therapy Association. (2000). *OT and community mental health.* Retrieved from http://www.aota.org/About-Occupational-Therapy/Patients-Clients/MentalHealth/Community/OTandCommunityMentalHealth.aspx.

American Occupational Therapy Association. (2010). Standards of practice for occupational therapy. *American Journal of Occupational Therapy, 64*(Suppl.), S10-S11.

American Occupational Therapy Association. (2014) Occupational therapy practice framework: Domain & process (3rd ed.). *American Journal of Occupational Therapy, 68*(Suppl. 1), S1-S48.

American Psychiatric Association. (2013). *Diagnostic and statistical manual of mental disorders* (5th ed.). Washington, DC: Author.

Arbesman, M., & Logsdon, D.W. (2011). Occupational therapy interventions for employment and education for adults with serious mental illness: A systematic review. *American Journal of Occupational Therapy, 65*(3), 238-246.

Barber (2013). Spirituality and mental health: Applications for HCAs. *British Journal of Healthcare Assistants, 7*(2), 64-68.

Baum, C.M., Connor, L.T., Morrison, T., Hahn, M., Dromerick, A.W., & Edwards, D.F. (2008). Reliability, validity, and clinical utility of the Executive Function Performance Test: A measure of executive function in a sample of people with stroke. *American Journal of Occupational Therapy, 62*(4), 446-455.

Bayley, N. (2005). *Bayley Scales of Infant and Toddler Development* (3rd ed.). San Antonio, TX: Pearson Assessments.

Bazyk, S. (2011). *Mental health promotion, prevention, and intervention with children and youth: A guiding framework for occupational therapy.* Bethesda, MD: American Occupational Therapy Association.

Bonder, B.R. (2010). Cultural and sociological considerations in health promotion. In M.E. Scaffa, S.M. Reitz, & M.A. Pizzi (Eds.), *Occupational therapy in the promotion of health and wellness* (pp. 96-109). Philadelphia, PA: F.A. Davis.

Bonder, B.R., Bazyk, S., Reilly, B., & Toyota, J. (2005). Women's work in Guatemala. *Work: A Journal of Prevention, Assessment & Rehabilitation, 24,* 3-10.

Bonder, B., & Martin, L. (2013). *Culture in clinical care: Strategies for competence* (2nd ed.). Thorofare, NJ: Slack Incorporated.

Brown, C., & Dunn, W. (2002). *Adolescent/adult sensory profile.* San Antonio, TX: Pearson.

Brown, D.R., Carney, J.S., Parrish, M.S., & Klem, J.L. (2013). Assessing spirituality: The relationship between spirituality and mental health. *Journal of Spirituality in Mental Health, 15*(2), 107-122.

Carolan, M., Onaga, E., Pernice-Duca, R., & Jimenez, T. (2011). A place to be: The role of clubhouses in facilitating social support. *Psychiatric Rehabilitation Journal, 35*(2), 125-132.

Carriere, J.S.A., Cheyne, J.A., & Smilek, D. (2008). Everyday attention lapses and memory failures: The affective consequences of mindlessness. *Consciousness and Cognition, 17,* 835-847.

Chang, F., Helfrich, C.A., & Coster, W.J. (2013). Psychometric properties of the Practical Skills Test (PST). *American Journal of Occupational Therapy, 67,* 246-253.

Classen, S., & Velozo, C.A. (2014). Critiquing assessments. Evaluating clients. In B.A.B. Schell, G. Gillen, & M.E. Scaffa (Eds.), *Willard & Spackman's occupational therapy* (12th ed., pp. 302-321). Philadelphia, PA: Wolters Kluwer/Lippincott Williams & Wilkins.

Clemson, L., Bundy, A., Unsworth, C., & Singh, M.F. (2009). Validation of the modified assessment of living skills and resources, an IADL measure for older people. *Disability & Rehabilitation, 31*(5), 359-369.

Cornah, D. (2006). *The impact of spirituality on mental health: A review of the literature.* Mental Health Foundation. Retrieved from http://www.mentalhealth.org.uk/content/assets/PDF/publications/impact-spirituality. pdf?view=Standard.

Crepeau, E.B., Schell, B.A.B., Gillen, G., & Scaffa, M.E. (2014). Evaluating clients. In B.A.B. Schell, G. Gillen, & M.E. Scaffa (Eds.), *Willard & Spackman's occupational therapy* (12th ed., pp. 234-248). Philadelphia, PA: Wolters Kluwer/Lippincott Williams & Wilkins.

Doig, E., Fleming, J., Kuipers, P., & Cornwell, P.L. (2010). Clinical utility of the combined use of the Canadian occupational performance measure and goal attainment scaling. *American Journal of Occupational Therapy, 64,* 904-914.

Doucet, B.M., & Gutman, S.A. (2013). Quantifying function: The rest of the measurement story. *American Journal of Occupational Therapy, 67*(1), 7-9.

Dunn, W., Cox, J., Foster, L., Mische-Lawson, L., & Tanquary, J. (2012). Impact of a contextual intervention on child participation and parent competence among children with autism spectrum disorders: A pretest-posttest repeated-measures design. *American Journal of Occupational Therapy, 66*(5), 520-528.

Ellison, R., & Paloutzian, C. (1991). *Manual for the spiritual well-being scale.* Nyack, NY: Life Advance.

Erlandsson, L.K., Eklund, M., & Persson, D. (2011). Occupational value and relationships to meaning and health: Elaborations of the ValMO-model. *Scandinavian Journal of Occupational Therapy, 18,* 72-80.

Fazio, L.S. (2010). Health promotion program development. In M.E. Scaffa, S.M. Reitz, & M.A. Pizzi (Eds.), *Occupational therapy in the promotion of health and wellness* (pp. 195-207). Philadelphia, PA: F.A. Davis.

Fisher, A.G., & Bray Jones, K. (2012). *Assessment of motor and process skills: User manual* (Vol. 1, 7th ed. Rev. ed.). Fort Collins, CO: Three Star Press.

Folstein, M.F., Folstein, S.E., & McHugh, P.R. (1975). "Mini-mental state": A practical method for grading the cognitive-state of patients for the clinician. *Journal of Psychiatric Research, 12,* 189-198.

Forsyth, K., Salamy, M., Simon, S., & Kielhofner, G. (1998). *The assessment of communication and interaction skill* (ACIS) Version 4.0. Retrieved from http://www.cade.uic.edu/moho/productDetails.aspx?aid=1.

Fougeyrollas, P., & Noreau, L. (2003). *Assessment of life habits (LIFE-H, 3.0): General long form.* Quebec, Canada: International Network on the Disability Creation Process.

Gibson, R.W., DaAmico, M., Jaffe, L., & Arbesman, M. (2011). Occupational therapy interventions for recovery in the areas of community integration and normative life roles for adults with serious mental illness: A systematic review. *American Journal of Occupational Therapy, 65*(3), 247-256.

Gitlin, L.N., Schinfeld, S., Winter, L., Corcoran, M., Boyce, A.A., & Hauck, W. (2002). Evaluating home environments of persons with dementia: Interrater reliability and validity of the home environmental assessment protocol (HEAP). *Disability and Rehabilitation, 24*(1-3), 59-71.

Hemmingsson, H., Egilson, S., Hoffman, O., & Kielhofner, G. (2012). *School setting interview.* Retrieved from http://www.fsa.se/Global/Forlag/SSI%20affisch%20COTEC2012.pdf

Hilton, C.L., Ackermann, A.A., & Smith, D.L. (2011). Healthy habit changes in pre-professional college students: Adherence, supports, and barriers. *OTJR: Occupation, Participation & Health, 31*(2), 64-72.

Hwang, J.E. (2009). Reliability and validity of the health enhancement lifestyle profile (HELP). *OTJR: Occupation, Participation and Health, 30*(4), 158-168.

Iwasaki, Y., Coyle, C.P., & Shank, J. W. (2010). Leisure as a context for active living, recovery, health and life quality for persons with mental illness in a global context. *Health Promotion International, 25*(4), 483-494.

Javitt, D.C. (2009). Sensory processing in schizophrenia: Neither simple nor intact. *Schizophrenia Bulletin, 35*(6), 1059-1064.

Jensen, E. W., James, S.A., Boyce, W.T., & Hartnett, S.A. (1983). The family routines inventory: Development and validation. *Social Science and Medicine, 17,* 201-211.

Kållestad, H., Hansen, B., Langsrud, K., Ruud, T., Morken, G., Stiles, T.C., & Gråwe, R.W. (2012). Impact of sleep disturbance on patients in treatment for mental disorders. *BMC Psychiatry, 12,* 179.

Kasper, J.D., Black, B.S., Shore, A.D., & Rabins, P.V. (2009). Evaluation of the validity and reliability of the Alzheimer's disease-related quality of life (ADRQL) assessment instrument. *Alzheimer's Disease and Associated Disorders, 23*(3), 275-284.

King, G., Law, M., King, S., Hurley, P., Rosenbaum, P., Hanna, S., . . . Young, N. (2004). *Children's assessment of participation and enjoyment and preferences for activities of children.* San Antonio, TX: Pearson.

Kramer, J.M., Kielhofner, G., & Smith, E.V. (2010). Validity evidence for the child occupational self assessment. *American Journal of Occupational Therapy, 64,* 621-632.

Lai, M.H., Graham, J.W., Caldwell, L.L., Smith, E.A., Bradley, S.A., Vergnani, T., . . . Wegner, C. (2013). Linking life skills and norms with adolescent substance use and delinquency in South Africa. *Journal of Research on Adolescence, 23*(1), 128-137.

Law, M., Baptiste, S., Carswell, A., McColl, M.A., Polatajko, H., & Pollock, N. (2005). *Canadian occupational performance measure (COPM)* (4th ed.). Ottawa, ON: Canadian Association of Occupational Therapists.

Leahy, R.L. (2012). Introduction: Emotional schemas, emotion regulation, and psychopathology. *International Journal of Cognitive Therapy, 5*(4), 359-361.

Lloyd, C., & Williams, P.L. (2010). Occupational therapy in the modern adult acute mental health setting: A review of current practice. *International Journal of Therapy & Rehabilitation, 17*(9), 483-493.

Lorch, A., & Herge, E.A. (2007, May 28). Using standardized assessments in practice. *OT Practice, 12*(9), n.p.

Matuska, K. (2012). Description and development of the life balance inventory. *OTJR: Occupation, Participation, and Health, 32*, 220-228.

Moore, K., Merritt, B., & Doble, S.E. (2010). ADL skill profiles across three psychiatric diagnoses. *Scandinavian Journal of Occupational Therapy, 17*(1), 77-85.

Moos, R. (1995). Development and applications of new measures of life stressors, social resources, and coping responses. *European Journal of Psychological Assessment, 11*, 1-13.

Moos, R., & Moos, B. (1994). *Family environment scale manual: Development, applications, research* (3rd ed.). Palo Alto, CA: Consulting Psychologist Press.

Morris, R. (2012). Assessment of occupation and social performance. In J. Fox & K. Goss (Eds.), *Eating and its disorders* (pp. 61-74). New York, NY: Wiley-Blackwell.

Mundt, J.C., Freed, D.M., & Griest, J.H. (2000). Lay-person based screening for early detection of Alzheimer's disease: Development and validation of an instrument. *Journal of Gerontology: Psychological Sciences, 55B*, 163-170.

Munkholm, M., Berg, B., Löfgren, B., & Fisher, A.G. (2010). Cross-regional validation of the school version of the assessment of motor and process skills. *American Journal of Occupational Therapy, 64*, 768-775.

Neugarten, B.L., Havighurst, R.J., & Tobin, S.S. (1961). The measurement of life satisfaction. *Journal of Gerontology, 16*, 134-143.

Pescosolido, B.A., Medina, T.R., Martin, J.K., & Long, J.S. (2013). The "backbone" of stigma: Identifying the global core of public prejudice associated with mental illness. *American Journal of Public Health, 103*(5), 853-860.

Phillips, W.J., Hine, D.W., & Bhullar, N. (2012). A latent profile analysis of implicit and explicit cognitions associated with depression. *Cognitive Therapy and Research, 36*(5), 458-473.

Pierce, D., & Summers, K. (2011). Sleep: An exciting new frontier in occupation-based practice. In T. Brown & V. Stoeffel (Eds.), *Occupational therapy in mental health: A vision for participation* (pp. 736-754). Philadelphia, PA: F.A. Davis.

Potvin, M., Snider, L., Prelock, P., Kehayia, E., & Wood-Dauphinee, S. (2013). Children's assessment of participation and enjoyment/preference for activities of children: Psychometric properties in a population with high-functioning autism. *American Journal of Occupational Therapy, 67*, 209-217.

Prusti, S., & Bränholm, I. (2000). Occupational roles and life satisfaction in psychiatric outpatients with vocational disabilities, *Work, 14*, 145-149.

Reynolds, C.R., Richmond, B.O., & Lowe, P.A. (2003). *Adult manifest anxiety scale.* WPS. Retrieved from https://shop.psych.acer.edu.au/acer-shop/group/AMA.

Rogers, J.C., Weinstein, J.M., & Figone, J.J. (1978). The interest check list: An empirical assessment. *American Journal of Occupational Therapy, 32*(10), 628-630.

Rosenblum S., Sachs, D., & Schreuer, N. (2010). Reliability and validity of the children's leisure assessment scale. *American Journal of Occupational Therapy, 64*, 633-641.

Royal College of Psychiatrists. (2010). *Spirituality and mental health.* Retrieved from http://www.rcpsych.ac.uk/expertadvice/treatments/spirituality.aspx.

Schell, B.A.B., Scaffa, M.E., Gillen, G., & Cohn, E.S. (2014). Contemporary occupational therapy practice. In B.A.B. Schell, G. Gillen, & M.E. Scaffa (Eds.), *Willard & Spackman's occupational therapy* (12th ed., pp. 47-58). Philadelphia, PA: Wolters Kluwer/Lippincott Williams & Wilkins.

Schindler, V.P. (2010). A client-centred, occupation-based occupational therapy programme for adults with psychiatric diagnoses. *Occupational Therapy International, 17*(3), 105-112.

Shotwell, M.P. (2014). Evaluating clients. In B.A.B. Schell, G. Gillen, & M.E. Scaffa (Eds.), *Willard & Spackman's occupational therapy* (12th ed., pp. 281-301). Philadelphia, PA: Wolters Kluwer/Lippincott Williams & Wilkins.

Siedlecki, K.L., Manly, J.J., Brickman, A.M., Schupf, N., Tang, M.S., & Stern, Y. (2010). Do neuropsychological tests have the same meaning in Spanish speakers as they do in English speakers? *Neuropsychology, 24*, 402-411.

Social Security Disability Help. (2013). *Do mental disorders qualify for social security disability?* Retrieved from http://www.disability-benefits-help.org/blog/do-mental-disorders-qualify-social-security-disability.

Su, C., Chen, W., Tsai, P., Tsai, C., & Su, W. (2007). Psychometric properties of the Loewenstein occupational therapy cognitive assessment-second edition in Taiwanese persons with schizophrenia. *American Journal of Occupational Therapy, 61*, 108-118.

Tani, M.K., Ota, C., Yamada, H., Watanabe, T., Yokoi, H., Takayama, H., . . . Nobumasa, A. (2012). Mental and behavioral symptoms of person's with Asperger's syndrome: Relationships with social isolation and handicaps. *Research in Autism Spectrum Disorders, 6*(2), 907-912.

Tenback, D.E., van Harten, P.N., Slooff, C.J., & van Os, J. (2010). Incidence and persistence of tardive dyskinesia and extrapyramidal symptoms in schizophrenia. *Journal of Psychopharmacology, 24*(7), 1031-1035.

Vance, D.E., Dodson, J.E., Watkins, J., Kennedy, B.H., & Keltner, N.L. (2013). Neurological and psychiatric diseases and their unique cognitive profiles: Implications for nursing practice and research. *Journal of Neuroscience Nursing, 45*(2), 77-87.

Weiner, N.W., Toglia, J., & Berg, C. (2012). Weekly calendar planning activity (WCPA): A performance-based assessment of executive function piloted with at-risk adolescents. *American Journal of Occupational Therapy, 66*, 699-708.

Occupational Therapy Interventions in Mental Health

Learning Outcomes

By the end of this chapter, readers will be able to:

- Describe the domain of occupational therapy as it relates to intervention in mental health

- Discuss intervention strategies focused on occupations; client factors; performance skills; performance patterns; and contexts and environments, as these apply to mental health

- Identify the steps in the occupational therapy intervention process as described in the *Occupational Therapy Practice Framework, Third Edition* (American Occupational Therapy Association [AOTA], 2014), as these steps apply in mental health

- Discuss types of occupational therapy interventions including therapeutic occupations and activities; preparatory methods and tasks; education and training; and advocacy, as these interventions apply in mental health

- Describe occupational therapy intervention approaches that create and promote; establish and restore; maintain; modify; and prevent, as these approaches relate to mental health

- Describe desired outcomes of occupational therapy interventions in mental health

Bonder B.
Psychopathology and Function, Fifth Edition (pp 481-501).
© 2015 SLACK Incorporated.

KEY WORDS

- Supported employment
- Co-occupation
- Sensory room
- Sensory integrative intervention
- Occupational justice

- Self-advocacy
- Self-help
- Monitoring
- Collaborative consultation

CASE VIGNETTE, MR. SHIMBIR (PART 2)

In Chapter 22, you met Abdi Shimbir, a Somali refugee. Since we last met him, Mr. Shimbir was diagnosed by a psychiatrist as having posttraumatic stress disorder. The occupational therapy evaluation revealed that Mr. Shimbir had the following problems and concerns:

OCCUPATIONAL PROFILE

Mr. Shimbir lacks a constellation of meaningful occupations. He has not found gainful employment and misses his role as a farmer, work from which he derived both satisfaction and income. He has difficulty articulating a set of meaningful roles for himself.

OCCUPATIONS

Mr. Shimbir has no difficulty with activities of daily life, but he struggles with a number of instrumental activities of daily life. He does not understand the U.S. banking system, so he cannot manage his finances very well. He also finds U.S. stores, including grocery stores, confusing, thus making shopping difficult. His uncle has helped him to find local sources of familiar foods so that Mr. Shimbir is able to cook some familiar meals. He has no leisure activities and is not currently working. His social interactions are limited to his uncle and a few neighbors, in part because he does not speak much English and in part because he cannot manage transportation, so he does not go out much. His sleep is poor because of frequent nightmares.

BODY SYSTEMS AND BODY FUNCTIONS

Mr. Shimbir's physical health is good. He is somewhat deconditioned as a result of inactivity while he was in the various refugee camps, but he has no major deficits in body systems or body functions.

PERFORMANCE SKILLS

Mr. Shimbir's motor and process skills show no deficits. It is somewhat difficult to assess his cognitive skills due to his limited English; however, he clearly seems to have difficulty with emotional regulation and with social interaction.

HABITS, ROLES, AND PATTERNS

This is an area of significant difficulty for Mr. Shimbir. His life is without structure, and he seems aimless and has been unable to identify a set of roles for himself in his new life.

(continued)

CASE VIGNETTE, MR. SHIMBIR (PART 2) (CONTINUED)

THOUGHT QUESTIONS

1. Looking back at Chapter 9, what intervention plan do you think the psychiatrist might identify for Mr. Shimbir?
2. What do you see as Mr. Shimbir's most pressing concerns in terms of his occupational performance?
3. What are the strengths in Mr. Shimbir's occupational performance and the positive aspects of the context in which he lives?
4. What else might you want to know before framing an intervention plan?

Chapter 22 focused on how occupational therapy (OT) conceptualizes occupation and gathers information about client performance. It outlined the ways in which the OT view of mental health differs from that discussed in the fifth edition of the *Diagnostic and Statistical Manual of Mental Disorders* (DSM-5; American Psychiatric Association [APA], 2013). This difference guides intervention as well as assessment. The combination of approaches can benefit clients greatly. Psychopharmacology, psychotherapy, cognitive behavioral therapy, and other treatments offered by psychiatrists, psychologists, social workers, and nurse practitioners have tremendous value and are essential to ameliorating the symptoms of mental disorders.

However, without the focus on occupational performance that is the centerpiece of OT, clients may not experience the quality of life and life satisfaction that are vital to well-being (cf., Chou et al., 2012; Rizk, Pizur-Barnekow, & Darragh, 2011). There is growing recognition of this in the mental health literature. DSM diagnostic criteria frequently include dysfunction in daily activities. Occupational therapy is uniquely positioned to provide interventions that address the specific occupational issues that characterize mental disorders. In doing so, it improves the health of the individual, the family, and the community.

This chapter focuses on OT interventions as they relate to the areas that represent the domain of OT. It will briefly review the steps in the intervention process, types of interventions, intervention approaches, and, finally, desired outcomes of OT. You will see throughout this discussion that the material is familiar from your study of OT in working with clients with other kinds of disorders. It bears repeating that this is because of OT's unique perspective on health and wellness; the goal of OT is to support and facilitate occupational performance, regardless of the client's medical diagnosis.

Domain of Occupational Therapy in Mental Health

The domain of OT in mental health is actually the domain of OT. As you saw in Chapter 22, an emphasis on occupational performance does not require making a distinction between physical and mental disorders. It is the individual's performance patterns, occupations, and skills that are the focus of concern, not the medical diagnostic label, except insofar as that diagnosis contributes to skill or performance deficits. Remember that, as shown in Table 2-1 in Chapter 2, the domain of OT in mental health, as in all OT, includes the following:

- Occupations
- Client factors

- Activity demands
- Performance skills
- Performance patterns
- Context and environment

One study of the factors identified by therapists as being most central in mental health found eight areas perceived as most important (Casteleijn & Graham, 2012):

1. Process skills
2. Motivation
3. Communication and interaction skills
4. Self-esteem
5. Balanced lifestyle
6. Affect
7. Life skills
8. Role performance

These findings are consistent with a growing international emphasis on quality of life as an essential outcome of care (Diener, 2006). The Organization for Economic Co-operation and Development (OECD, n.d.) has issued guidelines on measuring internal cognitions, feelings, and appraisals that constitute quality of life; OT quite appropriately emphasizes occupations that lead to positive outcomes.

The Process of Occupational Therapy

Chapter 22 described strategies for evaluating a client's occupational profile and occupations, emphasizing needs, strengths, and abilities in each of these areas as described in the *Practice Framework* (AOTA, 2014). The first step in the OT process is evaluation; specifically, development of an occupational profile and analysis of occupational performance. Here we consider how to use that information to frame a plan for intervention to address issues related to occupational performance, particularly focused on occupations, client factors, performance skills, and performance patterns.

The second phase of the process is the actual intervention (AOTA, 2014), which involves creating an intervention plan, implementing the intervention, and reviewing the progress. The final phase in the OT process is measuring the outcomes.

Designing an intervention plan involves identifying goals based on the individual's strengths and deficits; the activities the individual needs and wants to perform; and the social, economic, and environmental resources available to the individual (AOTA, 2014). As goals are identified, types of intervention and intervention approaches must be selected based on the best available evidence about which strategies are most likely to support the individual's occupation. From the perspective of OT, it is not essential to know whether the client has a diagnosis of schizophrenia or bipolar disorder, but only to know what symptoms are affecting his or her occupational performance. It is vital to know whether the individual can accomplish what is expected of him or her, has valued goals, and derives satisfaction from his or her occupations. We first consider the ways in which various aspects of performance can be affected by mental disorders.

Occupations

OT intervention focuses on what clients need and want to do. These occupations include activities of daily living (ADL), instrumental activities of daily living (IADL), rest and sleep, education, work, play, leisure, and social participation. Each of these can be affected by the characteristic deficits of various mental disorders, and each can be the focus of intervention emphasizing improved performance.

Work is an occupation that is compromised in a number of mental disorders, ranging from intellectual disabilities and autism to schizophrenia, bipolar disorder, neurocognitive disorders, and others. Occupational therapy interventions such as supported employment (SE) focused on work performance can improve prospects for employment for individuals with serious mental disorders (Arbesman & Logsdon, 2011; Baxter et al., 2012). **Supported employment** is a process of placing clients in work that interests them, assessing their performance, and providing consultation as they integrate into their worker roles. Further, Arbesman and Logsdon found that there is evidence that SE intervention can enhance performance in other occupations, including IADL. Supported employment also affects self-efficacy and quality of life (Chan, Tsang, & Li, 2009).

In the same vein, supported education can enhance performance in educational occupations (Best, Still, & Cameron, 2008; Gutman, Kerner, Zombek, Dulek, & Ramsey, 2009). A variety of instructional interventions enhance educational attainment (Dirette & Kolak, 2004; Schindler & Kientz, 2013). A variety of barriers, such as fears and anxieties, lost motivation, and inability to concentrate, can be addressed through individualized interventions. Identifying barriers and practicing coping strategies for each may be helpful.

Basic daily living skills are a frequent focus of OT intervention (Ammerall & Coppers, 2012; Gibson, D'Amico, Jaffe, & Arbesman, 2011). There is a moderate amount of evidence for the effectiveness of such interventions (Gibson et al., 2011; Helfrich, Chan, & Sabol, 2011). An example of the kind of life skills that can be addressed is a focus on diet and nutrition. Educational strategies that enhance understanding of nutrition, in concert with skill-based interventions like sensory integration, can aid individuals with eating disorders (Gardiner & Brown, 2010). At a more general level, OT can positively impact the diet and eating habits of individuals with mental disorders by enhancing knowledge (Mahony, Haracz, & Williams, 2012). Occupational therapists recognize that their domain does not extend into specific dietary recommendations; however, support for development of healthy eating patterns can complement the role of the nutritionist, as can intervention to teach shopping skills (Figure 23-1).

It is well established that meaningful occupations include not only self-care, work, and education, but also opportunities for creativity (Fowler, 2011). Painting, drama (Javaherian-Dysinger & Freire, 2010), and creative writing all offer considerable therapeutic benefit, including opportunities to build confidence, experience a sense of accomplishment, and express emotions. This last outcome is particularly important for clients who are less verbal and have difficulty addressing emotional issues. For example, Seth Chwast, a young man with autism who has become known for his artwork (Chwast, 2014), says on his blog "I am standing next to the Artwork by Seth Chwast LED screen! I feel proud and enthusiastic!" While verbal expression is not his strength, his paintings are a testament to a rich and satisfying life. Creative occupations as interventions can be helpful for individuals with widely varying circumstances, including immigrants, whose mastery of English may impede their ability to benefit from verbal therapies (Pooremamali, Persson, & Eklund, 2011), and the homeless (Lloyd & Bassett, 2012; Thomas, Gray, McGinty, & Ebringer, 2011).

Therapeutic leisure activities include a wide array of options. Gardening is beneficial for some clients (Wagenfeld, 2013), as are outdoor activities like hiking and biking (DeAngelis,

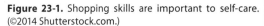

Figure 23-1. Shopping skills are important to self-care. (©2014 Shutterstock.com.)

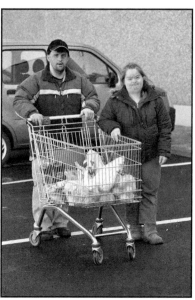

2013). There is very strong evidence that physical activity can reduce depression (Lyne, Moxon, & Valios, 2008), and at the same time promote health and well-being.

Likewise, play is essential for children and for adults. For children, play offers opportunities for enjoyment and for acquiring social, motor, and cognitive skills that contribute to many aspects of performance (Cordier, 2011).

Spirituality and religion are essential, but sometimes overlooked, occupations (Bassett, Lloyd, & Tse, 2008). Spiritual activities can provide a sense of hope and calm as the process of recovery moves forward. Such activities are not limited to religious participation and, therefore, may include various complementary and alternative strategies (like meditation and yoga). Helping a client to identify a religious congregation, plan transportation to attend a worship service, or connect with a church organization are also strategies to support the individual's ability to address his or her spiritual needs.

Many occupations involve more than the individual. The individual may participate in a variety of social occupations. There is a category for **co-occupation** (AOTA, 2014), that is, occupations that rely on more than one person in order to exist. It is not possible to be a parent without having children (or child-equivalents in the case of godparents or other kin-equivalent relationships). In order to be a care provider for someone with a psychosocial dysfunction, one must have that care recipient. Given the many psychosocial conditions in which family relationships have a contributory role, both in the emergence of the illness and in its eventual resolution, these co-occupations may require careful attention.

Client Factors

Once the therapist and client have established the occupations that are important and would benefit from intervention, either to enhance strengths or to remediate deficits, it is necessary to determine the specific client factors and performance skills that contribute to occupational performance. As you saw in Chapter 22, there are a large number of assessments that facilitate understanding of the factors that should be the focus of intervention. Client factors include values, beliefs, and spirituality; body functions; and body structures.

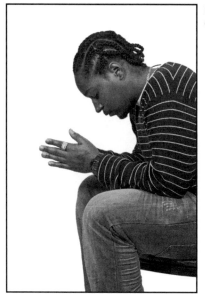

Figure 23-2. Spiritual occupations can be central to emotional coping. (©2014 Shutterstock.com.)

Client values, and particularly spirituality, can be a central source of mental distress or comfort, as well as a resource for recovery or a focus for intervention (Bassett et al., 2008). As Bassett and colleagues point out, spirituality:

> …is the individualized need to understand the purpose of life and underpins the meaning of everyday activities. It is the essence of the person and their inner motivator. The concept of spirituality is, therefore, an important consideration in recovery from mental illness. (p. 255)

Recovery, after all, requires the individual to find meaning and purpose in the face of anxiety, depression, and stress (Figure 23-2).

Intervention focused on body functions and body structures has been well described in other texts (cf., Schell, Gillen, & Scaffa, 2014). It is beyond the scope of this book to cover these in detail. Keep in mind, as we've discussed frequently, that individuals with mental disorders may also be dealing with the whole array of body function and body structure variables that affect performance. Individuals dealing with specific concerns about body function and body structure (e.g., someone who is visually or hearing impaired, or who has a broken bone) may have coexisting mental disorders or may develop a mental disorder in concert with a particular body function or body structure issue. It may be necessary, for example, to address issues of visual impairment while also addressing concerns about depression. In some sense, it doesn't really matter which came first.

Performance Skills

Individuals with mental disorders often demonstrate significant performance skill deficits in a number of areas that are vital to effective occupational performance. Intervention to address those deficits can greatly enhance performance. As described in the *Practice Framework* (AOTA, 2014), performance skills include motor and process skills, sensory-perceptual skills, emotional regulation skills, cognitive skills, and communication and social skills. These skills are the external expression of internal body systems and body functions that underlie them.

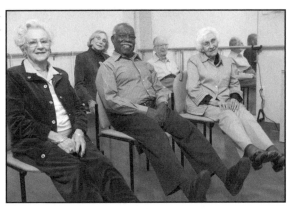

Figure 23-3. Physical activity has numerous benefits for older adults. (©2014 Shutterstock.com.)

Motor and process skill deficits accompany a number of mental disorders. For example, individuals with autism, intellectual deficits, and neurocognitive disorders often have motor impairments that affect function. Likewise, those with tic disorders may struggle with activities that require motor skills. Some interventions structured to provide motor practice may also enhance social and other skills, such as an intervention for individuals with autism that made use of motor learning to enhance social awareness (Gutman et al., 2010). Motor practice in the context of meaningful play can be extremely helpful in disorders like motor coordination disorder that have motor skills deficits as a defining characteristic (Morgan & Long, 2012). Increasingly, technological innovations like the Nintendo Wii are being used to address not only motor skills deficits, but also cognitive skills and other aspects of performance (Gil-Gomez, Llorens, Alcaniz, & Colomer, 2011). In working with older adults, physical activity can enhance physical capacity and also provide a source of socialization and pleasure (Figure 23-3).

A variety of strategies can address sensory-perceptual skills, some of which have been implemented with clients with problematic anger or substance issues (Stols, van Heerden, van Jaarsveld, & Nel, 2013). Sensory modulation and sensory discrimination can be enhanced through activities such as listening to ocean sounds as part of a mindfulness activity to improve auditory modulation or using scents to increase olfactory discrimination (Champagne & Koomar, 2011). An environmental intervention using a **sensory room** (Loukas, 2011) can enhance self-organization. Sensory rooms are therapeutic spaces designed to "promote self-organization, healing, and positive change through opportunities to interact with context, objects and people" (Loukas, p. 2). Typically, these spaces are designed to allow for control of sensory input to meet specific client needs. Activity opportunities in these spaces might include swings, ramps, ropes, ladders, and an array of objects for manipulation, each of which offers unique sensory input. In some instances, this kind of intervention may acquire a sensory-motor component in the kinds of movement that are encouraged (Woo & Leon, 2013).

Sensory integrative interventions have benefits in improving sensorimotor skills and motor planning, social skills, attention, behavioral regulation, and participation in active play, as well as improving achievement in academic performance (May-Benson & Koomar, 2010). These interventions involve creating a therapeutic environment that offers activities that enrich sensory experiences in a planned and controlled fashion.

Emotional regulation skills are almost by definition deficient or distorted in individuals with mental disorders. A variety of activities can promote emotional regulation. Bazyk (2011) describes a mental health promotion program of after school activities for disadvantaged children that encourage appropriate expression of anger and frustration as well as coping skills. Activities can include, among many others, drumming, woodworking, and gross motor play to reduce tension and stress. Adults also benefit from opportunities to develop coping skills and express emotion appropriately. For example, dog-assisted therapy in long-term care facilities may afford elders opportunities to experience unconditional approval that reduces feelings of anxiety and frustration (Cipriani et al., 2013). Activities that promote perceived control contribute to effective emotional regulation (Eklund, 2007).

There is a vast amount of literature on enhancing cognitive skills. Because cognitive skills deficits can occur in so many disorders throughout the life span, and because they have the potential to be so damaging to function, a wide array of strategies have been implemented to remediate them. Activities focused on enhancing play, language, and social interactions can have positive impact (Frolek Clark & Schlabach, 2013). Nintendo Wii games and other technological interventions can address multiple skill areas concurrently (Gil-Gomez et al., 2011). Cognitive remediation can improve cognitive skills and reduce cognitive distortions in people with schizophrenia (Cordier & Scanlan, 2012).

Likewise, there is strong evidence for the effectiveness of social skills training in remediating social skills deficits (Gibson et al., 2011). Such deficits are found in individuals with quite varied mental disorders, ranging from schizophrenia to autism to intellectual disabilities. Social skills training, for example, involves very concrete instruction on how to greet someone, creating a list of conversation topics, and practice of these social interactions through role-playing. Direct training, accompanied by practice and feedback, is most effective.

Performance Patterns

It is evident that, in addition to the therapeutic importance of individual occupations, maintaining or developing occupational habits also plays an important role in mental health (Davidson, 2003). Davidson suggests thinking about recovery in terms of developing effective habits, a strategy that can offer options even in the context of continuing symptoms. Such strategies encourage a strength-based model for mental health intervention, enabling clients to focus on their interests and abilities as they create lives they choose. Opportunities to build habits provide clients with a sense of perceived control (Eklund, 2007), which has been correlated with enhanced occupational performance in individuals with long-term mental illness.

Individuals with mental disorders often struggle with time use (Edgelow & Krupka, 2011). They may find it difficult to identify meaningful occupations and to find the energy and motivation to engage in those occupations. For such individuals, a focus on performance patterns and roles is essential (see Case Vignette on p. 490).

Overview of Intervention

The OT process involves several skills and strategies that must be applied throughout evaluation, intervention, and outcome assessment. These include effective clinical reasoning, therapeutic use of self, and activity analysis. These skills must be mastered and applied regardless of the setting or type of dysfunction the therapeutic process is addressing.

Clinical Reasoning

Clinical reasoning involves gathering necessary information, interpreting it in helpful and meaningful ways, and using that information to frame the most helpful possible interventions (Kuipers & Grice, 2009). Kuipers and Grice suggest that such reasoning can be promoted through the use of protocols and algorithms. In mental health, it appears that both intuitive and analytical abilities yield the most helpful results (Chaffey, Unsworth, & Fossey, 2012). The most important aspect of clinical reasoning is the awareness that the therapist must,

CASE VIGNETTE, MR. SHIMBIR (PART 3)

The therapist and Mr. Shimbir agree on several initial goals as the focus of intervention:
1. Improve self-care skills, with an emphasis on financial management, shopping, and using public transportation.
2. Improve English language skills.
3. Identify a job category that fits Mr. Shimbir's skills and develop a plan for securing work.
4. Develop coping skills to manage anxiety, depression, and sleep difficulties.

The therapist and Mr. Shimbir agree that the ultimate goal is to develop a satisfying occupational profile that supports Mr. Shimbir's function and also improves his quality of life and life satisfaction. The therapist then begins to frame an intervention plan based on the goals that have been developed.

THOUGHT QUESTIONS

1. What other goals might be appropriate for Mr. Shimbir?
2. What are some components of the activities listed here that might be necessary steps in achieving these goals?

in collaboration with the client, carefully consider options and approaches to maximize the potential for successful intervention. In Chapter 2, we reviewed a number of theoretical frameworks that can assist therapists in organizing information and making informed judgments. The use of these frameworks or models is of great value in structuring effective treatment strategies.

Therapeutic Use of Self

In mental health, the relationship between the therapist and client takes on particular salience (Taylor, 2014). Therapeutic use of self (Cole & McLean, 2003) emphasizes the important aspects of the relationship, including the experience of having another individual value and respect the client; opportunities for direct, clear feedback; emotional support; and opportunities to see, model, and practice effective communication. OT is certainly not alone in recognizing the importance of the therapeutic relationship. Effective therapists take advantage of opportunities to emphasize the positive aspects of their interaction with clients. As one example, a therapist was working with a family in which communication among members was vague and unclear. Family members did not trust one another. One day, as the family came into the session, the therapist noticed that the hem of the mother's skirt was torn. She pointed this out, and offered a safety pin as a temporary fix. This intervention served as the focus of the remainder of the session, since it had never occurred to the family members that they could say something so direct. They were impressed by the therapist's clear but supportive input, as well as her effort to offer a solution as she pointed out the problem. Such interventions can build effective interaction skills that enhance client satisfaction (Haertl, Behrens, Houtujec, Rue, & Haken, 2009).

Activity Analysis

In addition to understanding the client and building effective relationships, therapists must be able to understand the elements of particular activities (Thomas, 2012). As you have seen throughout this book, individuals with functional deficits may struggle with particular activities because of a mismatch between the needed abilities and the activity demands. Consider, for example, the activity of reading. To read this book, you have needed visual and perceptual skills to see and interpret the marks on the page, cognitive skills to make meaning of those marks and remember the information, and motor skills to hold the book and turn the pages. Some of those demands can be modified—perhaps minimizing the motor component by reading on a computer rather than from a book, or listening to an audio version to minimize the visual demands—while others cannot. You need to be able to understand the clusters of words, even if you substitute notes for memory. In working with individuals with mental disorders, understanding the characteristics of the activity can help ensure a good match between the client's therapeutic needs and the requirements of the activity, as well as the opportunities that activity may offer for remediation of a deficit or enhancement of a strength. For example, an individual who is dealing with depression may benefit from reduced work demands for a period of time through part-time work, work in a relatively structured environment, or engaging in simpler work tasks as a way to build confidence.

Intervention Process

Having constructed an occupational profile and completed an analysis of occupational performance, the next step in the OT process is to develop, in collaboration with the client, an intervention plan (AOTA, 2014). The plan will establish a set of goals for intervention, strategies for achieving those goals, and anticipated outcomes that can be measured periodically to see whether intervention is moving forward successfully. Keep in mind that many of these interventions can be provided by certified occupational therapy assistants (COTAs) with direction from occupational therapists. COTAs have considerable skill in implementing intervention and observing and reporting on the impact of the intervention.

Direct Interventions

Direct interventions are those provided to individuals or groups to address their needs. These include use of occupations and activities, preparatory tasks and methods, and, in some instances, education and training.

Therapeutic Use of Occupations and Activities

Examples of some of the many therapeutic occupations and activities were described previously. The possible range of activities is limited only by the therapist's creativity and the client's wishes. Occupation-based interventions provide not only the positive benefit of the activity itself, but a sense of accomplishment, self-esteem, and the acquisition of skills needed to perform needed and desired activities. So, for example, horticultural activities provide pleasure, the calming influence of nature, motor and sensory input, and a wide variety of other benefits (Parkinson, Lowe, & Vecsey, 2011; Willmott, Harris, Gellaitry, Cooper, & Horne, 2011). Creative arts offer optimal engagement and skill and confidence building (Griffiths, 2008). Physical exercise is beneficial to reduce stress, enhance motor skills and balance, and reduce depression (Alexandratos, Barnett, & Thomas, 2012).

Activities like cooking skills practice or SE (Lloyd, Bassett, & Samra, 2000) are additional examples of the therapeutic use of occupations. Practical experience, such as assigning a job in the clinic (e.g., organizing supplies, cleaning up after therapy sessions) is another example of use of occupation. This category also includes interventions that remediate underlying skills. These are interventions preparatory to activity (i.e., they are not in and of themselves meaningful occupations, but are skills necessary for participation in those occupations). For example, someone who would like to learn to cook must first be able to read and understand instructions, sequence actions, and keep track of steps in a process.

Feelings and attitudes can also be addressed through occupation. Inaccurate self-concept and lowered self-esteem, for example, are common among individuals with psychiatric disorders, regardless of specific diagnosis, and may lead to ineffective performance. Such individuals may not know that they can do particular activities, or they may feel a chronic sense of failure. Providing opportunities for success may bolster sagging self-esteem, and review of performance of a variety of activities may allow for more accurate self-assessment. One woman with quite severe depression noted that she had, at one time, enjoyed baking. The therapist encouraged her to bring cookies to the next activity group, at which the woman received considerable positive reinforcement for her efforts. That success gave her confidence to resume other valued activities that she had withdrawn from.

Activity-based interventions can be initiated both in individual therapy and in groups (Bullock & Bannigan, 2011; Champagne, 2012; Tokolahi, Em-Chhour, Brakwill, & Stanley, 2013). For some goals, groups have particular advantages. As an example, for a client concerned about self-concept, interaction in a group may provide valuable feedback about self-presentation and the impressions others have of the individual. Hearing about the experiences of others can be useful in learning to cope with an array of psychosocial deficits as well. Clients find that groups allow for transfer of experiences and knowledge from treatment to daily life (Undsteigen, Eklund, & Dahlin-Ivanoff, 2009). There is evidence that supportive socialization, in and of itself, is important in recovery from mental illness (Donohue, Hanif, & Berns, 2011). Because groups can also be a cost-effective and efficient way to provide care, it is important for occupational therapists to consider this strategy.

Preparatory Methods and Tasks

This category of interventions includes techniques that prepare a client for engagement in occupations. Such strategies as splinting, provision of mobility aids, and environmental modification are included in this group of interventions. They are less often employed in working with clients whose challenges are primarily social/emotional/cognitive, but they should not be overlooked. For example, clients with intellectual disabilities or any of the neurocognitive disorders may benefit from thoughtful modification of the environment. An individual with Alzheimer's disease may, during the middle stages of the disorder, be able to use pictures as cues to the contents of cabinets and closets, or to find his or her room if the door has a personal photo.

Education and Training

Educational approaches emphasize teaching of skills that then might be practiced and refined through therapeutic use of occupations (Berger, 2014). Educational interventions might focus on money management, coping strategies, and vocational exploration among many other topics. A particular area of concern is mental health literacy (Jorm, 2012). Many clients do not understand their own conditions very well and are unclear in general about mental health. Educational strategies that are structured for the client's level of comprehension and communication skills are most effective.

As an example of an educational approach, a therapist was facilitating a social skills group for several young women who were lonely and depressed. The women reported wanting to find friends and, perhaps, marriage partners. A quick survey of the group revealed that none of them could identify any strategies for meeting people other than going to bars, an activity they all found unpleasant. The therapist designed several informational sessions, with intervening "homework" (e.g., finding and trying one new activity each week), as a way to broaden the participants' horizons.

Training approaches tend to be more specific and concrete. For example, helping a child with autism learn social skills may require beginning with very specific instruction about how to make eye contact, or what constitutes an acceptable greeting. Instruction and practice can help hone those concrete skills.

Education and training may also be provided as indirect methods of intervention, as in cases where the input is provided to a parent or teacher, who then works with the client.

Advocacy

Not all interventions are provided directly to individuals or groups. A vital role for OT in mental health is in advocating for the needs of clients (Lohman, 2002). Advocacy involves providing information to those in decision-making positions such as, for example, in the case of the need for early intervention programs in schools (Jackson, Nanof, & Bowyer, 2013; Schleis & Daly, 2010). Children cannot speak with those managing public health departments or educational systems for themselves; therapists can help promote their best interests. In addition, it may be necessary to exert influence on legislators, as has been the case in establishing mental health parity (Gallew, Haltiwanger, Sowers, & van den Heever, 2004).

A number of leading thinkers in OT have emphasized the profession's role in promoting **occupational justice** (Townsend, 2012). Occupational justice suggests that it is every human's right to have access to and participate in meaningful occupations. While many individuals have limited power and lack the knowledge to work effectively in systems that can address their concerns, therapists are in a position to inform the public, contact policy makers, and promote the needs of the communities and individuals they serve. Because mental disorders are so often stigmatized, issues of occupational justice can be pronounced.

It is important to remember that **self-advocacy** is also important. Self-advocacy facilitates the individual's ability to address his or her needs through active participation in policy and through clear expression of personal requirements. In the long term, the individual's ability to undertake these activities can promote independence and long-term positive outcomes.

Consultation

Consultation is a growing area for OT practice (Holmes & Leonard, 2014). Although not specifically mentioned in the *Practice Framework* (AOTA, 2014), consultation is a strategy that enhances advocacy activities, but also supports education (e.g., working with parents or teachers to support the needs of a child with an intellectual disability) and other intervention strategies. Consultation involves indirect intervention that assists individuals and systems to support the needs of the client.

Federal legislation, including the Americans with Disabilities Act of 1990 (ADA; ada.gov, n.d.) and the Individuals With Disabilities Education Act (IDEA; Office of Special Education and Rehabilitative Services [OSERS], 1997), has increased the importance of this form of intervention. The ADA specifies that employers must make reasonable accommodations in the workplace for individuals with disabilities, including those with mental disorders. The occupational therapist has valuable expertise to lend to this effort. Specifically, the therapist can help the individual identify the components or characteristics of the job that cause difficulty, then work with the individual and the employer to identify accommodations that are realistic for the situation. More frequent breaks, a less stimulating environment, more specific instructions, and frequent feedback are all examples of modifications that may help an individual with a mental disorder cope with a job.

IDEA requires that children with disabilities that might interfere with their education are provided with supportive services in the least restrictive environment. Important OT contributions in providing these services often involve consultation with classroom teachers about the best ways to manage particular kinds of behavioral challenges. As we've already seen, OT can be helpful in structuring the kinds of mental health promotion programs that can enhance student well-being (Bazyk, 2011).

Similarly, there are consultation roles for occupational therapists in substance abuse prevention programs (Peloquin & Ciro, 2013; Stoffel & Moyers, 2004), **self-help** programs (Moyers & Stoffel, 2001), employment training programs, and programs for parents. An example of the latter is coaching activities to improve mothers' self-competence (Graham, Rodger, & Zivani, 2013). In all of these settings, consultation might focus on management of a particular case, understanding the difficulty that led to the case, new program development, or organizational issues. Consultation services may also be provided to other health professionals, including case managers (Chapleau, Seroczynski, Meyers, Lamb, & Hayes, 2011). Consultation services have demonstrated value in improving client outcomes (Chapleau, Seroczynski, Meyers, Lamb, & Buchino, 2012).

Intervention Approaches

To provide these interventions, a number of specific intervention approaches have been identified (AOTA, 2014). These include health promotion (create, promote); remediation and restoration (establish, restore); maintaining (maintain); compensation and adaptation (modify); and disability prevention (prevent).

Health promotion has become increasingly important in OT practice (Parnell & Wilding, 2010). While many professions have a role in health promotion, the occupation-focused efforts of OT have significant benefits for clients. The "well-elderly" study by the University of Southern California group (Clark et al., 1997) demonstrated the value of occupation-based community group intervention in supporting the health and well-being of older adults, including their mental health.

Remediation and restoration is most likely to focus on the person (performance skills and patterns, client factors including body functions and structures). The category of compensation and adaptation, on the other hand, emphasizes context or activity demands and might include individual choices about task selection and/or the specific nature of the task. Thus, depending on category, the focus might be on helping the individual to enhance skills and abilities or on selecting different activities or different forms of the activity. A framework for thinking about these strategies is selection, optimization, and compensation (SOC; Baltes & Baltes, 1990). As described in Chapter 2, this model was originally developed with a focus on aging well. However, the model has relevance for individuals with occupational performance deficits associated with cognition, emotional regulation, and social impairments. Throughout this text, examples of prevention approaches have been discussed. Think back to the discussion in Chapter 2 of school-based approaches that can minimize future psychosocial issues for young children. Refer to Bazyk (2011) for more details.

Both direct and indirect mechanisms can be effective. Direct methods include individual and group sessions. Indirect methods include **monitoring** (design of an intervention that is provided by another professional, for example a classroom teacher) and **collaborative consultation** (team members jointly determine needs and intervention goals) (Golos, Sarid, Weill, & Weintraub, 2011).

Modification of occupational demand or context is another strategy for therapeutic use of occupation. Some individuals do not have great capacity to change their own performance (e.g., individuals with various neurocognitive disorders), but they may benefit from changes in the activity that reduce demand on themselves. Such occupational or environmental modification (i.e., alteration of context) can be an effective strategy for enhancing performance. Another way of viewing this kind of intervention is that many individuals do not know how to construct the most supportive environments for themselves and can benefit from learning how to do so.

It is important to be aware that intervention occurs in the context of an intervention team. Effective teams identify strategies for communicating, designing collaborative goals, and supporting the total plan that will best serve the client. Ideally, the client is at the center of the process, and several strategies have been developed to ensure that the client benefits from coordination of care and also learns how to advocate for him- or herself. One such intervention, Promoting Resilience, Independence, and Self-Management (PRISM; Arya, 2013), uses a checklist that the client develops and brings to each appointment with each caregiver as a way to monitor progress. These approaches can enhance interaction and give the client a sense of self-efficacy.

Using any of these intervention strategies, therapists focus on enhancing their client's abilities in occupations, skills, and patterns. The ultimate goal of OT, unlike medicine or psychology, is effective function in meaningful occupation. The belief of occupational therapists is that a balance of occupation in all occupations promotes the best possible quality of life for the individual (Meyer, 1922/1977).

Review and Outcomes

Final, essential steps in the OT process involve periodic review during the intervention process to ensure that the activities are having the desired impact and an evaluation of outcomes toward the end of the intervention period to determine whether goals and objectives have been met. These steps require a return to the evaluation measures used initially and a review of goals in consultation with the client to secure both quantitative and qualitative evidence of impact. Outcomes may include (AOTA, 2014) the following:

- Occupational performance (improvement or enhancement)
- Prevention
- Health and wellness
- Quality of life
- Participation
- Role competence
- Well-being
- Occupational justice

These goals address individual needs, family interaction, and community well-being. The identification of outcomes is situation-specific so that for some individual clients, the main focus might be on participation, while for other, the emphasis might be on role competence. These outcomes also include population-level emphases, including occupational justice. Note that these outcomes apply equally regardless of the individual's medical/mental disorder diagnosis.

Cultural Considerations

Culture affects every aspect of occupational performance, both in terms of underlying values that dictate what occupations are most important to a client and in terms of enactment of those values. Conflict among cultural values can have dramatic negative impact on mental health, as in the case of the challenges facing a second-generation female Turkish immigrant to the Netherlands (Pooremamali, Östman, Persson, Eklund, 2011). The young woman was torn between the cultural gender roles characteristic of Turkish culture and the more liberal roles that are found in the Netherlands. Ultimately, participation in creative arts provided an opportunity for her to express and explore her own values.

Design of intervention must be culturally sensitive (Mendez & Westerberg, 2012). For example, in planning a program for parents of Latino children, language, economic, and cultural barriers to involvement in occupations must be addressed if intervention is to be successful.

Lifespan Considerations

Occupational profiles are, to a large extent, age-related. While some occupations are important throughout life (e.g., self-care), the expected skills and enactment of these occupations differ. Young children are typically not expected to cook or to bathe themselves, and their self-care focus is on learning to dress and manage hygiene. Older adults, depending on their living situations, may or may not need to cook for themselves or manage home repairs, while such occupations are typical for adults in their middle years.

Some occupations characterize one life phase more than another. For example, while play is important throughout life, it is a central occupational focus in childhood, but less so in adulthood. Work is a core occupation during the middle years and may extend into old age, but children (at least in the present in most Western cultures) are less likely to be engaged in work.

Recognition of the changes that occur through the lifespan, as well as the cultural context for those changes, can be vital in framing effective intervention. We return now to Mr. Shimbir to see how his treatment was designed and what progress he has made (see Case Vignette).

Resources

American Occupational Therapy Association (AOTA)
aota.org
AOTA has numerous practice guidelines and evidence-based practice resources. It also has special interest groups that publish articles about practice.

Burson, K.A., Barrows, C., Clark, C., Gupta, J., Geraci, J., Mahaffey, L., & Cleveland, P.M. (2010). Specialized knowledge and skills in mental health promotion, prevention, and intervention in occupational therapy practice. *American Journal of Occupational Therapy, 64,* S30-S43.
An official AOTA document identifying the specific knowledge and skills most effective in OT in mental health.

Schell, B.A.B., Gillen, G., & M.E. Scaffa, M.E. (Eds.), *Willard & Spackman's occupational therapy* **(12th ed.). New York, NY: Wolters Kluwer/Lippincott Williams & Wilkins.**
An excellent resource for detailed discussion of various intervention strategies, including not only individual intervention, but group process, advocacy, consultation, and other mechanisms.

CASE VIGNETTE, MR. SHIMBIR (PART 4)

Mr. Shimbir and the therapist have decided that an important early step in the intervention process would be largely a matter of additional education and information. Mr. Shimbir needed to learn how to find resources (e.g., a bus schedule or an English as a second language [ESL] class), and to get information about the steps of various activities he wanted to pursue (e.g., financial management). With guidance from the therapist, Mr. Shimbir began to learn how to use the Internet to locate information. He and the therapist used each session to focus on a specific self-care area that Mr. Shimbir felt was important and to locate several resources for ways to find assistance in that area. The therapist then helped him practice making phone calls to ask for help. During the first session, Mr. Shimbir located an ESL class and, with the therapist's help, called to get information and to register.

During the second session, Mr. Shimbir reported back that he had gone to his first class and had been pleasantly surprised by how much he enjoyed it. He felt the teacher was supportive and helpful, and he discovered that two other students from Somalia were enrolled in the class. He acknowledged with a smile that he and those two students had spent the break speaking in Somali, but he indicated that they made a pact to speak only English thereafter.

The therapist assisted Mr. Shimbir in completing the Strong Interest Inventory (CPP, Inc., 2009). Rather than administer the tool as a standardized test, the therapist used it as a mechanism for helping Mr. Shimbir identify the work activities he might enjoy. The therapist and Mr. Shimbir then went to the U.S. Bureau of Labor Statistics *Occupational Outlook Handbook* (2013) to identify job titles that fit his interests and skills. The next step was to begin to look for job openings both online and in the newspaper.

An additional component of the intervention plan was a focus on coping strategies to help Mr. Shimbir reduce his anxiety and manage the flashbacks that were so troubling to him. Through a combination of meditation and guided-mental imagery, Mr. Shimbir practiced refocusing at moments when he began to feel anxious (Lang et al., 2012).

As Mr. Shimbir's skills and coping mechanisms improved, the therapist began to increasingly suggest "homework" tasks to be completed between sessions. These included activities such as making phone calls to potential employers, filling out job applications, meditating regularly, and engaging in the other activities that Mr. Shimbir wanted to master.

At the end of 3 months of weekly sessions, Mr. Shimbir secured a job at a community garden, to which he commuted daily by bus. He was continuing his ESL classes, and he met regularly with several friends from the class to practice English. He was able to do the grocery shopping and the laundry to help his uncle around the house. He still struggled with financial management tasks, but he found a community center that offered money management courses and planned to take the course when it was next offered. Although he also still struggled with periods of intense anxiety, he reported that the episodes were slightly less frequent and that his meditation skills helped him to manage them. Similarly, he still had insomnia and nightmares, but these had diminished in intensity and frequency.

References

Ada.gov (n.d.) *The Americans with Disabilities Act of 1990 and Revised ADA Regulations Implementing Title II and Title III.* Retrieved from http://www.ada.gov/2010_regs.htm.

Alexandratos, K., Barnett, F., & Thomas, Y. (2012). The impact of exercise on the mental health and quality of life of people with severe mental illness: A critical review. *British Journal of Occupational Therapy, 75*(2), 48-60.

American Occupational Therapy Association (AOTA; 2014) Occupational therapy practice framework: Domain & process (3rd ed.). *American Journal of Occupational Therapy, 68*(Suppl 1), S1-S48.

American Psychiatric Association (APA; 2013). *Diagnostic and statistical manual of mental disorders* (5th ed.). Washington, DC: Author.

Ammerall, M.A., & Coppers, J. (2012). Understanding living skills: First steps to evidence-based practice. Lessons learned from a practice-based journey in the Netherlands. *Occupational Therapy International, 19*(1), 45-53.

Arbesman, M., & Logsdon, D.W. (2011). Occupational therapy interventions for employment and education for adults with serious mental illness: A systematic review. *American Journal of Occupational Therapy, 65*(3), 238-246.

Arya, D.K. (2013). PRISM: Promoting resilience, independence and self-management—A strategy to manage chronic mental illnesses. *Asian Journal of Psychiatry, 6,* 303-307.

Baltes, P.B., & Baltes, M.M. (1990). Psychological perspectives on successful aging: The model of selective optimization with compensation. In P. B. Baltes & M. M. Baltes (Eds.), *Successful aging: Perspectives from the behavioral sciences* (pp. 1–34). New York: Cambridge University Press.

Bassett, H., Lloyd, C., & Tse, S. (2008). Approaching in the right spirit: Spirituality and hope in recovery from mental health problems. *International Journal of Therapy & Rehabilitation, 15*(6), 254-259.

Baxter, C., Prior, S., Forsyth, K., Maciver, D., Meiklejohn, A., Irvine, L., & Walsh, M. (2012). Mental health vocational rehabilitation—Occupational therapists' perceptions of individual placement and support. *International Journal of Therapy & Rehabilitation, 19*(4), 217-225.

Bazyk, S. (Ed.). (2011). *Mental health promotion, prevention, and intervention with children and youth: A guiding framework for occupational therapy.* Rockville, MD: American Occupational Therapy Association, Inc.

Berger, S. (2014). Educating clients. In B.A.B. Schell, G. Gillen, & M.E. Scaffa (Eds.), *Willard & Spackman's Occupational Therapy* (12th ed., pp. 353-363). New York, NY: Wolters Kluwer/Lippincott Williams & Wilkins.

Best, L.J., Still, M., & Cameron, G. (2008). Supported education: enabling course completion for people experiencing mental illness. *Australian Occupational Therapy Journal, 55*(1), 65-68.

Bullock, A., & Bannigan, K. (2011). Effectiveness of activity-based group work in community mental health: A systematic review. *American Journal of Occupational Therapy, 65,* 257-266.

Casteleijn, D., & Graham, M. (2012). Domains for occupational therapy outcomes in mental health practices. *South African Journal of Occupational Therapy, 42*(1), 26-34.

Chaffey, L., Unsworth, C.A., & Fossey, E., (2012). Relationship between intuition and emotional intelligence in occupational therapists in mental health practice. *American Journal of Occupational Therapy, 66*(1), 88-96.

Champagne, T. (2012). Creating occupational therapy groups for children and youth in community-based mental health practice. *OT Practice, 17*(14), 13-18.

Champagne, T., & Koomar, J. (2011). Expanding the focus: Addressing sensory discrimination concerns in mental health. *Mental Health Special Interest Section Quarterly, 34*(1), 1-4.

Chan, A.S.M., Tsang, H.W.H., & Li, S.M.Y. (2009). Case report of integrated supported employment for a person with severe mental illness. *American Journal of Occupational Therapy, 63,* 238-244.

Chapleau, A., Seroczynski, A.D., Meyers, S., Lamb, K., & Buchino, S. (2012). The effectiveness of a consultation model in community mental health. *Occupational Therapy in Mental Health, 28*(4), 379-95.

Chapleau, A., Seroczynski, A.D., Meyers, S., Lamb, K., & Haynes, S. (2011). Occupational therapy consultation for case managers in community mental health: Exploring strategies to improve job satisfaction and self-efficacy. *Professional Case Management, 16*(2), 71-79.

Chou, K., Shih, Y., Chang, C., Chou, Y., Hu, W., Cheng, J., . . . Hsieh, C. (2012). Psychosocial rehabilitation activities, empowerment, and quality of community-based life for people with schizophrenia. *Archives of Psychiatric Nursing, 26*(4), 285-294.

Cipriani, J., Cooper, M., DiGiovanni, N.M., Litchkofski, A., Nichols, A.L., & Ramsey, A. (2013). Dog-assisted therapy for residents of long-term care facilities: An evidence-based review with implications for occupational therapy. *Physical & Occupational Therapy in Geriatrics, 31*(3), 214-240.

Clark, F.A., Azen, S.P., Zemke, R., Jackson, J.M., Carlson, M.E., Mandel, D., . . . Lipson, L. (1997). Occupational therapy for independent-living older adults: A randomized controlled trial. *Journal of the American Medical Association, 278,* 1321-1326.

Cole, M.B., & McLean, V. (2003). Therapeutic relationships redefined. *Occupational Therapy in Mental Health, 19,* 33-56.

Cordier, R. (2011). No friends no fun: The importance of playmates in developing the play and social skills of children with ADHD. Occupational Therapy Australia, 24th National Conference and Exhibition, 29 June - 1 July 2011. *Australian Occupational Therapy Journal, 58*(Suppl.), 59.

Cordier, R., & Scanlan, J.N. (2012). Cognitive remediation has global cognitive and functional benefits for people with schizophrenia when combined with psychiatric rehabilitation. *Australian Occupational Therapy Journal, 59*(4), 334-335.

CPP (2009). *Strong interest inventory.* Retrieved from https://www.cpp.com/products/strong/index.aspx.

Davidson, L. (2003). *Living outside mental illness: Qualitative studies of recovery in schizophrenia.* New York, NY: New York University Press.

DeAngelis, T. (2013). Therapy gone wild. *Monitor on Psychology, 44*(8), 49-52.

Diener, E. (2006). Guidelines for national indicators of subjective well-being and ill-being. *Applied Research in Quality of Life, 1,* 151-157.

Dirette, D., & Kolak, L. (2004). Occupational performance needs of adolescents in alternative education programs. *American Journal of Occupational Therapy, 58,* 337-341.

Donohue, M.V., Hanif, H., & Berns, L.W. (2011). An exploratory study of social participation in occupational therapy groups. *Special Interest Section Quarterly: Mental Health, 24*(4), 1-3.

Edgelow, M., & Krupa, T. (2011). Randomized controlled pilot study of an occupational time-use intervention for people with serious mental illness. *American Journal of Occupational Therapy, 65*(4), 267-276.

Eklund, M. (2007). Perceived control: How is it related to daily occupation in patients with mental illness living in the community? *American Journal of Occupational Therapy, 61,* 535-542.

Fowler, M. (December 19, 2011). Waverly Place and MAOT 2001: Creative approaches to recovery for adults with mental health issues. *OT Practice, 16,* 25-26.

Frolek Clark, G.J., & Schlabach, T.L. (2013). Systematic review of occupational therapy interventions to improve cognitive development in children ages birth–5 years. *American Journal of Occupational Therapy, 67*(4), 425-430.

Gallew, H.A., Haltiwanger, E., Sowers, J., & van den Heever, N. (2004). Political action and critical analysis: Mental health parity. *Occupational Therapy in Mental Health, 20*(1), 1-25.

Gardiner, C., & Brown, N. (2010). Is there a role for occupational therapy within a specialist child and adolescent mental health eating disorder service? *British Journal of Occupational Therapy, 73*(1), 38-43.

Gibson, R.W., D'Amico, M., Jaffe, L., & Arbesman, M. (2011). Occupational therapy interventions for recovery in the areas of community integration and normative life roles for adults with serious mental illness: A systematic review. *American Journal of Occupational Therapy, 65,* 247-256.

Gil-Gomez, J.A., Llorens, R., Alcaniz, M., & Colomer, C. (2011). Effectiveness of a Wii balance board-based system (eBaViR) for balance rehabilitation: A pilot randomized clinical trial in patients with acquired brain injury. *Journal of Neuroengineering & Rehabilitation, 8,* 30.

Golos, A., Sarid, M., Weill, M., & Weintraub, N. (2011). Efficacy of an early intervention program for at-risk preschool boys: A two-group control study. *American Journal of Occupational Therapy, 65,* 400-408.

Graham F., Rodger, S., & Zivani, J. (2013). Effectiveness of occupational performance coaching in improving children's and mothers' performance and mothers' self-competence. *American Journal of Occupational Therapy, 67,* 10-18.

Griffiths, S. (2008). The experience of creative activity as a treatment medium. *Journal of Mental Health, 17*(1), 49-63.

Gutman, S.A., Kerner, R., Zombek, I., Dulek, J., & Ramsey, A. (2009). Supported education of adults with psychiatric disabilities: Effectiveness of an occupational therapy program. *American Journal of Occupational Therapy, 63,* 245-254.

Gutman, S.A., Raphael, E., Ceder, L.M., Khan, A., Timp, K.M., & Salvant, S. (2010). The Effect of a motor-based, social skills intervention for adolescents with high-functioning autism: Two single-subject design cases. *Occupational Therapy International, 17*(4), 188-197.

Haertl, K., Behrens, K., Houtujec, J., Rue, A., & Haken, R.T. (2009). Factors influencing satisfaction and efficacy of services at a free-standing psychiatric occupational therapy clinic. *American Journal of Occupational Therapy, 63,* 691-700.

Helfrich, C.A., Chan, D.V., & Sabol, P. (2011). Cognitive predictors of life skill intervention outcomes for adults with mental illness at risk for homelessness. *American Journal of Occupational Therapy, 65,* 277-286.

Holmes, W.M., & Leonard, C. (2014). Consultation. In B.A.B. Schell, G. Gillen, & M.E. Scaffa (Eds.), *Willard & Spackman's occupational therapy* (12th ed., pp. 1089-1097). New York, NY: Wolters Kluwer/Lippincott Williams & Wilkins.

Jackson, L.L., Nanof, T., & Bowyer, P. (2013). Health care reform and school-based and early intervention practice. *OT Practice, 18*(1), CE1-CE8.

Javaherian-Dysinger, H., & Freire, M.E. (2010). Drama: Still a tool for healing and understanding. *Special Interest Section Quarterly: Mental Health, 33*(4), 1-3.

Jorm, A.F. (2012). Mental health literacy: Empowering the community to take action for better mental health. *American Psychologist, 67*(3), 231-243.

Kuipers, K., & Grice, J.W. (2009). The structure of novice and expert occupational therapists' clinical reasoning before and after exposure to a domain-specific protocol. *Australian Occupational Therapy Journal, 56*(6), 418-427.

Lang, A.J., Strauss, J.L., Bomyea, J., Bormann, J.E, Hickman, S.D., Good, R.C., & Essex, M. (2012). The theoretical and empirical basis for meditation as an intervention for PTSD. *Behavior Modification, 36*(6), 759-786.

Lloyd, C., & Bassett, H. (2012). The role of occupational therapy in working with the homeless population: An assertive outreach approach. *New Zealand Journal of Occupational Therapy, 9*(1), 18-23.

Lloyd, C., Bassett, H., & Samra, P. (2000). Rehabilitation programmes for early psychosis. *British Journal of Occupational Therapy, 63*(2), 76-82.

Lohman, H. (2002). Perspectives. Becoming involved with advocacy. *OT Practice, 7*, 35-36.

Loukas, K.M. (2011). Occupational placemaking: Facilitating self-organization through use of a sensory room. *Special Interest Section Quarterly: Mental Health, 34*(2), 1-3.

Lyne, J., Moxon, S., & Valios, N. (2008). Help to reduce depression. *Community Care, 13*(1747), 34, 36.

Mahony, G., Haracz, K., & Williams, L.T. (2012). How mental health occupational therapists address issues of diet with their clients: A qualitative study. *Australian Journal of Occupational Therapy, 59*(4), 294-301.

May-Benson, T.A., & Koomar, J.A. (2010). Systematic review of the research evidence examining the effectiveness of interventions using a sensory integrative approach for children. *American Journal of Occupational Therapy, 64*, 403-414.

Mendez, J.L., & Westerberg, D. (2012). Implementation of a culturally adapted treatment to reduce barriers for Latino parents. *Cultural Diversity and Ethnic Minority Psychology, 18*, 363-372.

Meyer, A. (1922/1977). The philosophy of occupational therapy. Reprinted from the Archives of Occupational Therapy, 1, 1-10. *American Journal of Occupational Therapy, 31*(10), 639-642.

Morgan, R., & Long, T. (2012). The effectiveness of occupational therapy for children with developmental coordination disorder: A review of the qualitative literature. *British Journal of Occupational Therapy, 75*(1), 10-18.

Moyers, P. A., & Stoffel, V. C. (2001). Community-based approaches for substance use disorders. In M. Scaffa (Ed.), *Occupational therapy in community-based practice settings* (pp. 318-342). Philadelphia: F. A. Davis.

Office of Special Education and Rehabilitation Services (OSERS; 1997). IDEA '97. Retrieved from http://www2.ed.gov/offices/OSERS/Policy/IDEA/the_law.html.

Organization for Economic Co-operation and Development (OECD, n.d.). *Better life index.* Retrieved from http://www.oecdbetterlifeindex.org/.

Parkinson, S., Lowe, C., & Vecsey, T. (2011). The therapeutic benefits of horticulture in a mental health service. *British Journal of Occupational Therapy, 74*(11), 525-534.

Parnell, T., & Wilding, C. (2010). Where can an occupation-focussed philosophy take occupational therapy? *Australian Occupational Therapy Journal, 57*(5), 345-348.

Peloquin, S.M., & Ciro, C.A. (2013). Self-development groups among women in recovery: Client perceptions of satisfaction and engagement. *American Journal of Occupational Therapy, 67*(1), 82-90.

Pooremamali, P., Östman, M., Persson, D., & Eklund, M. (2011). An occupational therapy approach to the support of a young immigrant female's mental health: A story of bicultural personal growth. *International Journal of Qualitative Studies on Health & Well-Being, 6*(3), 1-15.

Pooremamali, P., Persson, D., & Eklund, M. (2011). Occupational therapists' experience of working with immigrant clients in mental health care. *Scandinavian Journal of Occupational Therapy, 18*(2), 109-121.

Rizk, S., Pizur-Barnekow, K., & Darragh, A.R. (2011). Leisure and social participation and health-related quality of life in caregivers of children with autism. *OTJR: Occupation, Participation & Health, 31*(4), 164-171.

Schell, B.A.B., Gillen, G., & Scaffa, M.E. (Eds.). (2014). *Willard & Spackman's occupational therapy* (12th ed.). New York, NY: Wolters Kluwer/Lippincott Williams & Wilkins.

Schindler, V.P., & Kientz, M. (2013) Supports and barriers to higher education and employment for individuals diagnosed with mental illness. *Journal of Vocational Rehabilitation, 39*(1), 29-41.

Schleis, R., & Daly, N. (2010). Current Early Intervention Trends and Advocacy in Illinois. *Communique, 3*, 1-11.

Chwast, S. (2014). *Seth Chwast blog*. Retrieved from http://growyourbrainblog.blogspot.com/search?updated-max=2014-04-25T12:16:00-07:00&max-results=1&start=4&by-date=false.

Stoffel, V.C., & Moyers, P.A. (2004). An evidence-based and occupational perspective of interventions for persons with substance use disorders. *American Journal of Occupational Therapy, 58*(5), 570-586.

Stols, D., van Heerden, R., van Jaarsveld, A., & Nel, R. (2013). Substance abusers' anger behaviour and sensory processing patterns: An occupational therapy investigation. *South African Journal of Occupational Therapy, 43*(1), 25-34.

Taylor, R.R. (2014). Therapeutic relationship and client collaboration. In B.A.B. Schell, G. Gillen, & M.E. Scaffa (Eds.), *Willard & Spackman's occupational therapy* (12th ed., pp. 425-436). New York, NY: Wolters Kluwer/Lippincott Williams & Wilkins.

Thomas, H. (2012). *Occupation-based activity analysis*. Thorofare, NJ: SLACK Incorporated.

Thomas, Y., Gray, M., McGinty, S., & Ebringer, S. (2011). Homeless adults engagement in art: First steps towards identity, recovery and social inclusion. *Australian Occupational Therapy Journal, 58*(6), 429-36.

Tokolahi, E., Em-Chhour, C., Brakwill, L., & Stanley, S. (2013) An occupation-based group for children with anxiety. *British Journal of Occupational Therapy, 76*(1), 31-36.

Townsend, E.A. (2012). Boundaries and bridges to adult mental health: Critical occupational and capabilities perspectives of justice. *Journal of Occupational Science, 19*(1), 8-24.

Undsteigen, B., Eklund, K., & Dahlin-Ivanoff, S. (2009). Patients' experience of groups in outpatient mental health services and its significance for daily occupations. *Scandinavian Journal of Occupational Therapy, 16*(3), 172-180.

U.S. Bureau of Labor Statistics (2013). *Occupational outlook handbook*. Retrieved from http://www.bls.gov/oco

Wagenfeld, A. (2013). Nature: An environment for health. *OT Practice 18*(15), 15–19.

Willmott, L., Harris, P., Gellaitry, G., Cooper, V., & Horne, R. (2011). Effects of expressive writing following first myocardial infarction: A randomized controlled trial. *Health Psychology, 30*, 642-650.

Woo, C.C., & Leon, M. (May 20, 2013). Environmental enrichment as an effective treatment for autism: A randomized controlled trial. *Behavioral Neuroscience, 127*(4), 487-97.

Appendix

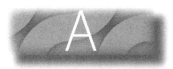

Psychotropic Medications by Class

TABLE A-1				
ANTIPSYCHOTICS DRUG CHART				
BRAND NAME	*GENERIC NAME*	*U.S. FOOD AND DRUG ADMINISTRATION (FDA)–APPROVED INDICATION*	*DOSAGE FORM*	*COMMON ADVERSE EFFECTS*
First-Generation Antipsychotics				
Thorazine	Chlorpromazine	Schizophrenia Manifestations of mania associated with bipolar disorder Intractable hiccups	Tablet Short-acting intramuscular injection	Extrapyramidal reactions (e.g., Parkinson-like symptoms, dystonia, akathisia, tardive dyskinesia), drowsiness, dizziness, skin reactions or rash, dry mouth, orthostatic hypotension, amenorrhea, galactorrhea, weight gain
				(continued)

Bonder B.
Psychopathology and Function, Fifth Edition (pp 503-532).
© 2015 SLACK Incorporated.

TABLE A-1 (CONTINUED)				
ANTIPSYCHOTICS DRUG CHART				
BRAND NAME	*GENERIC NAME*	*FDA–APPROVED INDICATION*	*DOSAGE FORM*	*COMMON ADVERSE EFFECTS*
Prolixin	Fluphenazine	Psychotic disorders	Tablet Oral solution Short-acting intramuscular injection Long-acting intramuscular injection	Extrapyramidal reactions (e.g., pseudo-Parkinsonism, dystonia, dyskinesia, akathisia, oculogyric crises, opisthotonos, hyperreflexia), drowsiness, lethargy, weight gain
Haldol	Haloperidol	Psychotic disorders Control of tics and vocal utterances of Tourette's disorder	Tablet Oral solution Short-acting intramuscular injection Long-acting intramuscular injection	Difficulty with speaking or swallowing; inability to move eyes; loss of balance control; mask-like facies; muscle spasms, especially of the neck and back; restlessness or need to keep moving (severe); stiffness of the arms and legs; trembling and shaking of the fingers and hands; twisting movements of the body; weakness of the arms and legs
Adasuve Loxitane	Loxapine	Schizophrenia Acute treatment of agitation associated with schizophrenia or bipolar I disorder	Capsule	Difficulty with speaking or swallowing; lip smacking or puckering; loss of balance control; mask-like facies; rapid or fine worm-like movements of the tongue; restlessness or desire to keep moving; shuffling walk; slowed movements; trembling and shaking of the fingers and hands; uncontrolled chewing movements; uncontrolled movements of the limbs

(continued)

TABLE A-1 (CONTINUED)

ANTIPSYCHOTICS DRUG CHART

BRAND NAME	GENERIC NAME	FDA–APPROVED INDICATION	DOSAGE FORM	COMMON ADVERSE EFFECTS
Trilafon	Perphenazine	Schizophrenia	Tablet	Extrapyramidal reactions (e.g., Parkinson-like symptoms, dystonia, akathisia, tardive dyskinesia), drowsiness, muscular weakness, dry mouth, blurred vision, weight gain, skin reactions, amenorrhea, galactorrhea
Mellaril	Thioridazine	Schizophrenia, in patients who fail to respond adequately to treatment with other antipsychotic medications	Tablet	Agitation, constipation, diarrhea, dizziness, drowsiness, dry mouth, enlarged pupils, jitteriness, nausea, stuffy nose, vomiting
Navane	Thiothixene	Schizophrenia	Capsule	Drowsiness, dystonia, akathisia, and other extrapyramidal effects; tardive dyskinesia; neuroleptic malignant syndrome
Stelazine	Trifluoperazine	Schizophrenia	Tablet	Extrapyramidal reactions (e.g., Parkinson-like symptoms, dystonia, akathisia), drowsiness, fatigue, muscular weakness, insomnia, blurred vision, skin reactions or rash, anorexia, dry mouth, hypotension, amenorrhea, galactorrhea

(continued)

TABLE A-1 (CONTINUED)

ANTIPSYCHOTICS DRUG CHART

BRAND NAME	GENERIC NAME	FDA–APPROVED INDICATION	DOSAGE FORM	COMMON ADVERSE EFFECTS
Second-Generation Antipsychotics				
Abilify Abilify Discmelt Abilify Maintena	Aripiprazole	Schizophrenia Acute treatment of manic or mixed episodes associated with bipolar I disorder as monotherapy and as an adjunct to lithium or valproate Maintenance treatment of bipolar I disorder, both as monotherapy and as an adjunct to lithium or valproate Adjunctive treatment of major depressive disorder Treatment of irritability associated with autistic disorder Acute treatment of agitation associated with schizophrenia or manic/mixed episodes of bipolar I disorder	Tablet Orally dissolving tablet Oral solution Short-acting intramuscular injection Long-acting intramuscular injection	Difficulty with speaking; drooling; loss of balance control; muscle trembling, jerking, or stiffness; restlessness; shuffling walk; stiffness of the limbs; twisting movements of the body; uncontrolled movements, especially of the face, neck, and back
Saphris	Asenapine	Schizophrenia	Sublingual tablet	Abnormal or decreased touch sensation; inability to sit still; increase in body movements; rapid or worm-like movements of the tongue; restlessness

(continued)

TABLE A-1 (CONTINUED)

ANTIPSYCHOTICS DRUG CHART

BRAND NAME	GENERIC NAME	FDA–APPROVED INDICATION	DOSAGE FORM	COMMON ADVERSE EFFECTS
Saphris (continued)		Acute treatment as monotherapy or adjunctive therapy with lithium or valproate of manic or mixed episodes associated with bipolar I disorder		Shakiness in the legs, arms, hands, or feet; trouble with breathing, speaking, or swallowing; twitching; twisting; uncontrolled chewing movements; uncontrolled twisting movements of the neck, trunk, arms, or legs; weakness of the arms and legs
Clozaril Fazaclo	Clozapine	Treatment-resistant schizophrenia; Reducing suicidal behavior in patients with schizophrenia or schizoaffective disorder	Tablet; Orally dissolving tablet	Blurred vision, confusion, dizziness, faintness, or lightheadedness when getting up suddenly; fast, pounding, or irregular heartbeat or pulse; fever; shakiness in the legs, arms, hands, or feet; sleepiness; sweating; unusual tiredness or weakness
Fanapt	Iloperidone	Schizophrenia	Tablet	Fast, pounding, or irregular heartbeat or pulse
Latuda	Lurasidone	Schizophrenia; Depressive episodes associated with bipolar I disorder as monotherapy and as adjunctive therapy with lithium or valproate	Tablet	Absence of or decrease in body movement; difficulty with swallowing; drooling; inability to sit still; incremental or ratchet-like movement of the muscles; loss of balance control; mask-like facies; muscle discomfort; muscle trembling, jerking, or stiffness; shuffling walk; slow movements; slow reflexes; slurred speech; uncontrolled movements, especially of the face, neck, and back

(continued)

TABLE A-1 (CONTINUED)

ANTIPSYCHOTICS DRUG CHART

BRAND NAME	GENERIC NAME	FDA–APPROVED INDICATION	DOSAGE FORM	COMMON ADVERSE EFFECTS
Symbyax	Olanzapine and Fluoxetine	Treatment of depressive episodes associated with bipolar I disorder Treatment-resistant depression	Capsule	Bloating or swelling of the face, arms, hands, lower legs, or feet; body aches or pain; confusion; congestion; cough; delusions; dementia; dryness or soreness of the throat; fever; hoarseness; rapid weight gain; runny nose; shakiness in the limbs; tender, swollen glands in the neck; tingling of the hands or feet; trouble with swallowing; unusual weight gain or loss; voice changes
Zyprexa Zyprexa Relprevv Zyprexa Zydis	Olanzapine	Schizophrenia Acute treatment of manic or mixed episodes associated with bipolar I disorder Adjunct to valproate or lithium in the treatment of manic or mixed episodes associated with bipolar I disorder Maintenance treatment of bipolar I disorder Treatment of acute agitation associated with schizophrenia and bipolar I mania	Tablet Orally dissolving tablet Short-acting intramuscular injection Long-acting intramuscular injection	Bloating or swelling of the face, arms, hands, lower legs, or feet; blurred vision; change in vision; change in walking and balance; clumsiness or unsteadiness; difficulty with speaking; difficulty with swallowing; drooling; impaired vision; inability to sit still; loss of balance control; mask-like facies; rapid weight gain; restlessness; shuffling walk; slowed movements; slurred speech; tic-like (jerky) movements of the head, face, mouth, and neck; tingling of the hands or feet; unusual weight gain or loss

(continued)

TABLE A-1 (CONTINUED)				
ANTIPSYCHOTICS DRUG CHART				
BRAND NAME	GENERIC NAME	FDA–APPROVED INDICATION	DOSAGE FORM	COMMON ADVERSE EFFECTS
Invega Invega Sustenna	Paliperidone	Schizophrenia Treatment of schizoaffective disorder as monotherapy and as an adjunct to mood stabilizers and/or antidepressants	Extended-release tablet Long-acting intramuscular injection	Difficulty with speaking; drooling; fast, pounding, or irregular heartbeat or pulse; increase in body movements; loss of balance control; muscle trembling, jerking, or stiffness; restlessness; shuffling walk; stiffness of the limbs; uncontrolled movements, especially of the face, neck, and back
Seroquel Seroquel XR	Quetiapine	Schizophrenia Acute treatment of manic or mixed episodes associated with bipolar I disorder; both as monotherapy and as an adjunct to lithium or divalproex Acute treatment of depressive episodes associated with bipolar disorder Maintenance treatment of bipolar I disorder, as an adjunct to lithium or divalproex Adjunctive therapy to antidepressants for the treatment of major depressive disorder	Tablet Extended-release tablet	Chills; cold sweats; confusion; dizziness, faintness, or lightheadedness when getting up suddenly from a lying or sitting position; sleepiness or unusual drowsiness
				(continued)

TABLE A-1 (CONTINUED)				
ANTIPSYCHOTICS DRUG CHART				
BRAND NAME	GENERIC NAME	FDA–APPROVED INDICATION	DOSAGE FORM	COMMON ADVERSE EFFECTS
Risperdal Risperdal Consta Risperdal M Tabs	Risperidone	Schizophrenia Acute manic or mixed episodes associated with bipolar I disorder alone or in combination with lithium or valproate Treatment of irritability associated with autistic disorder	Tablet Orally dissolving tablet Oral solution Long-acting injection	Aggressive behavior; agitation; anxiety; changes in vision; decreased sexual desire or performance; difficulty concentrating; difficulty speaking or swallowing; inability to move the eyes; loss of balance control; mask-like facies; memory problems; menstrual changes; muscle spasms of the face, neck, and back; problems with urination or increase in the amount of urine; shuffling walk; skin rash or itching; stiffness or weakness of the arms or legs; tic-like or twitching movements; trouble sleeping
Geodon	Ziprasidone	Schizophrenia Acute treatment as monotherapy of manic or mixed episodes associated with bipolar I disorder Maintenance treatment of bipolar I disorder as an adjunct to lithium or valproate Acute treatment of agitation associated with schizophrenia	Capsule Short-acting intramuscular injection	Cough; difficulty with speaking; drooling; fear or nervousness; fever; inability to sit still; loss of balance control; muscle trembling, jerking, or stiffness; restlessness; shuffling walk; sneezing; sore throat; stiffness of the limbs; twisting movements of the body

TABLE A-2				
MOOD STABILIZERS DRUG CHART				
BRAND NAME	GENERIC NAME	FDA-APPROVED INDICATION	DOSAGE FORM	COMMON ADVERSE EFFECTS
Carbatrol Epitol Equetro Tegretol Tegretol XR	Carbamazepine	Acute manic or mixed episodes of bipolar 1 disorder Partial seizures Generalized tonic–clonic seizures Mixed-seizure patterns Trigeminal neuralgia Glossopharyngeal neuralgia	Tablet Chewable tablet Extended-release tablet Extended-release capsule Suspension	Blurred vision or double vision, continuous back-and-forth eye movements
Lamictal Lamictal ODT Lamictal XR	Lamotrigine	Maintenance treatment of bipolar 1 disorder Adjunctive therapy in treatment of generalized seizures of Lennox-Gastaut syndrome, primary generalized tonic–clonic seizures, and partial seizures Conversion to monotherapy in patients with partial seizures who are receiving treatment with a single antiepileptic drug (AED)	Tablet Chewable tablet Orally dissolving tablets Extended-release tablets	Blurred vision, changes in vision, clumsiness or unsteadiness, double vision, poor coordination, skin rash
Lithobid	Lithium	Manic episodes of bipolar disorder Maintenance therapy of bipolar disorder	Tablet Capsule Oral solution Extended release tablet	Confusion, poor memory, or lack of awareness; fainting; fast or slow heartbeat; frequent urination; increased thirst; irregular pulse; stiffness of the arms or legs; troubled breathing, especially during hard work or exercise; unusual tiredness or weakness; weight gain

(continued)

TABLE A-2 (CONTINUED)

MOOD STABILIZERS DRUG CHART

BRAND NAME	GENERIC NAME	FDA-APPROVED INDICATION	DOSAGE FORM	COMMON ADVERSE EFFECTS
Trileptal Oxtellar XR	Oxcarbazepine	Monotherapy or adjunctive therapy of partial seizures in patients with epilepsy	Tablet Oral suspension Extended-release tablet	Change in vision, walking or balance, clumsiness or unsteadiness, cough, fever, sneezing, sore throat, crying, dizziness, double vision, false sense of well-being, feeling of constant movement of self or surroundings, mental depression, sensation of spinning, uncontrolled back-and-forth and/or rolling eye movements
Depacon	Valproate sodium	Monotherapy and adjunctive therapy for patients with complex partial seizures, simple and complex absence seizures Adjunctive therapy for multiple seizure types, which include absence seizures	Intravenous solution	Black, tarry stools; bleeding gums; bloating or swelling of the face, arms, hands, lower legs, or feet; blood in the urine; confusion; cough; crying; delusions; dementia; depersonalization; diarrhea; difficult breathing; dysphoria; euphoria; fever or chills; headache; loss of appetite; lower back or side pain; depression; nausea; nervousness;

(continued)

TABLE A-2 (CONTINUED)

MOOD STABILIZERS DRUG CHART

BRAND NAME	GENERIC NAME	FDA-APPROVED INDICATION	DOSAGE FORM	COMMON ADVERSE EFFECTS
Depacon (continued)				Painful urination; paranoia; rapid weight gain; rapidly changing moods; runny nose; shakiness or tingling in the limbs; shivering; sleepiness; tightness in the chest; trouble with sleeping; unusual bleeding or bruising
Depakene	Valproic acid	Monotherapy and adjunctive therapy for patients with complex partial seizures and simple and complex absence seizures Adjunctive therapy for multiple seizures types, which include absence seizures	Capsule Oral solution Oral syrup	Same as Valproate sodium
Depakote	Divalproex sodium	Monotherapy and adjunctive therapy for complex partial seizures and simple and complex absence seizures Adjunctive therapy for multiple seizures types, which include absence seizures Mania associated with bipolar disorder Migraine prophylaxis	Tablet Sprinkle capsules	Same as Valproate sodium

(continued)

	TABLE A-2 (CONTINUED)			
	MOOD STABILIZERS DRUG CHART			
BRAND NAME	*GENERIC NAME*	*FDA-APPROVED INDICATION*	*DOSAGE FORM*	*COMMON ADVERSE EFFECTS*
Depakote ER	Divalproex sodium extended-release	Monotherapy and adjunctive therapy for complex partial seizures and simple and complex absence seizures Adjunctive therapy for multiple seizures types, which include absence seizures Mania associated with bipolar disorder Migraine prophylaxis	Extended-release tablet	Same as Valproate sodium
Stavzor	Valproic acid	Monotherapy and adjunctive therapy for complex partial seizures and simple and complex absence seizures Adjunctive therapy for multiple seizures types, which include absence seizures Mania associated with bipolar disorder Migraine prophylaxis	Capsule	Same as Valproate sodium

TABLE A-3

ANTIDEPRESSANTS DRUG CHART

BRAND NAME	GENERIC NAME	FDA-APPROVED INDICATION	DOSAGE FORM	COMMON ADVERSE EFFECTS
Serotonin Reuptake Inhibitors				
Celexa	Citalopram	Treatment of depression	Oral solution	Decrease in sexual desire or ability, sleepiness or unusual drowsiness, agitation, blurred vision, confusion, fever, increase in the frequency of urination or amount of urine produced, lack of emotion, loss of memory, menstrual changes, skin rash or itching, trouble with breathing
Lexapro	Escitalopram	Treatment of major depressive disorder Generalized anxiety disorder	Tablet Oral solution	Constipation, decreased interest in sex, diarrhea, dry mouth, ejaculation delay, heartburn, inability to have or keep an erection, sleepiness or unusual drowsiness, trouble sleeping
Luvox Luvox CR	Fluvoxamine	Treatment of obsessive-compulsive disorder	Tablet Extended-release capsule	Change in sexual performance or desire, constipation, headache, trouble with sleeping, unusual tiredness
Brisdelle Paxil Paxil CR Pexeva	Paroxetine	Treatment of generalized anxiety disorder Major depressive disorder Obsessive-compulsive disorder Panic disorder Posttraumatic stress disorder Premenstrual dysphoric disorder	Tablet Capsule Oral suspension Extended-release tablet	Acid or sour stomach, decreased appetite, decreased sexual ability or desire, heartburn, pain or tenderness around the eyes and cheekbones, gas, problems in urinating, runny or stuffy nose, sleepiness or trouble sleeping, stomach discomfort or upset stomach

(continued)

TABLE A-3 (CONTINUED)				
ANTIDEPRESSANTS DRUG CHART				
BRAND NAME	*GENERIC NAME*	*FDA-APPROVED INDICATION*	*DOSAGE FORM*	*COMMON ADVERSE EFFECTS*
Brisdelle Paxil Paxil CR Pexeva (continued)		Social anxiety disorder Vasomotor symptoms of menopause		
Prozac	Fluoxetine	Treatment of major depressive disorder Treatment of binge eating and vomiting in patients with moderate to severe bulimia nervosa Obsessive-compulsive disorder Premenstrual dysphoric disorder Panic disorder with or without agoraphobia In combination with olanzapine for treatment-resistant depression or bipolar depression	Tablet Capsule Delayed-release capsule Oral solution	Hives, inability to sit still, itching, restlessness, skin rash, decreased appetite
Zoloft	Sertraline	Treatment of major depression Obsessive-compulsive disorder Panic disorder Posttraumatic stress disorder Premenstrual dysphoric disorder Social anxiety disorder	Tablet Oral concentrate	Decreased sexual desire or ability, acid or sour stomach, decreased appetite or weight loss, diarrhea or loose stools, heartburn, abdominal pain, sleepiness or trouble sleeping

(continued)

TABLE A-3 (CONTINUED)

ANTIDEPRESSANTS DRUG CHART

BRAND NAME	GENERIC NAME	FDA-APPROVED INDICATION	DOSAGE FORM	COMMON ADVERSE EFFECTS
Serotonin-Norepinephrine Reuptake Inhibitors				
Cymbalta	Duloxetine	Acute and maintenance treatment of major depressive disorder Generalized anxiety disorder Diabetic peripheral neuropathic pain Management of fibromyalgia Chronic musculoskeletal pain	Capsule	Body aches or pain, cough, difficulty having a bowel movement (stool), difficulty with breathing, dry mouth, ear congestion, frequent urination, headache, lack or loss of strength, loss of appetite, loss of voice, muscle aches, nausea, sleepiness or sleeplessness, sneezing, sore throat, increased sweating, weight loss
Effexor Effexor XR	Venlafaxine	Treatment of major depressive disorder Generalized anxiety disorder Social anxiety disorder Panic disorder	Tablet Extended-release tablet Extended-release capsule	Changes in vision; headache; high blood pressure; abnormal dreams; chills; constipation; decrease in sexual desire or ability; diarrhea; drowsiness; dry mouth; loss of appetite; nausea; stomach pain or gas, stuffy or runny nose; tingling, burning, or prickly sensations; trembling or shaking; fatigue; vomiting; weight loss
Pristiq	Desvenlafaxine	Treatment of major depressive disorder	Extended-release tablet	Decreased appetite; loss of sexual ability, desire, drive, or performance; sleepiness
Tricyclic Antidepressants				
Asendin	Amoxapine	Treatment of depression	Tablet	Dry mouth
Anafranil	Clomipramine	Treatment of obsessive-compulsive disorder	Capsule	Bladder symptoms, blurred vision, body aches or pain, confusion, cough, dizziness, dry or sore throat, excessive muscle tone, fear or nervousness

(continued)

	TABLE A-3 (CONTINUED)			
	ANTIDEPRESSANTS DRUG CHART			
BRAND NAME	GENERIC NAME	FDA-APPROVED INDICATION	DOSAGE FORM	COMMON ADVERSE EFFECTS
Anafranil (continued)				Fever, hearing loss, hoarseness, lack of appetite, loss of interest or pleasure, poor concentration, rhythmic movement of muscles, trouble concentrating, trouble sleeping
Elavil	Amitriptyline	Treatment of depression	Tablet	Numerous adverse effects possible but incidence not known
Norpramin	Desipramine	Treatment of depression	Tablet	Numerous adverse effects possible but incidence not known
Pamelor	Nortriptyline	Treatment of depression	Capsule Oral solution	Numerous adverse effects possible but incidence not known
Silenor	Doxepin	Depression Insomnia	Tablet Capsule Oral concentrate	Numerous adverse effects possible but incidence not known
Pamelor	Nortriptyline	Treatment of depression	Capsule Oral solution	Numerous adverse effects possible but incidence not known
Tofranil	Imipramine	Treatment of depression Nocturnal enuresis in children	Tablet Capsule	Numerous adverse effects possible but incidence not known
Vivactil	Protriptyline	Treatment of depression	Tablet	Numerous adverse effects possible but incidence not known
Monoamine Oxidase Inhibitors				
Marplan	Isocarboxazid	Treatment of depression	Tablet	Constipation, dry mouth
Nardil	Phenelzine	Treatment of depression	Tablet	Chills; confusion; faintness; overactive reflexes; shakiness in the limbs; sudden jerky movements of the body; swelling, trembling, or shaking of hands or feet

(continued)

	TABLE A-3 (CONTINUED)			
ANTIDEPRESSANTS DRUG CHART				
BRAND NAME	GENERIC NAME	FDA-APPROVED INDICATION	DOSAGE FORM	COMMON ADVERSE EFFECTS
Parnate	Tranylcypromine	Treatment of major depressive disorder	Tablet	Numerous adverse effects possible but incidence not known
Miscellaneous Antidepressants				
Brintellix	Vortioxetine	Treatment of major depressive disorder	Tablet	Nausea, diarrhea, dizziness, dry mouth, constipation, vomiting, flatulence, abnormal dreams
Desyrel Oleptro	Trazodone	Treatment of major depressive disorder	Tablet Extended-release tablet	Blurred vision, confusion, dizziness, faintness, sweating, unusual tiredness
Fetzima	Levomilnacipran	Treatment of major depressive disorder		Nausea, vomiting, constipation; blurred vision, increased sweating, fast heart rate, sexual effects
Remeron Remeron SolTab	Mirtazapine	Treatment of depression	Tablet Orally dissolving tablet	Constipation, dizziness, drowsiness, dry mouth, increased appetite, weight gain
Serzone	Nefazodone	Treatment of depression	Tablet	Blurred vision, clumsiness or unsteadiness, lightheadedness or fainting, ringing in the ears, skin rash or itching
Viibryd	Vilazodone	Treatment of major depressive disorder	Tablet	Diarrhea, dizziness, dry mouth, nausea, trouble sleeping
Aplenzin Budeprion SR Buproban Forfivo XL Wellbutrin Wellbutrin SR Wellbutrin XL Zyban	Bupropion	Treatment of major depressive disorder, including seasonal affective disorder Adjunct in smoking cessation	Tablet Extended-release tablet	Anxiety, dry mouth, hyperventilation, irregular heartbeats, irritability, restlessness, shaking, shortness of breath, trouble sleeping

TABLE A-4				
ANXIOLYTICS DRUG CHART				
BRAND NAME	*GENERIC NAME*	*FDA-APPROVED INDICATION*	*DOSAGE FORM*	*COMMON ADVERSE EFFECTS*
Benzodiazepines				
Niravam Xanax Xanax XR	Alprazolam	Generalized anxiety disorder Panic disorder with or without agoraphobia	Tablet Orally dissolving tablet Extended-release tablet Liquid	Being forgetful, clumsiness or unsteadiness, feelings of discouragement, sleepiness, feeling sad or empty, irritability, lack of appetite, lightheadedness, loss of interest or pleasure, shakiness and unsteady walk, slurred speech, trouble concentrating
Librium	Chlordiazepoxide	Short-term relief of symptoms of anxiety Withdrawal symptoms of acute alcoholism	Capsule	Numerous adverse effects possible but incidence not known
Klonopin Klonopin Wafers	Clonazepam	Panic disorder with or without agoraphobia	Tablet Orally dissolving tablet	Being forgetful, clumsiness or unsteadiness, feelings of discouragement, sleepiness, feeling sad or empty, irritability, lack of appetite, lightheadedness, loss of interest or pleasure, shakiness and unsteady walk, slurred speech, trouble concentrating

(continued)

TABLE A-4 (CONTINUED)

ANXIOLYTICS DRUG CHART

BRAND NAME	GENERIC NAME	FDA-APPROVED INDICATION	DOSAGE FORM	COMMON ADVERSE EFFECTS
Tranxene T-Tab	Clorazepate	Short-term relief of symptoms of anxiety Withdrawal symptoms of acute alcoholism	Tablet	Several adverse effects but are few common
Diastat Valium	Diazepam	Short-term relief of symptoms of anxiety Withdrawal symptoms of acute alcoholism Skeletal muscle relaxant	Tablet Liquid Intramuscular or intravenous injection Rectal gel	Shakiness and unsteady walk, trembling or other problems with muscle control or coordination
Ativan	Lorazepam	Short-term relief of symptoms of anxiety	Tablet Intramuscular or intravenous injection	Drowsiness, sleepiness
Versed	Midazolam	Preoperative sedation Induction and maintenance of general anesthesia	Intramuscular or intravenous injection	Numerous adverse effects but most are uncommon
Serax	Oxazepam	Short-term relief of symptoms of anxiety Withdrawal symptoms of acute alcoholism	Capsule	Numerous adverse effects but most are uncommon

5HT 1A (5HT$_{1A}$) Partial Agonist

BuSpar	Buspirone	Generalized anxiety disorder	Tablet	Restlessness, nervousness, or unusual excitement

Histamine (H$_1$) Antagonist/Antihistamine

Atarax Vistaril	Hydroxyzine hydrochloride Hydroxyzine pamoate	Symptomatic relief of anxiety in organic disease states in which anxiety is manifested	Tablet Capsule Liquid Intramuscular injection	Drowsiness, dry mouth

(continued)

TABLE A-4 (CONTINUED)

ANXIOLYTICS DRUG CHART

BRAND NAME	GENERIC NAME	FDA-APPROVED INDICATION	DOSAGE FORM	COMMON ADVERSE EFFECTS
Barbiturates				
Luminal	Phenobarbital	Indicated for use as a sedative	Tablet Liquid Intramuscular or intravenous injection	Residual sedation, drowsiness, lethargy, vertigo, nausea, vomiting, headache
Anticonvulsants				
Neurontin	Gabapentin	Adjunct treatment of partial seizures Postherpetic neuralgia Restless legs syndrome	Tablet Capsule	Clumsiness or unsteadiness; continuous, uncontrolled, back-and-forth, or rolling eye movements
Lyrica	Pregabalin	Adjunct treatment of partial seizures Diabetic peripheral neuropathy pain Postherpetic neuralgia Fibromyalgia	Capsule	Bloating of the limbs, blurred vision, numbness or pain in the limbs, clumsiness, delusions, dementia, difficulty speaking, dry mouth, headache, hoarseness, painful or difficult urination, weight gain, sleepiness, stabbing pain, tingling of the limbs
Sympatholytics				
Minipress	Prazosin	Hypertension	Capsule	Dizziness or lightheadedness, especially when getting up from a lying or sitting position; fainting (sudden)

(continued)

TABLE A-4 (CONTINUED)

ANXIOLYTICS DRUG CHART

BRAND NAME	GENERIC NAME	FDA-APPROVED INDICATION	DOSAGE FORM	COMMON ADVERSE EFFECTS
Inderal Inderal LA InnoPran XL	Propranolol	Hypertension Angina pectoris Migraine prophylaxis Hypertrophic subaortic stenosis Atrial fibrillation Essential tremor Adjunct treatment for pheochromocytoma Mortality reduction of postmyocardial infarction	Tablet Liquid Extended-release capsule Intravenous solution	Numerous, but incidence is unknown

TABLE A-5

HYPNOTICS DRUG CHART

BRAND NAME	GENERIC NAME	FDA-APPROVED INDICATION	DOSAGE FORM	COMMON ADVERSE EFFECTS
Nonbenzodiazepine Receptor Agonists				
Lunesta	Eszopiclone	Treatment of insomnia	Tablet	Confusion and clumsiness that is more common in older adults, daytime anxiety and/or restlessness, mood or mental changes
Sonata	Zaleplon	Short-term treatment of insomnia	Capsule	Dizziness, headache, muscle pain, nausea
Ambien Ambien CR Intermezzo	Zolpidem	Short-term treatment of insomnia Treatment of insomnia when waking in middle-of-the-night is followed by difficulty returning to sleep	Tablet Extended-release tablet Sublingual tablet	Drowsiness, headache, muscle aches, stuffy or runny nose

(continued)

TABLE A-5 (CONTINUED)

HYPNOTICS DRUG CHART

BRAND NAME	GENERIC NAME	FDA-APPROVED INDICATION	DOSAGE FORM	COMMON ADVERSE EFFECTS
Benzodiazepines				
ProSom	Estazolam	Short-term treatment of insomnia characterized by difficulty in falling asleep, frequent nocturnal awakenings, and/or early morning awakening	Tablet	Decrease in body movement, clumsiness, dizziness, unusual drowsiness
Dalmane	Flurazepam	Treatment of insomnia characterized by difficulty in falling asleep, frequent nocturnal awakenings, and/or early morning awakening	Capsule	Numerous adverse effects but unknown frequency
Doral	Quazepam	Treatment of insomnia characterized by difficulty in falling asleep, frequent nocturnal awakenings, and/or early morning awakening	Tablet	Drowsiness
Restoril	Temazepam	Short-term treatment of insomnia	Capsule	Several adverse effects but most uncommon or rare
Halcion	Triazolam	Short-term treatment of insomnia	Tablet	Lightheadedness
Melatonin Receptor Agonist				
Rozerem	Ramelteon	Treatment of insomnia characterized by difficulty with sleep onset	Tablet	Dizziness, sleepiness

(continued)

TABLE A-5 (CONTINUED)

HYPNOTICS DRUG CHART

BRAND NAME	GENERIC NAME	FDA-APPROVED INDICATION	DOSAGE FORM	COMMON ADVERSE EFFECTS
Psychostimulants				
Nuvigil	Armodafinil	Improves wakefulness in patients with excessive sleepiness associated with obstructive sleep apnea, narcolepsy, or shift-work disorder	Tablet	Several adverse effects but most uncommon or rare
Focalin Focalin XR	Dexmethylphenidate	Attention-deficit/hyperactivity disorder	Tablet Extended-release capsule	Stomach upset or discomfort, loss of appetite, weight loss
Dexedrine Dexedrine Spansule	Dextroamphetamine	Attention-deficit/hyperactivity disorder Narcolepsy	Tablet Liquid Extended-release capsule	Several adverse effects but generally uncommon or rare
Adderall Adderall XR	Dextroamphetamine and amphetamine	Attention-deficit/hyperactivity disorder Narcolepsy	Tablet Extended-release capsule	Several adverse effects but generally uncommon or rare
Vyvanse	Lisdexamfetamine	Attention-deficit/hyperactivity disorder	Capsule	Decreased appetite, headache, nausea, upper abdominal or stomach pain, vomiting
Concerta Daytrana Metadate CD Metadate ER Methylin Ritalin Ritalin LA Ritalin SR	Methylphenidate	Attention-deficit/hyperactivity disorder Narcolepsy	Tablet Chewable tablet Liquid Extended-release tablet Extended-release capsule Transdermal patch	Fast heartbeat

(continued)

TABLE A-5 (CONTINUED)

HYPNOTICS DRUG CHART

BRAND NAME	GENERIC NAME	FDA-APPROVED INDICATION	DOSAGE FORM	COMMON ADVERSE EFFECTS
Provigil	Modafinil	Improves wakefulness in patients with excessive sleepiness associated with obstructive sleep apnea, narcolepsy, or shift-work disorder	Tablet	Anxiety, headache, nausea
Central Nervous System Depressant				
Xyrem	Sodium oxybate	Cataplexy or excessive daytime sleepiness associated with narcolepsy	Liquid	Numerous adverse effects but uncommon, rare, or unknown incidence
Anticonvulsant				
Horizant	Gabapentin enacarbil	Restless legs syndrome	Extended-release tablet	Dizziness, drowsiness, dry mouth, gas, headache, nausea, weakness, weight gain
Dopamine Agonists				
Mirapex Mirapex ER	Pramipexole	Restless legs syndrome Parkinson's disease	Tablet Extended-release tablet	Dizziness; drowsiness; hallucinations; nausea; twitching, twisting, or other unusual body movements
Requip	Ropinirole	Restless legs syndrome Parkinson's disease	Tablet Extended-release tablet	Confusion, dizziness, drowsiness, falling, nausea, hallucinations, sleepiness, swelling of legs, twitching or other unusual body movements, worsening of Parkinsonism

TABLE A-6

DEMENTIA MEDICATIONS DRUG CHART

BRAND NAME	GENERIC NAME	FDA-APPROVED INDICATION	DOSAGE FORM	COMMON ADVERSE EFFECTS
Acetylcholinesterase Inhibitors				
Aricept Aricept RDT	Donepezil	Treatment of mild, moderate, or severe dementia of the Alzheimer's type	Tablet Orally dissolving tablet	Diarrhea, loss of appetite, muscle cramps, nausea, insomnia, fatigue
Razadyne Razadyne ER	Galantamine	Treatment of mild to moderate dementia of the Alzheimer's type	Tablet Liquid Extended-release capsule	Bladder problems, diarrhea, feeling sad or empty, irritability, anorexia, anhedonia, pain, fatigue, nausea, weight loss, trouble concentrating
Exelon	Rivastigmine	Treatment of mild, moderate, or severe dementia of the Alzheimer's type Treatment of mild to moderate dementia associated with Parkinson's disease	Capsule Liquid Transdermal patch	Diarrhea, indigestion, anorexia, weakness, weight loss, nausea
Cognex	Tacrine	Treatment of mild to moderate dementia of the Alzheimer's type	Capsule	Clumsiness, diarrhea, anorexia, nausea
N-Methyl-D-Aspartate (NMDA) Receptor Antagonist				
Namenda Namenda XR	Memantine	Treatment of moderate to severe dementia of the Alzheimer's type	Tablet Liquid Extended-release capsule	Confusion, many other less common adverse effects

	TABLE A-7			
	PSYCHOSTIMULANTS DRUG CHART			
BRAND NAME	**GENERIC NAME**	**FDA-APPROVED INDICATION**	**DOSAGE FORM**	**COMMON ADVERSE EFFECTS**
Adderall	Dextroamphetamine and amphetamine (mixed amphetamine salts)	Attention-deficit/hyperactivity disorder Narcolepsy	Tablet	Bladder problems, irregular heartbeat, lower back pain
Adderall XR	Dextroamphetamine and amphetamine (mixed amphetamine salts)	Attention-deficit/hyperactivity disorder and narcolepsy	Extended-release capsule	Same as dextro-amphetamine
Catapres	Clonidine	Hypertension Attention-deficit/hyperactivity disorder treatment (off label)	Tablet Transdermal patch	Constipation, numerous but less common
Concerta	Methylphenidate	Attention-deficit/hyperactivity disorder	Extended-release tablet	Rapid heart rate, abdominal or stomach pain, headache, loss of appetite, nervousness, insomnia
Daytrana	Methylphenidate	Attention-deficit/hyperactivity disorder	Transdermal patch	Same as Concerta
Dexedrine	Dextroamphetamine	Attention-deficit/hyperactivity disorder Narcolepsy	Tablet Extended-release capsule Oral solution	Numerous but less common
Focalin	Dexmethylphenidate	Attention-deficit/hyperactivity disorder	Tablet	Rapid heart rate, abdominal or stomach pain, headache, loss of appetite, nervousness, insomnia
Focalin XR	Dexmethylphenidate	Attention-deficit/hyperactivity disorder	Extended-release capsule	Same as Focalin

(continued)

TABLE A-7 (CONTINUED)

PSYCHOSTIMULANTS DRUG CHART

Brand Name	Generic Name	FDA-Approved Indication	Dosage Form	Common Adverse Effects
Intuniv	Guanfacine	Attention-deficit/hyperactivity disorder	Extended-release tablet	Blurred vision, confusion, dizziness, sweating, fatigue
Kapvay	Clonidine	Attention-deficit/hyperactivity disorder	Extended-release tablet	Numerous but less common
Metadate CD	Methylphenidate	Attention-deficit/hyperactivity disorder	Controlled-delivery capsule	Fast heart rate, abdominal or stomach pain, headache, anorexia, nervousness, insomnia
Metadate ER	Methylphenidate	Attention-deficit/hyperactivity disorder Symptomatic management of narcolepsy	Extended-release capsule	Same as Metadate CD
Methylin	Methylphenidate	Attention-deficit/hyperactivity disorder Symptomatic management of narcolepsy	Tablet Chewable tablet Oral solution	Same as Metadate CD
Nexiclon XR	Clonidine	Treatment of hypertension	Tablet Extended-release tablet Extended-release oral suspension	Same as Kapvay
Quillivant XR	Methylphenidate	Attention-deficit/hyperactivity disorder	Extended-release oral suspension	Same as Metadate CD
Ritalin	Methylphenidate	Attention-deficit/hyperactivity disorder Symptomatic management of narcolepsy	Tablet	Same as Metadate CD

(continued)

	TABLE A-7 (CONTINUED)			
	PSYCHOSTIMULANTS DRUG CHART			
BRAND NAME	*GENERIC NAME*	*FDA-APPROVED INDICATION*	*DOSAGE FORM*	*COMMON ADVERSE EFFECTS*
Ritalin LA	Methylphenidate	Attention-deficit/hyperactivity disorder	Long-acting capsules	Same as Metadate CD
Ritalin SR	Methylphenidate	Attention-deficit/hyperactivity disorder Symptomatic management of narcolepsy	Sustained-release tablet	Same as Metadate CD
Strattera	Atomoxetine	Attention-deficit/hyperactivity disorder	Capsule	Stomach problems, change in menstrual periods, bladder problems, cough, sexual changes, bowel changes, dizziness, dry mouth, shortness of breath, fatigue, insomnia
Tenex	Guanfacine	Management of hypertension Attention-deficit/hyperactivity disorder (not officially approved)	Tablet	Blurred vision, confusion, dizziness, fatigue
Vyvanse	Lisdexamfetamine	Attention-deficit/hyperactivity disorder	Capsule	Decreased appetite, headache, nausea, stomach pain, weight loss

TABLE A-8

SUBSTANCE-RELATED DISORDERS DRUG CHART

BRAND NAME	GENERIC NAME	FDA APPROVED INDICATION	DOSAGE FORM	COMMON ADVERSE EFFECTS
Campral	Acamprosate calcium	Maintenance of abstinence from alcohol in patients with alcohol dependence who are not currently consuming alcohol	Delayed-release tablet	Severe depression, irritability, anorexia, weakness, anhedonia, insomnia, fatigue, difficulty concentrating
Butrans	Buprenorphine	Management of moderate to severe chronic pain in patients requiring a continuous, around the clock opioid analgesic for an extended period of time	Transdermal patch	Back pain, cough or hoarseness, bowel or bladder changes, fever, headache, insomnia, vomiting
Subutex	Buprenorphine	Treatment of opioid dependence	Sublingual tablet	Same as Butrans
Antabuse	Disulfiram	Aid in the management of selected patients with chronic alcohol dependence who want to remain in a state of enforced sobriety so that supportive and psychotherapeutic treatment may be applied to best advantage	Tablet	Drowsiness
Dolophine	Methadone	Management of moderate to severe pain when a continuous, around-the-clock opioid analgesic is needed for an extended period of time Detoxification treatment of opioid addiction Maintenance treatment of opioid addiction	Tablet Liquid Dispersible tablet	Numerous adverse effect but each is uncommon, although individuals often have one or more

(continued)

TABLE A-8 (CONTINUED)

SUBSTANCE-RELATED DISORDERS DRUG CHART

BRAND NAME	GENERIC NAME	FDA APPROVED INDICATION	DOSAGE FORM	COMMON ADVERSE EFFECTS
Revia Vivitrol	Naltrexone	Treatment of alcohol dependence Blockade of the effects of exogenously administered opioids	Tablet Long-acting intramuscular injection	Abdominal or stomach cramping, anxiety, insomnia, headache, joint pain, nausea, fatigue, nervousness, restlessness and/or trouble sleeping
NicoDerm CQ	Nicotine	Reduces withdrawal symptoms, including nicotine craving, associated with smoking cessation	Transdermal patch	Stomach problems, cough, stuffy nose
Nicorette	Nicotine polacrilex gum	Reduces withdrawal symptoms, including nicotine craving, associated with smoking cessation	Gum	Same as NicoDerm CQ
Nicotrol	Nicotine	Aid to smoking cessation for the relief of nicotine withdrawal symptoms	Inhaler	Same as NicoDerm CQ
Nicotrol NS	Nicotine	Aid to smoking cessation for the relief of nicotine withdrawal symptoms	Nasal spray	Same as NicoDerm CQ

Note: The common adverse effects are shown for the medications listed. However, care providers should be alert to some of the less common, but severe, adverse effects, such as liver damage or suicidal ideation, and should report signs of these to the coordinating physician.

Appendix

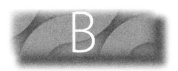

B

Assessments of Elements of Occupational Performance for Individuals With Mental Disorders

The table provides examples of assessment instruments that occupational therapists (OTs) may use to evaluate aspects of client performance as described in the Practice Framework (American Occupational Therapy Association [AOTA], 2008). The list includes some of the many instruments that OTs use; some were developed by OTs and others were developed by psychologists, educators, neurologists, and others.

Bonder B.
Psychopathology and Function, Fifth Edition (pp 533-542).
© 2015 SLACK Incorporated.

TABLE B-1

ASSESSMENTS OF ELEMENTS OF OCCUPATIONAL PERFORMANCE FOR INDIVIDUALS WITH MENTAL DISORDERS

PERFORMANCE AREA AND APPLICABLE INSTRUMENT NAME	AGE GROUP	AREA ASSESSED
Occupational Profile		
Canadian Occupational Performance Measure (COPM), 4th ed. (Law et al., 2005)	7 years and older	Self-care, leisure, productivity
Occupational Circumstances Assessment Interview and Rating Scale (OCAIRS; Forsyth et al., 2005)	Adolescents to adults	Causation, values, goals, interests, roles, skills, previous experiences, overall participation and adaptation
Occupational Self Assessment (OSA), Version 2.2 (Baron, Kielhofner, Iyenger, Goldhammer, & Wolenski, 2006)	14 years and older	Volition, habituation, performance, values, personal causation, interests, roles, habits, and skills
Client Assessment of Strengths, Interests, and Goals (CASIG): Self Report (SR) and Informant (I; Wallace, Lecomte, Wilde, & Liberman, 2004)	Adults	Overview of community functioning, social and instrumental activities of daily living (IADL), medication management, quality of life, psychiatric symptoms and behaviors
Child Occupational Self Assessment (Kramer, Kielhofner, & Smith, 2010).	Children and adolescents 6 to 17 years	Range of everyday activities
Areas of Occupation		
ADL		
Executive Function Performance Test (EFPT; Baum et al., 2008)	Adults	ADL, IADL
Bay Area Functional Performance Evaluation, 2nd ed. (Williams & Bloomer, 1987)	Adults	ADL, IADL, Social interaction, cognitive, emotional, and performance skills
IADL		
Instrumental Activities of Daily Living Scale (Lawton & Brody, 1969)	Older adults	IADL

(continued)

TABLE B-1 (CONTINUED)

ASSESSMENTS OF ELEMENTS OF OCCUPATIONAL PERFORMANCE FOR INDIVIDUALS WITH MENTAL DISORDERS

PERFORMANCE AREA AND APPLICABLE INSTRUMENT NAME	AGE GROUP	AREA ASSESSED
Kohlman Evaluation of Living Skills (KELS; McGourty, 1999)	Adults with cognitive impairments	ADL, IADL, community mobility, work, leisure
Assessment of Living Skills and Resources-Revised 2 (Clemson, Bundy, Unsworth, & Fiatarone Singh, 2008)	Adults	IADL interview
Life Skills Assessment (Helfrich, Chan, & Sabol, 2011)	Adults	Food and money management, community participation, self-care
Health Enhancement Lifestyle Profile (Hwang, 2009)	Adults	Health-related behaviors
Rest and Sleep		
Epworth Sleepiness Scale (Johns, 1991)	Adults	Daytime sleepiness
Occupational Profile of Sleep (Pierce & Summers, 2011)	Adults	Sleep
Education		
Academic Performance Rating Scale (DuPaul, Rapport, & Perriello, 1991)	School age	Academic success, productivity, impulse control
Miller Assessment for Preschoolers (MAP; Miller, 1988)	2 to 6 years	Sensory, motor, and cognitive skills associated with academic performance
Work		
Strong Interest Inventory (CPP, Inc., 2009)	Adolescents and adults	Career interests
Self-Directed Search (Holland, 1995)	14 years and older	Career interests
Play		
Interest Checklist (Matsutsuyu, 1969, revised by Rogers, Weinstein, & Figone, 1978)	Adolescents and older	Interests
Play History (Takata cited in Behnke & Fetkovich, 1984)	Children and adolescents	Interests, experiences, opportunities for play

(continued)

TABLE B-1 (CONTINUED)

ASSESSMENTS OF ELEMENTS OF OCCUPATIONAL PERFORMANCE FOR INDIVIDUALS WITH MENTAL DISORDERS

PERFORMANCE AREA AND APPLICABLE INSTRUMENT NAME	AGE GROUP	AREA ASSESSED
Child Behaviors Inventory of Playfulness (Rogers et al., 1998)	Children	Play and leisure
Assessment of Preschool Children's Participation (Law, King, Petrenchik, Kertoy, & Anaby, 2012)	2 to 6 years	Play skills, recreation, social activities
Leisure		
Activity Card Sort (Baum & Edwards, 2008)	Adults	Social, leisure, ADL
Leisure Satisfaction Scale (Trottier, Brown, Hobson, & Miller, 2006)	Adolescents and adults	Leisure
Leisure Competence Measure (Kloseck & Crilly, 1997)	All ages	Leisure awareness and skills
Children's Leisure Assessment Scale (Rosenblum, Sachs, & Schreuer, 2010)	12 to 18 years	Leisure preferences
Social Participation		
Child and Adolescent Scale of Participation (Bedell, 2009)	3 to 22 years	Participation in home, school, community
Meaningful Activity and Participation Assessment (MAPA; Eakman, Carlson, & Clark, 2010)	Older adults	Meaningfulness of occupations
Community Integration Questionnaire (Willer, Rosenthal, Kreutzer, Gordon, & Rempel, 1993)	Adults	IADL, leisure, social and productive activities
Clinical Assessment of Modes (Taylor et al., 2013)	Adults	Focus on client's perceptions of therapeutic relationship, with four separate formats, for varying times and modes of administration

(continued)

TABLE B-1 (CONTINUED)		
ASSESSMENTS OF ELEMENTS OF OCCUPATIONAL PERFORMANCE FOR INDIVIDUALS WITH MENTAL DISORDERS		
PERFORMANCE AREA AND APPLICABLE INSTRUMENT NAME	*AGE GROUP*	*AREA ASSESSED*
Client Factors		
Values, Beliefs, Spirituality		
Activity Index and Meaningfulness of Activity Scale (Gregory, 1983)	Older adults	Activity, leisure meanings
Pediatric Volitional Questionnaire (Basu, Kafkes, Schatz, Kiraly, & Kielhofner, 2008)	2 to 7 years	Motivation, values, interests
Body Functions		
Action Research Arm Test (Lyle, 1981)	Adolescents, adults, and older adults	Upper extremity functioning
Arm Motor Ability Test (Kopp et al., 1997)	Adults	Upper extremity functioning in the context of ADL and IADL
Performance Skills		
Sensory Perceptual Skills		
Adolescent/Adult Sensory Profile (Brown & Dunn, 2002)	Adolescents and adults	Sensory processing, behavioral and emotional response
Motor-Free Visual Perception Test (Colarusso & Hammill, n.d.)	4 to 11 years	Visual perception
Sensory Integration and Praxis Test (Ayers, 1975)	4 to 9 years	Praxis and sensory processing
Test of Visual and Perceptual Skills (Martin, n.d.)	4 to 19 years	Visual and perceptual skills
Motor and Praxis Skills		
Assessment of Motor and Process Skills (Fisher & Bray Jones, 2012)	3 years and older	Motor and process skills in the context of meaningful activities
Peabody Developmental Motor Scales, 2nd ed. (Folio & Fewell, n.d.)	Birth to 7 years	Gross and fine motor
Emotional Regulation Skills		
Functional Emotional Assessment Scale (Greenspan, DeGangi, & Weider, 2001)	7 months to 4 years	Emotional and social functioning

(continued)

TABLE B-1 (CONTINUED)		
ASSESSMENTS OF ELEMENTS OF OCCUPATIONAL PERFORMANCE FOR INDIVIDUALS WITH MENTAL DISORDERS		
PERFORMANCE AREA AND APPLICABLE INSTRUMENT NAME	*AGE GROUP*	*AREA ASSESSED*
Adult Manifest Anxiety Scale (Reynolds, Richmond, & Lowe, 2003)	Adults	Anxiety
Beck Depression Inventory-II (Beck, Steer, & Brown, 1996)	13 to 80 years	Depression
Coping Inventory (Zeitlin, 2007)	3 to 16 years (observation) 17 to adult (self-rated)	Coping with self, environment, use of resources
Child Behavior Checklist-Preschool, Child Behavior Checklist-School Age, Child Behavior Checklist-Multicultural (Achenbach, 2000)	Preschool: 1.5 to 5 years School: 6 to 18 years Multicultural: 1.5 to 5 years	Psychological symptoms
Cognitive Skills		
Clinical Dementia Rating Scale (Morris, 1993)	Older adults	Memory, orientation, judgment, problem solving
Cognitive Assessment Interview (Ventura et al., 2010)	Adults	Cognition
Allen Diagnostic Module, 2nd ed. (Earhart, 2006)	All	Problem solving, following directions
Lowenstein Occupational Therapy Cognitive Assessment, 2nd ed. (Itzkovich, Elazar, Averbuch, & Katz, 2000)	6 years and older	Cognitive processing
Weekly Calendar Planning Activity (WCPA; Weiner, Toglia, & Berg, 2012)	Adolescents	Executive function (can also assess patterns)
Awareness Interview (Anderson & Tranel, 1989)	Older adults	Recognition of cognitive, visual perception, and speech and language problems
MacNeill-Lichtenberg Decision Tree (MacNeill & Lichtenberg, 2000)	Older adults	Screening for cognitive, psychosocial, and emotional factors

(continued)

TABLE B-1 (CONTINUED)

ASSESSMENTS OF ELEMENTS OF OCCUPATIONAL PERFORMANCE FOR INDIVIDUALS WITH MENTAL DISORDERS

PERFORMANCE AREA AND APPLICABLE INSTRUMENT NAME	AGE GROUP	AREA ASSESSED
Communication and Social Skills		
Assessment of Communication and Interaction Skills (Forsyth, Salamy, Simon, & Kielhofner, 1998)	Adults	Communication, social interaction
Matson Evaluation of Social Skills for Individuals With Severe Retardation (Matson, 1995)	All ages	Social skills
Performance Patterns		
Habits		
Assessment of Life Habits (Fougeyrollas, & Noreau, 2003)	Adults	Habits related to nutrition, fitness, ADL, IADL, mobility, employment, relationships, and other performance areas
Assessment of Occupational Functioning, Second Revision (Watts, Brollier, Bauer, & Schmidt, 1989)	Adults	Volition, habits, values, roles, personal causation skills
Routines		
Life Balance Inventory (Matuska, 2012)	Adults	Balance in health, relationships
Roles		
Adolescent Role Assessment (Black, 1976)	Adolescents	Occupational role participation
Rituals		
Spiritual Well-Being Scale (Ellison & Paloutzian, 1991)	Adults	Individuals' interpretations of the meaning of spirituality
Context and Environment		
Analysis of Cognitive Environmental Support (Ryan et al., 2011)	Adults	Environment as related to cognition
Home Environment Assessment Protocol (Gitlin et al., 2002)	Older adults	Evaluation of the home environment for individuals with dementia
Family Environment Scale (Moos & Moos, 1994)	Children and adults	Family dynamics and interaction
Child and Adolescent Scale of Environment (Bedell, 2009)	3 to 22 years	Physical, social, attitudinal environment

References

Achenbach, T. (2000). *Child behavior checklist—Preschool.* Retrieved from http://www.aseba.org/preschool.html.

American Occupational Therapy Association (2008). *Occupational therapy practice framework: Domain and process* (2nd ed.). *American Journal of Occupational Therapy, 62*(6), 625-683.

Anderson, S.W., & Tranel, D. (1989). Awareness of disease states following cerebral infarction, dementia, and head trauma: Standardized assessment. *The Clinical Neuropsychologist, 3,* 327-339.

Ayers, J.J. (1965). *Sensory Integration and Praxis Test.* Torrance, CA: Western Psychological Services.

Baron, K., Kielhofner, G., Iyenger, A., Goldhammer, V., & Wolenski, J. (2006). *Occupational self-assessment* (OSA), Version 2.2. Retrieved from http://www.cade.uic.edu/moho/productDetails.aspx?aid=2.

Basu, S., Kafkes, A., Schatz, R., Kiraly, A., & Kielhofner, G. (2008). *Pediatric Volitional Questionnaire* (PVQ), Version 2.1. Retrieved from http://www.cade.uic.edu/moho/productDetails.aspx?aid=7.

Baum, C.M., & Edwards, D. (2008). *Activity card sort* (2nd ed.). Bethesda, MD: AOTA Press.

Baum, C., Connor, L.T., Morrison, T., Hahn, M., Dromerick, A.W., & Edwards, D.F. (2008). Reliability, validity, and clinical utility of the Executive Function Performance Test: A measure of executive function in a sample of people with stroke. *American Journal of Occupational Therapy, 62*(3), 446-455.

Beck, A.T., Steer, R.A., & Brown, G.K. (1996). *Beck Depression Inventory-II.* San Antonio, TX: Pearson.

Bedell, G. (2009). Further validation of the Child and Adolescent Scale of Participation (CASP). *Developmental Neurorehabilitation, 12,* 342-351.

Behnke, C., & Fetkovich, M. (1984). Examining the reliability and validity of the Play History. *American Journal of Occupational Therapy, 38,* 94-100.

Black, M.M. (1976). Adolescent role assessment. *American Journal of Occupational Therapy, 30,* 73-79.

Brown, C., & Dunn, W. (2002). *Adolescent/Adult Sensory Profile.* San Antonio, TX: Pearson.

Clemson, L., Bundy, A., Unsworth, C., & Fiatarone Singh, M. (2008). ALSAR-R2: *Assessment of living skills and resources-Revised.* Retrieved from http://www.sydney.edu.au/health-sciences/documents/assessment-living-skills.pdf.

Colarusso, R.P., & Hammill, D.D. (n.d.). *Motor-Free Visual Perception Test* (3rd ed.). Novato, CA; Academic Therapy Publications.

CPP, Inc. (2009). *Strong Interest Inventory.* Retrieved from https://www.cpp.com/products/strong/index.aspx.

DuPaul, G.J., Rapport, M.D., & Perriello, L.M. (1991). Teacher ratings of academic skills: The development of the Academic Performance Rating Scale. *School Psychology Review, 20,* 284-300.

Eakman, A., Carlson, M., & Clark, F. (2010). The Meaningful Activity Participation Assessment: A measure of engagement in personally valued activities. *International Journal of Aging and Human Development, 70,* 299-317.

Earhart, C.A. (2006). *Allen Diagnostic Module* (2nd ed.). Colchester, CT: S&S Worldwide.

Ellison, R., & Paloutzian, C. (1991). *Manual for the Spiritual Well-Being Scale.* Nyack, NY: Life Advance.

Fisher, A.G., & Bray Jones, K. (2012). *Assessment of Motor and Process Skills: User manual* (Vol. 1, 7th ed., rev. ed.). Fort Collins, CO: Three Star Press.

Folio, M.R., & Fewell, R.R. (n.d.). *Peabody Developmental Motor Scales* (2nd ed.). Novato, CA: Academic Therapy Publications.

Fougeyrollas, P., & Noreau, L. (2003). *Assessment of Life Habits* (LIFE-H, 3.0): General long form. Quebec, Canada: International Network on the Disability Creation Process.

Forsyth, K., Deshpande, S., Kielhofner, G., Henriksson, C., Haglund, L., Olson, L., . . . Kulkarni, S. (2005). *Occupational Circumstances Assessment—Interview Rating Scale* (OCAIRS), Version 4.0. Retrieved from http://www.cade.uic.edu/moho/productDetails.aspx?aid=35.

Forsyth, K., Salamy, M., Simon, S., & Kielhofner, G. (1998*). The Assessment of Communication and Interaction Skill* (ACIS), Version 4.0. Retrieved from http://www.cade.uic.edu/moho/productDetails.aspx?aid=1.

Gitlin, L.N., Schinfeld, S., Winter, L., Corcoran, M., Boyce, A.A., & Hauck, W.W. (2002). Evaluating home environments of persons with dementia: Interrater reliability and validity of the Home Environmental Assessment Protocol (HEAP). *Disability and Rehabilitation, 23,* 59-91.

Greenspan, S., DeGangi, G., & Wieder, S. (2001). *Functional Emotional Assessment Scale.* Interdisciplinary Council on Developmental and Learning Disorders. Retrieved from http://www.icdl.com/research/functional-emotional-assessment-scale.

Gregory, M.D. (1983). Occupational behavior and life satisfaction among retirees. *American Journal of Occupational Therapy, 37,* 548-553.

Helfrich, C.A., Chan, D., & Sabol, P. (2011). Cognitive predictors of life skill interventions: Outcomes for adults with mental illness at risk for homelessness. *American Journal of Occupational Therapy, 65,* 277-286.

Holland, J. (1995). *Self-directed search.* Retrieved from http://www.self-directed-search.com/.

Hwang, J.E. (2009). Reliability and validity of the Health Enhancement Lifestyle Profile (HELP). *OTJR: Occupation, Participation and Health, 30*(4), 158-168.

Itzkovich, M., Elazar, B., Averbuch, S., & Katz, N. (2000). *Loewenstein Occupational Therapy Cognitive Assessment* (2nd ed.). Wayne, NJ: Maddak.

Johns, M.W. (1991). A new method for measuring daytime sleepiness: The Epworth Sleepiness Scale. *Sleep, 14*, 540-545.

Kloseck, M., & Crilly, R. (1997). *Leisure Competence Measure (LCM): Professional manual and user guide.* London, United Kingdom: Leisure Competence Measure Data System.

Kopp, B., Kunkel, A., Flor, H., Platz, T., Rose, U., Mauritz, K.H., . . . Taub, E. (1997). Arm Motor Ability Test: Reliability, validity, and sensitivity to change in an instrument for assessing disabilities in activities of daily living. *Archives of Physical Medicine and Rehabilitation, 78*, 615-620.

Kramer, J.M., Kielhofner, G., & Smith, E.V., Jr. (2010). Validity evidence for the Child Occupational Self Assessment. *American Journal of Occupational Therapy, 64*, 621-632.

Law, M., Baptiste, S., Carswell, A., McColl, M.A., Polatajko, H., & Pollock, N. (2005). *Canadian Occupational Performance Measure (COPM;* 4th ed.). Ottawa, Ontario, Canada: Canadian Association of Occupational Therapists.

Law, M., King, G., Petrenchik, T., Kertoy, M., & Anaby, D. (2012). The assessment of preschool children's participation: Internal consistency and validity. *Physical & Occupational Therapy in Pediatrics, 32*, 272-287.

Lawton, M.P., & Brody, E.M. (1969). Assessment of older people: Self-maintaining and instrumental activities of daily living. *Gerontologist, 9*, 179-186.

Lyle, R. (1981). A performance test for assessment of upper limb function in physical rehabilitation treatment and research. *International Journal of Rehabilitation Research, 4*, 483-492.

MacNeill, S.E., & Lichtenberg, P.A. (2000). The MacNeill-Lichtenberg Decision Tree: A unique method of triaging mental health problems in older medical rehabilitation patients. *Archives of Physical Medicine and Rehabilitation, 81*(5), 618-622.

Martin, N. (n.d.). *Test of Visual and Perceptual Skills* (3rd ed.). Novato, CA: Academic Therapy Publications.

Matson, J.L. (1995). *Matson evaluation of social skills for individuals with severe retardation.* Baton Rouge, LA: Disability Consultants, LLC.

Matuska, K. (2012). Description and development of the Life Balance Inventory. *OTJR: Occupation, Participation, and Health, 32*, 220-228.

McGourty, L.K. (1999). *Kohlman Evaluation of Living Skills* (KELS). Annapolis Junction, MD: AOTA Products.

Miller, L.J. (1988). *Miller Assessment for Preschoolers.* San Antonio, TX: Pearson Assessments.

Moos, R. & Moos, B. (1994). *Family Environment Scale manual: Development, applications, research* (3rd ed.). Palo Alto, CA: Consulting Psychologist Press.

Morris, J.C. (1993). The Clinical Dementia Rating (CDR): Current version and scoring rules. *Neurology, 43*, 2412-2414.

Pierce, D., & Summers, K. (2011). Rest and sleep. In C. Brown & V.C. Stoffel (Eds.), *Occupational therapy in mental health: A vision for participation* (pp. 736-754). Philadelphia: F.A. Davis.

Reynolds, C.R., Richmond, B.O., & Lowe, P.A. (2003). *Adult Manifest Anxiety Scale.* Torrance, CA: WPS. Retrieved from https://shop.psych.acer.edu.au/acer-shop/group/AMA.

Rogers, C.S., Impara, J.C., Frary, R.B., Harris, T., Meeks, A., Semanic-Lauth, S., & Reynolds, M.R. (1998). Measuring playfulness: Development of the Child Behaviors Inventory of Playfulness. In M.C. Duncan, G. Chick, & A. Aycock (Eds.), *Play & culture studies: Diversions and divergences in fields of play* (Vol. 1; pp. 121-135). Greenwich, CT: Ablex.

Rogers, J., Weinstein, J.M., & Figone, J.J. (1978). The Interest Checklist: An empirical assessment. *American Journal of Occupational Therapy, 32*, 628-630.

Rosenblum, S., Sachs, D., & Schreuer, N. (2010). Reliability and validity of the Children's Leisure Scale. *American Journal of Occupational Therapy, 64*, 633-641.

Ryan, J.D., Polatajko, H.J., McEwen, S., Peressotti, M., Young, A., Rummel, K., . . . Baum, C. (2011). Analysis of cognitive environmental support (ACES): Preliminary testing. *Neuropsychological Rehabilitation, 21*, 401-427.

Taylor, R.R., Wong, S., Fan, C.W., Kjelberg, A., Alfredsson-Agren, K., Andersson, E., & Zubel, B. (2013). *Clinical assessment of modes—Client time 1 (CAM-C1): Communicating with your therapist.* Retrieved from http://ahs.uic.edu/cl/irm/assessments/.

Trottier, A.N., Brown, G.T., Hobson, S.J., & Miller, W. (2006). Reliability and validity of the Leisure Satisfaction Scale (LSS-short form) and the Adolescent Leisure Interest Profile (ALIP). *Occupational Therapy International, 9*(2), 131-144.

Ventura, J., Reise, S.P., Keefe, R.S., Baade, L.E., Gold, J.M., Green, M.F., . . . Bilder, R.M. (2010). The Cognitive Assessment Interview (CAI): Development and validation of an empirically derived, brief interview-based measure of cognition. *Schizophrenia Research, 121*, 24-31.

Wallace, C.J., Lecomte, T., Wilde, J., & Liberman, R.P. (2004). *Client Assessment of Strengths, Interests, and Goals (CASIG)-Self Report (SR) and Informant (I)*. Northridge, CA: Psychiatric Rehabilitation Consultants.

Watts, J.H., Brollier, C., Bauer, D., & Schmidt, W. (1989). Assessment of occupational functioning: The second revision. In J.H. Watts & C. Brollier (Eds.), *Instrument Development in Occupational Therapy* (pp. 61-88). New York, NY: Haworth.

Weiner, N.W., Toglia, J., & Berg, C. (2012). Weekly calendar planning activity (WCPA): A performance-based assessment of executive function piloted with at-risk adolescents. *American Journal of Occupational Therapy, 66,* 699-708.

Willer, B., Rosenthal, M., Kreutzer, J., Gordon, W., & Rempel, R. (1993) *Community Integration Questionnaire.* Thorold, Ontario, Canada: Centre for Research on Community Integration at the Ontario Brain Injury Association.

Williams, S.L., & Bloomer, J. (1987). *Bay Area Functional Performance Evaluation* (2nd ed.). Palo Alto, CA: Consulting Psychologists Press.

Zeitlin, S. (2007). *Coping Inventory.* Bensonville, IL: Scholastic Testing Service.

Index